Fundamentals of

Paramedic Practice

Fundamentals of Paramedic Practice

A Systems Approach

Third Edition

EDITED BY

Sam Willis

Course Co-ordinator for Paramedicine, Charles Darwin University,
Teaching Fellow of the Higher Education Academy, PhD Candidate

Ian Peate

Editor in Chief *British Journal of Nursing*;
Consultant Editor *Journal of Paramedic Practice*;
Consultant Editor *International Journal for Advancing Practice*;
Visiting Professor Northumbria University;
Visiting Professor St Georges University of London and Kingston University, London;
Professorial Fellow Roehampton University;
Visiting Senior Clinical Fellow University of Hertfordshire

WILEY Blackwell

This third edition first published 2024

Edition History
Wiley-Blackwell (1e, 2015), Wiley-Blackwell (2e, 2020)

Registered Offices
John Wiley & Sons, Inc., 111 River Street, Hoboken, NJ 07030, USA
John Wiley & Sons Ltd, The Atrium, Southern Gate, Chichester, West Sussex, PO19 8SQ, UK

For details of our global editorial offices, customer services, and more information about Wiley products visit us at www.wiley.com.

Wiley also publishes its books in a variety of electronic formats and by print-on-demand. Some content that appears in standard print versions of this book may not be available in other formats.

Library of Congress Cataloging-in-Publication Data applied for

Paperback: 9781394164790

Cover Design: Wiley
Cover Image: © Courtesy of Charles Darwin University (CDU)

Set in 9.5/12.5pt Source Sans Pro by Straive, Chennai, India

Contents

List of Contributors

Elicia Austin
Elicia previously worked as Research Paramedic for South Central Ambulance Service. Following this she entered Higher Education as a lecturer at Coventry University. She currently works as Senior Lecturer of Paramedic Science and is Research Fellow at the University of Hertfordshire. Elicia will begin her PhD part-time in the academic year 2023/2024 and stills enjoys working clinically as Bank Paramedic for the ambulance service.

Craig Barlow
Craig is Consultant Practitioner (Paramedic) in Emergency Medicine at St Georges University Hospital, London, UK. He is also Associate Lecturer in Advanced Clinical Practice at St Georges University Hospital and a member of NHS England Workstream 3 (Hospitals) Clinical Advisory Group. Craig has a specialist interest and background in advanced clinical practice, primary, urgent and emergency care, governance, and quality assurance, where he is Specialist Professional Advisor to the Care Quality Commission.

He began his career within a UK NHS ambulance service, where he later developed a portfolio career in advanced clinical practice within primary and urgent care, but most recently has returned to emergency care. Craig has worked at both local and regional levels for Health Education England in the faculty for advancing practice. He holds a BSc (Hons) in Paramedic Practice, Post Graduate Certificate in Education, Post Graduate Certificate in Professional Practice, and MSc in Advanced Clinical Practice and Professional Education. Craig is an active and longstanding instructor for the Resuscitation Council UK.

Seán Bolger
Seán is an experienced healthcare professional whose passion for nursing has taken him on a dynamic journey through various facets of the field. With a strong foundation in emergency nursing, Seán currently serves on the frontline as an Emergency Department nurse as well as a Clinical Educator. Currently based in Western Australia, Seán has experience in healthcare delivery in Ireland and the United Kingdom.

In addition to his work in the hospital setting, Seán has made a meaningful impact in community healthcare. As a Nurse Practitioner, he has worked closely with diverse populations, ensuring access to quality care and promoting health and wellness. Seán's experiences extend beyond traditional healthcare settings, as he has provided nursing services in police custody environments, as well as resource-poor areas such as music festivals and cruise ships.

Jemmima Bowd
Jemmima is an ambulance paramedic working in Geelong, Victoria, Australia. She graduated with a Bachelor of Paramedicine at Griffith University in 2021 and previously worked in event medicine and the Covid-19 vaccination programme.

Janie Brown
Janie is an Associate Professor in Curtin School of Nursing, a Senior Research Fellow at St John of God Midland Public Private Hospital and Lead of the International Consortium for Occupational Resilience (ICOR). She is a Registered Nurse and has been a nurse educator within many adult education sectors throughout Australia. Janie is a nurse researcher who responds to demand driven research, continually striving to contribute in meaningful ways to the national and international health care community of practice. She does this through reflexive and effective nursing leadership and academic excellence in teaching and research. The nexus between her leadership, teaching and research roles engages Janie with nursing students, clinicians, higher education specialists and researchers to work collaboratively and collectively for better health outcomes for all Australians.

Marie Boulianne
Marie works at Bethesda Clinic as the Clinical Nurse Manager providing specialised mental health assistance to Defence Personnel, Veterans and First Responders. Her working experience includes a mixture of community mental health nursing, private practice, and academic positions in undergraduate and postgraduate nursing. She is a Credentialed Mental Health Nurse. She completed her PhD at the University of Notre Dame researching the role played by humour in the development of resilience and well-being in nursing.

Matt Campbell
Matt is a registered paramedic with St John WA in Australia. His work involves frontline pre-hospital care in

metropolitan Perth as well as working as an industrial paramedic in remote sites across Western Australia. Matt has also worked as a registered paramedic for the London Ambulance Service. Prior to his career as a paramedic he studied at the University of Adelaide and completed a Bachelor of Health Sciences with a major in Pathology. He has since completed a Bachelor of Paramedic Science and a Graduate Certificate in Healthcare in Remote and Extreme Environments. Matt has a passion for teaching and education and has held various positions at Flinders University and Curtin University.

Vince Clarke
Vince is Programme Lead for the BSc(Hons) in Paramedic Science at the University of Hertfordshire, UK, where he has been employed since 2016. He joined the London Ambulance Service in 1996, qualified as paramedic in 1998 and entered the Education and Development Department in 2001. He worked as part of the Higher Education team and developed in-house paramedic programmes as well as working closely with higher education partner institutions.

A Health & Care Professions Council partner since 2006, Vince has been involved in the regulatory approval of a wide range of paramedic educational programmes across the United Kingdom as well as assessing Continuing Professional Development submissions and sitting on Conduct and Competence Fitness to Practise panel hearings.

Vince is Trustee for Education for the College of Paramedics, the UK's professional body for paramedics, having previously held the position of Head of Endorsements. He maintains clinical currency and works for the London Ambulance Service as a Bank Paramedic. Vince also works as an independent paramedic expert witness for the Court and prepares reports on breach of duty for both claimants and defendants.

Vince's Professional Doctorate in Education focused on the theory-practice relationship in paramedic undergraduate education. This work informed the development of university accredited ambulance service paramedic Practice Educator courses and forms the basis for the College of Paramedics approach to practice-based learning with Vince having edited the College publication *'Paramedic Practice-based learning: A Handbook for Practice Educators and Facilitators'*.

Derek Collings-Hughes
Derek is a registered paramedic BParamed(Hons), MACPara originally from New Zealand who now resides in Western Australia. He holds a clinical role as an Ambulance Paramedic for St John Ambulance and an academic role as Lecturer in Paramedicine and Co-course Co-ordinator for the BSc-Paramedicine degree at Curtin University, Western Australia. Derek has a strong interest in the non-technical skills within paramedic practice. As such, his research interests include paramedic identity and professionalism, ethical and clinical decision-making, and using evidence to inform system improvements within paramedicine.

Joe Copson
Joe is a final-year PhD Student at the University of Hertfordshire and Lecturer in Paramedic Science at the University of East Anglia. He graduated in 2019 with a BSc (Hons) in Paramedic Science, following which he began his paramedic career working for the East of England Ambulance Service. He commenced his PhD full-time in 2021 – with funding from the University of Hertfordshire and the College of Paramedics – and is due to complete his PhD in 2024. His PhD is exploring the transition to practice experiences of newly qualified paramedics.

Clare Davies
Dr Clare Davies is a Registered Nurse and Registered Sick Children's Nurse (UK), and currently the Director of Postgraduate Studies at Sydney Nursing School, The University of Sydney. She has over 30 years' experience in nursing and has practiced in nursing leadership positions in the UK and Australia in the specialty of paediatrics and child health. She is a Master of Philosophy and Doctor of Philosophy graduate of The University of Sydney. Clare's research interests are aimed at improving the experiences of infants, children and adolescents who are admitted to hospital. Her current research investigates the rights and voice of children in healthcare and improving their experiences during medical procedures.

Michael Fanner
Michael is Postdoctoral Researcher at the Department of Social Policy and Intervention, University of Oxford, Honorary Assistant Professor in Community Child Health at the School of Health Sciences, University of Nottingham, and works one day a week as Health Visitor for Dorset HealthCare University NHS Foundation Trust. Michael is currently establishing an England-wide NIHR funded Supporting Early Minds Research Network to identify, facilitate and support the research infrastructure focusing on the development of accessible, acceptable, and targeted interventions aimed at the cognitive and mental wellbeing of infants, toddlers, and pre-schoolers and their families from diverse backgrounds. In 2012–2013, Michael graduated as a Registered Nurse (Adult) and Specialist Community Public Health Nurse (Health Visitor) at King's College London and maintains registration with Nursing and Midwifery Council through clinical, educational and

research practice. In addition, Michael is a Queen's Nurse and a Fellow of AdvanceHE/Higher Education Academy. Michael holds a PhD in social policy and has research interests in how social policy and clinical practice 'caters for' ethically complex social issues and evidence translation in infant mental health. Michael is an experienced educator and has lectured in nursing, paramedic science, social work and specialist community and public health nursing across a number of universities.

Matthew Faulkner
Anaesthetics North/Western Training Scheme, Melbourne, Victoria, Australia.

Sarah Fulford
Sarah is an Australian Historian and award-winning teacher. She holds a BA and MPhil and is Lecturer/MCASI in the Faculty of Health Science and Humanities at Curtin University. Through teaching, she is able to join the students' journey as they understand the sociological impact of marginalisation on vulnerable groups. Her Higher Degree by Research work focuses on a concept of camaraderie as evidenced throughout Australian military history and through this brings to the forefront the voices of Australian nurses who are marginalised within the context of Australian warfare.

Charlie Gadd
Charlie is an ambulance paramedic working in Melbourne, Victoria, Australia. He graduated with a Bachelor of Paramedicine from Griffith University in 2021 and has previous experience in event medicine and community education.

Emma Geis
Emma is the Award Lead and Lecturer in Paramedic Science at Keele University. Emma's background is as a London-based front-line paramedic, she then developed into being a training officer for the London ambulance service and has since completed her BSc in Leadership and Management in Healthcare, PGCE, Post Grad Certificate in Mental Health, and MSc in Medical Education. Due to her passion of mental health and well-being, Emma now works as the Co-academic Lead for the College of Paramedics' Future Workforce Mental Health Project since July 2021 and is starting her Professional Doctorate in Health Education in September 2023.

Justin Honey-Jones
Justin is a Specialist Lecturer Practitioner (Paramedic) and Designated Safeguarding Lead for East of England Ambulance Service. He is Associate Lecturer in Paramedic Science and Medical and Healthcare Education at Anglia Ruskin University and External Examiner in Paramedic Degree Apprenticeships at the University of Cumbria.

Justin is also Partner (Fitness to Practice Registrant Panel Member) at Health and Care Professions Council.

He began his career as a combat medical technician with the British Army Reserves and at the London Ambulance Service NHS Trust, initially as an emergency medical technician and later progressing to be a paramedic after completing the LAS Paramedic Academy programme. He holds a BSc (Hons) in Paramedic Practice from St George's Hospital Medical School, University of London, an MA in Education and Training from the University of Wales, Trinity St Davids and is currently undertaking a Post Graduate Diploma in Advanced Paramedic Practice at the University of Hertfordshire.

Jack Howard
Jack is an intensive care paramedic at Ambulance Victoria in Melbourne, Australia. Jack has been working across Victoria, predominantly in the northern suburbs of Melbourne, as a front-line paramedic for the past 13 years. Jack has a BSc in Health Science (Paramedicine) from Victoria University and an MSc in Specialist Paramedic Practice from Monash University.

Jane Jennings
Jane is a registered paramedic working in Australia. Prior to working as a paramedic she worked as a management accountant in the building industry. Jane's love of people, learning, and community has allowed her to contribute to projects like this, encouraging further learning and development in the field of paramedicine.

Netta Lloyd-Jones
Netta is Associate Lecturer, Oxford Brookes University. She has extensive experience of working in nursing and healthcare practice education within higher education institutions, working in partnership with the NHS, private, voluntary, and independent sectors. Practice education expertise includes implementing professional regulatory body standards (for nursing, paramedics, occupational therapy, physiotherapy, and osteopathy), quality assurance, and Standards of Conduct: Fitness to Practice. Since retiring from being full time, Netta is Associate Lecturer supporting the Masters' programmes in Hong Kong (nursing, management, and leadership), including MSc modules in advanced research design, dissertation supervision, and module lead for the Mastering Professional Nursing Practice module (advanced and culturally safe practice). As Intensive Care Lecturer Practitioner at Oxford Radcliffe Hospitals NHS Trust, she was seconded to the Department of Health as Nursing Officer, within the

NHS Executive for two years before returning to Oxford Brookes University. Posts held include Head of Department, School Executive Projects Officer, and Collaborative Provision Lead, before taking up post as Head of Practice Education.

Jack Matulich
Intensive Care Unit, Gold Coast University Hospital, Southport, Queensland, Australia.

Jennie McGowan
Jennie is a registered paramedic and registered nurse, working in Western Australia. Her background in nursing has given her a solid foundation for clinical and non technical skills as a paramedic. Jennie graduated with a bachelor of Nursing from Notre Dame University in 2015. Jennie specialised in emergency nursing, particularly in rural areas, completing a Graduate certificate in Emergency Nursing from the University of Tasmania in 2018. This inspired her interest in out of hospital care. Jennie then begun working as a road based retrieval nurse, whilst begining her Paramedicine studies, graduating with a Bachelor of Paramedicine from Curtin University. Jennie works for a jurisdictional Ambulance service across rural, remote and metropolitan regions; providing clinical care along with education and support to ambulance volunteers and junior clinicians.

Melinda (Dolly) McPherson
Melinda (Dolly) is Advanced Clinical Practitioner at the University Hospital Southampton and HEMS Specialist Paramedic with the Hampshire and Isle of Wight Air Ambulance. She is a degree paramedic with an MSc in Advanced Practice and has obtained her prescribing qualification. She has experience in the NHS across a number of environments including the ambulance service, minor injuries, the emergency department and within GP practices. She has an interest in reading and writing academic literature with previous publications in the *Journal of Paramedic Practice*, *International Emergency Nursing Journal*, and *Standby CPD*. It is her aim to add to the evidence base that currently inspires paramedic practice whilst learning from it herself. She is currently furthering her interests in research, education and quality improvement working alongside the Royal College of Emergency Medicine (RCEM), the pre-hospital trainee operated research network (PHOTON), and Health Education England (HEE).

Nevin Mehmet
Nevin's is currently Deputy Head of School for Human Sciences, and a Senior Lecturer Applied Ethics for Health & Public Health and supports the paramedic and public health curriculum. Nevin gained an MA Medical Ethics and Law degree and her research interest are within Public Health and Healthcare Ethics in particularly with curriculum delivery within the health, paramedic and public health curriculum.

Simon Menz
Simon is a registered paramedic in Australia who is currently Clinical Support Paramedic with a state-based ambulance service. Simon commenced his paramedic career in 2011, graduating from Edith Cowan University with a BSc in Paramedic Science. After becoming fully qualified in 2014, he has undertaken a variety of paramedic roles within his service, including paramedic mentor, community paramedic, and paramedic trainer. In 2020, Simon completed a Masters in Specialist Care Paramedic Practice with Monash University. He has developed a passion for training with a special interest in critical care, de-escalation, obstetrics, and human factors.

Simon also works part time as Paramedic Lecturer at Notre Dame University. Prior to this, Simon was Assistant Lecturer at Curtin University for the undergraduate Paramedicine program. In his spare time, Simon is a board member of the *International Journal for Advancing Practice* where he advocates for the profession of paramedicine.

Sarah Neal
Sarah Neal qualified as an Adult Nurse in 1988 working at the Royal Free Hospital in London, firstly caring for people with neurosciences disorders and then transferring to care for those with HIV/AIDs. Sarah then moved to Oxford developing her skills over a number of years to become Lecturer Practitioner for Neuroscience Intensive Care, Oxford Radcliffe Infirmary NHS Trust. During this role she led and taught neuroscience post-qualifying education.

Sarah had a particular interest in clinical decision-making and medical ethics. She also contributed to the work of the local Nursing and Allied health professions research ethics committee. In 2004, Sarah became a Senior Lecturer at Oxford Brookes University, teaching across the curriculum for Bachelors and Masters Adult Nursing. Sarah developed expertise in practice education undertaking the role of Placement Lead for Adult Nursing (Oxford) from 2004-2015. Sarah is now the Head of Practice Education at Oxford Brookes University working in close partnership with leaders in the NHS and Private and Voluntary Sector to ensure high quality placement experiences for pre-registration Paramedic Science, Physiotherapy, Occupational Therapy, Nursing, Midwifery and Social work students. Her interests are fitness to practise and learning professional behaviour and suitability.

Alexander Olaussen
Dr Olaussen is a clinician-scientist in the field of pre-hospital emergency care. Clinically, he is a registered paramedic and medical doctor working as a rural emergency doctor.

Academically, he has published over 60 peer-reviewed articles, and 2 books, and is currently completing his PhD through Monash University and Alfred Hospital. In terms of education, Alex is an Adjunct Senior Lecturer at Monash University with in the Bachelor of Paramedicine, a Fellow with the Higher Education Academy, and has to date mentored 18 honours and masters students. He is a research fellow with the National Trauma Research Institute (NTRI) and Alfred Emergency Health Services, and on the ILCOR task force for education, implementation and teams.

Alexander Palmer
Alexander started his career as an Emergency Medical Technician for the London Ambulance NHS Trust and later progressed to Paramedic after completing the LAS Paramedic Academy programme. During the Covid-19 pandemic he worked as a Vaccination Centre Manager in the UK vaccination programme. He holds a BSc (Hons) in Management and Leadership in Health and Social Care from Anglia Ruskin University.

Katie Pavoni
Katie is Associate Professor and Course director/Pastoral Lead for the BSc in Paramedic Science, at St George's, University of London. Her area of passion and interest is practitioner, student ,and patient mental health and in her clinical work she works as a paramedic and mental health practitioner.

Katie is a member of the College of Paramedics Mental Health & Wellbeing Steering group and co-academic lead for the Future Workforce Mental Health Project where she has co-designed a national mental health and well-being curriculum for pre and post registration paramedics, a national well-being support tool and a mental health and well-being education package for mentors and preceptors for early career paramedics. In addition, Katie works with the British Red Cross.

She holds an MSc Advanced Practice (Mental Health) and is undertaking her PhD in Health & Social Care Research: Mental Health.

Georgina Pickering
School of Biomedical Sciences – Paramedicine, Charles Sturt University, Bathurst, New South Wales, Australia.

Rasa Piggott
Rasa specialises in developing evidence - based education content and curricula that serves to progress paramedic professionalisation nationally and internationally. Rasa's authorship and academic roles are founded in her continued currency of practice as a Registered Paramedic and Registered Nurse. Rasa's professional ambition aligns with industry and profession transformational change objectives, including paramedic capability advancement concerning holistic patient assessment, comprehensive biopsychosocial care, risk mitigation and clinical governance adherence. Rasa is a profession leader of industry equity, equality and human-rights compliance. She operates with unwavering dedication to improving conditions for marginalised cohorts amongst patient and provider consumer pools, with a view to improving societal health equity and outcomes.

Markus Pitter
Markus has in excess of 15 years of service as a front-line paramedic in Australia. Throughout his career he has worked in a variety of roles including solo response, remote clinical support, clinical incident review and analysis, human factors and interplay in paramedicine, and design and implementation of innovative clinical practice guidelines. In addition to his hands-on experience, Markus is a passionate educator having worked with several Universities as a sessional lecturer and delivered in-service training and education. Markus is currently a Senator in the Western Australian Clinical Senate which aims to improve clinical care across the health care system and working as an extended care paramedic.

Helen Pocock
South Central Ambulance Service NHS Foundation Trust, Bicester, UK.

Steven Poulton
Steve is Senior Lecturer in Paramedic Science at York St John University. He became a pracademic following the birth of his first son; having worked full-time in a UK ambulance service he continues to maintain clinical shifts on a monthly basis in addition to his full-time role. Steve's passion for educating people, from patients to students, has seen him become a part of the UK College of Paramedics CPD team, from concept to delivery. Steve is involved in creating clinical CPD events for all those seeking something to learn. Academically, Steve holds two degrees, a Post Grad Certificate in Academic Education, and is working towards an MSc.

Kieran Robinson
Kieran started his career in the East of England Ambulance Service after completing his BSc in Paramedic Science and worked on a mixture of ambulances, rapid response vehicles, and in the emergency operations centre doing telephone triage. Alongside this work, Kieran completed his MSc in Critical Care and a level 3 Award in Education and Training before undertaking some work as an associate lecturer with Anglia Ruskin University. He also completed a scholarship with the Healthcare Leadership Academy, subsequently contributing to the organisation as Cohort Director and achieving fellowship status with the Institute of Leadership and Management.

Broadening his experiences, Kieran spent some time working with a private ambulance service in a clinical leadership role. He also completed a temporary contract as Senior Operations Manager for the ambulance service in Qatar preparing for the FIFA World Cup. Most recently, he has been working in a new community team as Virtual Ward Senior Practitioner.

Simon Sawyer
Simon is Director of Education at Australian Paramedical College and Adjunct Senior Lecturer at Griffith University.

He has worked as an Advanced Life Support Paramedic in Victoria, Australia since 2012. He began designing and teaching paramedic programs as a lecturer at Monash University in 2015. Simon holds an Adjunct Senior Lecturer position with the Paramedicine Department at Griffith University where he studies family and domestic violence, paramedic education, and paramedic well-being. Simon completed a PhD on the paramedic response to family violence and teaches paramedics how to respond to patients experiencing family and domestic violence. He is currently the Director of Education at the Australian Paramedical College and still works as a Paramedic.

Marco Scarvaci
Marco is a registered paramedic working in Western Australia. He graduated with a Bachelor of Paramedicine at Curtin University and also has a previous degree in a Bachelor of Exercise and Sport Science. Marco previously worked in health and fitness but then changed to become an Emergency Medical Dispatcher which sparked his career in this field.

Brian J. Sengstock
Brian is the Associate Head of School (Healthcare Sciences) and Senior Lecturer in Healthcare Sciences at Charles Sturt University. Brian began his career working was a volunteer ambulance officer, before progressing into both clinical and ambulance communication centre roles, and finally paramedic and health leadership and management education in the university setting. He holds a Postgraduate Certificate in Intensive Care Paramedic Studies from Charles Sturt University, a Graduate Certificate in Emergency and Disaster Management from Queensland University of Technology, and a Master of Emergency Management from Charles Sturt University. Brian completed his PhD in 2008 through CQ University.

Ramon Z. Shaban
Professor Ramon Z. Shaban is Clinical Chair of Communicable Disease Control and Infection Prevention with the Sydney Infectious Diseases Institute of the Faculty of Medicine and Health at the University of Sydney and Western Sydney Local Health District. Professor Shaban is a leading internationally credentialed expert infection control practitioner with particular strengths in high-consequence infectious diseases, disease control, emergency care and health protection. As Clinical Chair he is Chief Infection Control Practitioner and District Director of Communicable Disease Control and Infection Prevention for Western Sydney Local Health District, where he provides strategic and operational leadership of infection prevention and disease control services. He is also Associate Director of the New South Wales Biocontainment Centre, Australia's first purpose-built state-of-the-art facility for the prevention, containment and management of high-consequence infectious disease located at Westmead Hospital in New South Wales.

Samantha Sheridan
School of Biomedical Sciences – Paramedicine, Charles Sturt University, Bathurst, New South Wales, Australia.

Jade Speed
Jade studied at St George's Hospital Medical School, University of London gaining a BSc (Hons) in Paramedic Science. Following this, she began her career as a paramedic with the London Ambulance Service. During the Covid 19 pandemic, Jade worked in conjunction with colleagues from the London Fire Brigade and trained three firefighters to work alongside paramedics to deliver care to patients across London. With a specific passion and interest in safeguarding, following the pandemic, Jade took a secondment with the Safeguarding Team within the Ambulance Service and after a year, Jade was fortunate enough to gain a full-time job as a Safeguarding Specialist for the London Ambulance Service.

Dan Staines
Department of Nursing, Midwifery and Healthcare Practice, Coventry University, Coventry, UK.

Clare Sutton
School of Biomedical Sciences – Paramedicine, Charles Sturt University, Bathurst, New South Wales, Australia.

Samantha Sweet
Samantha is a paramedic working with London's ambulance service. Having completed her degree at University of Hertfordshire, she returned to this university and completed a masters degree in emergency and critical care. Samantha is an associate lecturer at Anglia Ruskin University alongside her full time role. And also volunteers for a charity critical care system.

Renate Taylor
Renate began her journey working in primary schools as special educational assistant whilst undertaking BSc Psychology with the Open University. This followed with BSc in Mental Health Nursing, studying at the University of Hertfordshire, which was a passion to understand and help those experiencing serious mental health problems. As a newly qualified nurse she undertook a taught MSc in Cognitive Behavioural Therapy. Renate was awarded an accolade for service improvement in rolling out the SBARD in mental health services in Hertfordshire. Joining the University of Bedfordshire, she embraced her role of teaching in higher education with passion and interest to support mental health nursing students in their learning and clinical practice. Additionally, she is a founder member of the Recovery College in partnership with the NHS Trust and is currently working at the University of Roehampton as Senior Lecturer in Mental Health Nursing and Nurse Education.

Ruth Townsend
School of Biomedical Science, Charles Sturt University, Bathurst, New South Wales, Australia.

Jane Warland
Jane is Adjunct Associate Professor University of Adelaide. She began her midwifery career training as a midwife at Adelaide's Queen Victoria Hospital (now Women's and Childrens). She practised as a clinician midwife for 20 years before undertaking her PhD. She has worked in Midwifery Education since 2008. Her key areas of teaching interest are facilitating normal birth and complex midwifery care. Jane has published widely. She is a senior researcher, with a research track record in Stillbirth where she is recognised as an international leader in this field.

Aimee Yarrington
Aimee has been a qualified midwife since 2003. She has worked in all areas of midwifery practice, from the high-risk consultant-led units to the low-risk stand-alone midwife-led units. She left full-time midwifery practice to join the ambulance service in 2009, starting as an emergency care assistant and working her way up to paramedic, while always keeping her midwifery practice up to date. She has worked in several areas within the ambulance service, including the emergency operations centre and the education and training department. Her work towards improving the education of prehospital maternity care has led to her being awarded a fellowship award from the College of Paramedics. Aimee strives to improve the teaching and education for clinicians in dealing with prehospital maternity care.

Preface

In this latest, third edition there is a lot to celebrate including significant revisions in almost all chapters that draw on the latest evidence, meaning students and practitioners can keep on top of growing trends in research and practice. This is complemented by fresh new ideas presented by new authors including clinical paramedics, medical doctors, academics and researchers, allowing those new ideas and perspectives to be brought to the text.

This edition also boasts new chapters in response to the changing face and dynamic world of paramedicine.

A new chapter on end-of-life care provides a narrative for paramedics who are faced with providing care to those individuals and families during this time of crisis, and a new chapter on de-escalation skills delivers frameworks for paramedics to consider using during cases involving heightened stress. Low acuity cases are also increasing in paramedic work and require the paramedic to be able to refer people to different services: this new chapter complements the existing chapter on minor injuries, both of which are written by those who have significant expertise in these areas.

When students enter work integrated learning (WIL) they are met with many opportunities for learning but also challenges relating to the world of practice. Therefore, a new chapter on practice-based learning provides hints and tips for students and mentors functioning in this complex environment. With an increase in cases of domestic violence and abuse, a new chapter is presented by a leading academic in their field, who studied domestic abuse at doctoral level, giving credibility to and confidence in the theories provided in the chapter.

We believe that by responding to the changing face of paramedicine through fully revised chapters, bringing fresh new perspectives and authors to the text, and writing new chapters to reflect modern paramedicine, *Fundamentals of Paramedic Practice: A Systems Approach* remains a contemporary text that meets the ongoing needs of the student paramedic, qualified clinicians, and the profession.

Sam Willis
Ian Peate

Acknowledgements

In this third edition, we would like to acknowledge the hard work of those delivering high quality, person-centred care and who strive to be the best paramedics they can be.

We would also like to acknowledge those staff who contribute to out-of-hospital (OOH) care through professional bodies such as the Australasian College of Paramedicine and the UK College of Paramedics. These organisations represent their members while striving for professional development of individuals and, more broadly, advancement of OOH care.

Additionally, we acknowledge the important work undertaken by those who participate in raising clinical standards through the regulatory bodies such as the Australian Health Practitioner Agency (AHPRA) and the UK Health and Care Professions Council. Through the monitoring of educational institutions and ensuring paramedics meet the exacting standards of the paramedic, standards of care are raised in turn leading to increased public confidence in paramedics.

Sam Willis
Ian Peate

About the Companion Website

This book is accompanied by a companion website:

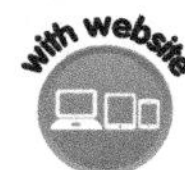

www.wiley.com/go/willis/paramedic3e

The website includes:

- Interactive multiple-choice questions
- Case studies to test your knowledge
- Glossary of terms used in each chapter
- Answers to activities

Scan this QR code to visit the companion website:

CHAPTER 1

Professionalism in paramedic practice

Sarah Neal

Faculty of Health and Life Sciences, Oxford Brookes University, Oxford, UK

Netta Lloyd-Jones

Faculty of Health and Life Sciences, Oxford Brookes University, Oxford, UK

Contents

LEARNING OUTCOMES

On completion of this chapter the reader will be able to:

- Discuss the importance of professionalism in relation to paramedic practice.
- Identify three key themes of professionalism.
- Describe concepts that influence professionalism.
- Describe how professionalism is learned.
- Describe the potential outcomes of behaving unprofessionally.

Fundamentals of Paramedic Practice: A Systems Approach, Third Edition. Edited by Sam Willis and Ian Peate.

Companion website: www.wiley.com/go/willis/paramedic3e

Case study

A student paramedic is halfway through their course. They have several months experience of working with registered paramedics treating and caring for patients in practice. The expectations are that they need to start using initiative to assess cases and suggest treatment and actions, whilst being supervised by the paramedic.

The paramedic they are working with is experienced, confident, and has impressed the student on many occasions. The registered paramedic is popular with their colleagues and often takes the lead when discussing difficult situations in work and is also a key member of the team when socialising outside of work. They enjoy pranks and often laugh about other colleagues' vulnerabilities.

They have assessed a patient and are planning to return to the emergency department with the patient. The plan is for the student to treat the patient in the back of the ambulance whilst the paramedic is driving. The student is feeling anxious and 'out of their depth' but they want to impress the paramedic. The student does not say anything about their concerns. The patient deteriorates on the return journey.

Introduction

Contemporary paramedics must not only demonstrate extensive clinical knowledge and skills for paramedic practice but also **professionalism** throughout their daily lives, both on and off duty. This chapter identifies and discusses key aspects of professionalism required for effective and safe paramedic practice.

Professionalism in paramedic practice

For the paramedic to demonstrate professionalism, they must know what is required of them by their professional statutory regulatory body. For example, in the UK this is the Health and Care Professions Council (HCPC), and in Australia this is the Australian Health Practitioner Regulation Agency (AHPRA). Regulatory bodies provide a professional code of conduct that applies to their registered paramedics. The principles that underpin such codes relate directly to professional knowledge, skills, behaviour, and attitude, as well as professional clinical performance by being the 'knowledgeable doer'. This refers to the integration of theory and practice (Benner 1984), and practising safely within the scope of education, training, and practice for the protection of the public. Practising safely is also embedded within the HCPC (2016) Standard 9.1, which states:

> *You must make sure that your conduct justifies the public's trust and confidence in you and your profession.*

Behaving professionally is a standard expected not only by the HCPC and regulatory bodies of other countries such as Australia, where legislation allows paramedics to be a regulated profession (Townsend 2017) but also by patients, co-workers, other healthcare professionals, and the public. Healthcare professionalism is currently under a great deal of scrutiny, with increasing numbers of fitness-to-practise cases being heard by most healthcare professional statutory regulatory bodies, where issues of inappropriate or unprofessional behaviour are cited. In 2021–2022, the number of registered paramedic fitness-to-practise cases in the UK was 367 (1.1% of all paramedic registrants). This continues the trend of paramedic cases being the second highest number of fitness-to-practise cases of all allied health and care professions in the UK (HCPC 2021) and appears to be a similar pattern to other countries. It is therefore important that all paramedics consider professionalism as a lifelong competence that will require continual demonstration (and development) throughout their careers. The resources that professional associations such as the College of Paramedics (UK) provide to support lifelong learning and professional development are continually developing (van der Gaag et al. 2017).

Defining professionalism

Defining professionalism is not easy, as it is diverse, multifaceted, and open to individual interpretation. Between 1990 and 2015, there was a plethora of literature on what constitutes professionalism in healthcare, and the concept continues to evolve according to societal changes.

Sociologists may define 'a profession' in terms of being a vocation with a specific body of knowledge, a defined range of skills, which is inherently trustworthy and ethical and provides a service to society (e.g. as usefully summarised in the seminal work by Hugman 1991, pp. 2–9 and Johnston and Acker 2016). Some healthcare literature has focused upon values of care and compassion held by the profession itself, and roles undertaken by its registered practitioners, for example, developing honest relationships with patients (e.g. Burges Watson et al. 2012), patient advocacy (e.g. Batt et al. 2017), and clinical excellence (Jauregui, J. et al. 2016).

More helpful detail is found in Bossers et al. (1999) schemata of professionalism, dividing the concept into three main themes:

- Professional parameters (e.g. legal and ethical aspects)
- Professional behaviours (e.g. discipline-related knowledge and skills)
- Professional responsibilities (e.g. responsibility to patients, oneself, employers, and the public)

Research commissioned by the HCPC in 2011 explored healthcare professionals' understanding of professionalism. It concluded that the key to professional behaviour is 'the interaction of person and context, and the importance of situational judgement' (HCPC 2014, p. 3). This is particularly relevant to paramedics, where responses to crisis, trauma, and emergency situations involving family and significant others, and the heightened emotion at such times, can result in misperceptions and miscommunications (van der Gaag et al. 2017).

Professionalism is now regarded as a meta-skill, comprising situational awareness and contextual judgement, which allows individuals to draw on the communication, technical, and practical skills appropriate for a given professional scenario (HCPC 2014), rather than it comprising of a set of discrete skills. Such professional judgement will be dependent upon the knowledge developed through logic; sensed intuitively; gained through experience, particularly prior experience of similar events; and influenced by education, socialisation, and the human resources of employing organisations (Johns 1992; Gallagher et al. 2016; Brown et al. 2005). In addition to this, the current focus is upon consistently demonstrating a set of identifiable, positive professional attributes, values, and behaviours. It is this challenge of embedding a discrete body of knowledge into the philosophy and values of a profession that the paramedic profession is exploring (Johnston and Acker 2016; Givati et al. 2017).

Professionalism as ethical practice

The nature and practice of a paramedic's role demand that they understand morals and ethics and utilise this understanding within their practise (Chapter 3, Legal and Ethical Aspects of Paramedic Practice details this more). As this chapter discusses, what paramedics view ethics to be is important within a professional context. Meta-ethics (what is meant by 'right' and 'wrong'), normative ethics (placing the concepts of 'right' and 'wrong' into professional practice situations), and applying ethics in specialised areas, such as healthcare or public health ethics, are all part of demonstrating professionalism. In a scoping review to outline scales for measuring professional behaviour amongst paramedics, Bowen et al. (2017) identified the key characteristics of professionalism. These include practising within a professional code of ethics. Key principles that underpin professionalism as ethical practice include integrity, honesty, trustworthiness, probity, objectivity, and fairness. These key professional characteristics are also applied as legal principles when determining cases of professional misconduct. Professionalism can thus be regarded as ethical competence in all aspects of professional activity. However, at times it can take courage to maintain professional ethical principles, to speak up, and/or to potentially demonstrate your own vulnerability for the overall gain of the people you have a duty to care for and the profession you represent.

Professional identity, socialisation, and culture

Professional identity, professional socialisation, and professional culture will all influence understanding of what professionalism is within particular professions.

Identity

Identification encompasses basic cognitive and social processes through which we make sense of and organise our human world (Monrouxe 2010), including behaviours, knowledge and skills, values and beliefs, the context in which we work, and its associated socialisation. Together with both personal and group identity, these are all key components (Fitzgerald 2020). Our thoughts, experiences, and reflections create a complex catalogue of who we are as individuals and members of groups (Fitzgerald 2020). Professional identity is assimilated with other aspects of a personal sense of identity including the variety of roles that you undertake in society, for example, within family, friendships, communities, as well as your profession. Paramedic professional identity involves being able to practise with knowledge and skill, demonstrating a commitment to the paramedic profession, and being accountable and responsible for one's own actions (and omissions) through exercising professional judgement. Whilst there are some widely perceived stereotypical 'identities' of paramedics (such as being a hero or a lifesaver), the key components of paramedic identity are best described as a professional expert in developing honest relationships with patients (Johnston and Acker 2016), where patients benefit from timely treatment of their complex clinical needs outside of the hospital environment.

Socialisation

Students learn to think critically within university and practice contexts. Professional socialisation is a combination of an individual's professional development and the extent to which an individual adopts, acquires, and adjusts to the professional group in the practice context (Ajjawi and Higgs 2008). Socialisation in a healthcare profession will depend on the individual's past experiences, reflection on practice, and learning experiences, which will change and develop throughout their career. Socialisation is therefore negotiated in both university and practice settings, which shapes individual and collective professional identity and work culture through shared challenges and the values of both educational and vocational experiences (Givati et al. 2017). It is important to be aware of the culture within practice so that socialisation does not negatively impact upon ability for inquiry into evidence base for clinical decision-making. For example, in an ethnographic study of nurses' socialisation upon graduation, Voldbjerg et al. (2021) found that they were inadvertently prevented from inquiring about evidence base because experienced colleagues were seen to be the main knowledge source. As experienced registrants may not all be confident in nurturing an inquiring approach in newly registered staff, the local culture of professional practice needs to be supportive of questioning practice, and must not see this as incompetence or insecurity. This could equally apply to paramedic practice and associated socialisation.

Practice insight

Make an effort to communicate professionally with those around you, such as other students, university lecturers, and ambulance service staff. This will increase your learning opportunities and improve your working relationships. Consider how building friendships with colleagues within the practice setting can enhance or detract from professional practice and your development.

Another aspect of becoming socialised in the paramedic community is the introduction to the knowledge and expertise of the range of practitioners working within the practice setting. For paramedics, this includes working with ambulance technicians, patient transport services and operational managers, education teams within ambulance services, and a range of professionals in hospital and other community healthcare settings such as primary care. The relevant hierarchical structure of the organisation of service delivery is also influential in determining the professional behaviour (and attitudes) expected. For example, the power and authority in an organisation (and/or profession) are embedded within job descriptions, forms of address, policies and procedures, and practice standards.

Professional culture

Historically, the paramedic professional culture has been one of training rather than education, there may be a juxtaposition of old and new professional cultures causing tensions and potential confusion for the emerging professional (e.g. confusion making decisions about what is an appropriate professional attitude or behaviour) (van der Gaag et al. 2017; Townsend 2017), and it has been regarded as 'the trainer's role' to 'instil' professionalism without opportunity for learners to question. A more facilitative, questioning, and reflective approach changes how students learn about professionalism. Professional culture can influence and be influenced by the challenges of change and its management. New students and employees are keen to 'fit in' to the work culture and are aware of being scrutinised by registrants when on placement (Givati et al. 2017). If this is not embraced a philosophical tension may be created between the old and the new thus hindering organisational change and the development of the profession (HCPC 2014; Gallagher et al. 2016). The university might be seen as the 'intruder' who has caused the 'loss of the communal occupational nature of paramedic practice'

(Givati et al. 2017, p. 367) but also as a key influencer in the development of professionalism (Givati et al. 2017). The influence of the professional culture may also have an impact upon the contribution to research in practice (Burges Watson et al. 2012). In addition, culture will be influenced by care being provided in out-of-hospital settings, which are high-risk environments (regarding patient safety) due to the unpredictable and increasingly complex nature of the paramedic interventions required (Hagiwara et al. 2019; Mallinson and Willis 2020).

Learning professionalism

Learning about the concept of professionalism and how to demonstrate competence is achieved throughout the paramedic educational curricula, both campus and practice based. This is in addition to taught components such as discussing cases of academic misconduct, developing clinical decision-making, or critical thinking. However, much of what paramedics learn is through working with mentors and registered paramedics, through role modelling in practice, and within the university setting. Positive and negative **role models** in practice can provide a great influence on the understanding of the concept. Positive role models are widely reported as having excellent interpersonal skills, enthusiasm, commitment to excellence and evidence-based practice, integrity, effective teaching skills, building rapport with students, and being committed to professional development, safe practice, and exceptional clinical skills. Where there are clear policy obligations for practice staff (e.g. mentors) to 'teach', connections between theoretical and practical knowledge are more likely to be made (Peiser et al. 2018). However, there are significant challenges for paramedic staff who support students in practice. In particular there may be conflict between supporting and assessor roles alongside heavy service delivery workloads (e.g. Johnston and Acker 2016; HCPC 2017) and, where there are only informal requirements for supporting students in practice, staff are 'inclined to attend to the development of contextual knowledge with a consequent disconnect between theory and practice' (Peiser et al. 2018, p. 16). In addition, campus-based teaching may only have a limited effect on learning compared to work-based learning, and role modelling professional attributes appears crucial to developing professionalism in students (Felstead and Springett 2016; Nevalainen et al. 2018). Humans unconsciously learn from their environment, and may not be aware that they are learning, so paramedic students might find it hard to appreciate their learning from working alongside registered paramedics in busy environments or may not assimilate learning until further on in their career. In addition, the wealth of knowledge, skill, and behaviours of an experienced role model is often difficult to verbalise until formal recording occurs in writing (Scott and Spouse 2013), and observation of behaviours and decision-making, for example, may be unconsciously integrated into the observer's practice (Hunter and Cook 2018).

Most people know more than they can ever put into words. This tacit knowledge (after Polyani 1958) is also conveyed to learners by positive role models offering solutions in complex and challenging encounters, which can be integrated into the existing knowledge of the paramedic.

Practice insight

Recognise the many different elements of paramedic practice and be aware that elements of expertise exist in part due to experience within the profession. Therefore, it is important to listen to and embrace aspects of practice that have been shared with you by more experienced clinicians. If you are unsure whether what you are being taught is correct, explore further with the practitioner, investigate research, policies, and protocols related to the issue, contact other staff for support (e.g. colleagues, lecturers), read your professional code of conduct/ethics, and investigate the matter further.

The earlier interest in the evidence base for learning professionalism (e.g. Roff and Dherwani 2011; Lloyd-Jones 2013; Carter et al. 2015) indicated that socialisation had the potential to erode professional attributes learned in the university and presented a rationale for increasing the focus upon professional parameters, behaviours, responsibilities, and values, so that public confidence in registered professionals is not compromised. Professionalism is therefore a competence that extends beyond registration, and all paramedic professionals must continue to demonstrate it throughout their career. To do this, it is still useful to consider the work of Carter et al (2016), which explored fifteen dimensions of professionalism. See Table 1.1 for an overview of the fifteen dimensions of professionalism.

This exploration resulted in six factors of professionalism being identified:

- Being valued by the public
- Appropriate behaviours
- Organisational and professional care

TABLE 1.1 The fifteen dimensions of professionalism.

Professional identity	Reliability
Professional status	Competence, knowledge and improvement
Normative elements such as regulation and social status	Pride in the profession
Comparative perceived status in relation to other professions	Appearance
	Flexibility
Adherence to ethical practice principles	Behaviour outside work
	Organisational context
Interactions with patients	Situational awareness
Interactions with staff	

Source: Carter et al. 2015.

- Positive/proactive professional behaviours
- Professional identity and pride
- Learning orientation

These six factors are fundamental to professionalism. Carter et al. (2015) found that the quality and provision of these factors (except feeling valued by the public) appear to diminish as the practitioner journeys through their career. It is important to be aware of how self-assessment of professionalism may be influenced by socialisation. Any potential dissonance between self-perception and actual outcomes needs to be identified. The impact of the culture of the organisation or the local work environment should be considered, as this can either enable or limit paramedic professionalism (Gallagher et al. 2016; HCPC 2014).

Consistent reflective practice throughout your career is a key aspect of professional development and professionalism. Your professional code of practice will be a useful quick guide to refer to in your reflections. It may also be useful to use the generic questionnaire as a reflective aid to guide discussions about complex professionalism constructs. For the full questionnaire, see Appendix A of Carter et al. (2015).

Reflective practice

Schön (1987) recommended both reflection in action and reflection upon action as ways of developing professional practice. For paramedic practice, it is often reflection after the event that is more prevalent, due to the emergency nature of the work, however, both approaches are useful in informing future practice. Howlett's (2019) qualitative study explored paramedics' intended use of reflection as they transitioned from students to newly registered professionals. The participants recognised that reflection was a positive tool that aided continual professional development and could influence the wider paramedic community. As newly registered practitioners progressed, they understood the need for an evidence base to underpin their reflections and actions. They did, however, express concern that not all opportunities for reflection were recognised or encouraged when they were in practice. Some of the participants indicated that where the reflection had been part of an assessment, they were more likely to have a negative experience or view of the outcome. For reflection to be experienced positively they needed to be supported by role models within the practice organisation. They needed their colleagues to recognise the effectiveness of reflection and to encourage consistent use. As the paramedic student enters practice as a novice, they require positive experiences of reflection supported by mentors to be able to develop their professional competence and take these skills into their future career.

There are several models of reflective practice that will help support learning through reflection in and on practice, for example, Gibbs (1988) (Figure 1.1), Driscoll (2007), Johns (2000), or Kolb (1994). All help to structure reflection and support learning from experience and encourage in-depth thinking and prompt use of alternatives (Paterson and Chapman 2013). It is important that students try different models, as this helps understanding of the overall process from which individual preference for model selection can be made for future practice.

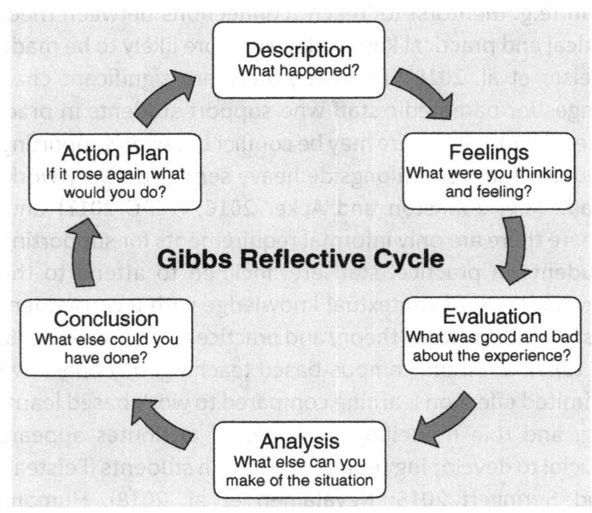

FIGURE 1.1 Gibbs' 1998 reflective cycle.

Practice insight

To ensure you advance your professional competence and benefit from reflective practice you need to think of it as a skill to be learned and developed over time. Explore the various models of reflection and ask for guidance and support from clinical and academic role models.

Assessment of professionalism

Demonstrating professionalism is determined by the assessment requirements of the educational programme, or once registered, the standards expected by the employer organisations, peers, professional regulatory body (e.g. HCPC, AHPRA), and professional associations, e.g. professional bodies such as the College of Paramedics (UK). Students are assessed by clinical mentors and other colleagues with whom they work in practice. Self and peer assessment, objective structured clinical examinations (OSCEs), simulation, direct observation by academic tutors, critical incident reports, and learner-maintained portfolios are some of the ways in which triangulations of assessment can be achieved. Such triangulation is important to reduce the subjectivity of a particular assessor, and any single measure alone is not sufficient (Reljić et al. 2017).

Addressing issues of lack of professionalism when employed as a registered paramedic will usually be undertaken by following relevant local policies (e.g. professional conversations and appraisal, application of bullying and harassment policies or grievance procedures, assessment against clinical skills and procedure policy documents).

Practice insight

Visit your university website and take a look at the student charter/code of conduct. Also visit your regulatory body website (e.g. HCPC) and read the student code of conduct, performance, and ethics, to recognise the standards that affect you as a student. You may also be aware of such standards laid out by the ambulance service/trust/organisation you practise with. Make sure you are aware of all of these standards from the start of your paramedic programme and continue to update yourself throughout your career (e.g. when reflecting upon your practice experiences).

Scope of practice and professional confidence

A professional must work within their scope of practice. This requires the ability to consider the context, personal professional competence, and ethical and legal frameworks. The decision to proceed with care or treatment will require professional judgement. The ability to practise safely and effectively will be reliant on education and maintaining clinical and professional competence and the environmental context. The paramedic's approach to scope of practice is likely to change as they develop through their career from novice to expert, moving from a supervised unregulated student who is responsible for their actions to becoming a registered professional who is accountable for the care and treatment they provide. From course commencement, student paramedics are required to be working towards the professional code of conduct and need to be supported in their learning to understand how their professional standards apply to them in their role as a student and as a future registrant. For example, the HCPC (2016b) has produced a guide to help support student learning in preparation for when they apply for registration. In addition to this, the different paramedic roles may vary (e.g. practitioner, manager, tutor) and therefore the scope of practice will alter, however, the practitioner must always work within their level of competence (AHPRA 2022).

Jackson et al. (2019) undertook a narrative review of the literature in relation to professional confidence and expertise across allied health disciplines. They suggest that professional confidence can be experienced by the practitioner across all stages of their career. To be professionally confident the paramedic requires a clear understanding of their role and scope of practice and must be able to practise effectively and competently. Experiences in practice and the way in which they overcome challenges and build upon success will impact their professional confidence. Jackson et al. (2019 p. 231) conclude that, 'Reflection-on-practice and reflexivity are recommended personal practices for increasing one's own professional confidence'.

Help-seeking behaviour

A professional (student or registered) may experience times when they are not competent in a skill or feel out of their depth in a situation. It is important that the individual is self-aware and able to recognise this. The professional will need to address this and seek appropriate support to develop their practise. It may be that the practitioner feels embarrassed or fearful about this, not wanting to portray themselves as anxious, risk averse, or over dependent on their supervisors (Sturman et al. 2020). This can pose a conundrum for the practitioner, how to maintain professional safety whilst not being seen negatively and/or as incompetent by their peers, seniors, and the patients in their care. Sturman et al. (2020) observe that some students can frame their help-seeking as safe and self-regulated. The ability to identify authoritative advice is an important skill for safe clinical practice. The point at which you raise this with a mentor will depend upon the context and environment, for example, immediate action and quick communication is required in emergency situations whereas less urgent settings may allow for more detailed explanation and exploration. Suggested tips for setting the scene, to allow for help-seeking behaviour, and promoting patient safety are included in the practice insights to help development.

Practice insight

Help-seeking behaviour in professional practice:

- Identify areas for development prior to commencing a placement/shift, categorising them into short- and long-term goals; you could use your practice assessment documentation, competency requirements, and professional codes as a guide.
- When you first meet your mentor, set 'ground rules' about how and when to address areas for development and/or highlight concerns. Aim for an open and ongoing dialogue.
- Frame your 'ground rule' discussions positively, e.g. identifying the need for patient safety, wanting to demonstrate self-awareness, and wanting to target self-development.
- If you are nervous about raising this with you mentor rehearse this, for example, with a peer or academic support person.
- Face your fear and 'speak up', especially when patient safety is likely to be compromised.
- Reflect upon how these discussions have gone and learn how to develop this aspect of your professionalism as you move forward in your career. You could ask for feedback from you mentor to inform your reflection.
- If you experience negativity when you ask for help (e.g. bullying behaviour) seek support from seniors either within practice or in the educational setting and address the concerns according to local policy.

Sturman et al. (2020) suggest that students appear to learn rapidly through their help-seeking encounters. It is therefore important for mentors to be aware of the potential reluctance of students to seek help, and to overcome this by developing supportive student–mentor relationships. These relationships can be managed by fostering an environment where it is safe to explore areas for development; listening to the students' fears and seeking resolution through positive action planning and offering feedback; responding promptly to student requests without compromising patient safety; providing opportunities to reflect together; encouraging students to seek assistance; and providing constructive feedback and role modelling help-seeking behaviour.

Health and well-being

One determinant of safe professional practice is the health and well-being of the practitioner. This is a common component of regulatory body fitness-to-practise requirements (AHPRA 2022; HCPC 2022; PHECC 2017). The AHPRA (2022) guidance indicates that the practitioner has a responsibility to reflect upon their own ability to practise safely and not rely on their own self-assessment; they must consult others appropriately should their judgement be impaired. There is a developing awareness for the need to support practitioners in raising concerns about their own or colleagues' health. This can be at the level of employment or by reporting to the professional regulatory body if the condition or impairment is likely to significantly impede safe practice long term. It is important to utilise occupational health services and well-being clinics and provide supportive one-to-one conversations to support employees to maintain their health and reinforce positive coping strategies. Professional bodies may also provide useful resources – for example, the Health and Well-being Framework (HCPC 2022), which outlines responsibilities not only for the individual professional but also their manager and employer, and employee representative groups.

Practice insight

You need to be aware of your own health and well-being, seeking appropriate support when necessary. Recognising that health and well-being is the professional responsibility of all, consider how you would support colleagues who raise concerns about their own health and well-being.

Professionalism whilst working under stress

Healthcare professionals work in stressful situations and emergency practitioners such as paramedics consistently have to navigate challenging and complex treatments, which at times are undertaken in dangerous environments. Maintaining professionalism and working within codes of practice are paramount to safe and effective care even when working under stress. Practitioners should be mindful of the potential for burn-out and therefore explore techniques to minimise this risk.

Mallinson and Willis (2020) recommend a performance-enhancing psychological strategy model for enabling readiness of practitioners in emergency situations. The model takes the professional through steps to become calm and focused ready for engagement (Table 1.2). To ensure positive outcomes the practitioner will need to practise the activities within the model aiming for them to become embedded and utilised effortlessly within the practice setting.

Cultural safety

The educational preparation of the paramedic profession is mainly focused on clinical knowledge and skills; however, it is argued that this needs to be balanced with appropriate preparation in other aspects of patient care to effectively practise in uncertain, changing, and diverse professional environments (Ebbs and Gonzalez 2019). Practising in diverse environments is related to providing culturally safe care.

TABLE 1.2 Performance-enhancing psychological strategies.

B	Breathe (tactical breathing)	Slow, deep inhalations and exhalations e.g. square-box breathing
T	Talk (to self)	Motivational positive internal self-talk prior to or during a challenging activity (e.g. I can do this, I will be calm, I have the skills to manage this)
S	See (mental rehearsal)	Visualise the situation and mentally rehearse the activity about to be undertaken
F	Focus using a trigger word	Preparation of a personal trigger word which has been developed and practised over time to move the practitioner quickly towards engaging with the patient/activity in calm and focused manner

Source: *adapted from* Mallinson and Willis 2020 (after Lauria et al. 2017).

A key principle of safe practice is to understand that only the patient and/or relevant colleagues can determine whether or not actions are culturally safe. Since the 1990s, cultural safety has gained increasing focus in the preparation of other healthcare professions, however, as yet little has been produced directly addressing paramedic preparation for working in a diverse population in a culturally safe manner. Culture can be defined as incorporating ethnicity, social background and socio-economic status, gender or sexual orientation, spiritual and health beliefs, age, and level of education (Holland 2018; Westenra 2018). As cultural safety is determined by the recipient of care, the experience of anyone involved in the care (e.g. patient, family, carers, significant others) may identify that the cultural identity and/or well-being of the patient has been 'diminishe[d], demean[ed] or disempower[ed]' in any manner (NCNZ 2011, p. 7).

There are various theoretical models and frameworks to inform developing culturally safe practice in healthcare. It is suggested that those utilised by other healthcare professions can be adapted and applied to paramedic practice. For example, Papadopoulos et al.'s (1998) transcultural skills development model is underpinned by the recognition of oppression that exists in society and mitigation is needed against the effects this has with the goal of equalising any imbalances of power between individuals and/or groups of people (Aqil et al. 2021). The model focuses upon the development of skills in four stages (Figure 1.2).

Each stage of this model has its own components, for example:

- Cultural awareness: including our personal values and beliefs, and the nature of cultural identity.
- Cultural knowledge: as derived from various disciplines including anthropology, psychology, sociology medicine, healthcare, and traditional and folk practices.
- Cultural sensitivity: developing appropriate relationships with patients by considering how we view their cultural beliefs and values, approaching each patient as an equal partner in decision-making, and respecting their individuality. This includes meeting the specific language, cultural, and communication needs of patients and their families.
- Cultural competence: this is the synthesis and application of the previous three stages: awareness, knowledge, and sensitivity.

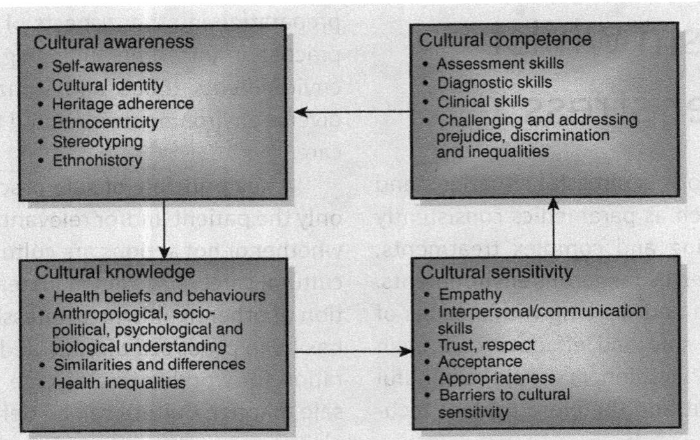

FIGURE 1.2 Transcultural skills development model. Source: Papadopoulos et al. 1998.

The above components of culturally safe practice also apply to professionalism when working within a multicultural workforce. To provide culturally safe and respectful practice, how best to prepare for culturally safe paramedic practice needs to be considered.

Practice insight

Do you know what your code of professional practice states about culturally safe practice?

Professional regulation

Professional regulation varies according to the laws of the country in which the paramedic practices. There are country-specific administrative schemes for addressing health, performance, and conduct (e.g. AHPRA 2021; HCPC 2021), however, the principles that underpin these processes are similar. The function of a professional regulatory body is to maintain the standards of the profession and to protect the public. Registrants of a profession are required to adhere to their code of professional conduct. If a registrant breaches the professional code through an act or omission the professional regulatory body may need to take action. This will be determined by whether the error in practice is minor and a learning opportunity or more severe malpractice that requires investigation according to local policy with potential for escalation. These principles apply to actions and behaviour within work or outside of the workplace. As a result, investigation of the registrant's fitness to practise and decisions about their suitability to continue as a registrant will be made.

The impact of a paramedic's actions and behaviour outside of the workplace may have consequences for their professionalism and registration. For example, some professional regulatory bodies specify serious or grave criminal offences that would be automatically referred directly to a professional regulatory body fitness-to-practise committee. Examples of cases include hate crimes, sexual offences, extortion, blackmail, murder/manslaughter, causing death by dangerous driving, or serious drug-related offences. In addition to these offences, less serious or non-criminal activity occurring outside of work may still impact upon fitness to practise being called into question at a more local level (e.g. by the employer).

The outcome of fitness-to-practise investigations and hearings will vary depending upon the individual case and circumstances, the most significant may lead to suspension or termination of employment and/or removal of the practitioner from the register, and in extreme cases potential criminal investigation.

As emerging professionals, student paramedics have a responsibility to enact the professional codes even when they are not yet registered and accountable. There are four main areas of regulation that apply to student paramedic programmes:

- Academic misconduct
- Unprofessional behaviour within university-based settings (including social media)
- Unprofessional behaviour in practice settings (including social media)
- Health-related issues

As a process for maintaining the ethical practice of students, universities are required to have established fitness-to-practise procedures and processes for determining the fitness to practise of students. Such procedures tend to mirror professional statutory regulatory bodies' processes for hearing cases of professional misconduct. However, these processes are also designed to support students in learning professional behaviour. All cases will need to follow an approved process that allows each to be addressed on an individual basis. Every case will be different; however, panel decisions and outcomes from university hearings of alleged misconduct can be broadly classified as:

- No case to answer.
- Minor breaches of conduct.
- Significant breaches of conduct.
- Serious breaches of conduct, which may result in temporary suspension/withdrawal from practice and/or programme. This usually does not exceed twelve months. The individual will need to provide evidence of developments and remediation before being able to return to the programme.
- Major breaches of conduct, which may result in the individual being permanently withdrawn from their preregistration programme.

Practice insight

What advice would you give to another student paramedic if they had broken the law in their personal life activities? What policies and professional codes would apply?

Raising concerns

The codes of practice require the professional practitioner to raise and escalate concerns related to themselves or another individual or an organisation. The concern can relate to unsafe practice or behaviours (both within and outside of the practice setting) of a professional that breach the code.

The need for honesty and **candour** when things go wrong is a common component of professional codes. Professionals have a responsibility to understand when they need to declare their own changes in circumstance (e.g. health, impairment, behaviours, lawbreaking) to their employer and/or their professional regulatory body. The raising of concerns usually follows an escalation pathway and local policies should be identified and complied with. Minor and moderate concerns can be managed at a local level by addressing them with the individual and considering supportive action plans to improve behaviours, attitudes, or unsafe practice/lack of knowledge. Only significant concerns would be investigated and managed by the professional regulatory body.

The act of raising and escalating a concern can take courage (Wiisak et al. 2022) and may also cause significant stress for the person making the allegations. Healthcare professionals, registered or student, may be reluctant to raise concerns due to fear, avoidance of being seen as a troublemaker, financial loss, not wanting to declare a lack of skill/knowledge, and feeling disengaged or undervalued (Kirk et al. 2018; Yalçın et al. 2022).

A qualitative hermeneutic phenomenological study undertaken by Fisher and Kiernan (2019) explored the lived experience of student nurses to gain an insight into the factors influencing their ability to speak up or remain silent if they witnessed suboptimal care. They found that social identity and wanting to belong within the practice setting may inhibit their decision to raise the concern. This was exacerbated by the fear of reprisal and their junior status within the power structure of the setting. It was juxtaposed by the knowledge of professional responsibility and some students would raise their concerns. Fisher and Kiernan (2019, p. 5) suggest that 'Students require the assurance that robust and effective support mechanisms are in place as a safety net when they do raise their concerns'. This is supported by Yalçın et al. (2022) where registered professionals can be encouraged to raise concern when the work environment has a non-blame culture and supports feedback in a positive manner. The findings from Fisher and Kiernan (2019) could also apply to the paramedic setting.

Practice insight

What standards, policies, and processes would guide you if you needed to raise a concern about a professional you were working with?

Conclusion

Paramedics must demonstrate professionalism in all aspects of their practice. Guidelines exist that can help the paramedic to achieve this, and this chapter provides an overview of the key issues and principles to help the paramedic understand and demonstrate professionalism in all aspects of their lives, but most importantly in their role in providing patient care.

Activities

Now review your learning by completing the learning activities in this chapter. The answers to these appear at the end of the book. Further self-test activities can be found at **www.wileyfundamentalseries.com/paramedic/3e**.

Test your knowledge

1. What are the three main themes that constitute professionalism?
2. What may influence understanding of professionalism for paramedics?
3. Does behaving professionally apply when you are on duty or when you are off duty?
4. What are the five levels of outcome against which fitness-to-practise panels judge individual student cases proven to have behaved unprofessionally?

Activity 1.1

John, a registered paramedic, has just finished a shift and is completing his time sheet. He turns to you and tells you to make sure that you claim an extra hour of overtime even though you do not feel you are entitled to do so. He reassures you by saying: 'It's OK, everybody does, it happens all the time and nobody ever says anything.'

What would you say or do if you were in the coffee room listening to this conversation? What do you think about this?

Activity 1.2

In relation to the case study:

(a) Now the student is in the position where the patient is deteriorating, and they don't know the next steps in treating the patient. What actions should they take?
(b) What can the student do to prevent a similar situation arising again?

Activity 1.3

Think about when you have cared for a patient from a different cultural background to yourself. Use one of the transcultural care models to reflect upon your practice.

Glossary

Academic integrity: Honesty, responsibility, and rigour in scholarship and research, including avoidance of cheating or plagiarism.

Candour: Be open and honest when something goes wrong (HCPC, 2022b).

Fitness to practise: Fitness to practise means to practise in a safe, competent, knowledgeable way, demonstrating a professional attitude through behaviour, so that the public are protected.

Health and Care Professions Council (HCPC): The professional statutory regulatory body for paramedics in the UK.

Australian Health Professional Agency (AHPRA): The professional statutory regulatory body for paramedics in Australia.

Mentor: A mentor is a generic term to mean the person allocated to support the student in their learning in practice, (there may be different roles/titles for this role in different practice areas – such as preceptor, supervisor, clinical mentor).

Paramedic professional identity: Paramedic professional identity involves being able to practise with honesty, integrity, and trustworthiness, and with knowledge and skill. It includes demonstrating a commitment to the paramedic profession and being accountable and responsible for one's own actions (and omissions) through exercising evidence-based practice and professional judgement.

Professionalism: Knowledge, skills, and attitudes expected from a person on a professional register, incorporating:
Professional parameters (e.g. legal and ethical aspects)
Professional behaviours (e.g. discipline-related knowledge and skills)
Professional responsibilities (e.g. responsibility to patients, oneself, employers, and the public).

Role model: A role model is a person who demonstrates good practice and whose behaviour is replicated by others.

References

AHPRA (Australian Health Practitioner Regulation Agency) (2022) *Shared Code of Conduct*. Available at: https://www.ahpra.gov.au/Resources/Code-of-conduct/Shared-Code-of-conduct.aspx (accessed 3 December 2022).

AHPRA (Australian Health Practitioner Regulation Agency) (2021) *Regulatory Guide*. Available at: https://ahpra-search.clients.funnelback.com/s/redirect?collection=ahpra-websites-web&url=https%3A%2F%2Fwww.ahpra.gov.au%2Fdocuments%2Fdefault.aspx%3Frecord%3DWD21%252f30898%26dbid%3DAP%26chksum%3DbuR53aWtd9Hai7xs7Fbuqg%253d%253d&auth=pYrlyJ7fU2KUQftAUfnrpg&profile=paramedicine&rank=2&query=Regulatory+Guide (accessed 5 January 2023).

Ajjawi, R. and Higgs, J. (2008). Learning to reason: a journey of professional socialisation. *Advances in Health Sciences Education* **13**: 133–150.

Aqil, A.R., Malik, M., Jacques, K.A. et al. (2021). Engaging in anti-oppressive public health teaching: challenges and recommendations. *Pedagogy in Health Promotion* **7**: 344–353. doi: 10.1177/23733799211045407.

Batt, A.M., Ward, G., and Acker, J.J. (2017). Paramedic patient advocacy: a review and discussion. *Internet Journal of Allied Health Sciences and Practice* **15** (4): Article 8. https://nsuworks.nova.edu/ijahsp/vol15/iss4/8 (accessed 20 March 2018).

Benner, P. (1984). *From Novice to Expert: Excellence and Power in Clinical Nursing Practice*. Menlo Park, California: Addison Wesley.

Bossers, A., Kernaghan, J., Hodgins, L. et al. (1999). Defining and developing professionalism. *Canadian Journal of Occupational Therapy* **66**: 116–121.

Bowen, L.M., Williams, B., and Stanke, L. (2017). Professionalism among paramedic students: achieving the measure or missing the mark? *Advances in Medical Education and Practice* **8**: 711–719.

Brown, W.E., Margolis, G., and Levine, R. (2005). Peer evaluation of the professional behaviours of emergency medical technicians. *Prehospital and Disaster Medicine* **20**: 107–114.

Burges Watson, D.L., Sanoff, R., Mackintosh, J.E. et al. (2012). Evidence from the scene: paramedic perspectives on involvement in out-of-hospital research. *Annals of Emergency Medicine* **60** (5): 641–650.

Carter, M., Hesselgreaves, H., Rothwell, C. et al. (2015). *Measuring Professionalism* as a Multi-Dimensional Construct-Professionalism and Conscientiousness in Healthcare *Professionals (Study 2)*. London: Health and Care Professions Council. Available at: Available at: https://www.hcpc-uk.org/globalassets/resources/reports/measuring-professionalism-as-a-multi-dimensional-construct—professionalism-and-conscientiousness-in-healthcare-professionals—study-2.pdf?v=636785062220000000 (accessed 2 December 2022).

Driscoll, J. (ed.) (2007) *Practising Clinical Supervision: A Reflective Approach for Healthcare Professionals*. Edinburgh: Balliere Tindall.

Donaghy, J. (2013). The role of the Health Professions Council. *Journal of Paramedic Practice* **5**: 370–371.

Ebbs, P., and Gonzalez, P., (2019) A need to balance technical and non-technical skills. *Journal of Paramedic Practice* **11**: 98–99. doi: 10.12968/jpar.2019.11.3.98.

Eraut, M. (2007). Learning from other people in the workplace. *Oxford Review of Education* **33**: 403–422.

Felstead, I.S. and Springett, K. (2016). An exploration of role model influence on adult nursing students' professional development: a phenomenological research study. *Nurse Education Today* **37**: 66–70.

Fitzgerald, A. (2020) Professional identity: a concept analysis. *Nursing Forum* **55** (3): 447–472.

Fisher, M. and Kiernan, M. (2019) Student nurses' lived experience of patient safety and raising concerns. *Nurse Education Today* **77**: 1–5.

Gallagher, A., Vyvyan, E., Juniper, J. et al. (2016). Professionalism in paramedic practice: the views of paramedics and paramedic students. *British Paramedic Journal* **1**: 1–8.

Gibbs, G. (1988). *Learning By Doing: A Guide to Teaching and Learning Methods*. Oxford: Further Education Unit, University of Oxford.

Givati, A., Markham, C., and Street, K. (2017). The bargaining of professionalism in emergency care practice: NHS paramedics and higher education. *Advances in Health Sciences Education* **23**: 353–369.

Hagiwara, M.A., Magnusson, C., Herlitz, J. et al. (2019). Adverse events in prehospital emergency care: a trigger tool study. *BMC Emergency Medicine* **19**: 1–10.

HCPC (Health and Care Professions Council) (2014). *Professionalism in Healthcare Professionals*. London: HCPC. Available at: https://www.hcpc-uk.org/globalassets/resources/reports/professionalism-in-healthcare-professionals.pdf (accessed 5 January 2023).

HCPC (Health and Care Professions Council) (2016). *Standards of Conduct, Performance and Ethics*. London: HCPC.

HCPC (Health and Care Professions Council) (2016b). *Guidance on Conduct and Ethics for Students*. London: HCPC.

HCPC (Health and Care Professions Council) (2021). *Fitness to Practise Annual Report*. London: HCPC. Available at: https://www.hcpc-uk.org/globalassets/resources/reports/fitness-to-practise/fitness-to-practise-annual-report-2021-22.pdf (accessed 3 December 2022).

HCPC (Health and Care Professions Council) (2022). *Health and Wellbeing Framework: Helping You to Help Yourself*. London: HCPC. Available at: https://www.hcpc-uk.org/globalassets/resources/2022/health-and-wellbeing-framework-2022.pdf?v=637825094840000000 (accessed 3 December 2022).

HCPC (Health and Care Professions Council) (2022b). *The Duty of Candour in Practice*. London: HCPC. Available at: https://www.hcpc-uk.org/standards/meeting-our-standards/raising-concerns-openness-and-honesty/the-duty-of-candour/the-duty-of-candour-in-practice/ (accessed 9 January 2023).

Hilton, S.R. and Slotnick, H.B. (2005). Proto-professionalism: how professionalisation occurs across the continuum of medical education. *Medical Education* **39**: 58–65.

Holland, K. (2018). *Cultural Awareness in Nursing and Health Care: An Introductory Text. 3e*. New York, NY: Routledge.

Howkins, E.J. and Ewens, A. (1999). How students experience professional socialisation. *International Journal of Nursing Studies* **36**: 41–49.

Howlett, G. (2019) Nearly qualified student paramedics' perceptions of reflection and use in practice. *Journal of Paramedic Practice* **11**: 258–263.

Hugman, R. (1991). *Power in Caring Professions*. Basingstoke: Macmillan.

Hunter, K. and Cook, C. (2018) Role-modelling and the hidden curriculum: new graduate nurses' professional socialisation. *Journal of Clinical Nursing* **27** (15–16): 3157–3170.

Jackson, B., Purdy, S., and Cooper-Thomas, H. (2019). Role of professional confidence in the development of expert allied health professionals. *A Narrative Review Journal of Allied Health; Washington* **48**: 226–232.

Jauregui, J., Gatewood, M.O., Ingen, J.S. et al. (2016). Emergency medicine resident perceptions of medical professionalism. *The Western Journal of Emergency Medicine* **17** (3): 355–361.

Johns, C. (1992). Developing clinical standards. In: *Knowledge for Nursing Practice* (ed. K. Robinson and B. Vaughan), 54–62. Oxford: Butterworth Heinemann.

Johns, C. (2000). *Becoming a Reflective Practitioner*. Oxford: Blackwell.

Johnston, T. and Acker, J. (2016). Using a sociological approach to answering questions about paramedic professionalism and identity. *Australasian Journal of Paramedicine* **13**: 1–7.

Kirk, A. Armstrong, K., Nurkka, N. et al. (2018). The impact of blame culture on paramedic practice: a qualitative study exploring English and Finnish paramedic perceptions. *International Journal of Emergency Services* **7**: 214–227.

Kolb, D.A. (1984) *Experiential Learning: Experience as the Source of Learning and Development*. New Jersey: Prentice Hall.

Lauria M.J., Gallo I.A., Rush S. et al. (2017). Psychological skills to improve emergency care providers' performance under stress. *Ann Emerg Med.* **70**: 884–890. .doi: 10.1016/j.annemergmed.2017.03.018.

Lloyd-Jones, N. (2013). Enhancing the Oxford Brookes undergraduate fitness to practise governance with e-learning tools for professionalism. *Health and Social Care Annual Conference 2013 Post Event Resources – e-Resources*. Available at: https://www.advance-he.ac.uk/knowledge-hub/health-and-social-care-annual-conference-2013-post-event-resources-e-resources (accessed 5 January 2023).

Mallinson, T., and Willis, S. (2020) The zero point survey and egg-timer model combined for crew management. *Journal of Paramedic Practice* **12**: 430–435. doi: 10.12968/jpar.2020.12.11.430.

Monrouxe, L.V. (2010). Identity, identification and medical education: why should we care? *Medical Education* **44**: 40–49.

NCNZ (Nursing Council of New Zealand) (2011). *Guidelines for Cultural Safety, the Treaty of Waitangi and Maori Health in Nursing Education and Practice*. Wellington: NCNZ. Available at: https://online.flippingbook.com/view/960779225/ (accessed 25 February 2023).

Nevalainen, M., Lunkka, N., and Suhonen, M. (2018). Work-based learning in healthcare organisations experienced by nursing staff: a systematic review of qualitative studies. *Nurse Education in Practice* **29**: 21–29.

Papadopoulos, I., Tilki, M. and Taylor, G. (1998). *Transcultural Care: A Guide for Health Care Professionals*. Dinton: Quay Books.

Papadopoulos, I. (2006). *Transcultural Health and Social Care: Development of Culturally Competent Practitioners*. London: Elsevier Health Sciences.

Paterson, C. and Chapman, J., (2013). Enhancing skills of critical reflection to evidence learning in professional practice. *Physical Therapy in Sport* **14**: 133–138.

Peiser, G., Ambrose, J., Burke, B. et al. (2018). The role of the mentor in professional knowledge development across four professions. *International Journal of Mentoring and Coaching in Education* **7**: 2–18. doi: org/10.1108/IJMCE-07-2017-0052.

PHECC (2017). *Code of Professional Conduct & Ethics*. Naas Co Kildare, Ireland: Pre-Hospital Emergency Care Council.

Polyani, M. (1958). *Personal Knowledge: Towards a Postcritical Philosophy*. New York: Harper Torchbooks.

Reljić NM, Lorber M, Vrbnjak D, et al. (2017). Assessment of clinical nursing competencies: literature review. In: *Teaching and Learning in Nursing* (ed. Pajnkihar, M., Vrbnjak, D., and Stiglic, G. (2017), pp. 49–68. IntechOpen. Available at: https://www.intechopen.com/books/teaching-and-learning-in-nursing (accessed 25 February 2023).

Roff, S., Chandratilake, M., McAleer, S. et al. (2012). Medical student rankings of proposed sanction for unprofessional behaviours relating to academic integrity: results from a Scottish medical school. *Scottish Medical Journal* **57**: 76–79.

Roff, S. and Dherwani, K. (2011). Development of inventory for polyprofessionalism lapses at the protoprofessional stage of health professions education together with recommended responses. *Medical Teacher* **33**: 239–243.

Schön, D. (1987). *Educating the Reflective Practitioner. San Francisco*: Jossey-Bass.

Schon, D. (2003). *The Reflective Practitioner. How Professionals Think in Action*. London: Ashgate.

Scott, I. and Spouse, J. (2013). *Practice-based Learning in Nursing, Health and Social Care: Mentorship, Facilitation and Supervision*. Chichester: Wiley.

Sturman, N., Jorm, C., and Parker, M. (2020). With a grain of salt? Supervisor credibility and other factors influencing trainee decisions to seek in-consultation assistance: a focus group study of Australian general practice trainees *BMC Family Practice* **21**: 28.

Townsend, R.M. (2017). What Australian and Irish paramedic registrants can learn from the UK: lessons in developing professionalism. *Irish Journal of Paramedicine* **2**: Available at: http://irishparamedicine.com/index.php/ijp/article/view/69 (accessed 20 March 2018).

van der Gaag, A., Gallagher, A., Zasada, M. et al. (2017). People like us? Understanding complaints about paramedics and social workers. London: HCPC. Available at: https://www.hcpc-uk.org/resources/reports/2017/people-like-us-understanding-complaints-about-paramedics-and-social-workers/ (accessed 25 February 2023).

Voldbjerg, S.L., Wiechula, R., Sørensen, E.E. et al. (2021). Newly graduated nurses' socialisation resulting in limiting inquiry and one-sided use of knowledge sources—An ethnographic study. *Journal of Clinical Nursing* **30**(5–6): 701–711.

Westenra, B. (2019) A framework for cultural safety in paramedic practice. *Whitireia Nursing and Health Journal* **26**: 11–17.

Wiisak, J., Suhonenhttps, R., and Leino-Kilpi, H. (2022) Whistleblowers – morally courageous actors in health care? *Nursing Ethics* **29**: 1321–1544.

Yalçın, B., Baykal, Ü., and Türkmen, E. (2022). Why do nurses choose to stay silent? A qualitative study. *International Journal of Nursing Practice* **28**: 1–7.

CHAPTER 2

Professional health regulation for paramedicine

Ramon Z. Shaban

Faculty of Medicine and Health, University of Sydney, Sydney, New South Wales, Australia; Nursing, Midwifery and Clinical Governance Directorate, Western Sydney Local Health District, Westmead, New South Wales, Australia

Ruth Townsend

School of Biomedical Science, Charles Sturt University, Bathurst, New South Wales, Australia

Markus Pitter

Registered Paramedic, MACPara, BsC

Contents

LEARNING OUTCOMES

On completion of this chapter, the reader will be able to:

- Demonstrate an understanding of the key concepts underpinning professionalism.
- Demonstrate an awareness of the contemporary issues relating to professional regulation of paramedicine and out-of-hospital (OOH) care.
- Appraise the recent development of paramedic health professional regulation.

Fundamentals of Paramedic Practice: A Systems Approach, Third Edition. Edited by Sam Willis and Ian Peate.

Companion website: www.wiley.com/go/willis/paramedic3e

Case study 1

Donald, a paramedic who attended an emergency call to a patient having a seizure, was the subject of a complaint. The investigating panel received evidence about Patient A's health condition and how it affected her behaviour. One sign was that her behaviour could be disinhibited. Whilst being interviewed during the investigation, the registrant's crewmate, George, said that the patient was singing 'You Sexy Thing' in the company of the paramedics. Also, George noted that Patient A was abnormally loud in her speech when getting out of the ambulance at the hospital. When they returned to the ambulance George had said, 'Oh my God, she's a total nutjob, crackers, mental.' It should have been apparent to Donald that the patient was vulnerable. Despite this, after her release from hospital Donald visited the patient at her home. She had made him a drink, they had chatted, followed by sex. This sequence of events happened a further two times. A complaint was lodged. An investigation into Donald's inappropriate relationship of an intimate and/or sexual nature with a vulnerable patient led to a hearing into possible breaches of professional boundaries. This constituted misconduct, which represented impaired fitness to practise. The complaint was proven, and Donald was struck off the register.

Introduction

Paramedics comprise an increasingly critical and sizeable component of advanced emergency healthcare systems worldwide. Their actions and practice as health **professionals** are fundamental to the health and well-being of individuals and society. This chapter examines professional regulation, the leading global contemporary issue within ambulance and out-of-hospital (OOH) emergency care, and the implications for professional practice. It reports the findings of leading contemporary research into the global regulation of paramedics; discusses these findings, considers other evidence about health professional regulation; and explores the challenges for paramedicine as an emerging profession.

Principles for paramedic professional health regulation

Globally, there is an increasing unprecedented demand for high-quality and safe healthcare. This demand, particularly for emergency healthcare (Shaban, 2011; Considine et al. 2019; Williams et al. 2021), drives reform in the healthcare sector (Institute of Medicine 2000; Shaban 2018). Healthcare reform, changes in healthcare philosophy, shifting patient demographics, and increasing costs associated with healthcare mean there is a push to increase healthcare safety, efficiency and quality (Australian Commission on Safety and Quality in Health Care [ACSQHC] n.d.).

In line with advances in the availability of **information** and education, patients have pushed and been encouraged to be 'partners in their health care' (ACSQHC n.d.). The vision for quality medical care championed by luminaries such as Florence Nightingale, Avedis Donabedian (Donabedian 1966, 1988), and many others over the last hundred years has been realised in ways they could not have imagined. The rise of evidence-based practice and ever-increasing patient and consumer voices are constant reminders to health professionals of patients' need for, and fundamental right to, high-quality and safe healthcare and involvement in their own care decisions.

Such changes can be seen in Australia, for example, by the creation of the National Registration and Accreditation Scheme in 2010, which champions an overarching goal to protect the public and ensure all health practitioners provide high-quality professional standards (Australian Government Department of Health and Aged Care 2021). At the core of high-quality and safe healthcare, particularly emergency healthcare, is a highly skilled, trained, experienced, and professional workforce. Globally there is a mixture of professional and paraprofessional roles performed by healthcare workers in emergency healthcare systems. Some occupational groups such as medicine and nursing have established universally as a profession. For other groups such as paramedics this establishment is varied. However, there is a strong global drive to ensure that all occupational groups who operate in the emergency healthcare sphere establish themselves and serve as health professionals (Considine et al. 2019).

Health professional regulation for paramedic professionalism

The terms 'profession', 'professional', and 'professionalisation' are contested and carry different meanings. For this chapter we will be discussing 'professionalism' as defined by Freidson (2001, p. 1) to refer to 'a knowledge base of abstract theories and complex skills acquired through higher education, relative self-regulation supported by professional bodies and associations, the need to exercise personal judgement, and perhaps most importantly, a commitment to public service' (see also Kreber 2017). Professionalism is acting 'within a set of norms, principles and standards of conduct and competency' that places the interests of others before oneself (Evetts 2014). The manner in which a group develops as a profession is called professionalisation (Abbott 1988; Professional Standards Council 2018). Australia's Professional Standards Council (2018) specifies the importance of the core elements of integrity, ethics, trust, and expertise as key reference points in developing emerging professional groups and professions.

The nature of regulation by professionalism adds an extra layer of regulatory responsibility to some occupational groups but not others. For example, the whole population is regulated by criminal and civil laws, but healthcare professionals are also regulated by laws that relate specifically to their work. These laws provide special privileges in exchange for health practitioners meeting particular responsibilities. For example, the laws protect the group from unwanted members, protect the profession's name, and provide the profession the power to establish independent standards of conduct and competence. The privilege can extend to safeguard their independence to judge, criticise, or refuse 'employers, patrons and the laws of the state' if it is necessary to protect the patient's best interest (Freidson 2001). This duty exists even in the face of opposition from powerful factions, including the state. If a practitioner fails to meet the required standards of conduct and competence established by the profession – which often reflect community standards – then conditions may be placed on their ability to practice their profession. That is, they may be compelled to undertake additional training and supervision. At worst, the practitioner may have their ability to practise rescinded either temporarily or permanently.

The best way for paramedics to avoid falling into the latter categories is to act with professionalism (see Table 2.1). In short, paramedics must remain current with best practice, education, and training to maintain their competence to practise to the required standard to deliver quality and safe care. Additionally, professionalism requires them to work according to a set of agreed values and to put their patients' interests ahead of their own. These expectations are codified in the various laws that regulate paramedics in the UK and Australia (Health and Care Professions Council [HCPC] 2001; Paramedicine Board of Australia – Professional Capabilities for Registered Paramedics, n.d.). The objective of the legislation is the same in both the UK (Secretary of State for Health 2007) and Australia – to improve patient safety and to increase the flexibility of the healthcare workforce. However, there are differences between the two regulatory models that have different implications for the paramedic profession in each of those jurisdictions.

TABLE 2.1 The five Es of professionalisation.

Education	• Formally accredited, entry-level formal qualifications or certification exist based on identified, specific technical and professional requirements to practise in a discrete area. • There is a requirement for ongoing education and continuing professional development.
Ethics	• Published, prescribed professional and ethical standards that clients can expect their professional to demonstrate, including specific expectations of practice and conduct, and a commitment to a higher duty. • A transparent process through which the professional and ethical standards are generated by the professional community that governs their conduct, with a clear mandate to improve consumer protection that goes beyond reiterating the relevant statutory expectations.
Experience	• The requirement for personal capabilities and experience required to practise as a professional in the discrete area.
Examination	• A fair, transparent, and independent mechanism by which education, ethics, and experience are assessed, validated, and assured to the community. This mechanism includes not only qualification or certification requirements and traditional examinations, but also the requirement for regular validation and assurance, such as by compliance and professional audit expectations.
Entity	• An independent, capable entity to oversee and administer professional entry, professional standards, and compliance expectations on behalf of the public, which should comprise individuals who are regulated participants in that profession.

The UK experience

As Chapter 1 has documented, in the UK, paramedics have been regulated for over a decade. The drive towards regulation shared a similar genesis to that in Australia following a number of high-profile cases that resulted in the primary focus of safe, high-quality care for patients, being prioritised in a new regulatory model (Smith 2004). The regulatory process was designed to be removed from the government, the employer, and notably the profession (Chamberlain 2014). A secondary focus was on the development of a responsive, flexible healthcare workforce. The UK model is more bureaucratic in its structure than the Australian model and does not accommodate self-regulation by the profession. The nature of a bureaucratic model of regulation is that it attempts to generalise and flatten out skill sets and roles amongst professionals, in order to reduce silos of specialisation and increase flexibility within the healthcare workforce (Secretary of State for Health 2007; Townsend 2018). This model has some advantages and it has certainly facilitated the extension of the scope of practice of paramedics beyond just the traditional emergency prehospital ambulance response (College of Paramedics 2015). However, it also has some weaknesses. For example, it blunts several elements typically associated with a profession, including having a unique purpose, specialised knowledge and skill that are not usually practised by others, and a distinct professional identity and thus political power (Brown et al. 2000). The bureaucratic model is contrary to the notion of specialisation and the division of labour along specialised lines.

As work has become more complex over time, specialisation has increased in several fields, particularly in healthcare. The division of labour in this way recognises that not every practitioner can know everything or indeed do everything well – 'a jack of all trades is a master of none'. This is especially true in complex and highly technologically advanced healthcare fields like paramedicine. Understanding that some healthcare regulatory systems are designed to divide labour in terms of speciality and others, like the UK, are designed to blend and generalise some healthcare roles allows for some examination of the way in which each system supports the exercise of professionalism.

Townsend (2018) undertook a study of the role of the law in paramedic professionalism internationally and has observed that professionals share a number of traits, including specialised knowledge and the legal authority to use discretion in the application of that knowledge. This is consistent with the notion of self-regulation of the professions because their knowledge is too specialised for anyone other than those in the profession itself to understand. This principle is recognised in civil law where, in cases determining professional negligence, members of the professional peer group, not members of other health professions, are called to give evidence as to whether another member has breached professional standards of care (NSW Parliamentary Counsel's Office 2002).

Additionally, the exercise of professional discretion allows for practitioners to manage the complexity and variety of unique cases that they encounter and that are common to human healthcare. That is, there is a recognition that health practitioners who have met education, fitness to practise, and other standards sufficient to be registered as a member of the health profession are adequately well trained and responsible to be able to exercise professional discretion in the interests of their patient. However, the UK regulatory model limits specialisation and instead promotes generalisation. Townsend observes:

> *Discretionary specialisation associated with professionals allows for flexibility in the practice of specialised skills for a unique purpose. This notion of flexibility and the valuing of specialisation has been lost in the UK's restructure of the workforce that was implemented as an attempt to increase the skills mix of the healthcare workforce. The adoption of a bureaucratic regulatory regime that values uniformity in the form of generic standards of conduct and assessment of professional behaviour has hampered the ability of paramedics as professionals to regulate themselves and has not recognised the unique role and responsibilities that paramedics have and that set them apart from other health professionals. (Townsend 2018)*

The unintended consequences, Townsend (2018) argues, are significant, particularly in terms of the identity of paramedics and the control, or otherwise, that they have over their work:

> *Instead, paramedics in the UK are regulated the same way as art therapists. They are subject to a generic code of conduct. They do not have control over the nature of their work, which is evidenced by their lack of control over their curriculum. Their work performance is judged not by their peers but by outsiders. All of these elements have contributed to a lack of professional development for paramedics in the UK, despite the introduction of regulation to facilitate professionalisation over a decade ago. This demonstrates the paradox of the bureaucratic model of regulation that, prima facie*

appears to give paramedics professional status but has had the effect of leading them to believe that they have not fully professionalised because they do not have control over their own work.

The bureaucratic model of regulation in the UK has led to the generalisation of paramedic work in some areas. The question then becomes: Why be a paramedic at all? What is it that distinguishes paramedics from other similar health professionals like nurses? This blurring of professional roles and identities has the added effect of contributing to those sitting in judgement of paramedic performance not fully understanding who paramedics are or what paramedics do. This may not matter given that many paramedics appear to be happy to have extended opportunities to practise beyond the traditional paramedic role, but it has been noted by others that there is a risk that having 'knowledge or doctrine which is too general and vague or too narrow and specific provides a weak base for an exclusive jurisdiction' (Wilensky 1964, p. 150). This suggests that it is necessary for each profession to find what Townsend (2018) refers to as its 'Goldilocks zone') – the position where the profession maintains its authority over its unique role and specialised knowledge whilst also providing a useful service to a broad marketplace. There is some evidence that this generalised rather than specialised division of labour and blurring of professional roles and identities have implications for paramedics, including contributing to those sitting in judgement of paramedic performance not fully understanding who paramedics are or what paramedics do.

Brady argues that UK paramedics are being sanctioned by the regulator, the HCPC, for perceived deviations from guidelines – working outside their scope of practice – because the disciplinary panel does not know what paramedics actually do. This is consistent with Freidson's suggestion that professional practitioners are likely to view administrators who do not do or have not undertaken the daily work of the profession as being unable to understand their work. Also the practitioner's work is made more difficult by 'abstract technical norms and bureaucratic requirements designed to guide and record their activities' but that do not necessarily cohere with or prioritise the moral intention of the work they do (Freidson 1983). This misunderstanding by bureaucrats can occur when paramedics apply their specialised discretionary decision-making in the best interests of the patient, as do other health professionals (Brady 2013). Peer review, however, is a fundamental element of professional practice and is consistent with a self-regulatory framework rather than a bureaucratic framework. Thus, peer review (self-regulation) allows for assessment of the specialisation and expertise of the professional group by members of the professional group who hold the same knowledge and skill and have knowledge of the profession's role, purpose, and values. The confusion over role, identity, purpose, and values is consistent with the lack of clarity about who paramedics are in terms of their educational programmes, their gradually expanding range into nontraditional areas of practice, and their lack of a profession-specific code of conduct. Indeed, in a report commissioned by the regulator and conducted by the University of Surrey into the high number of complaints received by the regulator concerning paramedics, the authors suggested that the HCPC should clarify the criteria by which paramedics are held to account (van der Gaag et al. 2017).

The report did not recommend a change to the regulatory structure, but interestingly paramedics interviewed for it suggested a shift to a regulatory model such as that operated by the General Medical Council. This is a self-regulatory model similar to the Australian model, in that at least half the members of the professional standards review panel must be registered paramedics. Some commentators suggested this would provide better outcomes for paramedics, in part because there is a belief amongst paramedics that the current regulator does not know what paramedics do and does not understand the particularities of their practice (van der Gaag et al. 2017). Lovegrove and Davis (2013), in a review of paramedic education in the UK, identified that a major driver of the paramedic push to professionalisation was a desire to raise awareness of the capabilities of paramedics amongst others. Townsend (2018) argues that although UK paramedics are referred to as professionals under the current bureaucratic regulatory model, they are not regulated like professionals; that is, they do not self-regulate, as with a professionalism model. Townsend argues that this form of regulatory approach is paternalistic in the sense that it does not allow the paramedic profession to grow and develop to maturity as a full profession by not permitting independent regulation. This is consistent with the finding in the 'People like us?' report, which suggested that the profession was still evolving (Lovegrove and Davis 2013).

Admittedly, the regulatory model currently in place in the UK was developed over two decades ago, when paramedics worked differently and the expectations and understanding of what paramedics did amongst the public, law and policymakers, and the regulator were different. It is time for a review of the regulatory mechanism to allow paramedics to regulate their education and accreditation standards and to set a minimum paramedic curriculum.

The curriculum should encompass paramedicine's unique and specialised skills and knowledge and reflect its current minimum scope of practice, so that all registered paramedics share this same minimum standard. Setting such a standard would address issues of confusion, particularly amongst the regulators, who are also responsible for disciplining paramedics. Although the paramedic scope of practice has become quite broad, and this has allowed them to work in areas they have traditionally not occupied, the broadening and flattening of their specialised role as OOH emergency responders have not correlated with other aspects of their professional development. Indeed, there is even evidence that paramedics in the UK have called for 'guidance and limitations' to their practice via practice guidelines to ensure the protection of the public, as they consider themselves not 'professionals' but rather an 'aspirant and emergent group of people trying to understand what it is to be professional' (Donaghy 2013). An examination of some of the complaints made against paramedics regarding their practice and conduct can provide practitioners and educators with some information that may assist with the development of a culture and ethos of paramedic professionalisation in both the UK and Australia.

Paramedics misbehaving

Paramedics in the UK have been regulated for over a decade. There is a wealth of data available on the types and frequency of misconduct in which they have engaged. An examination of that data in 2015–2016 shows that 239 allegations of a breach of a paramedic's 'fitness to practise' were made against UK paramedics by the HCPC. The total number of registrants in that year was 22,380. Paramedics constitute only 6.55% of the total number of registrants, yet they made up the second-highest number of complaints (1.07%) of all the professions registered (HCPC 2016). The group with the largest number of concerns against paramedics was the public (42.8%), followed by the employer (25.2%), and then self-referral (20.2%) (HCPC 2016). Townsend (2018) argues that the UK results cannot be explained simply because of the number of paramedics and the intimate type of work that they do: 'Physiotherapists are the second-largest profession, yet have a much lower rate of concerns raised than paramedics or social workers in England' (HCPC 2016, p. 16). Although the numbers for social workers and paramedics are higher than for other health professions, the proportion of paramedics who were formally sanctioned by the regulator represented less than 0.3% of the total registered paramedic population, and this proportion is consistent with numbers across all registered health practitioners (HCPC 2016). One conclusion that can be drawn from this is 'that there continue to be so few allegations largely because the vast majority of registrants are committed to their job and vocation to help others . . . they therefore maintain their competence, continue to develop professionally and do not misbehave' (Health Professions Council 2012, p. 49). This suggests that paramedic professionalism is quite high.

However, there were some misconduct matters. The most common included:

> *attending work under the influence of alcohol; bullying and harassment of colleagues; breach of professional boundaries with service users or service user family members; breach of confidentiality; misrepresentation of qualifications and / or previous employment; failure to communicate properly and effectively with service users and / or colleagues; posting inappropriate comments on social media; acting outside scope of practice; falsifying service user records; and failure to provide adequate service user care (HCPC 2016, p. 46)*

Lack of competence examples included 'failure to provide adequate service user care; inadequate professional knowledge; and poor record-keeping' (HCPC 2016, p. 48). The third most common matters related to criminal convictions or cautions and included:

> *theft; fraud; shoplifting; possession of drugs and / or possession of drugs with the intent to supply; receiving a restraining order and breach of a restraining order; driving under the influence of alcohol; failure to provide a specimen; assault (common or by beating); possession of pornographic images; and sexual offences (HCPC 2016, p. 50)*

The type of behaviour complained about included assault, criminal damage, drink driving, drugs possession, fraud, possession of child pornography, attending work under the influence of alcohol, bullying and harassment of colleagues, engaging in a sexual relationship with a service user, failing to provide adequate care, false claim to qualifications, and self-administration of medication.

The reason the regulator has sanctioned practitioners for these behaviours is because their actions represent an

The Australian experience Case study 2

Jessica, a paramedic working alone in remote Australia went to several drug safes in her jurisdiction. She was able to steal restricted medication and conceal her actions for some time. Once discovered she was counselled and provided with rehabilitation. As there was no centralised means of registration or tracking of concerning behaviours, she was free to travel and work in across the country.

abuse of trust or power, amounting to an exploitation or deception of a vulnerable person for personal gain, as in Case Study 1 at the beginning of this chapter. Some of the actions also represent a failure to respect the rights of patients to make choices for themselves about their own care, and/or pose a risk to the safety of the patient that is contrary to the purpose of the profession. Some of the actions demonstrate a failure to act legally, but in all cases, there has been a failure to act ethically and professionally. This not only compromises patient safety but it also reflects low-quality care and has the potential to undermine the public's confidence in the profession.

December 2018 saw the inaugural registration of the paramedicine profession in Australia (Paramedicine Board of Australia, n.d.). The newly constituted Paramedicine Board of Australia and the Australian Health Practitioner Registration Agency (AHPRA) established registration and other standards for paramedics as registered health professionals (Paramedicine Board of Australia 2018). The new registration period included a three-year grandparenting scheme for those lacking formal qualifications under the newly established registration requirements. These paramedics could prove capability through alternative training and experience. Since 2022, this scheme has ended, and all OOH providers seeking to use the title of paramedic must adhere to the professional registration standards and requirements, thus protecting the profession's name.

The historical lack of uniform national regulation of paramedicine as a health profession in Australia means that there are relatively few publicly available records of paramedics' misconduct. Since registration, there are publicly available records of four cases involving the tribunal and deregistration of the individual. Part of the benefit of being regulated under the national law is that this information is publicly available (consider Case Study 2 in this context). This also ensures that the regulator will hear matters in accordance with the principles of natural justice and procedural fairness. AHPRA, the administrative body of the regulator, provides support to the national boards by administering the registration process. Part of this duty includes accepting and investigating complaints about professional conduct, performance, or the health of registered health practitioners and students; and working with the Health Care Complaints Commission in each state and territory to ensure community concerns are dealt with appropriately. (The exceptions are New South Wales, where complaints are investigated by the Health Professional Councils Authority and the Health Care Complaints Commission; and Queensland, where investigation is undertaken by the Queensland Health Ombudsman.)

AHPRA provides the associated material and a preliminary assessment to the respective board for consideration by a professional standards panel or a tribunal. The board may take several actions depending on the type and seriousness of the allegation against a practitioner or student and risk of harm to the public. This means that the knowledge, skill, or judgement of, or care exercised by, the practitioner in the health profession is to the standard reasonably expected of a health practitioner of an equivalent level of training or experience (Paramedicine Board of Australia n.d.).

Other regulatory requirements codify standards of professional practice or professionalism, such as mandatory reporting of **notifiable conduct** by practitioners. Mandatory notifications must be made to the regulator if a health practitioner forms a reasonable belief that another health practitioner has behaved in a way that constitutes notifiable conduct. A mandatory notification must also be made if a student has an impairment that may place the public at substantial risk of harm in the course of the student undertaking clinical training. There are four grounds that constitute notifiable conduct:

1. Impairment is defined under the national law as 'a physical or mental impairment, disability, condition or disorder (including substance abuse or dependence) that detrimentally affects or is likely to detrimentally affect the person's capacity to practise the profession' (AHPRA n.d., p. 8).

2. Practicing while intoxicated (meaning practising under the influence of drugs (either illegal or prescription) or alcohol).
3. A significant departure from accepted professional standards (including the code of conduct and guidelines relating to the profession).
4. Sexual misconduct (including sexual relations with a patient with or without consent).

As discussed, there are to date only four published cases resulting in deregistration of Australian paramedics since 2018. Therefore, an examination of the types of behaviours that were sanctioned by the performance and professional standards panel against registered medical practitioners and nurses in Australia may give some idea of likely issues that could arise in paramedic practice because the work of those professions is the most similar to that of paramedics.

The most common behaviours that have been noted include:

- Boundary violations, including inappropriate sexual comments and inappropriate sexual conduct; breaches of confidentiality; or inappropriate collection or use of patient information.
- Failures regarding consent, including failure to provide adequate or accurate information; or failure to assess a patient's capacity to consent.
- Inappropriate behaviour, like aggression towards a service user and even assault.
- Conflicts of interest.
- Health impairments, including the misuse or abuse of drugs or alcohol (AHPRA n.d.).

The common thread across all these behaviours is the failure to adhere to the bedrock of professionalism, putting the patient's interest and safety first.

Professionalism is increasingly regarded and valued as a meta-skill, comprising situational awareness and contextual judgement. Individuals can draw on the communication, technical, and practical skills appropriate for each given professional scenario (HCPC 2014), rather than a set of discrete skills. Such professional judgement will depend on the knowledge developed through logic, sensed intuitively, gained through experience, particularly prior experience of similar events, and influenced by education and socialisation (Johns 1992). Regulation by professionalism involves consistently demonstrating a set of identifiable, positive professional attributes, values, and behaviours, and being held to these standards by your professional peer group and others. Paramedicine is still evolving as a profession and there have recently been changes that have facilitated the process of professionalisation for paramedicine, including legal recognition and regulation of the profession.

Conclusion

Paramedics have a significant role in the provision of emergency and, in recent times, non-emergency OOH care. We have evolved to become highly skilled clinicians, working in high-risk environments, performing high-risk interventions, and charged with administering high-risk medications with little immediate oversight. As a result, paramedics possess enormous responsibilities to act in the patient's best interest. Yet there is an absence of professional self-regulation of paramedics globally (Shaban 2011; Considine et al. 2019). Unlike physicians, pharmacists, nurses, psychologists, and other recognised health professionals (who are often regulated by profession-based statutory authorities), paramedics and their practice in many jurisdictions are often regulated by individual, organisational requirements.

In practice this may mean paramedics are restricted to what the organisation's level of care or guideline will allow. Paramedics have to continue to develop their own culture and ethos of professionalism through the development of their identity, which embodies the group's values and ideals. Individual paramedics must develop and demonstrate professionalism in all aspects of their practice. Regulation by professionalism works to protect patients where a conflict of laws may operate and subjugate a patient's interests to those of another, for example, an employer or even the state (World Medical Association 1948). This power is one that must be used judiciously because as autonomously registered health practitioners – legal entities separate from an employer – paramedics will be held responsible by their professional body for their decisions and actions. Whilst paramedics continue to work with practice guidelines, as the profession continues to grow, the expectations on the individual may create conflict between employer and professional. This chapter provides an overview of the key issues and principles to help paramedics understand and demonstrate professionalism in all aspects of their lives, but most importantly, in their role in providing high-quality professional and safe emergency patient care.

Activities

Now review your learning by completing the learning activities in this chapter. The answers to these appear at the end of the book. Further self-test activities can be found at **www.wileyfundamentalseries.com/paramedic/3e.**

Test your knowledge

1. Describe in classic terms the standard that paramedicine should attain to be deemed a regulated health profession.
2. Describe three key drivers of health professional regulation in paramedicine.
3. Define practice as it applies to health professional regulation for paramedics.
4. What are the benefits of regulation by professionalism (Australia) versus bureaucracy (UK)?
5. What behaviour or conduct by paramedics is deemed notifiable as determined by the AHPRA?

Activity 2.1

Consider Case Study 1 at the beginning of this chapter. What are the issues you can identify regarding Donald's professionalism?

Should paramedics in remote communities, who no longer have a relationship with a patient, be able to commence a relationship with that patient?

Consider Case Study 2. Should Jessica be able to continue to practice autonomously without the availability of knowledge surrounding her difficulties with addiction?

Activity 2.2

For each of the following questions, state whether it is true or false:

1. Despite doing very different jobs, paramedics in the UK are regulated the same way as art therapists – true or false?
2. Paramedics in Australia will self-regulate – true or false?
3. Paramedic professionalism involves acting 'within a set of norms, principles and standards of conduct and competency' that places the interests of others before oneself – true or false?
4. The most common area of paramedic misconduct is clinical competence – true or false?
5. Paramedic misconduct does not include a breach of professional boundaries with service users or service user family members – true or false?

Glossary

Notifiable conduct: Conduct that breaches the professional code and expectations of a health profession and poses public risk such as practising whilst under the influence of intoxicants.

Professional: An individual who adheres to relevant ethical standards and holds themselves out as, and is accepted by, the public as possessing special knowledge and skills in a widely recognised body of learning derived from research, education, and training at a high level, and who is prepared to apply this knowledge and exercise these skills in the interest of others (Professions Australia 2018; Professional Standards Councils 2018).

References

Abbott, A. (1988). *The System of Professions: An Essay on the Division of Expert Labour*. Chicago: University of Chicago Press.

Australian Commission on Safety and Quality in Health Care (ACSQHC) (n.d.). *National Safety and Quality Health Service Standards*. 2e. Sydney: ACSQHC.

Australian Commission on Safety and Quality in Health Care (ACSQHC) (2017). *Annual Report 2016–17*. Sydney: ACSQHC.

Australian Health Practitioner Regulation Agency (AHPRA) (n.d.). *Panel decisions*. Available at: www.ahpra.gov.au/Publications/Panel-Decisions.aspx (accessed 19 March 2019).

Australian Health Practitioner Regulation Agency (AHPRA) (n.d.). Making a mandatory notification.

Brady, M. (2013). Health and care professions council: protecting whom? *Journal of Paramedic Practice* **5** (5): 246–247.

Brown, B., Crawford, P., and Darongkamas, J. (2000). Blurred roles and permeable boundaries: the experience of multidisciplinary working in community mental health. *Health & Social Care in the Community* **8** (6): 425–435.

Chamberlain, M. (2014). Reforming medical regulation in the United Kingdom: from restratification to governmentality and beyond. *Medical Sociology Online* **8** (1): 32–44.

College of Paramedics (2015). *Paramedic Career Framework. 3e*. Bridgwater, UK: College of Paramedics.

Considine, J., Shaban, R.Z., Fry, M. et al. (2019). Patient safety and quality in emergency care. In: *Emergency and Trauma Care for Nurses and Paramedics, 3e* (ed. K. Curtis, C. Ramsden, J. Considine, et al.). Sydney: Elsevier.

Donabedian, A. (1966). Evaluating the quality of medical care. *Milbank Quarterly* **83** (4): 691–729.

Donabedian, A. (1988). The quality of care. How can it be assessed? *Journal of the American Medical Association* **260** (12): 1734–1738.

Donaghy, J. (2013). The role of the Health and Care Professions Council. *Journal of Paramedic Practice* **5** (7): 370–371.

Evetts, J. (2014). The concept of professionalism: professional work, professional practice and learning. In: *International Handbook of Research in Professional and Practice-based Learning* (ed. B. Stephen, C. Harteis and H. Gruber), 29–56. Springer.

Freidson, E. (1983). The reorganization of the professions by regulation. *Law and Human Behavior* **7** (2/3): 279–290.

Freidson, E. (2001). *Professionalism: The Third Logic*. Cambridge: Polity Press.

Health and Care Professions Council (HCPC) (2001). *Health and Social Work Professions Order 2001 (UK)*. London: HCPC.

Health and Care Professions Council (HCPC) (2014). *Professionalism in healthcare professionals*. Available at: http://www.hpc-uk.org/assets/documents/10003771Professionalisminhealthcareprofessionals.pdf (accessed June 2014).

Health and Care Professions Council (HCPC) (2016). *Fitness to Practise Annual Report 2016*. London: HCPC.

Health Professions Council (HPC) (2012). *Regulating Ethics and Conduct at the Council for Professions Supplementary to Medicine – 1960–2002*. London: HPC.

Institute of Medicine (2000). *To Err Is Human: Building a Safer Health System*. Washington DC: National Academies Press.

Johns, C. (1992). Developing clinical standards. In: *Knowledge for Nursing Practice* (ed. K. Robinson and B. Vaughan), 59–72. Oxford: Butterworth Heinemann.

Kreber, C. (2017). The idea of a 'decent profession': implications for professional education. *Studies in Higher Education* **44**: 1–12.

Lovegrove, M. and Davis, J. (2013). *Paramedic Evidence Based Education Project (PEEP): Executive Summary and Summary of Recommendations*. Allied Health Solutions & Buckinghamshire New University.

NSW Parliamentary Counsel's Office (2002). Civil Liability Acts 2002 (NSW).

Office of Queensland Parliamentary Counsel (2009). *Health Practitioner Regulation National Law Act 2009*. Available at: https://www.legislation.qld.gov.au/view/pdf/2017-09-13/act-2009-hprnlq (accessed 19 March 2019).

Paramedicine Board of Australia (n.d.). *Fact Sheet: Managing Risk to the Public – How the Complaints and Concerns Process Works*. Melbourne: AHPRA.

Paramedicine Board of Australia (2018). *Registration Standards*. Melbourne: AHPR.

Professional Standards Council (2018). *What is a profession?* Available at: http://www.psc.gov.au/what-is-a-profession (accessed 5 February 2018).

Professions Australia (2018). *What is a profession?* Available at: www.professions.com.au/about-us/what-is-a-professional (accessed 2 February 2018).

Secretary of State for Health (2007). *Trust, Assurance and Safety – The Regulation of Health Professionals in the 21st Century*. London: Stationery Office.

Shaban, R.Z. (2011). *Paramedic clinical judgment of mental illness: a case study of accounts of practice*. PhD thesis. Brisbane: Arts, Education and Law Group, Griffith University.

Shaban, R.Z. (2018). Tackling errors in health care: the rise of financial penalties for preventable hospital-acquired complications. *Australian Hospital and Healthcare Bulletin* **2018**: 22–23.

Smith, J. (2004). *The Shipman Inquiry: Fifth report – Safeguarding patients: lessons from the past – proposals for the future*. **CM** 6394-1. London: Stationery Office.

Townsend, R. (2018). *The role of law in the professionalisation of paramedics in Australia*. PhD thesis. Canberra: School of Law, Australian National University.

van der Gaag, A., Gallagher, A., Zasada, M. et al. (2017). *People like us? Understanding complaints about paramedics and social workers*. Final report. Guildford: University of Surrey.

Wilensky, H.L. (1964). The professionalization of everyone? *American Journal of Sociology* **70** (2): 137–158.

World Medical Association (WMA) (1948). *Declaration of Geneva*. Geneva: WMA.

CHAPTER 3

Legal and ethical aspects of paramedic practice

Nevin Mehmet

School of Human Sciences, University of Greenwich, London, UK

Contents

LEARNING OUTCOMES

On completion of this chapter the reader will be able to:

- Discuss the importance of law in relation to paramedic practice.
- Discuss the importance of ethics in relation to paramedic practice.
- Identify ethical principles as frameworks that can be supported in practice.
- Identify legal principles as frameworks that can be supported in practice.
- Understand how the legal aspects that underpin ethical principles relate to paramedic practice.

Case study

An ambulance has been despatched to a high street where there are reports of an intoxicated male. This is the fourth call in the shift involving alcohol as a reason for ambulance attendance. The paramedic assesses the patient and it is clear that they cannot be left alone due to their intoxicated state. The patient cannot provide any information pertaining to a friend or family member, and as a final resort they are taken to the local emergency department.

Fundamentals of Paramedic Practice: A Systems Approach, Third Edition. Edited by Sam Willis and Ian Peate.

Companion website: www.wiley.com/go/willis/paramedic3e

Introduction

The paramedic role has evolved greatly in the last two decades, with paramedics needing to have an in-depth clinical knowledge base, to be highly skilled, and to be evidence-based practitioners (Eaton et al. 2018). With the increasing complex environments, paramedics often find themselves working with people in vulnerable and distressing situations. Therefore, today's paramedic must also demonstrate extensive knowledge of ethics and law that may impact their decision-making. Ethical decision-making is pivotal within the role of everyday practice for paramedics and at times they are required to make decisions within very complex settings that can often be unclear or unpredictable. It is therefore vital that paramedics have a core foundational understanding of how the key ethical principles can fuse with legislation or legal precedents to support decision-making within their practice.

Although this is a fundamental subject area and whole books have been written just focusing on the law and ethics for paramedic practice, it is not possible to prepare the reader for every eventuality. However, this chapter aims to introduce some key areas of focus on law and ethics within paramedic practice.

Legal aspects of paramedic practice

In the UK and Australia, paramedics are regulated by a particular piece of legislation that provides authority to an overarching regulator to manage the practice of practitioners. This regulatory regime applied *in addition to* other legal frameworks also regulate paramedic behaviour, these include civil laws (e.g. trespass, negligence, privacy, and confidentiality), criminal laws (e.g. assault, fraud), and employment laws (e.g. contract of employment with the employer). In this way, it could be argued that health professionals like paramedics are often subject to extra layers of law that may not apply to some other workers.

In the UK, that regulatory body is referred to as the Health and Care Professions Council (HCPC). In Australia, the regulatory body is the Paramedicine Board of Australia, which receives administrative assistance from the Australian Health Practitioner Regulation Agency (AHPRA). These two regulatory systems are slightly different in structure, although their objective is largely the same. The objective of both these regulatory agencies is to ensure public protection and safety by requiring paramedics to be suitably educated, competent, and able to work according to a set of conduct standards that place patient interests first.

The HCPC (2016) *Standards of Conduct, Performance and Ethics* establishes the ethical framework and professional standards expected of paramedics in practice. This includes the recognition that paramedics, as a matter of professionalism, must work within their limits of knowledge and skills, whilst maintaining their own health and well-being as well as their patients', as the practitioner may place a patient at risk if they are impaired whilst practising their profession. Breaches of these standards can result in paramedics being sanctioned in a number of ways by the HCPC. These sanctions can include restrictions on practice, investigations, civil litigation, or in extreme cases criminal charges and the loss of registration.

The Australian regulatory model differs from the UK model to the extent that paramedics in Australia have their own regulatory body – the Paramedicine Board of Australia – that will not only establish education, registration, conduct, and competence standards but also create disciplinary panels comprising members of the profession and the community to assess the performance of paramedics who may have breached their professional standards. A similar range of sanctions apply to paramedics who breach those standards. The important point for paramedics to remember regarding this regulatory regime is that it is designed to ensure that patients stay safe and that their interests are placed ahead of other interests, including those of the paramedic.

Consent to treatment

Department of Health (2001) state it is a legal and ethical principle that valid consent must be obtained prior to starting treatment or physical examination. This principle reflects the ethical principle of autonomy whereby all individuals have a fundamental right to determine what happens to their own bodies. Essentially, to respect a patient's autonomy and for consent to be valid Gillon (1994) states consent relies on:

- Patient capacity
- Consent being provided voluntarily
- The nature of the treatment being understood (broadly) by the patient

Therefore, the paramedic must ensure the patient is sufficiently informed about the proposed treatment in order to weigh up the benefits and risks, to be able to comprehend the procedure and then communicate their willingness to accept those benefits and risks or any concerns they may have to the treating paramedic. The term 'informed' means just that: there must be enough information available for someone who has the decision-making capability to be able to make a judgement. Gaining consent to treat a patient is an important aspect of paramedic practice. Implied (implicit) and informed consent are the two most commonly occurring forms of consent that affect the paramedic.

Informed consent

For the most part, prior to the commencement of treatment, a practitioner is legally required, as part of their duty of care, to inform the patient about the broad nature and effect of any proposed treatment. If the paramedic plans to give the patient an injection, then it is enough to inform the patient what drug they plan to give, why they are giving it, and importantly, what the side effects may be, both good and bad, as patients may not be aware of how unwell the administered drugs might make them feel. This is as much about good practice as it is about lawful practice. **Informed consent** is consistent with the overarching legal and ethical principle of individual autonomy, or the right to self-determination.

Often in paramedic practice the patient is not able to give any form of consent because they are unconscious, incompetent, or otherwise incapable of doing so. The paramedic must be able to assess the patient's decision-making capability accurately. If the patient does not have the capacity to consent to treatment, then this should be documented by the paramedic. Consent may be given by an authorised surrogate decision-maker, for example, someone who has been authorised to make such decisions in a formal legal instrument like a guardianship order or a spouse, a carer, or other family member. The law around surrogate decision-making differs in each jurisdiction. The same overriding principle of a 'patient's **best interest**' still applies in cases where there is a surrogate decision-maker.

If there is no other decision-maker around to act for the patient, then the paramedic can make decisions based on necessity, provided the decisions are made in the patient's best interest. Paramedics are able to rely on the legal principle of necessity to support their interventions. Necessity is the principle whereby the provision of treatment without consent can be justified on the basis that it is not practicable to communicate with the person you are assisting, *and* the action is one a reasonable person would take in the best interest of the assisted person. The basis of the provision of treatment is that it is necessary and in the patient's and society's best interests to do so.

Implied (implicit) consent

Implied consent is consent that is not explicitly given by the individual but is inferred from the person's actions or inactions. Picture the scene. You are the paramedic looking after a patient and you have them settled in the back of the ambulance. You move towards the patient with a blood pressure cuff and the patient extends their arm for you to apply it. This is **implied consent**.

This kind of consent is valid in a court of law, as the patient has expected the paramedic to treat them since they observed the paramedic approaching them with the blood pressure cuff. The patient has accepted the treatment by extending their arm. As a rule, the more serious the potential consequence of a treatment may be, the more important it is to have a higher level of consent. Implied consent is low-level consent and is usually reserved for low-level interventions. If the paramedic was considering performing an intervention with serious consequences, then it would be better practice to receive verbal or written consent for the treatment. There are some exceptions to a reliance on implied consent, and that is where the wishes of the patient are known (e.g. refusal of treatment stipulated in an advanced care directive or other equivalent instrument) or where there is a surrogate decision-maker (i.e. someone other than the patient who knows the patient well and would be able to make decisions as if they were the patient). However, another example of implied consent is with unconscious patients who require an emergency intervention to save life. Paramedics can assume that the patient would have consented to the treatment they provide to save the patient's life or limb and can proceed. Unless stated otherwise prior to losing consciousness.

There may be occasions where patients are happy to allow the paramedic to make decisions for them and assent to any treatment pathways offered. Paramedics can obtain a large degree of patient trust and maintaining public trust is the integrity of paramedic practice. This is essential, as trust brings the responsibility to ensure it is in the patient's best interest.

Best interest

The term 'patient's best interest' is routinely used in out-of-hospital care. This is because the nature of the professional power that paramedics have is particular to the work they do. Paramedics commonly work with very vulnerable people in extreme situations where the stakes are often high, sometimes literally life and death (Carver et al. 2020). As such, it is imperative that paramedics wield this professional power responsibly. The law does codify this principle in that the regulation of paramedics in both the UK and Australia is set up to protect the public. For example, standard one of the HCPC standards of conduct, performance, and ethics relates to promoting and protecting the interests of service users and carers.

It is therefore both an ethical and a legal obligation for paramedics to act in the patient's best interest. This may sound contrary to principles of autonomy, because it suggests that a paternalistic, 'paramedic-knows-best' attitude applies. However, acting in the patient's best interest does not allow a paramedic to override the choices of a competent patient. It does provide guidance for paramedics in decision-making where there is an incompetent patient (a patient who is unable to make decisions for themselves) or a conflict of choices. For example, the paramedic may have been directed by their employer to perform a certain task that is contrary to the wishes or interests of the patient. For example, this might mean taking the patient directly to a specialist treatment centre that can more appropriately deal with the patient's condition, rather than to a routine emergency department (ED) that may not always be equipped to do so. The paramedic as an independently regulated, autonomous professional may have an obligation in an instance like this to breach their employer's guidelines if it is in the best interest of the patient to do so. At all times the overriding principle informing the paramedic's decision-making should be how an action can best benefit a patient and do the least amount of harm. This may be difficult, particularly if the action the patient wants to take is harmful. For example, if a terminally ill patient refuses transport to hospital because they want to die at home, it would be a matter for the paramedics to help facilitate this request because, although it may be harmful, it could potentially be more harmful to override the patient's wishes as presented in the Mental Capacity Act (MCA) (2005).

All patients have a right to decide what they do and what happens to them, and unless the patient lacks the capacity to consent to treatment, they must be allowed to make that decision proactively. Take the example of a patient who presents to the paramedic with cardiac-related chest pain. The paramedic's role is to perform a thorough patient assessment and take an in-depth history in order to identify what treatments the patient should receive from the paramedic, and also to decide whether the patient should travel to the local ED or whether they should be taken directly to the cath lab for cardiac catheterisation. However, not all patients want to go to hospital or travel to a cath lab for treatment. This is when acting in the patient's best interest can become controversial. The paramedic must inform the patient in clear terms why they think the patient must travel for treatment, highlighting the possible effects of refusal, but they must also respect the decisions of the patient if they refuse; otherwise, the paramedic will be susceptible to claims of **battery**.

Battery

If a paramedic touches a patient without first gaining their consent to do so, it may be considered battery. It is good practice to get into the habit of simply asking the patient to obtain consent throughout the process and before it is done, which adds no extra burden to the paramedic in the execution of their usual business, from taking a pulse to performing a much more invasive intervention. This simple communication skill not only facilitates the paramedic meeting their legal obligations but also allows them to meet their ethical and professionalism standards as well. Asking the patient for permission to perform interventions lets the patient know what the paramedic is planning to do, which can help reduce anxiety and allow the patient to be a participant in their own care.

Negligence

Negligence occurs when the paramedic falls short of providing the standard of conduct and competence established by their peers as being a 'reasonable standard' for a paramedic with equivalent knowledge and training, and that results in harm being done to the patient. The standard is established from educational standards that inform the scope of practice, along with codes of conduct, clinical guidelines, and policy documents. These all help to establish the standard of care expected of a 'reasonable' paramedic. The legal standard of negligence is therefore very high because in most cases where negligence has been claimed against a practitioner, the peer group has provided evidence that they would have behaved in a similar way given the circumstances of a case. In order to be found negligent several elements need to be established, including that the paramedic owed the patient a duty of care, that the paramedic breached their duty by providing treatment that was below the reasonable standard, *and* that as a result of that breach of duty a harm was caused. The nature of civil liability law and the complexities of healthcare mean that it is quite difficult to prove that an act or omission to act by a practitioner was the direct cause of harm to a patient because usually patients are already harmed by some other process.

Duty of care

Wherever there is a practitioner–patient relationship, there is a duty of care. The paramedic employer might also have a duty of care that is separate from that of the paramedic. For example, an ambulance service owns the duty once telephone contact has been established. The term 'duty of care' was defined in the legal case *Donoghue v Stevenson* (1932) AC 562 at 580. It means that a person with a duty of care has an obligation to take care of, and prevent harm occurring to, another individual that may be 'so closely and directly affected by my acts that I ought reasonably to have them in contemplation as being so affected'. This duty extends to 'the examination, diagnosis and treatment of the patient and the provision of information in an appropriate case' (*Rogers v Whitaker* [1992] 109 ALR 625).

Breaching a duty of care

Whether or not a paramedic has breached their duty of care will be established by examining the standard expected of a 'reasonable paramedic' of equivalent knowledge and training faced with a similar situation. This is sometimes referred to as the **Bolam principle** (from the UK case *Bolam v Friern Hospital Management Committee* [1957] 1 WLR 582, where the principle was first elucidated) and it applies in both the UK and with only minor modifications in Australia (e.g. the standard cannot be irrational). Provided a practitioner can find a peer and other evidence (e.g. codes, guidelines, policies, educational standards) that would support the action of the paramedic, then it is probable that a breach will be unable to be established. The significance of this standard for paramedics is that now they are regulated as autonomous professionals, the peer standard will be established by paramedics, not practitioners from other disciplines like emergency medicine. This is because the Bolam principle is that the practitioner is assessed as meeting the standard of care of their peers, 'the reasonable paramedic', not the reasonable 'emergency doctor', who is trained to a different standard and has different skills.

Capacity to make decisions

To uphold the rights of the patient and to act in the patient's best interest, the paramedic should gain consent from the patient before commencing treatment. Paramedics must understand the MCA (2005), and paramedics are among the professional groups named in the MCA Code of Practice (Department of Constitutional Affairs 2007) who are required to have regard to the Act when carrying out their duties. The MCA (2005) confirms that it can be assumed that adults (legally classified as aged 16 years or over) have full legal capacity to make decisions for themselves unless it can be shown that they lack capacity to make a decision for themselves at the time it needs to be made.

It is up to the practitioner to prove that the patient was not competent to make decisions for themselves if the practitioner does not get consent from their patient for treatment (unless the practitioner is able to rely on the principle of necessity as a defence). The nature of paramedic work means that there are commonly occasions when the patient does not have the mental capacity to give valid consent to treatment, because the patient is unable to take in, retain, weigh up, and convey an understanding of the information shared by the paramedic about the proposed treatment. Establishing competence in patients is important, particularly if the consequences of decision-making are high. Within law, *competent* patients have a legal right to refuse medical treatment and under the MCA, a person is not to be treated as though unable to decide, merely because they make what is perceived as an unwise decision, even if it may result in their death.

In the instance of an acutely suicidal patient, establishing the competence of the patient becomes even more difficult because of the high stakes and often extreme time pressures that are placed on paramedics in those situations. It should be noted that there are no instances of paramedics having been prosecuted for treating an acutely suicidal patient, even when the patient has an objection to treatment. There are provisions within the criminal and mental health law that provide protection for those who offer help and treatment to acutely suicidal patients. It is important to note that this exception does not mean that the court would find *all* suicidal patients to be lacking in competence just by virtue of the fact that they are suicidal. Indeed, the court has commented many times that having suicidal thoughts can be an entirely rationale response to particularly stressful events (Townsend and Luck 2013). However, in the case of an emergency where there are time-critical factors and the stakes are high, there are protections afforded to paramedics against a charge of battery for treating a patient where there is some doubt about the patient's competence to give or refuse consent for treatment. As already noted, there are provisions within mental health law, which is particular to each jurisdiction (i.e. the UK and each state and territory in Australia) but largely similar in nature, allowing for the treatment of those patients who pose a risk of harm to self or others and have a mental illness or disorder.

Mental capacity in children and young people

For people under the age of 18 years, capacity is not presumed, and it is incumbent upon the child or young person to demonstrate that they have capacity to give or refuse consent for treatment. The Gillick principle, or Gillick *competence* as it is sometimes known, which applies in both the UK and Australia, established that a person under 18 years may be able to make decisions for themselves, provided they can demonstrate an ability to weigh up and use information to make a decision in the same way a competent adult would. This applies for consent to treatment. It does not generally apply to refusal of treatment. The Department of Health (2018) states young people aged 16 and 17 years are presumed to have competence to give consent for themselves. Younger children who have capacity and demonstrate full understanding of the proposed procedure/treatment can also give consent.

There is a sliding spectrum of capacity depending on the seriousness of the action being consented to or refused. For example, if a paramedic were to approach a 4-year-old child to put on a plaster for a superficial wound and the child started to scream, then it would be acceptable for the paramedic to consider this a refusal of treatment that would have little benefit in being pursued and perhaps create a greater harm (i.e. to the child's relationship with paramedics in the future). However, a young person under 18 years cannot refuse life-saving treatment, and neither can their parents or guardians. Only the court can decide if a person under 18 years can refuse life-sustaining treatment.

Often paramedics are called to children and young people of couples who are no longer together or where there are step-parents involved in the child's care. The legal particularities of the care of children in our society is that we *all* have an obligation to care for children, because they are considered vulnerable people unable to care for themselves. It may be that a paramedic is able to get consent from a parent about the treatment of their child, but if they are not, or if there is some disagreement as to which parent has decision-making powers that is unduly delaying treatment to the detriment of the child or young person, then paramedics can act without the consent of a parent, provided their action is in the child's best interest. This is again an example of acting under the principle of necessity for a person who is unable to give or refuse consent to treatment for themselves.

It should be noted that there are limits to the authority that parents must consent or refuse consent to treatment for their children. For example, a parent does not have the authority to refuse life-sustaining treatment nor can a parent override consent that is provided by a *'competent child'*. If a paramedic is placed in the difficult situation of assessing that the parent is not making decisions in the child's best interest, the paramedic can and should step in to treat the child in the child's best interest because the paramedic's professional, legal, and ethical responsibility involves protecting vulnerable patients of all ages.

Ethical aspects of paramedic practice

Before we can discuss what we mean by ethics as a term, we should consider why ethics is important to paramedic practice. Duncun (2010) claims that everyone involved in healthcare should have a fundamental concern with issues of values and ethics. Whatever aspect of healthcare one is in, and regardless of the specific engagements within a role, the nature and practice of healthcare demand that professionals are concerned with ethics. Paramedics are by no means an exception. However, in the last decade we have seen an increase of healthcare ethics literature move away from ethical issues in a clinical hospital setting and shift in recent years to incorporate ethical issues within emergency care, with more and more examples being used to illustrate ethical dilemmas within everyday paramedic practice. It must be noted that ethical texts cannot provide the answers for any given eventuality (Clarke et al. 2018) that may occur across the healthcare setting. Nevertheless, what ethical texts can provide is key ethical and legal frameworks that are integral to professional practice.

Paramedics often meet people in extremely difficult and distressing situations and at a time of heightened vulnerability for the patient(s) (Clarke et al. 2018). It is thus critical that paramedics have an understanding of the ethical issues that can have an impact on their decision-making in respect of patients and their families. In support of this, paramedics are still required to be registered with the HCPC and to adhere to the professional and ethical standards it prescribes. In addition, the paramedic has to be in a position to make informed decisions and judgements regarding patient care in cases where the standards and codes may not provide specific guidance. Therefore, the teaching and understanding of ethics are integral to paramedic education, and it is crucial that paramedics have a strong understanding of the ethical principles and legal precedents that apply to their practice, in order to be in a position to apply these principles to any changes within practice, procedures, or polices. The use of reflection within practice supports paramedics in developing a foundation of basic knowledge and experience into expert knowledge and skills, to enable them to recognise and acknowledge the effects of their actions (Carver et al. 2020)

Howlett (2019) provides the paramedic with clear directions for considering their ethical behaviours within a given situation and enables them to question whether the treatment they have provided is in line with ethical practice.

Ethics and morality

Ethics is often considered to be a branch of philosophy that addresses questions about morality; therefore, when ethics is used in the context of moral philosophy, it is often concerned with the study of morality, moral problems, and moral judgements. Ethics also attempts to define what is good and evil, right and wrong, justice and virtue (Mehmet 2011). There are three key aspects that support our understanding of what we mean by ethics:

- *Meta-ethics* provides analytical thinking about the source of the meaning of words or concepts; it can be considered as the theoretical side of ethics. Examples would be the term 'morals' and the source of 'morality', or questioning the meaning of terms such as 'right', 'wrong', 'good', or 'evil' within the context of morals.
- *Normative ethics* attempts to give answers to moral questions and problems in relation to what might be the morally right thing to do in a given situation, or whether someone is a morally good person.
- *Applied ethics* attempts to apply the concepts of ethics and to answer difficult moral questions that people face in their lives, such as whether assisted suicide is morally wrong, or whether individuals have the right of self-determination.

The combination of all three aspects of what we understand as ethics is important within a professional context. Meta-ethics allows us to question these terms and to obtain a greater understanding of the concept and ideas of what we mean by 'right' and 'wrong' in particular, within the professional context. Normative ethics allows us to place these concepts into real situations and apply their meanings. For example, if lying is considered morally wrong and this is taken to be a moral norm, then the application of this norm would be the question: Should patients *always* be told the truth? Applied ethics provides the platform to apply ethics to specialised areas such as healthcare ethics, public health ethics, or business ethics.

Utilitarianism and deontology

Modern philosophers or ethicists have contributed to two main ethical theories: utilitarianism and deontology. A third theory, virtue ethics, although arguably the oldest in origin, is rarely used within healthcare as it is not action guiding in the same sense as utilitarianism and deontology. However, in recent times, virtue theory is starting to be applied across social work and some aspects of healthcare.

Utilitarianism is a doctrine proposed by Jeremy Bentham (1748–1832) and later by John Stuart Mill (1806–1876), whereby an action is morally good if it produces the greatest amount of good or pleasure for the greatest amount of people. Deontology (*deon* meaning 'duty') proposes that it is the moral intention of the agent that makes an action right or wrong. According to Immanuel Kant (1734–1804), we have a moral duty within society to act in a morally permissible way. Kant articulated a set of universal laws, whereby moral rules were applicable to all, so that if something is right for one, it is right for all. It is from deontology and the idea of set moral norms that 'codes of ethics' originated, since deontology provides fixed rules about what is right and wrong universally. Beauchamp and Childress (2019) consider that deontology provided the foundations for building a simpler and more effective way of supporting people in what is considered morally right and wrong within society, and developed four ethical principles – autonomy, **beneficence**, **nonmaleficence**, and justice – that arose from deontological theory (see the next section).

Virtue ethics stems from the work of the ancient philosopher Socrates and was further developed by Plato and then more extensively by Aristotle. This theory focuses on the attention of the character rather than their actions as the focus of moral concern, and someone who shows virtues such as kindness, generosity, respect for persons, honesty, and compassion is the model of moral conduct.

Although it does not consider actions – i.e. rather than 'what I ought to do' the focus is 'what type of person ought I be' – someone's intentions and character will be reflected in their actions. Campbell et al. (1997) and Macintyre (2007) have supported the adoption of virtue theory in medical and nursing ethics, and paramedic practice should be no exception. The adoption of virtue ethics in education on ethics may support students in recognising that virtues are an extension of what we consider professionalism to be, and it encourages them to consider their own character.

Ethical principles: an ethical framework

The ethical principles proposed by Beauchamp and Childress (2019) are often used as an ethical framework within healthcare, as these four main principles are considered to govern every aspect in healthcare and to support decision-making. This is also referred to as principlism, which is not designed as a moral theory but rather a framework for determining what to do. The four principles are taken to be *prima facie* rather than absolute duties. This means that it is permissible to break or diminish one or more ethical principles to meet a more pressing requirement from another *prima facie* duty. For example, if you were to respect an individual's autonomy by carrying out their requests, but it may cause the individual a degree of harm (physical or psychological), then it would be permissible to diminish their autonomy, as that would be in their best interest.

The four ethical principles are as follows:

- *Respect for autonomy:* respect the capacity of individuals to choose their own definition of a 'good' life and to act accordingly. An autonomous decision (act) is one that is made (performed) intentionally, with understanding, and without controlling influences. Fundamentally, it is respecting the individual's decision regarding their treatment and this must be respected.
- *Beneficence:* maximise benefits and account for all the actions of a health professional to ensure they are in the individual's best interest.
- *Nonmaleficence:* 'do no harm', or do not cause any 'undue' harm, which must be balanced in particular against the potential benefits of a course of action. Leaving a vulnerable patient at home may address the autonomy of the patent, but they may require hospitalisation, leading the paramedic to need to weigh the potential harm against the potential benefits.
- *Justice:* consideration of what is fair and equitable or what is owed to each person. Each individual's rights are accounted for, such as allocation of resources and time spent on scene with patients that may limit the time spent with other patients.

Although these four principles provide a framework and foundation of support for actions and decisions within healthcare practice, it also has to be recognised that principlism does have its limitations. First, it can lend itself to being presented in the form of a checklist ensuring all principles have been met. It may be not only unsuitable but also detrimental to advocate the adoption of all four principles in a given situation. In addition, the principles can conflict. For example, vaccinations are administered with the aim of providing a potential benefit to an individual, yet simultaneously impart a degree of physical harm and risk. When ethical principles are in conflict, the use of specifying and balancing may provide a foundation for obtaining the right course of action that must be ethically justified. Specification requires the person to spell out where, when, why, how, by what means, to whom, or by whom the action is to be done or avoided. Alternatively, balancing the principles against each other to determine which is the more pressing may determine the right course of action.

Conclusion

Paramedics must provide ethical healthcare to their patients; this is not a nicety, but a necessity. All patient interactions must be both ethical and have respect for the law. Guidelines exist that can help the paramedic to achieve this, and this chapter provides an overview of the key ethical and legal theories and principles to help the paramedic provide legal and ethical healthcare.

Activities

Test your knowledge

Now review your learning by completing the learning activities in this chapter. The answers to these appear at the end of the book. Further self-test activities can be found at **www.wileyfundamentalseries.com/paramedic/3e.**

1. What are the three key components set by Gillon (1994) to obtain consent?
2. What is a duty of care?
3. What does the term 'patient's best interest' mean? How is this applied to the HCPC and/or AHPRA?
4. What are the four main ethical principles?

Activity 3.1

Answer the following questions relating to consent to treatment:

1. Which two kinds of consent are most likely to affect paramedic practice?
2. How does a patient imply their consent to the paramedic?
3. What information do patients require to be able to make informed consent?

Activity 3.2

Imagine you attend a 26-year-old who drank antifreeze (a poison) with the intention of suicide. The patient called an ambulance as they wished to die in hospital rather than die alone at home. Consider the legal and ethical issues this raises working as paramedic.

Glossary

Autonomy: The right of self-determination or the right to make one's own choices. The autonomous individual must be competent to make decisions affecting their life and welfare.

Battery: When a patient is touched by a health professional without giving prior consent.

Beneficence: A moral obligation to act in the benefit of others. The principle of beneficence requires us to enable others by preventing or limiting harm.

Best interest: Doing what is right for the patient rather than for any other reason.

Bolam principle: A test used to recognise if a paramedic or medical professional has breached a duty of care.

Competence: Used to describe a situation of capability and capacity. For example, the patient has the competence to make their own decision about treatment.

Implied consent: Taking physical gestures and body language as an indication of agreement; for example, a patient's extended arm when a paramedic approaches with a blood pressure cuff.

Informed consent: Consent that is based on reliable and fully understood information.

Nonmaleficence: The moral obligation to 'do no harm', often balanced with the principle of beneficence.

References

Australian Health Practitioner Regulation Agency (AHPRA) (2022). Code of Conduct AHPRA.

Beauchamp, T.L. and Childress, J.F. (2019). *Principles of Biomedical Ethics. 8e*. Oxford: Oxford University Press.

Campbell, A.V., Charlesworth, M., Gillet, G. et al. (1997). *Medical Ethics*. Oxford: Oxford University Press.

Carver, H., Moritz, D., and Ebbs, P. (2020). Ethics and law in paramedic practice: boundaries of capacity and interests. *Journal of Paramedic Practice* **12** (10): 1–10.

Clarke V., Harris G., and Cowland S. (2018). Ethics and law for the paramedic. In: *Foundations for Paramedic Practice: A Theoretical Perspective, 2* (ed. A.Y. Blaber), 39–56. Buckingham: Open University Press.

Department of Health (2001). *Consent: What You Have a Right to Expect. A Guide for Adults*. London: Department of Health.

Department of Health and Social Care (2018). *Reference Guide to Consent for Examination on Treatment of Children.* 2e. London: Department of Health.

Department of Constitutional Affairs (2007). Mental Capacity Act 2005 code of practice. London: The Stationery Office.

Duncun, P. (2010). *Values, Ethics and Healthcare*. London: Sage.

Eaton, G., Mahtani K., and Catterall M. (2018). The evolving role of paramedics – a NICE problem to have? *Journal of Health Services Research & Policy* **23** (3): 193–195.

Gillon, R. (1994). *Principles of Health Care Ethics*. Chichester: John Wiley & Sons.

Health and Care Professional Council (HCPC) (2016). *Standards of Conduct, Performance and Ethics*. London: HCPC.

Howlett, G. (2019). Newly qualified student paramedics perception of reflection and use in practice. *Journal of Paramedic Practice* **11** (6): 258–263.

Macintyre, A. (2007). *After Virtue: A Study in Moral Theory.* 3e. London: Gerald Duckworth.

Mehmet, N. (2011). Ethics and wellbeing. In: *Understanding Wellbeing: An Introduction for Students and Practitioners of Health and Social Care* (ed. A. Knight and A. McNaught), 37–49. Banbury: Lantern Press.

Townsend, R. and Luck, M. (2013). *Applied Paramedic Law and Ethics*. Sydney: Elsevier.

CHAPTER 4

The impact of professional culture on paramedics and students

Sarah Fulford

Faculty of Humanities, Curtin University, Perth, Australia

Derek Collings-Hughes

Faculty of Health Sciences, Curtin University, Perth, Australia

Contents

LEARNING OUTCOMES

On completion of this chapter, the reader will be able to:

- Demonstrate an understanding of what 'organisational culture' and 'professional culture' are and how they relate to 'paramedic culture'.
- Understand how culture can impact individuals and organisations as it relates to their behaviour, patient care, and organisational morale.
- Be able to critically reflect upon local ambulance culture and how this will impact future clinical practice.

Fundamentals of Paramedic Practice: A Systems Approach, Third Edition. Edited by Sam Willis and Ian Peate.

Companion website: www.wiley.com/go/willis/paramedic3e

Case study

As part of their curriculum, a paramedic student is on placement in an ambulance with a qualified paramedic. While at a call, as they approach their patient, the patient makes derogatory comments to the student against their gender and tells them with expletives not to go near the patient. The student is shocked and feels unable to answer back to the slur, as this may taint their professionalism, but they also feel that they should not have to endure such language in the workplace.

When the student returns to the station, they find it difficult to report what has just occurred.

They also discover, when they do bring it up with their paramedic mentors, that there seems to be an acceptance that verbal and physical violence towards staff 'is just part of the job' and 'nothing ever happens' if it is reported. The student feels uncomfortable with this and wonders if this response has something to do with the organisational culture.

As we explore the role of culture in paramedicine and its impact on ambulance services, paramedics, and patients, consider this example and how you think the existing culture may have affected this student's experience.

Introduction

The concept of culture within a workplace is not new and yet it is something that is not given the attention it deserves. Professional culture can be easily overlooked during routine practice, and especially during times of stress, for example, as recently seen with a once in a 100-years pandemic when frontline workers were exposed to a level of working stress previously unseen. While people can look towards the policies and procedures of a workplace for guidance and an understanding what the culture is, there can also be an awareness on an individual level that things need to change, especially when a problem has been identified but the professional culture itself is not changing alongside it. The concept of culture includes the context of the people who work in the organisation – their training, their personal views, and their context – and it is often dependent on the parameters leaders within the organisation will allow to provide colleagues the safety to explain, explore, and reinforce their own ideas.

The pandemic challenged us all culturally and socially. While some people embraced lockdown and the isolation, many others struggled without human connectivity. From a world that moved quickly towards technology, where we spoke to each other via phone message rather than a phone call, we now understand how important it is to be relatable to other humans, and to have that social contact (Matos 2021). For paramedics, the impact of the pandemic might be immeasurable. While many people were able to move their work to the online space or take their work home, paramedics had to be on the frontline; there was no choice. A culture of 'getting on with it' and putting the public first was vital to the continued work of paramedics. Other aspects of culture such as camaraderie and storytelling (explained below) likely also played a part in dealing with the stresses of frontline ambulance work during a pandemic.

But how is culture relevant for the individual paramedic or student paramedic? Understanding the organisational and professional culture as a student is important, as both will place social pressure on a student to develop as a professional in line with the existing culture. As we will see throughout this chapter, culture can be an excellent tool for learning, but individuals must reflect on the effects of that culture (which can be both positive and negative) to ensure they are growing in accordance with their personal values and the broader professional expectations as well.

Defining culture

Culture is a word that is prevalent in everyday language, yet it is a word with several meanings. Originally used to define the producing or nurturing of a thing such as the culturing of bacteria or a crop, culture has since been adopted by the social sciences, particularly in anthropology, to describe a broad social concept (Jahoda, 2012). In the late twentieth century, the word culture gained popularity in the thriving corporate world and improving 'corporate culture' has since been touted as the business executive's path to success. Although we may all assume that everyone means the same thing when using the term 'culture', Jahoda (2012) explains that what is meant by culture varies greatly, even within the social sciences. Several acceptable definitions exist, and agreeing on one clear definition is a difficult, if not impossible, task.

With this in mind, as we discuss the effects of culture on paramedic practice, it will be helpful to start with a shared definition of culture. So, within this chapter, we will use the definition of culture laid out by Hong as being:

> *[a] network of knowledge, consisting of learned routines of thinking, feeling, and interacting with other people, as well as a corpus of substantive assertions and ideas about aspects of the world (Hong 2009, p. 4)*

Culture has several important characteristics. It is shared among the group's individuals; it is externalised through symbols, rituals, folklore, and social constructs; it creates a shared language and social expectations between members; and it is passed down between 'generations' of the group's members (Hong 2009). Importantly, culture is not static. Hong explains that culture is constantly under development as new generations accept and reject the knowledge passed down to them. Therefore, while culture is rooted in shared knowledge, it has deep connections with identity, language, action(s) and belief. We encounter several types of culture in our daily lives. However, the two most relevant to the paramedic's professional life are organisational and professional culture. These two forms of culture are intertwined, with some overlap, and together they make up 'paramedic culture'.

Stop and Reflect

Can you think of examples of the different cultures in your own life? How do you think these have influenced the following:

- Your beliefs
- Your values, morals, and ethics
- Your behaviour
- Your knowledge and learning
- The decisions you have made

Organisational culture

Organisations have their own policies and procedures governing the workplace, and there are often overarching hierarchies or governance systems that help maintain the organisation's functioning. This ensures that employers and employees are kept safe and within organisations, and that customers or patients are interacted with safely.

In an organisational context, this can also embody a folklore, which can develop outside of, or due to, the parameters put in place by the policies and processes (Michalopoulos and Xue 2021). Folklore becomes the lived experiences of working in an environment, it is the stories told, the symbols used, and the collegiality shared (Tangherlini 2000). Sometimes this results in a camaraderie growing between employees. In a negative capacity, this camaraderie can grow as employees bond together against the machinations they face within the workplace. A positive folklore can exist when this sense of camaraderie is based on loyalty, respect, and empowerment.

Stop and Reflect

We have all heard terms such as 'bad work culture' or a 'toxic office culture':

- Where do you think these phrases evolve from in the workplace?
- How do you think this affects the workers within an organisation?
- Conversely, what makes a 'great workplace culture'?
- How does this affect workers?

Culture is important as it helps with job satisfaction, feeling of collegiality, and sense of belonging in an organisation. Often within an organisation, the culture historically in place will be perpetuated by those who commence work there, and when the system is questioned the standard response can be: 'That is how we have always done it.' Thus, if a person is unable to question what or why they are doing a task or do not feel empowered to ask questions and receive feedback, this directly affects job satisfaction, and within paramedicine, positive patient outcomes. It then becomes the responsibility of both employer and employee to call out parts of the culture that need to be improved. It also requires that those in power pay attention to the issues faced by their staff.

Tsai and colleagues highlighted that organisational culture is the values and beliefs that have existed in an organisation and that importantly: 'Administrators usually adjust their leadership behavior to accomplish the mission of the organisation, and this could influence the employees' job satisfaction' (Tsai 2011). These values (and priorities) can also vary within the organisation and may create organisational subcultures. Wankhade (2012) noted that within an unnamed UK ambulance service there were three separate subcultures – all with differing priorities. These were the executive culture (middle/upper management), the engineering culture (communications and dispatch staff), and the operator culture (frontline/operational staff). Wankhade (2012) also noted significant conflict between each subculture and described an 'us vs them' culture among paramedics – who often thought managers were 'out to get them'. However, this conflict often did not result from malice or ill intent. Rather, it was likely generated from differing priorities of what was most important to each area. Conflict due to different organisational cultures (or subcultures) has also been noted among emergency services, where it arises due to differing priorities and cultural expectations (Van Scotter and Leonard 2022).

Stop and Reflect

- Can you think of an experience when you have seen an 'us vs them' mentality between workers and management?
- Do you think this resulted from one party making decisions deliberately to annoy or harm the other?
- Do you think the 'us vs them' mentality helped or hampered progress/compromise?
- How do you think an internal 'us vs them' culture between workers and management affects morale?

Professional culture

If organisational culture is the culture created within an organisation or by an employer, then professional culture is the shared knowledge, worldviews, and expectations created by a profession. Although professional and organisational culture may be closely linked, they are not necessarily the same. This shared culture can be seen between members of that profession regardless of where they work. This does not mean that the culture within a profession must be identical in every location. It is likely that just as paramedic practice differs geographically, paramedic culture also differs widely between jurisdictions (Reynolds 2008). Like organisational culture, professional culture can influence behaviour and beliefs. As such, it is paramount to understand the role of professional culture and how it interacts with organisational (or ambulance service) culture in paramedic practice.

One of the defining traits of a profession is that it encompasses a unique culture that has a specific role in guiding the behaviour of its members. Adherence to these cultural norms is not just due to social pressure; it is core to being a 'professional'. Wilensky (1964, p. 138) states that what separates the professional from the non-professional (in addition to a unique body of knowledge) is that 'the professional man [sic] adheres to a set of *professional norms*'. A professional culture sets these norms and plays a unique role within the profession.

Stop and Reflect

- As a student on placement, have you noticed an expectation of how a paramedic should act or behave? Particularly in their interactions with colleagues and patients?
- How do you think these expectations differ from those present in other forms of employment, for instance, a job in sales or retail?

Non-professions (such as the trade occupations) or semi-professions (such as assistant occupations) may also have a form of occupational culture. One would be hard-pressed, for instance, to argue that construction workers do not possess a form of culture based on shared knowledge and folklore (Greenwood, 1957). What differs, though, is that this type of culture does not necessarily guide behaviour, influence values and, most importantly, does not always embody a need to place the public interest ahead of one's own. Townsend (2017, p. 192) states: 'a feature distinguishing between a non-profession and a profession is the obligation on the professional to act with professionalism, which, at its core, is about putting the patient's interests before the practitioner's'. This form of professional culture, one that places public interest first, separates a professional culture from a non-professional one. Consequently, the norms and culture of the profession are essential to guiding behaviour in all professional situations.

Culture is also instrumental in structuring the profession. It often sets the standards of how one enters the profession, acts while within it, and advances through its structures. Furthermore, it determines how one would acceptably challenge existing values, knowledge, or techniques within it (Greenwood 1957). As such, professional culture is laden with shared etiquette, knowledge, symbols, and folklore, which members must adhere to if they wish to enter and remain within the profession. Culture, then, also plays an integral role in inducting new members of a profession into it. It does this by teaching not only the knowledge required to perform the technical aspects of the role but also the profession's norms, values, and behavioural expectations. These values and norms are additionally communicated to members of a profession through a written code, such as a code of conduct or ethics (another defining feature of a profession). Although codes should contain the moral aspects of a profession, members often learn these through the professional culture instead (Collings-Hughes et al. 2021).

Examples demonstrating how culture can influence behaviour, shape norms, and educate new entrants into the paramedic profession can be found in the section 'How can culture in paramedicine affect your clinical practice?' But first, we should consider the history of paramedic culture because, as we outlined in the 'Introduction', culture is not static and is constantly evolving.

Paramedic culture

Paramedicine history

Paramedicine has evolved from a history of a strict 'uniformed' or paramilitary culture. This likely ties closely with paramedicine's deep history stemming from the Knight's Hospitaller, the Order of St John, and the more recent birth of modern prehospital emergency care from military trauma care (Reynolds 2008). From this historical perspective, a specific structure has governed paramedics (previously ambulance officers) as military or paramilitary organisations (such as the police or fire service). These structures include hierarchical ranking systems, epaulettes, and uniforms (McCann 2022). Beneath the surface, they include a 'command and control' power structure, where senior or ranking officers are respected and obeyed unquestionably (McCann 2022). Operationally this resulted in a culture where uniform and presentation were prioritised, senior ranking members were to be obeyed, and time served was valued far more than new and innovative thinking (Van Scotter and Leonard 2022). This also created a culture of what it means to be 'a good paramedic' being akin to one's presentation and ability to fit into the colonially based, male-dominated archetypes of a strong male who shows little emotion and is not 'affected' by the emotional aspects of the role (Reynolds 2008; Devenish 2014; McCann 2022).

Stop and Reflect

- How do you think a culture based on 'masculine' traits of 'being tough' and 'unaffected by the job' affects the ability of a student or paramedic to speak up when they are affected by an experience at work or placement as per the Case study?
- What effect does this have on a paramedic's well-being, mental health, and career longevity?

Clinical guidelines had been structured similarly. They were 'protocols' based on 'doctors-orders' and strict adherence to the protocols was paramount (Maria 2021). Stepping outside the protocols was cause for reprimand, but so too could be failing to follow a protocol when it was indicated, even if it did not make sense to do so. From the 1980s to the early 2000s, however, paramedicine saw significant increases in clinical skill and autonomy. The UK achieved regulation of the paramedic profession akin to other well-established health professions such as nursing and physiotherapy (Townsend 2017). Education standards began to increase (Williams et al. 2009) and during this time other areas of paramedicine such as Ambulance Victoria's Mobile Intensive Care Ambulance paramedics were being viewed as 'cutting edge' in out-of-hospital emergency care (Willis and McCarthy 1986).

These education changes, coupled with a change in the type of work that a paramedic undertakes, and decades of work towards the 'professionalisation' of paramedicine have led to a change in culture. Paramedicine is now moving beyond the strictly paramilitary culture of its history to a new, emerging 'professional' culture. For the individual entering a profession such as paramedicine, the professional culture is an integral part of their education. Culture is an invaluable way of learning 'how to be a paramedic' and through culture, students also learn 'what it means to be a paramedic' or what the moral and behavioural expectations of a paramedic are (Devenish 2014). Consequently, culture is also instrumental for students in developing their professional identity, noting that defining paramedic identity remains difficult (Long et al. 2018).

Paramedicine culture now and into the future

There is no single accepted model of paramedicine culture. The seminal work by Reynolds (2008) provides an ethnographic analysis of the organisational structure and culture in a state-wide ambulance service within Australia (South Australian Ambulance Service). Reynolds (2008) notes there is significant cultural variance based on geographical and employer differences within paramedicine, often underpinned by organisational and political structures. An example of this would be to compare the growing emphasis on the Australian profession as a 'self-governing' profession to that of the US, which remains largely a medical-led and paramilitary structured occupation.

For paramedic students (and practising paramedics), the culture described above may still seem all too familiar.

However, modern paramedicine is evolving, as a new professional culture is replacing the previous militaristic structure. Some aspects of this historical culture remain within paramedicine and may always do so. For example, many healthcare professions are attempting to flatten hierarchies because this can improve patient safety (Kirk et al. 2018). As such, within paramedicine, although rank structures similar to the military are still present, the historically strict hierarchical power of this ranking structure is decreasing (McCann 2022). As this change occurs traits from the previous paramilitary or uniformed cultural structures are often held on to and perpetuated by older (in terms of service length) members of the profession (McCann 2022). Other aspects such as uniforms remain important to the culture and identity of paramedicine. The green uniform is synonymous with paramedicine in parts of the world, highlighted with the phrase 'family in green', despite this evolution away from militaristic or uniformed culture (McCann 2022; Van Scotter and Leonard 2022).

This evolving culture can be further highlighted by considering the evolution of clinical protocols, guidelines, and clinician responsibility. McCann (2022) reports that in the UK there is a changing culture within paramedicine towards a culture of professionalism, flexibility, and personal responsibility for clinical decisions. Paramedics in this study expressed feelings of pride in their significant clinical autonomy and personal responsibility, as clinical protocols have been replaced by clinical guidelines (McCann 2022). But while these paramedics understood guidelines as just that, guidance rather than strict rules for blind adherence, this was contrasted by a conflict experienced between this autonomy and the existing 'overbearing' or 'micromanaging' management styles (McCann 2022). This evolution has also been seen in Australia where protocols have largely been replaced with 'clinical guidelines', although to what extent they are 'guidelines' was questioned more among Australian paramedics (Maria 2021).

Stop and Reflect

- As a student learning from senior paramedics, how do you think it affects learning to see different paramedics express fundamentally different views?
- For example, if one more experienced clinician who trained in the day of 'strict protocols' still expects clinical guidelines to be treated this way but the next mentor expects them to be treated as a 'guide' with more grey than black and white answers, how might you negotiate this?

The current cultural change in paramedicine is partly linked to the changing nature of paramedic practice. There have been significant increases in paramedic educational standards with the expansion of a paramedic's role from 'stretcher bearers' to a fully fledged health profession (Williams et al. 2009; Gough 2018; Reed et al. 2021). Several countries now recognise paramedicine as a health profession through similar regulation processes to related professions such as nursing and medicine. Regardless of the direction of causation, as predicted by Hong (2009) (see above), paramedicine is experiencing change as newer members of the profession decide which parts of the existing culture to keep and which are no longer relevant.

Stop and Reflect

- How do you think paramedics should decide which parts of the existing culture to continue?
- What factors should be considered?
- How do we find the balance between 'this is how we've always done it', tradition, and progress?

How can culture in paramedicine affect your clinical practice?

We have explained what culture is, the emerging culture within paramedicine, and how both professional and organisational cultures contribute to 'paramedic culture', which is essential to paramedicine as a profession. However, how can culture influence the individual? This section will discuss the inescapable influence of culture, how it can be both positive and negative, and explain why self-reflection is integral to deciding if a cultural influence is positive or negative. These examples are taken from (informal and folkloric) conversations with practising paramedics around the aspects of paramedic culture they encounter regularly.

Influences of paramedic culture

Dark humour

The use of, and often the need for, dark or sardonic humour is especially important while working in a stressful environment. Although common amongst emergency services

(Christopher 2015; Devenish 2014), the use of humour to process and cope with tragic situations is not unique to them. However, students sometimes report that this type of humour is jarring if they have not been exposed to it before (Christopher 2015). The use of dark humour often creates a camaraderie between employees and builds loyalty. It is also a form of self-counselling where one is able to make 'light' of a situation. It aids in a paramedic's ability to distance themself from the tragedy that can be encountered in their role. While not being able to reduce the stressful experience itself, this form of coping may help increase resilience and the ability to deal with the stressors a paramedic faces (Christopher 2015).

However, the culture of dark humour can also have negative aspects. Dark humour can become an excuse for unprofessional behaviour and reinforce entrenched cultural negativity like hazing, misogyny, and racism. The overuse of dark humour, particularly in times of chronic stress, can lead to distancing oneself more and more from the humanity of patients (Christopher 2015; Olsthoorn and Thompson 2018).

Stop and Reflect

- Have you noticed this type of humour during placements?
- How did you feel about the use of dark humour?
- How do you think the overuse of dark humour and distancing oneself from patient(s) can affect patient-centred care?

Camaraderie

Camaraderie is a term often used in a warfare context, and within this is a masculine understanding of the concept, which focuses on 'mateship' (Dryrenfurth 2015). From an historical standpoint, mateship is synonymous with the masculine. However, this concept has continued to evolve to include everyone. Within this concept of camaraderie, loyalty and friendship emerge, literally taking care of your mate. Moreover, within the evolving parameters of this framework, a camaraderie that exists within the broader society and the importance of this connectivity can exist in the workplace. If there is loyalty towards your team, if there is loyalty towards each other, then the outcomes for the paramedic and those they are helping improve. This sense of collegiality is imperative for a paramedic workforce, which is often involved in stressful working conditions.

A particular way that paramedics often build camaraderie is through storytelling, sometimes referred to as sharing 'war stories' (linking again to camaraderie's roots in warfare). The use of storytelling is an integral part of paramedic culture, not only for building trust but also for teaching and as a coping mechanism, similar to dark humour (Olsthoorn and Thompson 2018). Paramedics use this storytelling to tell tales of tragedy, humour, and the storyteller 'just doing their job' as they describe events most non-paramedics would never encounter.

Stop and Reflect

- How do you think this culture of storytelling can aid new paramedics in bonding and joining the culture?
- Do you think the sharing of war stories can go too far?
- What about if all paramedics ever talk about, at work or home, are these tales of 'just doing their job' - how can this affect their well-being?

Flattening the hierarchy and improving patient safety

Amir and Pinto (2021, p. 72) stated: 'Paramedics are still taught and indoctrinated with the sentiment that a paramedic's role is to respond to high-acuity biological emergencies and rapidly transport patients to a hospital. The organisational culture and operational realities they operate within reinforce these ideas'. The culture of paramedicine works on a concept of previous understanding where the hierarchy in place continues to be reinforced. To ensure positive patient outcomes and positive working experiences for the paramedics, this intrinsic hierarchy needs to be flattened. This then incorporates a clear feedback focus between the executive team and all employees within the organisation and empowers members of any rank to feel comfortable sharing their ideas. If paramedics are empowered to voice their concerns and know they will be listened to within these parameters, then the hierarchy, which is an enculturated aspect of paramedicine, will start to flatten.

Stop and Reflect

- As a student on placement, would you feel comfortable speaking up if you noticed something that was missed by the treating paramedic?
- Can you consider why it would be important that the culture allowed for all members to feel like they can speak up?

A 'no-blame' culture and improving reporting of clinical concerns

Along with the importance of flattening hierarchies is the need to move away from 'blame culture'. A blame culture is one where the result of reporting and investigating a mistake will be the blame of (and often punitive action towards) an individual person. Health has been fraught with a history of blame culture, and paramedicine is no exception (Kirk et al. 2018). The previous strict nature of clinical protocols may have only worsened this within paramedicine – any deviation could be seen as an 'error' or 'breach'. However, what happens when someone needs to think outside of these parameters and move into a 'grey' area to ensure patient safety? Within health services the fear of the potential loss of registration or employment for not adhering to these guidelines evolves into distrust and a constant fear that paramedics will lose their jobs if they make a mistake (Maria 2021). Modern health systems encourage a non-blame reporting culture where clinicians are encouraged to self-report mistakes so systems can be improved. Hospitals now have open and blame-free presentations/audits of cases, and lessons learned are shared between clinicians to reduce error in a blame-free way. A positive blame-free culture is important for enabling clinicians to discuss queries they have, share lessons they have learned, and be transparent when a mistake is made (Kirk et al. 2018).

Stop and Reflect

- Suppose a paramedic made a medication error but no harm came to the patient. Do you think they would self-report this incident if they felt punitive punishment would follow?
- What if reporting that error improved the system and, consequently, the reporting paramedic prevented another clinician from making the same mistake, but this time it may harm a patient?

Being 'cut out to be a paramedic'

There can exist an idea of what it is to be 'cut out to be paramedic' or an expectation that some things are 'just part of the job'. This also means there may be an expectation that being a paramedic involves dealing with scenarios often unthinkable in other occupations (Credland and Whitfield 2021; Mausz et al. 2022). Sometimes this is defended through comments like 'that's just how it is' or 'that's the way we've always done it'. This becomes a mantra that is then self-perpetuated as new people join the profession. With no one questioning it, the existing culture is reinforced and the expectation to 'just deal with it' is maintained. This can be demonstrated when considering the issue of assault upon healthcare/emergency workers. Mausz et al. (2022) found that a paramedic culture of accepting that assault was 'part of the role' further perpetuated this within the ambulance service. This meant paramedics were less likely to report assault as they felt it was pointless to do so, which in turn meant there were often no consequences for perpetrators of assault.

Stop and Reflect

- How do you think this acceptance of 'being cut out for paramedic work' and 'it's just part of the job' affected our student in the Case study?
- Do you think this can affect paramedics in other areas of their work such as managing fatigue, dealing with stress/emotions, and the physical toll of manual handling in an ambulance environment?

'If we're all doing it, then who tells us it's wrong'

Culture plays an integral role in teaching new entrants the expected behavioural and moral norms of the profession. The professional culture will also reinforce these norms with existing members. This form of learning is beneficial, and creating cultural norms is an important part of a profession. However, if left unchecked, this can have a negative impact. In a study involving Australian paramedics, when paramedics were asked how they learn and judge what acceptable professional behaviour of a paramedic is, most indicated they tend to learn the accepted moral behaviours expected of them through a combination of existing moral standings and their peers or senior paramedics (Collings-Hughes et al. 2022). This was often in favour of more formal means such as a written professional code. Some even felt that culture is such a powerful method of learning that even if they disagreed with an aspect of the culture, eventually, they would 'just fall in line' with their peers. One participant reflected on the power of culture and realised this could be a problem. To paraphrase their response: If it is part of the culture and everyone is doing it, who will pick up that what is happening (and what everyone is doing) is wrong?

Stop and Reflect

- How do you determine your ethical and moral expectations – of not only being an employee but also a health professional?
- Do you feel emboldened to speak up if you see behaviour you disagree with?
- How do you think you will notice if something is not right if 'everyone is doing it'?

Cultural expectations and personal lives

Cultural expectations mean that a professional is expected to act a certain way, which is decided on and reinforced by the profession. In some instances, this is not just during hours of employment, as the elevated social role that professionals are privileged to have extends beyond their employment (Greenwood 1957; Wilensky 1964). An example of this can be seen when a profession, and by extension its regulators, enforces public behaviour outside of employment that is inconsistent with the employee's personal beliefs (for example, anti-vaccination messaging). However, this entry of professional culture into personal lives is not without risk. In 2020, a now-retracted, peer-reviewed journal article was published in a respected journal that judged the 'professionalism' of trainee surgeons' private social media material (Hardouin et al. 2020). While the study was presented as rating the 'professionalism' of the trainees, this publication was met with outcry from the medical community, as what was really being judged was the trainees' conformity to an outdated cultural expectation of how a medical practitioner should present themselves to the public. The result of this paper was a viral Twitter tag '#medbikini' – where respected medical practitioners from across the globe posted photos of themselves in swimwear (something that was judged 'unprofessional' by the paper's authors), dispelling the idea that a professional medical practitioner cannot have an everyday personal life too.

Stop and Reflect

- Can you think of behaviour that would be frowned upon by a health professional's peers if displayed in their personal lives?
- Can you think of ways this is both positive and sometimes negative?
- What determines the difference?

Culture as a tool for learning

Culture is specifically important for education and reinforces the practical knowledge and ethical concepts of 'being a paramedic'. The passing on of knowledge is an integral part of what makes up a culture – this includes the professional knowledge of 'how to do' paramedicine. Having an area or domain of expert knowledge is also important to what it means to be a 'profession', and the tradition of passing this knowledge from one generation of professionals to the next is important in maintaining this area of expertise (Greenwood 1957). Trusting, safe, mutually beneficial relationships are important to learning, and this bond is often created by way of culture. A mentor and mentee can exchange ideas through shared values and beliefs (encompassed in the culture). Negative aspects of a culture can exist, though, and mentalities of 'sink or swim' or 'learning by fire' can harm the learning process (Devenish 2014). Creating a trusting relationship, a no-blame and flattened hierarchy coupled with storytelling can create the conditions for meaningful learning.

Stop and Reflect

- What type of experiences have you had as a student?
- Were you thrust into the work with little support to 'learn by fire'? Or were you guided more carefully to build confidence and collaborative learning with your mentors?
- Which do you think is likely to help students learn?

Conclusion

What is the point of focusing on culture in an organisation or paramedic context? Is it important?

Within the changing aspects of healthcare, there is a growing need to move away from the 'older' (paramilitary) culture to a newer (professional) culture of self-reflection where paramedics can focus on their collegiality and within the parameters of where they are working. This is not to say that everything must be removed or overhauled. What it does mean is that negative aspects of culture should be recognised and addressed, and from there both ambulance services and the paramedic profession can move forward. This can be achieved, not by stopping the camaraderie that has developed into folklore but by reinforcing the positive aspects of the culture and not emulating the harmful components.

Culture must be recognised as having both positive and negative aspects. While the use of humour and story sharing is an important way of building rapport, the negative overtones can turn into a toxic workplace and harm patient outcomes. This is important while remembering that empathy is required to ensure patient-centred care, while also managing the intersection of paramedic burnout and pandemic-related overload. Some professional expectations will find their way into a paramedic's personal life, along with the stories and folklore of being a paramedic. However, it is essential that identifying as a paramedic does not totally absorb one's identity. While culture is an important method of learning both the technical and moral expectations of a profession, self-reflection is an essential aspect of professionalism. This includes reflecting on the professional culture and how it influences one's clinical practice, for better or worse.

Activities

Now review your learning by completing the learning activities in this chapter. The answers to these appear at the end of the book. Further self-test activities can be found at **www.wileyfundamentalseries.com/paramedic/3e.**

Test your knowledge

1. What is culture?
2. How does culture affect positive health outcomes for patients?
3. How can a positive culture be fostered for paramedics?

Activity 4.1

For each of the following questions, state whether it is true or false:

1. No one should ever speak up against the understanding of culture in a paramedic workplace?
2. Just because 'we've always done it that way' we should continue doing it that way?
3. As a student paramedic should you be able to voice concerns you have?

References

Amir, A. and Pinto, A. (2021). Paramedica have untapped potential to address social determinants of health in Canada. *Healthcare Policy* **16** (3): 67–75. doi: 10.12927/hcpol.2021.26432.

Allana, A., Kuluski, K., Tavares, W. et al. (2022). Building integrated, adaptive and responsive healthcare systems – lessons from paramedicine in Ontario, *Canada. BMC Health Services Research* **22**. doi: 10.1186/s12913-022007856-z.

Bom, M. (2012). *Women in the Military Orders of the Crusades. The New Middle Ages*. New York: Palgrave Macmillan.

Christopher, S. (2015). An introduction to black humour as a coping mechanism for student paramedics. *Journal of Paramedic Practice: The Clinical Monthly for Emergency Care Professionals* **7** (12): 610–617. doi: 10.12968/jpar.2015.7.12.610.

Collings-Hughes, D., Townsend, R., and Williams, B. (2021). Professional codes of conduct: a scoping review. *Nursing Ethics* **29** (1): 1–16. doi: 10.1177/09697330211008634.

Collings-Hughes, D., Townsend, R., and Williams, B. (2022). Paramedic use and understanding of their professional code of conduct. *Nursing Ethics* **30** (2): 258–275. doi: 10.1177/096973 30221130607.

Credland, N.J. and Whitfield, C. (2021). Incidence and impact of incivility in paramedicine: a qualitative study. *Emergency Medicine Journal* **39** (1): 52–56. doi: 10.1136/emermed-2020-209961.

Devenish, A. (2014). Experiences in becoming a paramedic: a qualitative study examining the professional socialisation of university qualified paramedics. PhD Dissertation. Queensland University of Technology, Brisbane, Queensland.

Dryrenfurth, N. (2015). *Mateship: A Very Australian History*. Melbourne: Scribe.

Eckstein, H. (1996). Culture as a Foundation Concept for the Social Sciences. *Journal of Theoretical Politics* **8** (4): 471– 497. doi: 10.1177/0951692896008004003.

Gough, S. (2018). Welcoming paramedics into the National Registration and Accreditation Scheme. *Australasian Journal of Paramedicine* **15** (4). doi: 10.33151/ajp.15.4.675.

Green B., Oeppen R., Smith D. et al. (2017). Challenging hierarchy in healthcare teams – ways to flatten gradients to improve teamwork and patient care. *The British Journal of Oral Maxillofical Surgery* **55** (4): 449–453. doi: 10.1016/j.bjoms.2017.02.010.

Greenwood, E. (1957). Attributes of a profession. *Social Work* **2** (3): 45–55. doi: 10.1093/sw/2.3.45.

Hardouin, S., Cheng, T.W., Mitchell, E.L. et al. (2020). Prevalence of unprofessional social media content among young vascular surgeons. *Journal of Vascular Surgery* **72** (2): 667–671. doi: 10.1016/j.jvs.2019.10.069.

Hong, Y. (2009). A dynamic constructivist approach to culture: moving from describing culture to explaining culture. In: *Understanding Culture: Theory, research, and application* (ed. R.S. Wyer, C. Chiu, and Y. Hong), pp. 709–720. Washington, DC: Psychology Press.

Jahoda, G. (2012). Critical reflections on some recent definitions of 'culture'. *Culture & Psychology* **18** (3): 289–303. doi:10.1177/1354067X12446229.

Kirk, A., Armstrong, K., Nurkka, N. et al. (2018). The impact of blame culture on paramedic practice: a qualitative study exploring English and Finnish paramedic perceptions. *International Journal of Emergency Services* **7** (3): 214–227. doi: 10.1108/IJES-10-2017-0052.

Long, D.N., Lea, J., and Devenish, S. (2018). The conundrum of defining paramedicine: more than just what paramedics 'do'. *Australasian Journal of Paramedicine* **15** (1). doi: 10.33151/ajp.15.1.629.

Maria, S. (2021). Paramedics' clinical reasoning and decision-making in using clinical protocols and guidelines. PhD Dissertation. Charles Sturt University, New South Wales, Australia.

Matos, M., McEwan, K., Kanovský, M. et al. (2021). The role of social connection on the experience of COVID-19 related post-traumatic growth and stress. *PLOS ONE* **16** (12). doi: 10.1371/journal.pone.0261384.

Mausz, J., Johnston, M., and Donnelly, E.A. (2022). The role of organizational culture in normalizing paramedic exposure to violence. *Journal of Aggression, Conflict and Peace Research* **14** (2): 112–122. doi: 10.1108/JACPR-06-2021-0607.

McCann, L. (2022). *The Paramedic at Work: A Sociology of a New Profession*. Oxford: Oxford University Press.

Michaelopoulous, S. and Xue, M. (2021). Folklore. *The Quarterly Journal of Economics*. doi: 10.1093/qje/qjab003.

Olsthoorn, M., and Thompson, S. R. (2018). Stretchers and stories: the importance of stories in paramedic education. *Whitireia Nursing & Health Journal* **25** (25): 10–17. doi: 10.3316/informit.280841847620177.

Reed, B., Cowin, L., O'Meara, P. et al. (2021). Perceptions and knowledge of self-regulation of paramedics in Australia. *Australasian Journal of Paramedicine* **18**: 1–12. doi: 10.33151/ajp.18.963.

Reynolds, L.C. (2008). Beyond the front line: an interpretative ethnography of an ambulance service. PhD Dissertation. University of South Australia, Adelaide, South Australia.

Tangherlini, T. (2000). Heroes and lies: storytelling tactics among paramedics. *Folklore* **111** (1): 43–66. doi: 10/1080/00155 8700360889.

Townsend, R. (2017). The role of law in the professionalisation of paramedicine in Australia. PhD Dissertation. The Australian National University, Canberra, Australia.

Tsai, Y. (2011). Relationship between organizational culture, leadership behaviour and job satisfaction. *BMC Health Services Research* **11** (98): 1– 9. doi: 10.1186/1472-6963-11-98.

Van Scotter, J.R., and Leonard, K.M. (2022). Clashes of cultures during crises: coordinating firefighter, police and paramedic interactions. *Disaster Prevention and Management* **31** (4): 374–386. doi: 10.1108/DPM-09-2021-0273.

Wankhade, P. (2012). Different cultures of management and their relationships with organizational performance: evidence from the UK ambulance service. *Public Money & Management* **32** (5): 381–388. doi: 10.1080/09540962.2012.676312.

Wilensky, H. L. (1964). The professionalization of everyone? *American Journal of Sociology* **70** (2): 137–158. doi: 10.1086/223790.

Williams, B., Onsman, A., and Brown, T. (2009). From stretcher-bearer to paramedic: the Australian paramedics' move towards professionalisation. *Australasian Journal of Paramedicine* **7** (4): 1–12. doi: 10.33151/ajp.7.4.187.

Willis, E., and McCarthy, L. (1986). From first aid to paramedical: ambulance officers in the health division of labour. *Community Health Studies* **10** (1): 57–67. doi: 10.1111/j.1753-6405.1986.tb00080.x.

CHAPTER **5**

Human factors in paramedicine

Sam Willis

School of Medicine, Charles Darwin University, Darwin, Northern Territory, Australia

Helen Pocock

South Central Ambulance Service NHS Foundation Trust, Bicester, UK

Contents

LEARNING OUTCOMES

On completion of this chapter the reader will be able to:

- Define human factors.
- Recognise a model of error minimisation.
- Identify several environmental factors specific to prehospital care that may allow error to occur.
- Identify numerous behaviours that mitigate error.
- Use the egg-timer model to identify and manage disagreement.

Fundamentals of Paramedic Practice: A Systems Approach, Third Edition. Edited by Sam Willis and Ian Peate.

Companion website: www.wiley.com/go/willis/paramedic3e

Case study

Tom is a newly qualified paramedic. He is keen to impress his patients and colleagues with his knowledge and skills and wants to fit in with his new crewmates. At the first job of the morning, Tom is required to administer aspirin to a patient suffering chest pain. He has heard in the crew room that 'every good paramedic knows their medicines protocols by heart' and so doesn't want to display any sign of weakness by checking his medicines protocol app. Fortunately for Tom, his technician crewmate spots that the patient is contraindicated for aspirin on account of his haemophilia. He advises Tom to check his protocols every time and not to listen to crew-room bravado. A medicine error is avoided this time and Tom learns a valuable lesson.

Introduction

As a paramedic you work within a complex system. Your performance is reflected through your knowledge, skills, and intentions, and is partly about 'the system'. Consequently, **human factors** research is the study of the interaction between humans and the system. A key driver of the system is safety; it is not enough simply to 'get things done'. These things must be done in a safe way to ensure each element of the system is concerned with preventing error. For instance, it is not enough simply to give a paramedic a new medicine to use; there are several errors that could occur as a consequence of this change. The paramedic must be educated about the medicine and when and how to use it to develop the knowledge and skill. They should also be provided with adequate tools to deliver the medicine, e.g. cannulation equipment. The environment is not always ideal for medicine administration: there should be sufficient warmth and lighting in the ambulance, for instance. The organisation's culture and objectives should positively influence the paramedic's use of the medicine.

This chapter discusses how the paramedic's environment, or the system in which they work, can contribute to unsafe practice, and provides an insight into how this can occur.

What are human factors?

Paramedic care is influenced by environmental, organisational, and personal influences. These influences are not controlled by the clinician and are termed human factors. Working definitions of human factors relevant to paramedic practice are scarce, but an effective definition is as follows: human factors are any matters in the paramedic's environment that may negatively affect safe clinical care. Such examples include poor communication, ambulance design, fatigue, role conflict between crews, and disparities in decision-making.

Human error in paramedicine

Errors are rarely exclusively the fault of the individual. Even a person with murderous intent *should* be unable to follow through with these intentions if they are working within a safe system. Blaming an individual for an error may seem to exonerate the organisation of responsibility, but it will do nothing to improve safety in the future. There would be no **onus** on the organisation to investigate its systems and processes to seek a safer solution. On the other hand, blaming 'the system' would take all responsibility away from the individual and negate the need for them to exhibit safe behaviour. The reality is more balanced, in which 'blame' rarely features and instead learning opportunities are presented.

Humans are **fallible**: everyone makes errors at some point. But in most cases, humans are the defence mechanism against **human error**. Ideally, we should be working within a multilayered system that allows other defence mechanisms to prevent an error of judgement becoming a clinical error. Reason's (1997) 'Swiss cheese' model illustrates this. Each piece of cheese represents a process designed to protect from error. According to this model, if all the holes line up there is no 'cheese' preventing the error (Figure 5.1). However, in the Case study at the beginning of this chapter, Tom's 'cheese layers' should involve consulting his medicines protocol, in addition to checking with his crewmate that he has read the protocol correctly.

For an error to occur there will inevitably be an environment or set of conditions that allows errors to occur. Table 5.1 identifies such conditions and associated errors in prehospital care.

To manage these environmental conditions, a model known as the Systems Engineering Initiative for Patient Safety (**SEIPS**) was designed to minimise error by examining the entire system. It goes beyond those individual processes put in place as barriers to error, instead adopting a

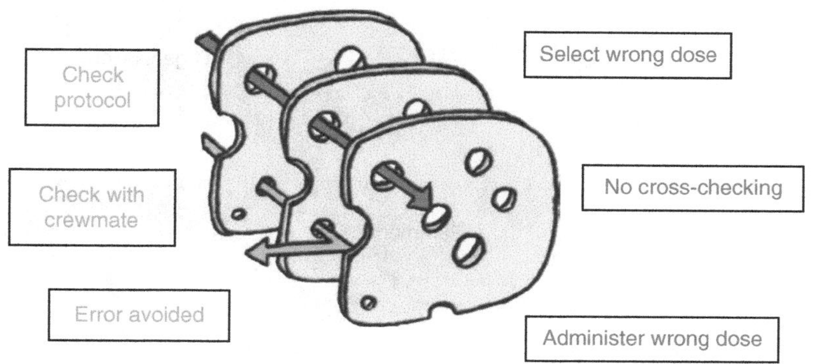

FIGURE 5.1 Error minimisation in prehospital care based on Reason's Swiss cheese model of errors. Source: Image courtesy of Abigail Milner.

TABLE 5.1 Summary of error-producing conditions in prehospital care.

Condition	Example
Unfamiliarity with the task	Paramedics are routinely faced with new situations, or medical conditions they have never experienced before, and are expected to safely triage and manage these cases in a timely manner.
Time shortage	During a time-critical situation every second counts. Examples include having to apply clinical skills much more quickly than in non-time-critical situations or being required to travel to an incident under emergency conditions.
Excessive noise	Typical background noises include relatives and family members, TV, police radios, or traffic (see discussion on background noise).
Poor human–system interface	A badly laid-out ambulance will prevent paramedics from treating their patients safely, and many paramedics may also place themselves at risk to help a patient.
Information overload	Receiving large volumes of personal information, such as a medical history from a patient, or being required to complete several complex tasks all at the same time.
Misperception of risk	Demonstrating a complacent attitude towards risky tasks.

Source: Adapted from Willis and Mellor (2018).

whole-systems approach (Carayon et al. 2006). In this model, an error is the product of the entire system. If a task is poorly defined, or the paramedic lacks the knowledge to operate the tools provided, the complexity of that task is increased and making an error becomes more likely. By considering the design of the various factors within a system and their impact on the other factors, the likelihood of error can be reduced. Figure 5.2 provides a diagrammatic representation of the SEIPS model. Consider yourself being the paramedic at the centre of the model and how your daily practice is influenced by each of the components, as well as how each component influences the others.

Tasks

Let us consider one of the riskiest paramedic tasks: handing over a patient at hospital. At first glance, this seems like a relatively straightforward process: we move the patient onto the hospital bed and tell the doctor/nurse why we have brought the patient to them. However, on closer inspection there are several processes involved, any of which presents risk if not performed effectively (see Figure 5.3).

What seems like one task is ultimately made up of numerous subtasks. Each of these subtasks could be further broken down into its **constituent** parts, each of which poses a risk. For instance, something as simple as handing over an accurate patient name may be more complicated if the patient has an alternative name by which they prefer to be known.

The handover of information should be a standardised process. However, an Australian study of patient handover from residential care to ambulance to emergency triage revealed disparities. The information included in each handover varied depending on the type of information imposed by the related document and the clinical role of the caregiver (Campbell et al. 2017). A UK comparison of ambulance service patient report forms and emergency

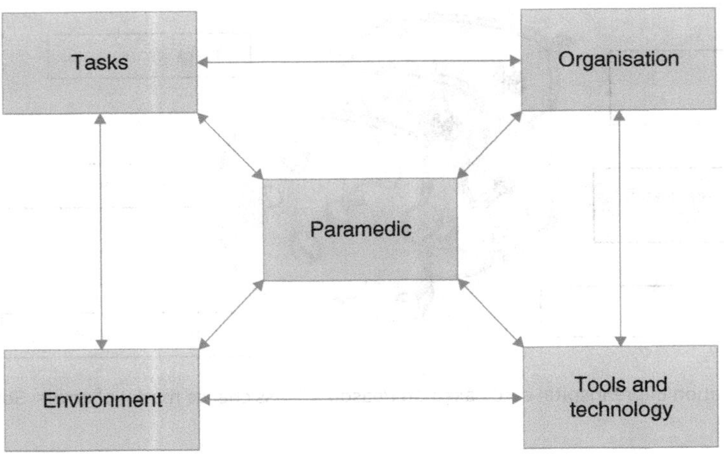

FIGURE 5.2 Diagrammatic representation of Carayon et al.'s (2006) SEIPS model.

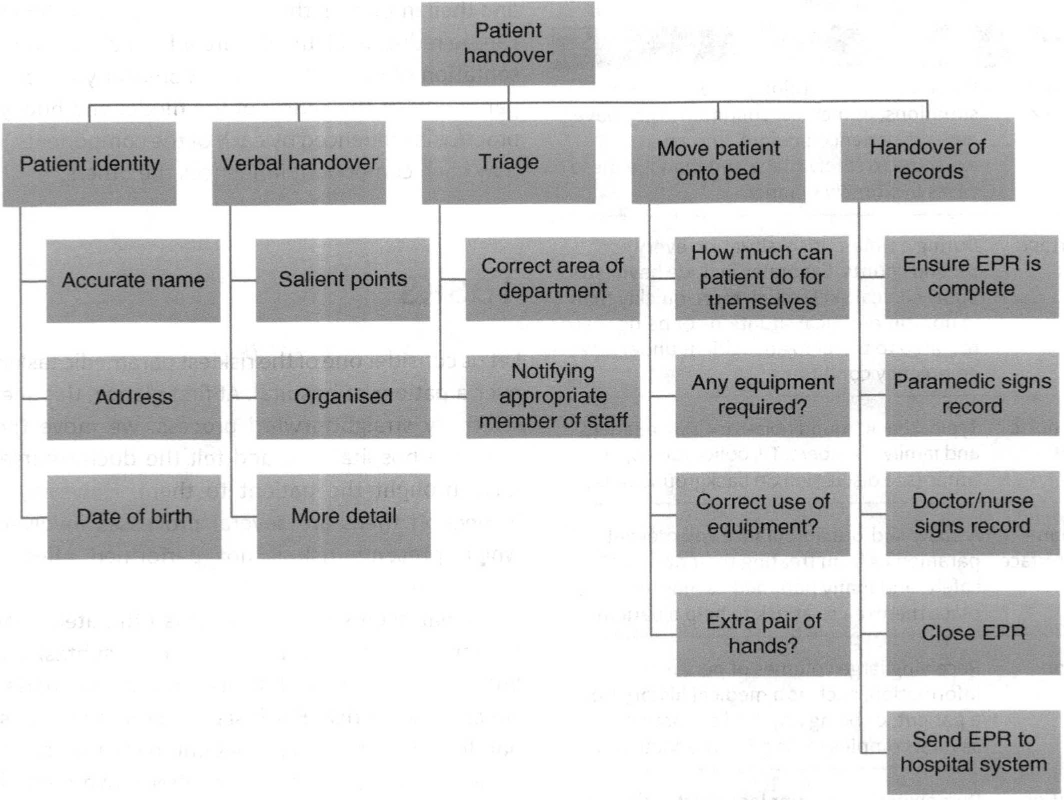

FIGURE 5.3 Flow diagram showing the true complexity of the patient handover process.

department documentation revealed that 26% of information is changed or lost at handover from ambulance to emergency department (Murray et al. 2012). The accuracy of information is bound to have an impact on patient care.

Also consider the effects of time pressure on the handover tasks shown in Figure 5.3. Might it make cutting corners more likely, if there is limited time in which to conduct the handover?

Organisation

The culture of an organisation is bound to have an influence over the behaviour of individuals working within it. This is likely to happen on (at least) two different levels. At a management level, safety may be taken very seriously, and systems may be put in place (for example, an internal near-miss reporting system) to support this. This may be available to all staff and its use encouraged, but if the local team do not see the point in undertaking this time-consuming activity, it may not be acted upon.

In the Case study at the beginning of the chapter, Tom did not consult the medicine protocol on his mobile app and so failed to notice that the patient fulfilled one of the **contraindications** for aspirin. His employer may well have provided the app for staff use, but because the local team culture dictated that checking protocols was a sign of a weak paramedic, Tom did not check.

In a safe organisation, individuals are made aware of the organisation's goals, standards, and procedures. Ideally there is a two-way conversation between management and staff about processes, procedures, and expectations. In this way, unsafe attitudes can come to light and be challenged for the benefit not only of the patients but also of the staff.

Clinical scenario: learning from error

Sarah was faced with a situation she had not encountered before. She was about to draw up a dose of adrenaline for a paediatric patient. In the heat of the moment, she remembered the interactive case study that her manager had sent to crews only a few weeks before. She recalled the importance of double-checking medicines with her crewmate and held up the ampoule for her crewmate to confirm the medicine name and expiry date before she proceeded.

This scenario highlights an example of good organisational practice, where learning from errors/near misses is shared widely to help others avoid making such errors. This activity benefits not only staff and patients but also the organisation as a whole since a learning culture will foster openness and progressive attitudes.

Tools and technology

How many devices do you use daily as a paramedic? There are the obvious electronic devices such as the electronic patient record, the defibrillator, and the oxygen saturation monitor, as well as the less obvious but equally important nebulisation mask, safety cannula, and giving set. These are all designed to improve the care and safety of patients. As technologies develop, each of these devices is subject to improvements and adaptations.

Whilst the intention is to improve care through developing the technologies and tools, the unintended consequences of such changes can increase the complexity of a task, as the use of a new piece of equipment must be learnt. At best, this can slow a task; at worst, make it unsafe. This highlights the importance of daily vehicle checks. You may have a **Make Ready Centre** to prepare your vehicle and its staff will ensure that all necessary kits are in place, but they may not be there at the start of your shift to point out the new piece of equipment that has been added to your ambulance. Always ensure that you are familiar with all equipment and ask for guidance if you are not.

Consider some of the paper tools that you use (or their electronic equivalents). These may be essential to ensure the safe referral of your patient to another service, e.g. the falls referral form. If you are not familiar with how to complete and submit it, this tool is of no use to you or, more importantly, your patient.

Environment

The environment in which a paramedic works can be highly variable, which is part of the challenge of the role. Variety is also one of the factors that attracts people to paramedicine. You have to accept that there are some aspects of your environment you can control and others you cannot. For instance, you cannot control the weather but you can keep your vehicle saloon warm for your patient.

Your ambulance will be designed for optimal ergonomic benefit (Hignett et al. 2009). For instance, your defibrillator/electrocardiogram (ECG) monitor will be housed at around eye level and within easy reach so that you can respond to patient changes easily and quickly. Storage cupboards will have been carefully designed so that the most important equipment is within reach for quick access, and those that house the heaviest equipment are at floor level. Outside the ambulance, however, which is where a great deal of your work takes place, the environment is far less predictable and controllable. This can make even the simplest task feel less organised and therefore harder. If you are cannulating a patient at the roadside, the task will feel more complex than if it were being performed in the ambulance. You will need to make additional decisions such as where to place a sharps box and how best to position your patient and equipment. If you remove daylight from the situation, this further complicates the task. There are ways of organising your equipment and team members that can reduce some of the variability and make your tasks feel simpler and safer. Some of these will be revisited later in the chapter.

Interactions

Each of these factors in isolation will affect how you perform your duties but they will also have an impact on each other. We have already seen how the relatively straightforward *task* of cannulation can be complicated by the *environment* in which it is performed. Now consider the added complication that you are using a new type of *equipment:* a new safety cannula. Unfortunately, the *organisation* has not provided any training for staff. As each of these new factors is introduced to the scenario, the complexity of the task increases, as does the chance of error.

By changing one or more of these elements, the effect can be to make the task safer and simpler. For instance, if the organisation prioritises safety and provides training, this can **mitigate** the risks posed by the unfamiliarity of the equipment or the challenges of the environment. As a paramedic, you cannot control all these factors but having an awareness of how they interact and influence your performance can make you more self-aware and, ultimately, a safer clinician.

Human factors in paramedic practice

It is beyond the scope of this chapter to provide a full discussion of all the known human factors that affect paramedic practice, although it is possible to recognise and discuss common human factors that affect the paramedic on a daily basis, including crew or team working, paramedic fatigue, stress, and situational awareness.

Crew/team working

Being able to work within a team is a fundamental part of ambulance service work. Paramedics work a variety of shifts which cover a twenty-four-hour continuum, and there are occasions when ambulance crews working together have never met each other before.

> **Practice insight**
>
> When working with a new crew member, take some time to get to know them. Provide mutual respect by recognising the skills, knowledge, and personal qualities that each member brings into the ambulance.

Each person brings into the ambulance their own levels of experience and education, as well as their individual personality and preferences for how they want to get things done. This diversity can be a source of strength in a crew, but equally it can be a source of conflict. Such conflict can occur daily, arising from differences of opinion or clashes of personality, compounded by stress and worker fatigue. Summers and Willis (2010) recognise a pattern of decision conflict that might occur during a typical emergency call, termed the 'egg-timer model of disparity' (Figure 5.4). At the start of the call it is likely that the crew's thinking and consideration for the call whilst en route differ (point A), but then come to be more closely related during the journey and as a result of discussion. Upon arrival at the scene there is likely to be some element of consideration between the crew that matches up (point B), followed by a potential difference in opinions (point C), possibly over what the presenting complaint is or how the patient should be managed. If the ambulance crew

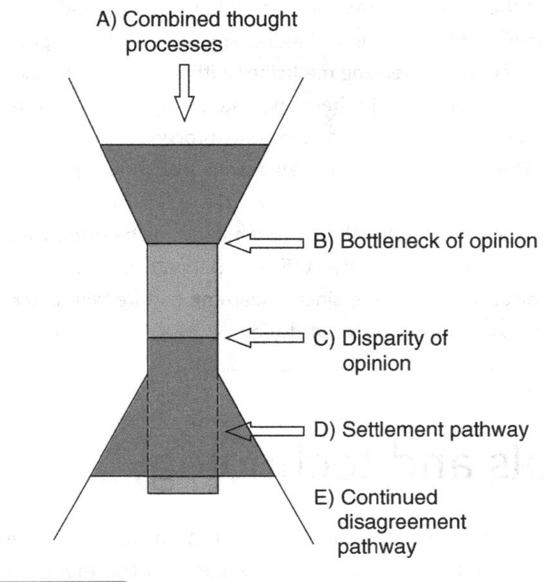

FIGURE 5.4 Egg-timer model of disparity.

communicate effectively there is likely to be a positive outcome (point D), but if not, the result will be a stark difference in opinion with the potential for adverse outcomes (point E). The key here is to make sure that with every disagreement the crew members communicate and work together as team players to ensure that there is a positive outcome and to reduce differences of opinion.

So what exactly are positive team-working characteristics? Table 5.2 identifies five qualities of team working, but the ability to exercise these qualities will be influenced by external matters such as paramedic fatigue and stress.

TABLE 5.2 **Positive team-working qualities.**

Positive team player qualities	Putting these into perspective
1. Creates enthusiasm and initiative to make things happen.	Motivation is everything. A motivated team can accomplish anything and can deal with any challenge they face. It is the responsibility of every team member to promote motivation and inspiration within their ambulance station and team.
2. Makes sure everyone clearly understands their roles.	There are many roles within the ambulance service such as emergency care assistant, emergency medical technician, emergency care practitioner, paramedic, advanced paramedic, paramedic level 1, and intensive care paramedic. Each of these roles differs slightly regarding its scope of practice. It is important to remember the limitations of practice and not undertake anything that extends beyond the scope of practice.
3. Listens to others and considers their suggestions and ways of working rather than dismissing them.	It is important to acknowledge the experience of other crew members and actively encourage team decision-making. Joint decisions made by team members can produce safer outcomes and promote a positive working environment, as well as increase worker motivation.
4. Becomes comfortable with disagreement.	We don't always get on with each other 100% of the time. Disagreement is inevitably going to occur at some stage. It is important to take a step back from any situation where a disagreement is taking place and not take the difference of opinion personally. Make every effort to resolve the conflict as soon as possible.
5. Has a positive attitude to and learns from setbacks.	The prehospital environment is fraught with complexities. There are going to be occasions where the practitioner is challenged beyond their normal coping mechanisms. It is important to embrace these moments and actively reflect upon them afterwards to learn how performance can be improved. This might involve liaising with others and giving/receiving feedback.

Situational awareness

The paramedic must maintain situational awareness for their own safety, the safety of their crew member, and the safety of the patient. Of the many definitions of situational awareness available, that provided by Endsley (1995, p. 36) is perhaps the clearest:

The perception of the elements in the environment within a volume of space and time, the comprehension of their meaning and the projection of their status in the near future.

A definition adapted for paramedic practice might be: situational awareness is having an awareness of an entire situation, taking note of all sources of information available to the paramedic, within the environment, which is inclusive of the sights, sounds, and smells of the given moment.

The paramedic must be aware of what is occurring around them at all times and they must actively gather information from a range of sources, including direct observation (seeing what is through the window of the ambulance) and sound (listening to information provided by crewmates and despatch, as well as the patient). This also extends to listening for external noises that might be pertinent to safety or situational analysis such as loud music. The situationally aware paramedic will use this information to plan, as well as preparing a course of action should something go wrong.

Having good situational awareness means taking note of and acting upon all available information (Endsley 1995). All this information needs to be processed for the paramedic to decide on the next step. Paramedics do not like surprises and good situational awareness will help to prevent a nasty surprise from materialising. Additionally, if something unexpected does occur, then a situationally aware paramedic will be able to plan alternative actions.

A hypothetical example could include the paramedic who is monitoring a patient in the back of the ambulance. Routinely, the alarms sound on the ECG/blood pressure monitor, which is sometimes caused by the parameters being set too sensitively. It is therefore easy to ignore the alarm when it sounds, and an immediate response is to silence it. The situationally aware paramedic, upon hearing the alarms, would recheck the patient and take note of the readings on the monitor. If en route to hospital, they would also check their location in case a pre-alert is required or consider diverting to a closer hospital.

The Resuscitation Council UK (2015) recognises that good situational awareness includes the following:

- Consideration of the location of the patient, which can give clues to the mechanism of injury.
- Obtaining information from any staff and/or family that might be present.
- Confirming the diagnosis with other staff members.
- Establishing and using those present, for example, identifying names, roles, and recognising who is leading.
- Taking note of any actions already established such as chest compressions during a cardiac arrest.
- Effectively communicating with the team and gathering information.
- Determining immediate needs.
- Implementing the necessary patient care.
- Considering the likely impact of any patient care.

Conclusion

Paramedics operate within unpredictable and complex environments where they are routinely faced with the unknown. Understanding how the environment in which they operate may influence their safe practice can contribute to error minimisation. Identifying human factors specific to paramedic care is an area requiring further research; meanwhile, this chapter identifies common human factor themes relevant to paramedic practice.

Activities

Now review your learning by completing the learning activities in this chapter. The answers to these appear at the end of the book. Further self-test activities can be found at **www.wileyfundamentalseries.com/paramedic/3e.**

Test your knowledge

1. What are human factors?
2. Identify five human factors that affect paramedic practice.
3. List six signs of stress.
4. Identify five causes of stress in the prehospital setting.
5. What causes paramedic fatigue?
6. What would you consider to be hazardous attitudes?

Activity 5.1

Consider the following scenario. Identify:

1. The task
2. Organisational factors
3. Environmental factors
4. Tools and technology

Jim is working as a solo responder in a rapid response car. At the start of his shift, a colleague points out that the new cardiac monitors have arrived on station and gives Jim a brief overview of how they work. Jim asks if he will be trained in operating the monitor but is told that it is quite easy to use and advised to 'have a play with it' when he gets a chance.

At that point Jim's radio sends an alarm and he is sent out on his first call, to an elderly patient who has collapsed in the street. The patient says that he is fine and that he has only fainted. Jim knows he should undertake a 12-lead ECG to rule out cardiac causes, but there are several factors that make this course of action unlikely.

Jim might choose to call for ambulance back-up to complete his patient assessment before deciding whether to convey the patient to hospital or discharge him on scene. Other factors may dictate that he opts to take the patient to hospital in the car, where a full assessment can be undertaken. In any case, clearly Jim is not in an ideal situation during his shift today.

Activity 5.2

Suggest how the scenario in Activity 3.1 could be made safer in the same four areas:

1. The task
2. Organisational factors
3. Environmental factors
4. Tools and technology

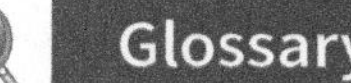

Glossary

Contraindication: A specific reason according to which a procedure, drug, or surgery is inappropriate due to the risk of harm it could pose to the patient.

Fallible: Able/likely to make an error.

Human error: An unintended action.

Human factors: The study of the interaction between people and other elements of a system.

Make Read Centre: A centre dedicated to cleaning, restocking, fuelling, and maintaining ambulances.

Mitigate: Lessening the severity of something (i.e. situation, pain, mistake).

Onus: Someone's duty, obligation, or responsibility.

SEIPS: Systems Engineering Initiative for Patient Safety.

References

Campbell, B., Stirling, C., and Cummings, E. (2017). Continuity matters: examining the 'information gap' in transfer from residential aged care, ambulance to emergency triage in southern Tasmania. *International Emergency Nursing* **32**: 9–14.

Carayon, P., Schoof Hundt, A., Karsch, B.-T. et al. (2006). Work system design for patient safety: the SEIPS model. *Quality & Safety in Healthcare* **15**: i50–i80.

Endsley, M.R. (1995). Toward a theory of situation awareness in dynamic systems. *Human Factors Journal* **37** (1): 32–64.

Hignett, S., Crumpton, E., and Coleman, R. (2009). Designing emergency ambulances for the 21st century. *Emergency Medicine Journal* **26**: 135–140.

Murray, S.L., Crouch, R., and Ainsworth-Smith, M. (2012). Quality of the handover of patient care: a comparison of pre-hospital and emergency department notes. *International Journal of Emergency Nursing* **20** (1): 24–27.

Reason, J. (1997). *Managing the Risks of Organizational Accidents*. Burlington, VT: Ashgate.

Resuscitation Council UK (2015). *Resuscitation Guidelines*. London: Resuscitation Council.

Summers, A. and Willis, S. (2010). Human factors within paramedic practice: the forgotten paradigm. *Journal of Paramedic Practice* **2** (9): 424–428.

Willis, S. and Mellor, G. (2018). That final fatal error: crew resource management. *International Journal of Paramedic Practice* **7** (2): 26–29.

CHAPTER **6**

Sociological aspects of paramedic practice

Kieran Robinson

Virtual Ward Clinical Coordinator, Central & North West London NHS Foundation Trust, Milton Keynes, UK

Contents

LEARNING OUTCOMES

On completion of this chapter the reader will be able to:

- Define sociology.
- Describe functionalism, conflict theory, and symbolic interactionism.
- Discuss the social context of health and ill health.
- Develop a sociological imagination.
- Apply sociological theory to analyse current paramedic practices.

Case study

An ambulance has been despatched to a private address for a female complaining of shortness of breath. Upon arrival at the two-bedroom flat, the paramedic crew notice that the flat is messy and there are four other people living there. All occupants are smoking and the patient in question owns three cats. The patient confirms that she is asthmatic and, upon further questioning, states that she has been a smoker since she was thirteen years old and that her parents were also smokers. The patient has lived away from her family since the age of sixteen due to falling out with her mother. Since then, she has disowned her family and has been unable to work due to stress-induced asthma.

Fundamentals of Paramedic Practice: A Systems Approach, Third Edition. Edited by Sam Willis and Ian Peate.

Companion website: www.wiley.com/go/willis/paramedic3e

Introduction

Sociology has an important place in paramedic education. Paramedics treat patients not in isolation but in the context of their homes, families, networks, and communities. Sociology – the scientific study of society, social structures, and social relationships – helps us to work with patients insightfully, respectfully, and with awareness of their social worlds. An understanding of sociology can help a paramedic to stay client centred and deliver culturally sensitive and personalised care. It can also help to broaden practitioners' awareness of the social causes of health and ill health; the imbalances in power, equality, and justice in the health and social care system; the way in which social interactions can shape our thoughts, feelings, and behaviours; and our own role within the health and social care sector. Changes in societal ideologies directly impact on clinical practice, as do our own views on these ideologies. Due to institutional racism, indigenous Australian people face a lower life expectancy and higher prevalence of disease, whilst being less likely to receive appropriate medical care, when compared to the general population (Elias and Paradies 2021). A further example is highlighted in a scoping review by Westwood (2022) who identifies a relationship between religious affiliation and negative attitudes towards LGBT people amongst healthcare professionals and students in the UK and provides examples of practice concerns raised in relation to this. These examples demonstrate how societal views and ideologies can have a wide-ranging impact on healthcare, patient experience, and outcomes.

Accordingly, this chapter will introduce the reader to some key principles in sociology that can help to illuminate our paramedic practice.

The sociological imagination

Our first key concept, the **sociological imagination,** was developed by American sociologist C. Wright Mills in the 1950s. Mills urged us not to view individuals and societies as distinct, suggesting instead that individuals both shape and are shaped by the society in which they live. He proposed that many personal problems are in fact caused by public influences – societal and political forces that are outside one's personal control (Mills 1959). He argued that learning to develop a sociological imagination or learning to see one's own and others' experiences in the context of history and social structures can bring liberation from personal problems (Mills 1959).

Practice insight

When talking to a patient, take some time to get to know them. Break down barriers by asking them about their family and social history (above and beyond what is required for the paperwork). Listen to what they have to say and empathise with them.

Three sociological paradigms

Having met this concept of the sociological imagination, now let us turn to three sociological **paradigms** (philosophical and theoretical frameworks for viewing the world) that can help to illuminate paramedic practice. Sociology contends that our social world is made up of numerous social units or subsystems that collectively create social structure. Social units can range from the interaction of two people to small groups, to large and complex social structures such as global organisations or political systems. Sociologists focus on three different social units or systems: social relationships (the microsystem), institutions (the mesosystem), and society as a whole (the macrosystem; Figure 6.1). For each of these social units, a different paradigm is applied: **functionalism, conflict theory,** and **symbolic interactionism.**

Functionalism

Functionalism was initially developed as a macro-level theory, though many sociologists believe it is better placed as a meso-level theory (OpenStax College 2012). Meso-level theories are focused on studying institutions and social structures, as these can both reflect and influence society as a whole.

Functionalism initially developed out of the writings of Herbert Spencer (1820–1903) and Émile Durkheim (1858–1917) and was one of the earliest theories of sociology. Functionalists argue that our lives are influenced by interrelated social structures and that each part of society has consequences for the function of society as a whole. Thus, Durkheim asserted that society is more than the sum

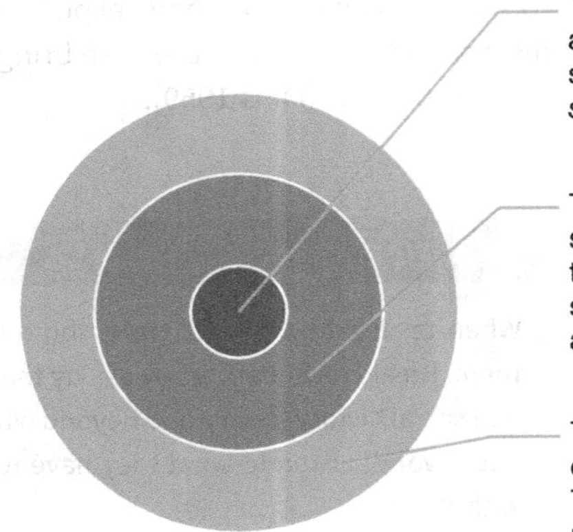

The microsystem: made up of individuals and social relationships. To discuss this social unit we use the paradigm known as *symbolic interactionalism*.
The mesosystem: made up of institutions such as the church, the political system, the economic system. To discuss this social unit we use the paradigm known as *functionalism*.
The macrosystem: made up of global organisations and the global community. To discuss this social unit we use the paradigm known as *conflict theory*.

FIGURE 6.1 The social system.

of its parts, whilst Spencer suggested that, just as the body has organs that need to work together for health, society has subsystems or institutions such as the economy, the media, political parties, the legal system, schools, and hospitals, and all these institutions need to work together in order to achieve optimal social functioning and social order (Spencer 1898 cited in OpenStax College 2012).

Durkheim argued that, in order for the constituent parts to work together, the system needs to have boundaries such as laws, customs, and rituals (Durkheim 1984), which reflect the 'collective consciousness' – or shared beliefs, values, and attitudes that persuade individuals to behave in accordance with social norms.

Durkheim followed a positivistic framework. This is a belief that observable reality within a society can lead to the production of generalisations, with a focus on factual information and data to avoid human bias (Alharahsheh and Pius 2020).

The views of idealism and interpretivism traditionally oppose this, stating that the human experience cannot be explored in the same way as physical phenomena (Alharahsheh and Pius 2020), and that the human ability to think is the true source of knowledge (Turyahikayo 2021).

In the twentieth century, Talcott Parsons synthesised these views, stating that both views could be accommodated in one 'action frame of reference' leading to the creation of his seminal book *The Structure of Social Action* and the foundation of modern functionalism as a concept (Ormerod 2020).

Conflict theory

Conflict theory is a macro-theory, meaning it focuses on the nature and structure of society as a whole. It explores how social structures create and perpetuate power imbalances, which in turn generate conflict (Ormerod 2020). Conflict theory highlights that there are finite resources within society; therefore individuals need to compete for power, resources, and opportunities, and those who have greatest access to these will seek to maintain their position (Ormerod 2020). Conflict theorists believe that social conflict is both normal and essential for change, adaptation, and survival.

Marx

Karl Marx (1818–1883), the most famous conflict theorist, argued that all elements of society are influenced by the economic system. He observed the industrial revolution and the rise of *capitalism* and drew attention to the significant inequalities between factory owners and factory workers. Marx predicted that capitalism would cause a rise in inequality as the *bourgeoisie,* or people who owned factories and therefore owned the means of production, would be motivated to maintain their social position by preventing the *proletariat,* or those who worked for factory owners, from advancing their social position. He argued that class inequalities occurred throughout history and naturally tended towards an end point of social revolution (Marx and Engels 2023).

Marx asserted that what we do defines who we are. He argued that capitalism caused alienation, since the proletariat worked for money and therefore the connection between worker and product was lost. His view was that this misalignment caused individuals to become isolated and detached from their occupations, society, and their own sense of self, leading to a feeling of disempowerment (Marx and Engels 2023).

Marxist theory suggests this alienation is perpetuated and reinforced by a 'false consciousness', where the beliefs of the dominant class could be imposed on the nondominant class (Marx and Engels 2023). For example, the bourgeoisie's preferences for social competition over social cooperation might create a cultural belief that hard work is rewarding. If this belief is accepted, then the proletariat are less likely to question their social position and may even assume individual responsibility for their social position.

Marx would have highlighted that class and health inequalities are a key determinant of health – a view supported by the World Health Organization (WHO) who state that social factors account for 30–55% of health outcomes (WHO 2023). A report by the WHO investigating the effect of social determinants of health on outcomes during the Covid-19 pandemic found significant inequalities in rates of hospitalisation and mortality. Possible reasons for this include higher rates of chronic disease that increase the risk of a poor outcome, greater exposure to the virus itself, difficulty in adhering to public health measures, and reduced access to health services (WHO 2021).

In England between 2018 and 2020, males living in the most deprived areas of the country had a life expectancy of 9.7 years lower than those in the least deprived areas. For females, this difference was 7.9 years. Females living in the most deprived areas lived 66.3% of their lives in good general health on average, compared to 82% of those in the least deprived areas (Office for National Statistics 2022).

Similarly, in Australia during 2017–2018, adults living in the most deprived areas were 1.6 times more likely to be obese and 1.2 times more likely to have uncontrolled high blood pressure. In 2020, they were 1.5 times more likely to die (Australian Institute of Health and Welfare 2022). These findings support the global concerns of the WHO and highlight the significance of social inequalities in healthcare.

Symbolic interactionism and microsociology

Our third main sociological view of the world is known as symbolic interactionism (sometimes called microsociology), which focuses on social interactions between individuals and studies how social interactions shape society (Giddens and Sutton 2017). This paradigm assumes that individuals play an active role in shaping reality.

Symbolic interactionism was developed by George Herbert Mead (1863–1931) and his student Herbert Blumer (1900–1987). This approach assumes that people develop meaning by interacting with others and with objects in society, and this meaning influences their behaviour, identity, and beliefs about what is normal, ethical, and fair (Giddens and Sutton 2017). This paradigm thus assumes that society is a product of social interactions, as reality is actively created and interpreted through our social interactions.

Goffman

Erving Goffman (1922–1982) suggested that social interaction follows a set of social rules that maintain social order. Goffman argued that people behave like actors, in that they use tactics to actively manage their social identities to protect themselves from negative evaluation by others (Goffman 1969).

Practice insight

Remember that it takes time to get to know a person. Even though you may be expected to work with someone for the first time in an ambulance or in an out-of-hospital setting, you won't really know that person until you have worked with them over time. Consider this when deciding how much of your own private life you wish to share during the shift (for further reading, look up the 'Johari window' model of self-awareness).

Goffman highlighted the importance of social integration. He suggested that people actively claim a social role, and that this role needs to be recognised and accepted by others (Goffman 1969). For example, to be an effective paramedic you need to assume the role behaviours and attitudes of a paramedic, and patients, carers, and other health professionals need to recognise that you are filling this role and play along with it. Goffman argued that when others recognise and play along with our roles, then communication runs smoothly as a shared understanding is established. Where our roles and behaviours are not clearly understood or accepted by others, there can be conflict and misunderstanding (Mishra and Masih 2023). For example, if a paramedic is called to a motor vehicle accident, they may need to resuscitate an individual, assess for spinal cord injuries, and attend to open wounds. By carrying out these activities the paramedic is able to signify to others that they are doing an important job, and they are doing it well. Other tasks may be less well understood. For example, if a paramedic is called to assess an older person who is having breathing difficulty, they may initially talk to the client and ask them about their day. Through this interaction they may be making clinically skilled observations about the patient's breathing, pallor, cognition, or mental state, but this may not be obvious to the patient, and any onlookers might believe the paramedic is simply chatting, wasting time, or failing to attend to the patient's needs (Béphage 1997).

Self-identification and an understanding of the role of a paramedic is important for job satisfaction, workplace cohesiveness, and self-actualisation. If paramedics don't have a clear sense of their identity, they're denied the ability to form character through their work (Furness et al. 2021). This supports the theory of social integration by highlighting the negative consequences of a lack of perceived identity and role within society.

Milling et al. (2022) found that social integration influenced the intensity of resuscitation efforts in cardiac arrest patients. The presence of bystanders other than family members was found to influence ambulance clinicians to prolong resuscitation efforts to demonstrate that they did all they could within their role and to look their best. Some clinicians were found to be frustrated at what they perceived to be 'unrealistic' expectations of some bystanders, yet many were still influenced to continue resuscitation. Where bystander CPR had been undertaken, clinicians felt a sense of obligation to continue, to assure the bystanders that they had done the right thing.

The sociocultural context of health

Several chapters in this text are focused on helping the reader to assess a patient's biological function and make judgements about their health. However, it is important to note that our understanding of health and ill health is *socially* constructed. Today we tend to believe in a bio-psycho-social model of health; in other words, we think that health is determined by our biology, psychological functioning, and social issues such as our lifestyle, socioeconomic status, and social support. Society has not always had this view. If we were to travel back in time we would be able to see how our perception of health and ill health has shifted because of social changes. Before we had microscopes we did not know about bacteria, or viruses. People believed that poor health was related to moral, spiritual, or supernatural causes, and treatments for ill health reflected these beliefs.

Goffman argued that the meaning of an illness is derived from social interaction. He suggested that certain illnesses, whether visible or hidden, could become **stigmatised,** and therefore labelling a person with a stigma could discredit and devalue the person, causing social alienation and exclusion (Goffman 1986).

In one scoping review, patients with mental disorders were found to be likely to have felt 'rejected' by healthcare staff (Sølvhøj et al. 2021), and this phenomenon appeared to be found globally, underscoring the effect of cultural beliefs and stigma on healthcare provision.

Symbolic interactionists argue that sociocultural beliefs can determine how we view health and ill health, whether an illness is subject to social **stigma,** and therefore how it is experienced and treated. Some diagnoses are considered controversial by health professionals; for example, patients suffering from psychogenic non-epileptic seizures frequently experience stigma from healthcare providers, leading to a poorer quality of care and an impact on mental well-being (Annandale et al. 2022). Many health professionals have demonstrated a lack of knowledge surrounding the condition and find patients presenting with it frustrating, whilst believing the symptoms to be of the patient's own volition (Rawlings and Reuber 2018). Asadi-Pooya et al. (2020) argue that even the terminology can impact on this and propose calling the condition 'functional seizures', as this is more neutral regarding aetiology and proved more popular with patients and clinicians alike.

Another example is highlighted by Quintner (2020), who explains that female patients with fibromyalgia struggle to have medical professionals believe them due to a complex set of social and philosophical factors including misogyny and a disbelief as to the level of pain the patient is experiencing.

Whilst stigma can and does affect patient well-being, it also has a direct impact on clinical outcomes (Ko et al. 2022). Patients with bipolar disorder who experienced stigma from people around them were more likely to experience greater functional impairment and anxiety (Perich et al. 2022).

Culture not only shapes beliefs about illness but can equally affect the way illness is experienced. Conrad and Barker (2010) highlight that illness can have an impact on people's occupations and their social network and may make a person's world feel smaller. Illness can be seen as an opportunity to re-evaluate values and for self-discovery, change, and personal growth. Interestingly, not all cultures around the world have a way of expressing illnesses that are relatively common in the West. For example, some cultures have no experience of eating disorders and others have no language for depression. Sarkissian and Sharkey (2021) highlight that ethnocultural groups are more likely to *somatise* signs of mental distress. This means that they may feel physical symptoms such as nausea or chest pain, rather than experiencing the low mood that we might associate with depression.

Several studies have shown that social values can have a significant impact on clinical decision-making. A seminal study by Sudnow (1967) indicated that health professionals engaged in *social rationing* – the withholding of potentially beneficial interventions based on their perceived social worth. For example, Sudnow found that individuals who were attributed with undesirable or deviant social roles were less likely to receive critical interventions – even resuscitation.

Whilst some researchers have debated the transferability of Sudnow's findings to today's healthcare system, there are several studies that support the view that perceived social worth can have a significant impact on the number and quality of interventions provided. Timmermans (1998) replicated many of Sudnow's findings. In his study, patients were more likely to receive lengthy and rigorous resuscitation if they were personally known to the treating health professionals, if they were a well-known person with a valued social role, if they were young, and if they were a patient whom the health professional had previously treated. Individuals were less likely to receive resuscitation, or resuscitation efforts might have been limited, if they were referred from a residential care facility, if they had overdosed or been intoxicated, or if they were perceived as elderly and frail. Timmermans (1998) and Sudnow (1967, 1983) reported that some of the individuals in the low social worth group were pronounced dead whilst still alive or whilst lifesaving interventions were still viable. In Nurok and Henckes's (2009) ambulance service study, it was found that perceived socioeconomic status and social worth could affect the efficiency and quality of treatment (Milling et al. 2022). Timmermans (1998) and Sudnow (1967, 1983) also found that if a health condition was considered to be 'self-inflicted', then care could be withheld or unnecessary invasive interventions prescribed. Similar findings have been reported more recently by Vela et al. (2022), who found that marginalised groups such as ethnic minorities, disabled people, and those with sexual or gender orientations other than heterosexual and cisgender are still more likely to have their care affected, including communication and clinical decision-making. These negative biases have been shown to lead to a worse quality of care (Motzkus et al. 2019).

Sociocultural views and expectations also affect the experience of healthcare providers and their satisfaction with their career. Student paramedics may experience role dissonance due to the societal view of paramedics as 'heroes' and 'rescuers' shaping their expectations of the role, with a subset of high-acuity and technically skilled incidents receiving the majority of media attention. This is then reinforced by educators wanting to inspire their students. As students or newly qualified professionals many view these high-acuity incidents as a right of passage and can be disappointed upon realising their frequency is insignificant when compared to incidents related to caring for those with chronic illnesses and the elderly (Rees et al. 2022).

Medicalisation and demedicalisation

Medicalisation is a process in which phenomena that were once viewed as normal or socially deviant become viewed as conditions that require medical attention. **Demedicalisation** is the opposite process, where an illness is no longer defined as an illness but comes to be seen as either normal or a condition of social deviance.

Ivan Illich argues that medicine has the potential to cause harm through medicalisation and demedicalisation, by leading people away from their natural coping mechanisms to become dependent on the medical system. For example, he saw that labelling someone as ill could lead them to believe that they were a 'victim', and this could disable them from coping with their environment, alienate them from their relationships, and increase their dependence on the health system (Illich 1976; Sheaff 2005).

Medicalisation can affect how people view personal responsibility for a condition and how other people respond to the person with the condition (Aslam et al. 2021; Grannell et al. 2021).

Women's health issues, including menstruation, pregnancy and childbirth, and menopause, are frequently cited as examples of medicalisation. The meaning and experience of menopause vary across cultures, and some cultures may not even recognise it as a medical concept. For example, Lock (1994) found the prevalence of women reporting issues with menopause is significantly less in Japan than in North America. A more recent literature review of global menopause studies found that in the US, vasomotor symptoms ('hot flashes', sweating) were less prevalent in Japanese American women than in white women (Monteleone et al. 2018), again suggestive of cultural differences and demonstrating the concept of medicalisation. Similarly, Fu et al. (2008) found large variations in menopause symptoms between Australian and Taiwanese women, although they also press for more research into other potential factors such as diet, oestrogen levels, and levels of regular exercise.

In some cultures, menopause is seen as an entirely normal biological transition, whilst in the West menopause can be viewed by some as a condition either to be endured or to be treated, with more negative terminology used such as 'ovarian failure' for early menopause (Namazi et al. 2022).

Healthy women may be advised to take hormones to manage the symptoms of menopause, maintain health, and increase their longevity. These treatments have evolved in recent years and are now more widely recommended, although they remain controversial (Flores et al. 2021; Mehta et al. 2021).

Conclusion

This chapter has shown the value of applying sociological concepts to paramedic practice. To do so helps us recognise how both health and ill health are to some extent socially constructed, as are interactions between health professionals and patients. Learning to see ourselves, our team, and patients in the context of the broader social environment can help us to take a patient-centred and culturally sensitive approach to care, advocate for clients who may find feel disempowered, and understand the full extent of our role within the broader social system.

Activities

Now review your learning by completing the learning activities in this chapter. The answers to these appear at the end of the book. Further self-test activities can be found at **www.wileyfundamentalseries.com/paramedic/3e.**

Test your knowledge

1. Define 'sociology'.
2. Describe what Mills meant by the 'sociological imagination'.
3. Identify social and cultural factors that can influence one's health beliefs and one's experience of health and ill health.
4. Consider the Case study at the beginning of the chapter and explain how social interaction can lead to stigmatisation and social rationing.
5. Describe the consequences of medicalisation.

Activity 7.1

Generate a discussion on station or with your crewmate. Ask them about their thoughts on conflict theory and about competition for power in the ambulance service. Specifically ask what action has been taken by paramedics to try to change their working conditions for the better.

Activity 7.2

Adopt a conflict perspective and consider how your social class, gender, age, or ethnicity might have an impact on your health and well-being. Consider what inequalities you may face if you were:

- A homeless single parent living in rural Australia.
- A widow with five children from war-torn Somalia who has just applied for refugee status.
- A twelve-year-old young carer who has taken on the responsibility for caring for her mother, who has schizophrenia, and three siblings.
- A ninety-five-year-old Bangladeshi women living on a council estate in West London.

How might your environment and your social situation influence your health and well-being, your access to healthcare, your power to gain access to social welfare and equal opportunity, and your ability to educate yourself and access resources to improve your social situation?

Activity 7.3

Consider how you behave in different social contexts. Do you exhibit the same behaviours when you are communicating and interacting with your family, flatmates, colleagues, practice educator, and lecturers? Consider how the social context affects your interactions with these people, and how the feedback you receive from them shapes your identity and your perception of what it means to be a paramedic student.

Activity 7.4

Consider the example of Winterbourne View, a care home for people with learning disabilities. Eleven staff working at Winterbourne View were convicted of abuse and neglect (Department of Health 2012; Flynn 2012). In a BBC (2011)

Panorama documentary, staff were observed punishing patients, wrestling patients to restrain them, and inciting aggressive games. In fact one of the staff members was heard saying, 'The only language she [one of the patients] understands is force' (Flynn 2012).

Consider how healthcare institutions might socialise staff to behave in ways that conflict with their perceived sense of self. How might healthcare institutions depersonalise patients? How might staff working in teams have a reduced sense of personal responsibility for their actions? How might a lack of training, reflection, supervision, and review of work practices prevent staff from seeing their actions as potentially abusive? How might team working make it difficult to be a whistle-blower?

Activity 7.5

Consider how you might react if you were diagnosed with an illness that is subject to a significant amount of social stigma, such as schizophrenia, chronic fatigue syndrome, or HIV. What would you think about your diagnosis? How would this make you feel? How would other people respond to you? How would other people's reactions affect you?

Activity 7.6

Consider your beliefs and values about health and ill health. How have you come to hold them and are they congruent with other cultural groups in your community and with mainstream medicine? How might your beliefs and values affect your ability to attend to a client who holds different beliefs? How might they affect your ability to work within a team when other professionals hold opposing beliefs?

Glossary

Conflict theory: A social paradigm that focuses on social competition and social inequalities.

Demedicalisation: A process in which a medical condition is no longer viewed as such and comes to be seen as either normal or a condition of social deviance.

Functionalism: The belief that society is like a system with subsystems that need to work together to create and maintain social order. It focuses on the way social structures and functions socialise us to conform to norms, role expectations, customs, and traditions.

Medicalisation: A process in which what was once viewed as normal or socially deviant comes to be viewed as a medical condition.

Paradigm: A framework containing assumptions about how the world can be interpreted, analysed, and understood.

Sociological imagination: Wright Mill's view that personal problems are often the result of public or social influences, and that by learning to view the social environment and the historical context one can free oneself from blame and become empowered to act on the system.

Stigma: A devalued social characteristic that identifies a person as being deviant or different.

Stigmatisation: The process by which one's identity can become 'spoiled' or devalued through social interaction with others.

Symbolic interactionism: A paradigm that focus on social interaction and social creation of meaning.

References

Alharahsheh, H.H., and Pius, A. (2020). A review of key paradigms: positivism vs interpretivism. *Global Academic Journal of Humanities and Social Sciences* **2** (3): 39–43.

Annandale, M.M., Vilyte, M.G., and Pretorius, C. (2022). Stigma in functional seizures: a scoping review. *Seizure* **99** (3): 131–152.

Asadi-Pooya, A.A., Brigo, F., Mildon, B. et al. (2020). Terminology for psychogenic nonepileptic seizures: making the case for 'functional seizures'. *Epilepsy & Behavior* **104** (Part A): 106895.

Aslam, I., Khalid, T., and Zafar, G. (2021). Over-medicalization: a modern problem divisible from medicalization. *Sys Rev Pharm* **12** (5): 236–238.

Australian Institute of Health and Welfare. (2022). *Health Across Socioeconomic Groups*. Available at: https://www.aihw.gov.au/reports/australias-health/health-across-socioeconomic-groups (accessed 30 April 2023).

BBC (2011). Undercover care: the abuse exposed. *Panorama*, 31 May 2011. Available at: http://www.bbc.co.uk/programmes/b011pwt6 (accessed 19 May 2023).

Béphage, G. (1997). *Social Science and Health Care: Nursing Applications in Clinical Practice*. London: Mosby.

Conrad, P. and Barker, K. (2010). The social construction of illness: key insights and policy implications. *Journal of Health and Social Behaviour* **51**: s67–s79.

Department of Health (2012). Department of Health review: Winterbourne View Hospital: interim report. Available at: http://www.humanrightsinhealthcare.nhs.uk/Library/whats_new/Department-of-Health-Review-Winterbourne-View-Hospital-Interim-Report.pdf (accessed November 2012).

Durkheim, É. (1984). *The Division of Labour in Society* (trans. W.D. Halls). London: Macmillan.

Elias, A. and Paradies, Y. (2021). The costs of institutional racism and its ethical implications for healthcare. *Journal of Bioethical Inquiry* **18** (1): 45–58.

Flores, V.A., Pal, L., and Manson, J.E. (2021). Hormone therapy in menopause: concepts, controversies, and approach to treatment. *Endocrine Reviews* **42** (6): 720–752.

Flynn, M. (2012). Winterbourne View Hospital: a serious case review. South Gloucestershire Safeguarding Adults Board. Available at: http://www.southglos.gov.uk/Pages/Article%20Pages/Community%20Care%20-%20Housing/Older%20and%20disabled%20people/Winterbourne-View-11204.aspx (accessed November 2012).

Fu, S.Y., Anderson, D., and Courtney, M. (2003). Cross-cultural menopausal experience: comparison of Australian and Taiwanese women. *Nursing & Health Sciences* **5** (1): 77–84.

Furness, S., Hanson, L., and Spier, J. (2021). Archetypal meanings of being a paramedic: A hermeneutic review. *Australasian Emergency Care* **24** (2): 135–140.

Giddens, A. and Sutton, P. (2017). *Sociology*. 8e. Cambridge: Polity Press.

Goffman, E. (1969). *The Presentation of Self in Everyday Life*. London: Allen Lane.

Goffman, E. (1986). *Stigma: Notes on the Management of Spoiled Identity*. London: Penguin.

Grannell, A., Fallon, F., Al-Najim, W. et al. (2021). Obesity and responsibility: is it time to rethink agency? *Obesity Reviews* **22** (8): e13270.

Illich, I. (1976). *Limits to Medicine: Medical Nemesis – the Expropriation of Health*. London: Marion Boyars.

Ko, C., Lucassen, P., van der Linden, B. et al. (2022). Stigma perceived by patients with functional somatic syndromes and its effect on health outcomes – a systematic review. *Journal of Psychosomatic Research* **154** (1): 5–6.

Lock, M. (1994). Menopause in cultural context. *Experimental Gerontology* **29** (3–4): 307–317.

Marx, K. and Engels, F. (2023). The Communist Manifesto. Kindle edition. Available at: https://www.amazon.co.uk/Communist-Manifesto-Karl-Marx-ebook/dp/B0BYMGP6P4/ref=sr_1_4?crid=1GPW7SBBBT1SC&keywords=the+communist+manifesto&qid=1684525745&rnid=341677031&s=digital-text&sprefix=the+communist+manifest%2Cdigital-text%2C124&sr=1-4(accessed 19 May 2023).

Mehta, J., Kling, J.M., and Manson, J.E. (2021). Risks, benefits, and treatment modalities of menopausal hormone therapy: current concepts. *Frontiers in Endocrinology* **12** (91): 1–4, 10–11.

Mills, C.W. (1959). *The Sociological Imagination*. New York: Oxford University Press.

Mishra, R., and Masih, E. (2023). To venture and confirm determinants responsible for role conflict: a critical review. *IJFMR-International Journal for Multidisciplinary Research* **5** (2): 1–3.

Monteleone, P., Mascagni, G., Giannini, A. et al. (2018). Symptoms of menopause – global prevalence, physiology and implications. *Nature Reviews Endocrinology* **14** (4): 199–215.

Motzkus, C., Wells, R.J., Wang, X. et al. (2019). Pre-clinical medical student reflections on implicit bias: implications for learning and teaching. *PLOS ONE* **14** (11): e0225058.

Namazi, M., Sadeghi, R., and Behboodi Moghadam, Z. (2019). Social determinants of health in menopause: an integrative review. *International Journal of Women's Health* **11** (1): 637–647.

Nurok, M. and Henckes, N. (2009). Between professional values and the social valuation of patients: the fluctuating economy of pre-hospital emergency work. *Social Science and Medicine* **68** (3): 504–510.

Office for National Statistics. (2022). Health state life expectancies by national deprivation deciles, England: 2018 to 2020. Available at: https://www.ons.gov.uk/peoplepopulationandcommunity/healthandsocialcare/healthinequalities/bulletins/healthstatelifeexpectanciesbyindexofmultipledeprivationimd/2018to2020 (accessed 30 April 2023).

OpenStax College. (2012). Introduction to sociology. https://cnx.org/contents/kHDrTlrv@1.14:_97x1rAv@2/Introduction-to-Sociology (accessed June 2017).

Ormerod, R. (2020). The history and ideas of sociological functionalism: Talcott Parsons, modern sociological theory, and the relevance for OR. *Journal of the Operational Research Society* **71** (12): 1873–1899.

Perich, T., Mitchell, P.B., and Vilus, B. (2022). Stigma in bipolar disorder: a current review of the literature. *Australian & New Zealand Journal of Psychiatry* **56** (9): 1060–1064.

Quintner, J. (2020). Why are women with fibromyalgia so stigmatized? *Pain Medicine* **21** (5): 882–888.

Rawlings, G.H. and Reuber, M. (2018). Health care practitioners' perceptions of psychogenic nonepileptic seizures: a systematic review of qualitative and quantitative studies. *Epilepsia* **59** (6): 1109–1123.

Rees, N., Williams, J., Hogan, C. et al. (2022). Heroism and paramedic practice: a constructivist metasynthesis of qualitative research. *Frontiers in Psychology* **13** (1): 1–17.

Sarkissian, A.D, and Sharkey, J.D. (2021). Transgenerational trauma and mental health needs among Armenian genocide descendants. *International Journal of Environmental Research and Public Health* **18** (19): 5–7.

Sheaff, M. (2005). *Sociology and Health Care: An Introduction for Nurses, Midwives and Allied Health Professionals*. Maidenhead: Open University Press.

Sølvhøj, I.N., Kusier, A.O., Pedersen, P.V. et al. (2021). Somatic health care professionals' stigmatization of patients with mental disorder: a scoping review. *BMC Psychiatry* **21** (1): 1–19.

Sudnow, D. (1967). *Passing On: The Social Organization of Dying*. Upper Saddle River, NJ: Prentice Hall.

Sudnow, D. (1983). Dead on arrival. *Trans-action* **5** (1): 36–43.

Timmermans, S. (1998). Social death as a self-fulfilling prophecy: David Sudnow's *Passing On* revisited. *Sociological Quarterly* **39** (3): 453–472.

Turyahikayo, E. (2021). Philosophical paradigms as the bases for knowledge management research and practice. *Knowledge Management & E-Learning* **13** (2): 209–224.

Vela, M.B., Erondu, A.I., Smith, N.A. et al. (2022). Eliminating explicit and implicit biases in health care: evidence and research needs. *Annual Review of Public Health* **43:** 477–501.

Westwood, S. (2022). Religious-based negative attitudes towards LGBTQ people among healthcare, social care and social work students and professionals: a review of the international literature. *Health & Social Care in the Community* **30** (5): 1449–1470.

World Health Organization (2021). COVID-19 and the social determinants of health and health equity: evidence brief. Available at: https://www.who.int/publications/i/item/9789240038387(accessed 30 April 2023).

World Health Organization (2023). Social determinants of health. Available at: https://www.who.int/health-topics/social-determinants-of-health#tab=tab_1 (accessed 30 April 2023).

CHAPTER 7

Communication competency in healthcare

Rasa Piggott

Academic, Author, Registered Paramedic, Registered Nurse, Advocate

Contents

LEARNING OUTCOMES

On completion of this chapter the reader will be able to:

1. Recall fundamental communication process models and communication theory.
2. Discuss provider–patient principles of effective communication in the context of patient-centred care.
3. Examine interdisciplinary communication techniques that foster safe healthcare.
4. Analyse barriers to effective communication in healthcare.
5. Identify effective, standardised, and replicable communication tools for healthcare communication.

Introduction

Healthcare communication is complex and multifactorial. Facilitating effective interpersonal communication between stakeholders is a core paramedic competency. Communication effectiveness is directly proportionate to the quality of care provided and patient outcomes. Diagnostic error, treatment error, and patient harm result when barriers to effective interdisciplinary and patient–provider communication exist. Up to 70% of adverse and sentinel healthcare events are caused by communication error (Guttman

Fundamentals of Paramedic Practice: A Systems Approach, Third Edition. Edited by Sam Willis and Ian Peate.

Companion website: www.wiley.com/go/willis/paramedic3e

et al. 2021). This chapter unpacks the intercultural and interpersonal communication skills required to uphold positive patient-safety culture and prevent patient harm.

Communication process

In its most elementary form, a communication process is a series of steps taken to send and receive information. Different communication process models exist to reflect the varying degrees of complexity within communication passages and circuits. In healthcare, sound application of a communication process model improves patient safety by improving provider–patient shared decision-making, disclosure accuracy, error mitigation, risk management, use of healthcare facilities, patient adherence to care regimens, and patient psychosocial support. Effective application of a communication process model reduces provider–patient uncertainty and lessens patient readmissions. Providers who understand and apply communication process models improve patient safety and clinical outcomes.

Transmission model of communication

Transmission communication depicts unidirectional information transfer. There is one 'sender' of information, and one passive 'receiver' of information. The receiver's role is limited to information 'absorption'. Success of information conveyance depends on the sender. Examples of transmission communication in healthcare include written patient documentation, discharge summaries, case dispatches via radio for ambulance paramedics, hospital 'code' announcements, and patient notification details sent from

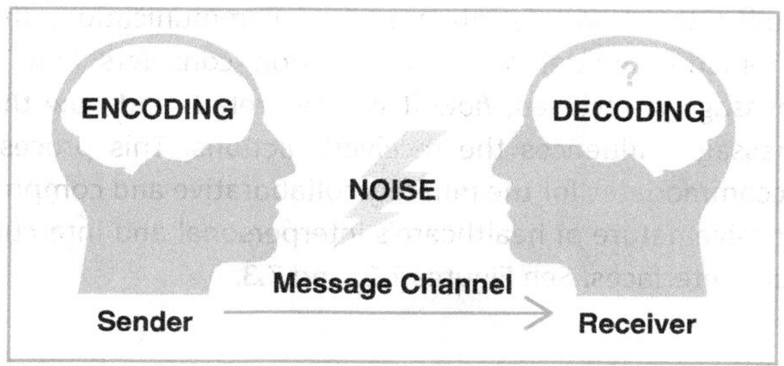

FIGURE 7.1 The transmission model of communication. Source: http://pressbooks.library.torontomu.ca/communication.

ambulance paramedics to hospital staff. Although communication linearity does at times hold purpose, for the most part it has unsafe limitations. Transmission communication does not consider *how* a message is received, *how* it is interpreted, nor *how* the message influences the receiver's actions. It is assumed that information 'meaning' is contained in the 'message' itself, whereas human communication and human meaning-making is more complex than this. Interdisciplinary and provider–patient information exchange should accommodate for human messaging variables that impact message interpretation and response, i.e. attitudes, expectations, knowledge base, environmental influences, personal values, and health literacy. See Figure 7.1.

Interaction model of communication

The interaction model of communication describes a cyclical communication process. Message 'sender' and 'receiver' roles alternate between participants. Physical and psychological communication cues are accommodated for, and purposeful feedback techniques are used to confirm message receipt, interpretation and meaning-making.

Case study 1

A doctor receives a page to attend a code/emergency call on a hospital ward. They respond immediately by physically relocating to the ward, in keeping with hospital process. In this instance, sender–receiver transmission communication has been effective.

Case study 2

Paramedics working for an ambulance service are caring for a patient in a busy, loud, public place. Paramedic A asks paramedic B if they can prepare analgesia in keeping with patient presentation. Paramedic B prepares medication as per their interpretation of Paramedic A's request/patient presentation. The incorrect medication is prepared and administered. In this instance, transmission communication in combination with internal and external 'noise' has resulted in incongruent meaning-making between colleagues, compromising patient safety.

Unlike the transmission model of communication, the interaction model of communication considers *how* a message is received, *how* it is interpreted, and *how* the message influences the receiver's actions. This process accommodates for the innately collaborative and comprehensive nature of healthcare's interpersonal and intercultural interfaces. See Figures 7.2. and 7.3.

Communication theory

Every provider–patient encounter is an interpersonal and intercultural experience. Healthcare providers are familiar with their 'healthcare environment', terminology, and processes. Patients and their support network may lack said familiarity. If a provider–patient exchange does not accommodate for provider–patient differences (health literacy, culture, values, goals), the patient is less likely to understand, interpret, and retain information. This hampers a patient's capacity to provide informed consent/refusal, which correlates with harm. Understanding communication theories and how they interplay with healthcare improves the paramedic's ability to accommodate for provider–patient differences and thus assure patient safety. Interaction and relationship-centred theories will be briefly reviewed in this chapter.

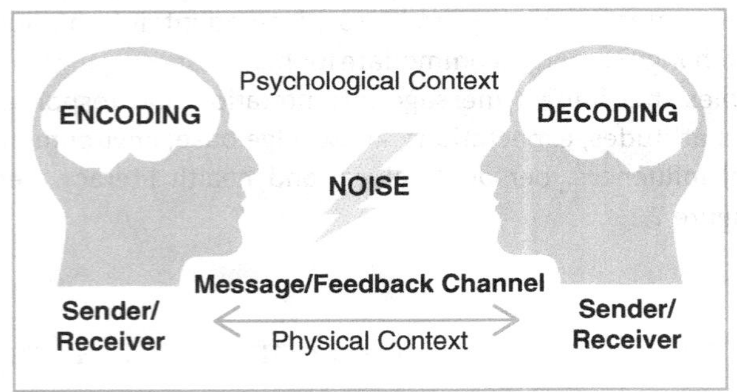

FIGURE 7.2 The interaction model of communication.
Source: http://pressbooks.library.torontomu.ca/communication

Interaction-centred theories

Interaction-centred theories unpack the cause-and-effect relationship between provider–patient communication.

Communication accommodation theory

The communication accommodation theory is an interaction-centred theory that explores sociolinguistic strategies underpinning communicative behaviours and interpersonal dynamics. This theory explains the human predisposition to engage in communication 'convergence' and/or 'divergence'; the phenomenon of adapting one's own communication cues such that they are similar or dissimilar to those involved in your communication exchange. In healthcare, variables that result in negative ramifications of communicative convergence include role relations, perceived power, and perceived status. Research tells us that patient's perceive providers as having power or authority over themselves. Steep authority gradients, actual or perceived, correlate with patient harm. As healthcare providers, recognising the potential for provider–patient authority gradients – and understanding that this may result in a patient partaking in communicative convergence as opposed to communicative behaviours

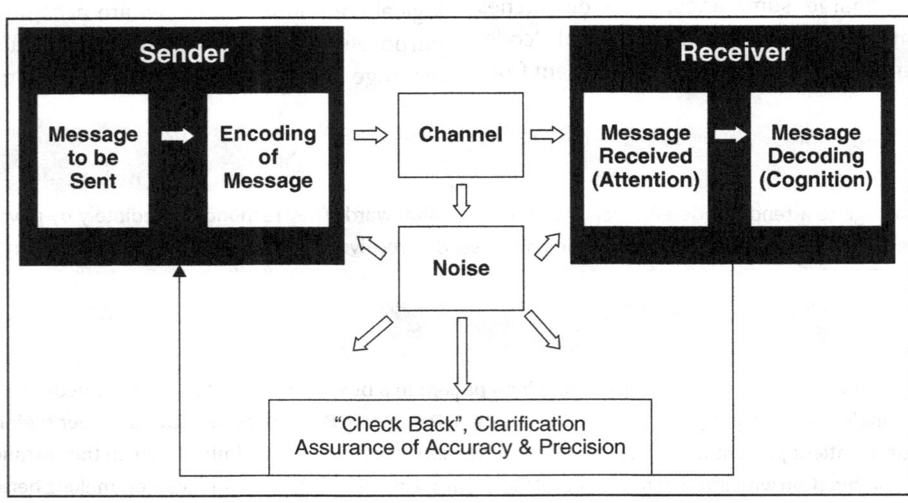

FIGURE 7.3 Interaction model of communication. Source: Guttman et al. 2021/Wolters Kluwer Health.

Case study 3

A paramedic working for an ambulance service is caring for a patient in a busy, loud public place.
It is 3 a.m.; both healthcare providers are tired.
Paramedic A: 'Are you happy to prepare analgesia for administration?'
Paramedic B: 'Yes, I agree analgesia is required. I believe medication X would be most appropriate. Do you agree?'
Paramedic A: 'Yes, medication X would be most appropriate. Are you comfortable with a 2.5mg starting dose?'
Paramedic B: 'I agree with a 2.5mg starting dose. I will dilute this 10mg/1mL vial of medication X into 10mL of normal saline.'
(Paramedic B physically shows Paramedic A the medication vial and normal saline ampoule. Paramedic A and Paramedic B read medication and saline label aloud to each other.)
Paramedic B hands Paramedic A labelled syringe: 'Here is 10mg in 10mL of medication X. Ready for you to provide 2.5mg.'
Paramedic A: '2.5mg, meaning 2.5mL being administered'"
Paramedic B: 'Yes, 2.5mL to be administered.'
By cyclically paraphrasing and summarizing verbal and written communication cues (i.e. communication feedback), Paramedic A and Paramedic B have mitigated internal and external 'noise', ensuring message interpretation has been understood as intended. Implementation of alternating sender and receiver roles has translated to safe patient care.

that allow them to construct messages reflective of their present biopsychosocial truth – is imperative for the provision of safe care. The interpersonally aware provider will use verbal and non-verbal communication behaviours that flatten authority gradients and prevent the negative ramifications of patient communicative convergence. The interpersonally aware provider will use communicative behaviours that create a working partnership with the patient to assure patient autonomy and safety.

Relationship-centred theories

Relationship Centred Theories unpack communication dynamics during information disclosure.

Social penetration theory

The social penetration theory explores the scaffolded approach to developing trust in a relationship. The human condition primes us to commence new relationships 'superficially'. Over time, some 'surface level' relationships are 'penetrated', allowing a relationship to access a 'central' layer. This is achieved by building trust and connection over time. A relationship that has accessed its 'central layer' comprises reciprocal disclosure of core values, beliefs, emotions, and concerns between parties. Healthcare providers are often required to ask probing and private questions that invade the 'central layer' of relationship scaffolding, whilst bypassing surface and peripheral relationship establishment. In addition, professional boundaries mitigate the ability for a provider–patient relationship to be truly reciprocal. Relationships in which disclosure is not reciprocated, i.e. one-sided relationships, place the person who is 'self-disclosing' at risk of emotional exhaustion and depersonalisation.

Health providers need to be equipped with interpersonally aware communicative tools that help patients to feel safe to self-disclose when participating in a patient interview. See Table 7.1 offers exemplar communication techniques that foster trust and rapport establishment.

Communication privacy management theory

The communication privacy management theory describes the process of concealing vs revealing private information. Individual and collective privacy boundaries exist in healthcare. 'Successful communication is more likely when those involved explicitly acknowledge the existence of private information and together determine privacy rules and boundaries' (Bylund et al. 2012, p. 265).

Communication modalities

Non-verbal communication

Non-verbal communication forms the majority of a communication exchange. 'Nonverbal communication (NVC) is defined as a variety of communicative behaviours that do not carry linguistic content and are the messages transmitted without using any words' (Wanko Keutchafo et al. 2020, p. 2). Patients are highly impacted by provider non-verbal communication. Regardless of words being spoken,

TABLE 7.1 Exemplar communication techniques that foster trust and rapport establishment.

Introduce self in a personal manner, maintain open body language, attempt to position self at patient's level (i.e. do not stand over the top of patient).	Explain that you might have to ask some personal questions, but it's the patient's choice as to what they wish to disclose. Empower them.
Explain your role and if in a team setting the names and roles of all present. Let the patient know who in their healthcare team is responsible for what and who will be communicating with them throughout their care episode.	Invite the patient to participate in their care throughout the episode. Let them know they are welcome to ask questions and raise concerns at any time.
Determine the patient's personal identifiers. What is their preferred name? How would they like to be addressed? Consider patient gender identity and preferred pronouns. Respect their true self.	Ask the patient if they have an Advanced Care Plan in place.
Determine if the patient needs assistance to communicate. Consider health literacy, language barriers, cultural and religious backgrounds.	Ask the patient what their goals of care are. Actively hear them.
Take steps to overcome communication barriers: interpreter service, avoid jargon, avoid complex medical terms.	Take into consideration family and carer concerns.
Direct communication to the patient, even if there is an interpreter or carer present.	Depending on setting and role, routinely re-check the patient's needs, concerns, preferences, goals, and questions.
Ask the patient if they have any concerns about sharing their information with their family or carer.	Always sincerely thank the patient for engaging with you and sharing their story with you.

non-verbal communication can illustrate empathy, respect, reassurance, support, disinterest, boredom, anger, or disbelief. Incongruency between verbal and non-verbal communication heightens patient anxiety, whereas congruency between verbal and non-verbal communication improves a patient's trust in a provider.

Kinesics

Kinesics refers to the role of hand, arm, body, and face movements in non-verbal communication. Positive use of body language is known to enhance provider–patient rapport and thus patient safety. Subtle head nods suggest that a healthcare provider is paying attention. It exhibits active listening. This can make a patient feel heard and understood, resulting in an increased likelihood of patients sharing pertinent information required for diagnoses. When a provider is seated, leaning slightly forward and keeping hands visible with an open chest indicates one is actively listening and interested in the patient's story. When standing, an upright physical appearance with one's 'shoulders back' as opposed to slumping communicates active listening and genuine provider interest. Conversely, standing with one's hands on hips is a subconscious non– verbal cue designed to make one look big, assertive, and intimidatory. Standing over a patient can also be interpreted as aggressive or intimidatory; doing so creates unwanted authoritarian division. Crossing of arms across one's chest suggests subconscious disinterest or frustration. Other body language cues that can be interpreted as disinterest include fidgeting, slumping or physically turning away.

Facial expressions are almost universally recognisable in terms of the non-verbal communication cues they portray, however, the triggers for different facial expressions and the social norms that influence facial expressions are culturally diverse. In healthcare, commencing provider–patient interactions whilst smiling is a powerful 'immediacy behaviour'. Immediacy behaviours are communicative behaviours that imply positivity such as liking a person. They create prompt psychosocial 'closeness' between parties. As the provider begins to undertake their patient interview, there is a need to tap into emotional intelligence and interpersonal awareness such that the provider can match their facial expression to the patient's current experience and storytelling.

Eye contact

Eye contact as a non-verbal communication tool differs depending on a person's cultural identity and norms. Where culturally appropriate, maintaining good eye contact can be interpreted as a willingness to listen, can help make a patient feel heard, and demonstrates respect. Typically, Western culture's view eye contact as a positive non-verbal communication cue, whilst some East Asian cultures consider too much eye contact as disrespectful. Similarly, eye contact amongst some Indigenous and First Nations persons makes said persons feel uncomfortable and can be viewed as rude or even aggressive. Some First Nation's persons interpret respect by the lowering of one's eyes during conversation. As a healthcare provider, managing the non-verbal communication behaviour of eye contact requisites educating oneself on cultural safety concepts, seeking cultural competency advice from experts, and accommodating for an individual's eye-contact needs by observing and responding to their cultural identity and body language.

Proxemics

Proxemics can be 'defined as the social meaning of space and interactive field, which determines how relationships occur' (Wanko Keutchafo et al. 2020, p. 8). Proxemics refers to 'four zones' of personal space. Healthcare staff typically work in the 'social space' zone; this respects a person's personal space and maintains professionalism. When physically assessing patients, providers may need to move into a person's 'personal' zone. Maintaining an awareness of the discomfort that this might create for some people, and understanding every human's fundamental right to bodily autonomy, is essential to providing a safe and consensual provider–patient exchange. When the need to physically assess a patient arises, creating a constant dialogue that explains what you would like to do, how it will occur, why you are suggesting it be undertaken, and securing informed consent before stepping into a person's personal space is bioethically and legally essential. The healthcare provider should also consider how they position themselves in space when talking to patients. i.e. consensually sitting at level with or kneeling before older populations when undertaking a patient interview demonstrates respect, active listening, and removes authority gradients. Figure 7.4 illustrates the concept of proxemics.

Active listening

Active listening forms an imperative part of the communication cycle. Active listening includes concentrating with sensitivity such that content, its intent, and any accompanying non-verbal cues can be interpreted by the provider. Active listening cannot occur in a 'hurried' situation. Even in 'emergency' situations, a healthcare provider can appropriately pace engagement to ensure active listening occurs. A provider who is actively listening will engage in postures, body movement, facial expressions, and eye contact in keeping with the patient's cultural ideologies such that the patient knows they are being heard. In addition, the competent active listener will minimise verbal encouragement and exemplify attentive silence. To round out evidence of active listening, a healthcare provider will typically paraphrase what they have been told and ask the patient to correct them if they have misinterpreted anything.

Verbal communication

Verbal communication is a complex and layered composition of language principles comprising more than words. It is influenced by culture, societal rules, regulative rules (how we arrange words in a sentence), attitudes, direct versus indirect verbal messaging, and context.

Vocalics

Paralanguage refers to the vocal components of communication that are not words but impact messaging and meaning making. Vocalics refers to speech rate, vocal quality, pitch, tone, intensity, pausing, and silence. Vocalics provide 'context' to the words being shared. In healthcare, speaking too quickly in a demeaning tone negatively impacts patients. Similarly, speaking too loudly and too quickly creates a barrier to effective communication with patients. Tone monotony, militaristic tone and soft tones can negatively impact patients depending on their cultural identity and personal experiences. Tone can be interpreted as persuasive, assertive, passive, condescending, and impatient, all of which influence how a patient may feel and thus react to a provider. Improper use of provider tone dissuades patients from sharing information. There are clear healthcare benefits when providers use empathetic and friendly tones, along with moderately paced speech. Pausing and using silence are important vocalic tools that invite patients to comprehensively tell their story.

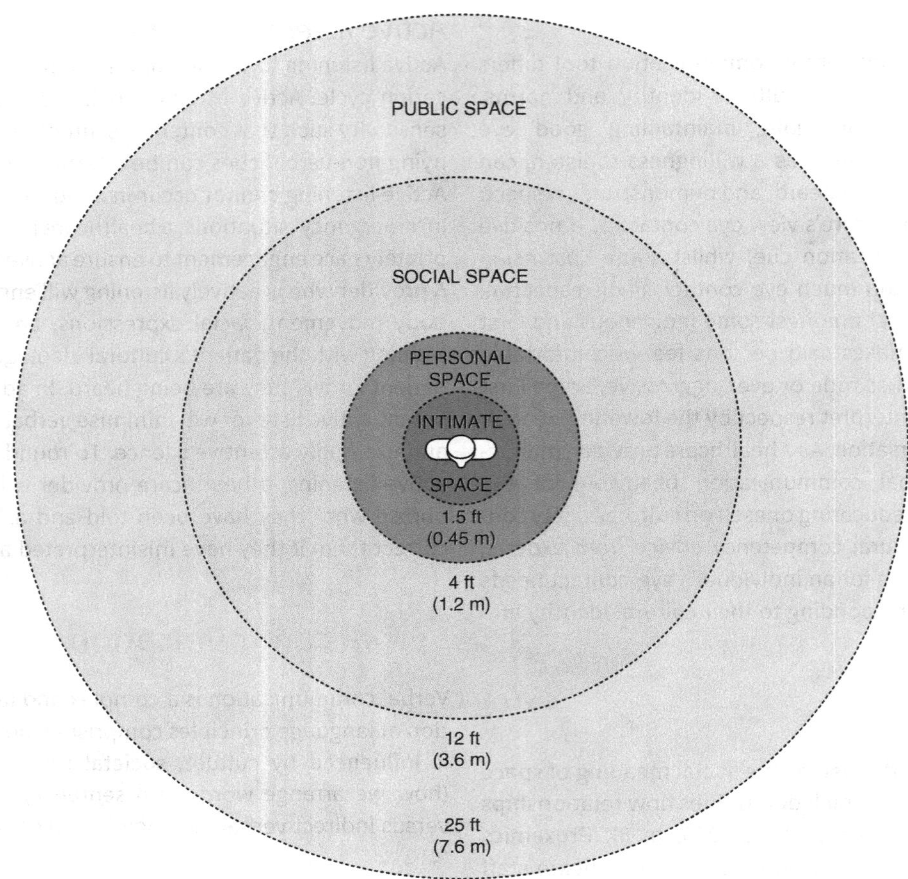

FIGURE 7.4 Concept of proxemics. Source: https://openeducationalberta.ca/foundationsforsuccessinnursing/chapter/2-2-basic-communication-concepts/ " /Alberta / CCBY 4.0 / Public.

Patient-centred communication

Historically, medical paternalism governed healthcare. Medical paternalism stipulates that the health professional knows what is best for the patient in the absence of shared decision-making. Medical paternalism stems from a 'bio-medical' model of healthcare. This biomedical paradigm views the patient as their disease and pathology, whilst imperative psychosocial determinants of a person's health are not considered. As twenty-first-century research and evidence-base has evolved, we have come to learn that a person's health is 'biopsychosocial'. The biopsychosocial model of healthcare responds to the interplay between a person's psychology, social health, economic health, emotional health, physical health, and innate biology, as well as their personal values and perspective, resulting in improved patient outcomes.

To facilitate biopsychosocial healthcare, patient-centred care via patient-centred communication is key. Patient-centred communication 'is a two-way dialogue between patients and care providers. In that dialogue, both parties speak and are listened to without interrupting; they ask questions for clarity, express their opinions, exchange information, and grasp entirely and understand what the others mean.' (Boykins 2014, as cited in Kwame and Petrucka 2021, p. 2).

Participating in patient-centred communication yields significant patient beneficence. It is evidenced to facilitate symptom resolution, improve patient care plan adherence, improve treatment outcomes, enhance patient satisfaction, and improve quality of life for patients, their families, and their communities.

Patient-centred interview

Open-ended questions

A patient-centred interview commences with open-ended questions and continues to use open-ended questions throughout its undertaking. Open–ended questions do not limit the patient's reply to a 'yes' or 'no'. They invite the patient to provide an in-depth response, creating space for them to safely disclose information in keeping with their own narrative. Using open-ended questions as a communication tool results in comprehensive, accurate, and relevant information collation, improving diagnoses accuracy and provision of patient-centred care. Traditionally, patient interviews were 'provider-centred' in that they comprised focussed or closed questions that routinely interrupted the patient. This correlates with poor patient satisfaction, misdiagnosis, and poor patient outcomes. Open-ended questions secure a collaborative dialogue between provider and patient in which all parties are equal, and they ensure the patient is assessed as a holistic, biopsychosocial being. See Table 7.2.

Probing questions

Probing questions help the patient elaborate on the information they've provided in response to open-ended questions. They can be framed as open or closed questions, though they should never 'lead' a patient to an answer. Probing questions help to summarise what the patient has discussed, thereby offering the patient an opportunity to correct the provider if any information has been misinterpreted. See Table 7.3.

TABLE 7.2 **Open-ended questions.**

Open-ended questions	How are you feeling today?
	How can we help today?
	What is worrying you today?
	What kind of problems have you been having recently?
	What are your goals for your care plan?

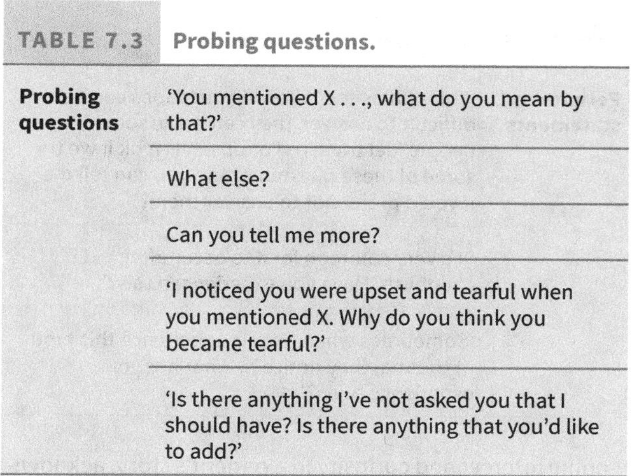

TABLE 7.3 **Probing questions.**

Probing questions	'You mentioned X . . ., what do you mean by that?'
	What else?
	Can you tell me more?
	'I noticed you were upset and tearful when you mentioned X. Why do you think you became tearful?'
	'Is there anything I've not asked you that I should have? Is there anything that you'd like to add?'

Paraphrasing

A provider who intermittently paraphrases what the patient has said and asks the patient to correct them if they have misunderstood anything is demonstrating active listening. This fosters patient trust, prevents medical error, and ensures a patient-centred experience. See Table 7.4.

Permission statements

Permission statements are a form of communication that combine statements with questions. Their intent is to iterate that the patient's experience is 'normal'. Doing so makes the patient feel more comfortable, and as such more likely to self-disclose important health information. See Table 7.5.

Empathy/emotional expression

Empathetic communicative behaviour is key to facilitating a patient-centred experience. A provider demonstrates empathy when they openly respect patient dignity, conduct themselves with warmth and compassion, demonstrate that they understand a patient's unique needs, display

TABLE 7.4 **Paraphrasing.**

Paraphrasing	'I've heard you say X. Are you able to tell me if I've missed anything or misinterpreted anything?'
	'Have I understood this correctly X?'

TABLE 7.5 Permission statements.

Permission statements	'Sometimes the following questions can be difficult to answer, they can make some people feel triggered or upset. Is it ok if we try some of these questions, and you can tell me if you'd prefer not to answer them?'
	'It's very common for X to occur after childbirth. Have you experienced this?'
	'Sometimes when people experience this type of trauma, they notice X. What has your experience been?'

genuine interest and curiosity in a patient's story, acknowledge the patient's truth, and demonstrate belief in a patient's story. A part of engaging in empathetic communication is allowing for flexibility within a patient interview, i.e. allowing the patient's narrative to guide patient interview structure, whilst still achieving all necessary aspects of said interview. Dependent on a patient's presenting symptoms, there are times when providers need to prioritise applying pre-determined physical assessment frameworks that expediate recognition and response to patient life-threats, whilst mitigating human error. Even so, an urgent, high-stress situation shouldn't detract from a provider's ability to display empathy whilst engaging with a patient. See Table 7.6.

Teach-back theory

Creating a patient-centred and safe healthcare experience requires the provider to evaluate a patient's level of insight into their current experience and proposed healthcare options. Insight equates to a patient having decision-making capacity, which equates to them being able to provide informed consent or informed refusal regarding their healthcare. If a health provider has not communicated in a manner that fits the health literacy and personal attributes of an individual, that individual may not have all the information they need to partake in informed decision-making. Legally and bioethically, there are very few circumstances in which a person can have care forced upon them, against their will, without it being an abuse of their human rights. A communication technique that allows providers to evaluate a person's level of insight and understanding is termed the teach-back method. This method serves to close communication gaps between provider and patient by asking the patient to restate what they have been told, what they believe is happening, what care they have been offered, and why. If a person cannot 'teach back', i.e. explain to the provider why certain care has been offered and the positives vs negatives of that care offer, then a provider may need to rephrase their communication. Accommodating for individuals when engaging in the 'teach-back' method is key. For example, does the provider need to use written material to ensure effective communication and patient understanding has occurred? Providers should always aim to appeal to the auditory, visual, and tactile needs of a person's cognition. See Table 7.7.

TABLE 7.6 Empathy.

Empathy	'That must be really difficult, thank you for sharing that with me. Do you feel like telling me more about this?'
	'How do you feel about that?'
	'I hear you. This is an incredibly challenging time for you and I'm so thankful that you've shared this information with me. Would you like to talk about this some more?'

Trauma-informed communication

The negative impact of trauma on biopsychosocial health is long-lasting. All healthcare providers should assume a history of trauma when engaging with patients. Doing so will ensure the provider engages with patients in a trauma-informed manner, thereby preventing re-traumatisation. When engaging with patients, a trauma-informed provider will habitually consider 'what has happened to you', as opposed to, 'what is wrong with you'. When a provider changes their inner dialogue to reflect trauma awareness,

TABLE 7.7 Teach back.

Teach back	'To make sure I've explained everything properly, are you able to tell me when you are going to take this medication, and how you are going to take this medication at home?'
	'I'd like to make sure I've explained the potential causes of your current symptoms to you properly, and their potential consequences. Are you able to tell me what your symptoms are, and what their consequences may be?'
	'We've discussed a lot today, and I want to make sure I've explained things clearly. Are you able to summarise . . . ?'

TABLE 7.8 Trauma-informed communication.

Trauma-informed communication	'If you feel comfortable . . .'
	'If you feel that you're ready . . .'
	Absence of judgement, absence of blame. Specific details regarding a traumatic experience should only be unpacked by those appropriately educated to do so, i.e. psychologists, psychiatrists.
	De-stigmatise language. i.e. don't label people. A person has been diagnosed with X. They themselves are not X. A person has a condition. They themselves are not the condition.
	Ask the patient if they feel comfortable in their current environment (with the provider). Is there anything the provider can do to help make a patient feel more comfortable i.e. an alternate space, a health provider of a different gender identity etc.
	Never minimise a person's experience in the urgency of managing symptoms. Always prioritise validating a person's experience.

it ensures the provider fosters the five principles of trauma-informed care: safety, choice, collaboration, trustworthiness, and empowerment. Trauma-informed care acknowledges the multifaceted and pervasive ramifications of trauma on all body systems, and it strives to create safe boundaries for all patients. One of the most important rules of a trauma-informed approach to communication is to never force a person to tell their story but rather to create a space in which they feel safe to self-disclose. See Table 7.8.

Culturally responsive communication

Table 7.9 gives some examples of culturally responsive communication. A helpful definition of the term is provided by Minnican and O'Toole (2020, p. 2):

> Culturally responsive communication can be defined as communicating with awareness and knowledge of cultural differences and attempting to accommodate those differences. This involves respect and an understanding that socio-cultural issues such as race, gender, sexual orientation, disability, social class and status can affect health beliefs and behaviours. Therefore, providing person- centred healthcare requires culturally responsive communication.

Honesty and complex conversations

Literature tells us that many healthcare providers self-identify that they struggle with conducting complex conversations. There exists confusion and nervousness about how to best approach difficult or emotive conversations with patients, i.e. end-of-life conversations, the delivery of bad news, topics that carry the potential to create conflict, etc. This can result in these conversations being avoided, despite patients wanting and needing to have these conversations in the setting of their lived experience. As a provider of healthcare, creating a therapeutically beneficial relationship with a patient involves pairing **honesty with compassion.** Information should be delivered in a straightforward manner whilst adopting previously discussed non-verbal communication techniques. Although difficult, developing one's communication skillset such that **false reassurance** and **distancing language** is avoided, is essential. See Tables 7.10 and 7.11.

TABLE 7.9 Culturally responsive communication.

Culturally responsive communication	'When there are troubles in your family, what do you do? Who do you turn to for help?'
	'Tell me about your beliefs and practices.'
	'What are some incorrect assumptions people have made about your beliefs?'
	'What traditions are important to you?'
	'How do you view your role in your family?'
	'What do you need from me to ensure I respect your culture and beliefs?'

TABLE 7.10 Honesty and complex conversations.

Honesty and complex conversations	Patient: 'I am scared I might die.' Provider: 'Tell me more.'
	Provider: 'Your partner (insert name) has died.'

TABLE 7.11 False reassurance and distancing language.

False reassurance	Patient: 'I am scared I might die'. Provider: 'Everything will be ok.' This is false reassurance. Dishonesty does not create space for open communication.
Distancing language	Provider: 'They didn't make it.' Provider: 'They have passed away.' This distancing language is a subconscious attempt to create false space from a perceived threat. It demonstrates dishonesty. In times of high stress, patients, family members, and bystanders need access to clear, direct, honest language in the context of compassion.

Closed-ended questions

Closed-ended questions limit a patient's response to yes or no and should only be used after the patient has had ample time to provide their information via open-ended questions. Closed-ended questions can help a provider ascertain specific information when it is needed, i.e. clarifying details about a patient's symptoms. Closed-ended questions do inherently carry the risk of 'leading' the patient if not crafted carefully, which can prevent essential patient information disclosure. See Table 7.12.

TABLE 7.12 Closed-ended question.

Closed-ended questions	**'Do you take your tablets?'** This limits the information the provider will receive from the information. Instead, as an example, ask 'How are you taking your medication'?
	'Have I understood correctly that you have a sharp pain your stomach?'
	'Do you have any other symptoms or concerns at present that are worrying you?'

Leading questions

Leading questions are questions that a provider subconsciously structures in a way that suggests they are searching for a pre-determined answer. These questions make the patient feel as though they should be answering a question in a specific way, preventing the patient from providing accurate detail. Leading questions should always be avoided when communicating with patients. See Table 7.13.

Why questions

'Why' questions as a communication tool risk making the patient feel judged, or as though they need to justify or defend their actions. This should be avoided in healthcare. Creating a judgement-free zone by crafting questions appropriately is imperative for gathering accurate patient information and providing patient centred care. See Table 7.14.

Silence

When used correctly, silence is a powerful communication tool in a patient interview. Moments of silence after a provider has asked a question or after a patient has answered a question allows the patient to reflect on the question and potentially add further detail. Creating silence is a balancing act, as too long of a 'silent' period leads to the patient feeling uncomfortable.

TABLE 7.13 Leading questions.

Leading questions (AVOID)	'. . . but it's not a cramping pain?'
	'You didn't miss your medication this morning, did you?'
	'. . . you don't have any chest pain?'
	'. . . you're not worried about that?'
	'Is it a stabbing pain?'

TABLE 7.14 Why questions.

Why questions (AVOID)	'Why didn't you take your medication?' Instead ask: 'What do you think caused you to miss you medication dose?'
	'Why do you use . . .?' Instead ask: 'How do you feel before you consume . . .?'

Barriers to effective communication

At the provider–patient interface, communication involves multifarious variables that challenge communication effectiveness, i.e. stakeholder opinion, education, culture, emotion, life circumstance, health literacy, aspiration, and cognitive bias. Healthcare settings often invoke competing priorities, distractions, stress, fatigue, and cognitive overload, further challenging communication effectiveness.

Linguistic barriers

- Language barriers.
- Cultural differences in non-verbal communication meaning (eye gaze, head nodding, touch).
- Vocabulary difference between stakeholders.
- Rate of speaking.
- Age of stakeholders.
- Education background of stakeholders.
- Familiarity with medical terminology/health literacy.
- Lack of trauma-informed language.

Institutional and system barriers

- Absence of workplace 'speak-up' culture.
- Ineffective healthcare policy.
- Negative workplace culture and incivility.
- Authoritarian, unsupportive management styles.
- Poor managerial leadership skills.
- Staff shortages.
- Unsafe roster configurations engendering healthcare provider health issues.
- Staff burnout.
- High workloads.
- Insufficient time to interact with patients.
- Task-focussed care.
- Management that emphasises rules, tasks, results instead of prioritising relationship building.
- Management that prioritises brand over people.
- Poor clinical governance frameworks and risk management capabilities.
- Poor provider team cohesion.
- Poor e-health infrastructure.
- Poor professional development opportunities.

Cognitive and behavioural barriers

- Cognitive biases.
- Human factors.
- Cognitive overload.
- Providers leading care by way of their own values, beliefs, and cultural background.
- Disrespectful, derogatory, patronising provider communication.
- Provider failing to listen to patient story.
- Patient disrespectful behaviour toward provider.
- System facilitated provider misconduct or unlawful provider action/inaction.

Environmental barriers

- Noisy surrounds
- Lack of patient privacy
- Poor ventilation
- Poor lighting
- Cramped spaces

Interdisciplinary communication

Communication between healthcare providers is a high-risk exercise. Its potential for perpetuating unsafe patient care is heavily evidenced both during care provision and when care is being transferred between providers.

Within healthcare teams, there are numerous variables that impede effective communication, most of which stem from outdated and unsafe hierarchical division. Some factors that affect a person's position within the 'hierarchy' of a team include a provider's sex, gender identity, personality, age, cultural background, job title, and an individual's unregulated control of another's career prospects.

Crew Resource Management (CRM) is an interdisciplinary education construct that aims to address the human factors contributing to team communication dysfunction and thus patient risk. CRM education focusses on situational awareness, decision-making, teamwork, leadership, and stress management. CRM education alone is not enough to mitigate patient risk in the healthcare industry (an industry that is still unlearning it's authoritarian and hierarchical origins). To mitigate patient harm, healthcare teams also require access to definitive communication processes such as structured communication algorithms and frameworks, and retribution free reporting systems.

Critical information communication

Delays in essential care occur when communication breaks down between healthcare providers. Every member of a healthcare team is responsible for patient advocacy. All members of a team should feel safe to voice patient-safety concerns, and all members in a healthcare team should be included in decision-making. This prevents human error.

When a health provider finds themselves aware of a patient-safety concern but team barriers are preventing that concern from being aptly communicated or responded to, they can use graded assertiveness communication models. See Figures 7.5, 7.6, and 7.7.

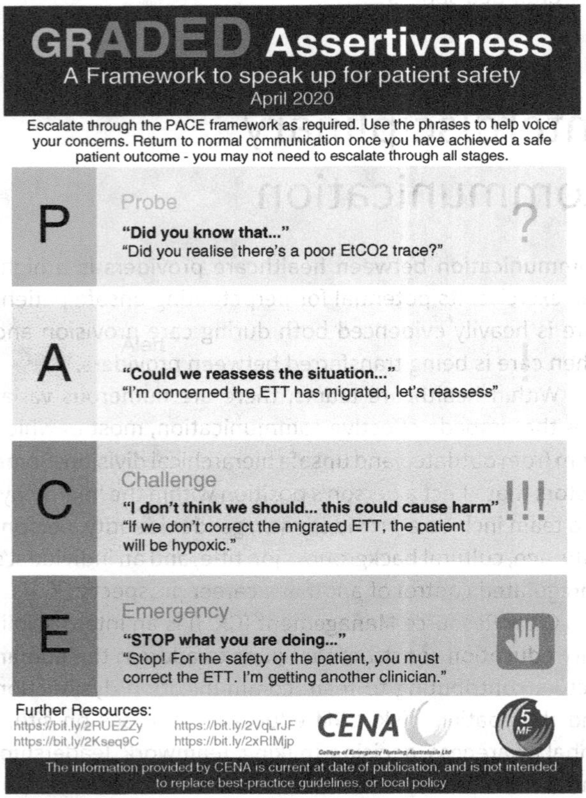

GRADED Assertiveness
A Framework to speak up for patient safety
April 2020

Escalate through the PACE framework as required. Use the phrases to help voice your concerns. Return to normal communication once you have achieved a safe patient outcome - you may not need to escalate through all stages.

P Probe
"Did you know that..."
"Did you realise there's a poor EtCO2 trace?"

A Alert
"Could we reassess the situation..."
"I'm concerned the ETT has migrated, let's reassess"

C Challenge
"I don't think we should... this could cause harm"
"If we don't correct the migrated ETT, the patient will be hypoxic."

E Emergency
"STOP what you are doing..."
"Stop! For the safety of the patient, you must correct the ETT. I'm getting another clinician."

Further Resources:
https://bit.ly/2RUEZZy https://bit.ly/2VqLrJF
https://bit.ly/2Kseq9C https://bit.ly/2xRIMjp

CENA College of Emergency Nursing Australasia Ltd

The information provided by CENA is current at date of publication, and is not intended to replace best-practice guidelines, or local policy

FIGURE 7.5 Graded assertiveness – PACE. Source: College of Emergency Nursing Australasia (CENA) / https://intensivenurse.wordpress.com/2020/04/24/graded-assertiveness/ / last accessed 22 July 2023.

No one team member should be afraid to point out a risk, a concern or an actual or potential error.

Five-step advocacy

An alternative approach is the advocacy approach:

1. **Get attention** - *'Excuse me, doctor!'*
2. **Raise your concern** - *'There is no end-tidal CO_2 trace.'*
3. **State the problem as you see it** - *'I'm concerned that the intubation was unsuccessful.'*
4. **Suggest a solution** - *'Why don't we remove the ETT and go back to bagging the patient?'*
5. **Obtain an agreement** - *'Does that sound like a safe thing to do?'*

FIGURE 7.6 Graded assertiveness – 5-step advocacy. Source: https://trauma.reach.vic.gov.au.

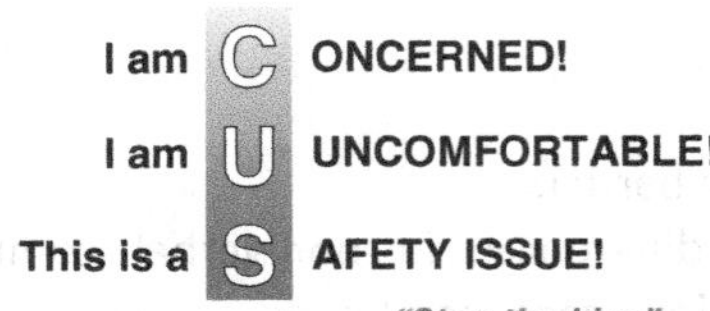
I am C ONCERNED!
I am U UNCOMFORTABLE!
This is a S AFETY ISSUE!
"Stop the Line"

FIGURE 7.7 Graded assertiveness – CNS. Source: https://www.ahrq.gov/teamstepps/instructor/essentials/pocketguide.html.

Closed loop communication

Throughout every episode of care, providers should aim to communicate in a manner that confirms they have received and understood information. Closed-loop communication involves referring to providers by their name, making eye contact, paraphrasing back to the provider what they have said and definitively asking if information has been received as intended. See Figure 7.8 and Table 7.15.

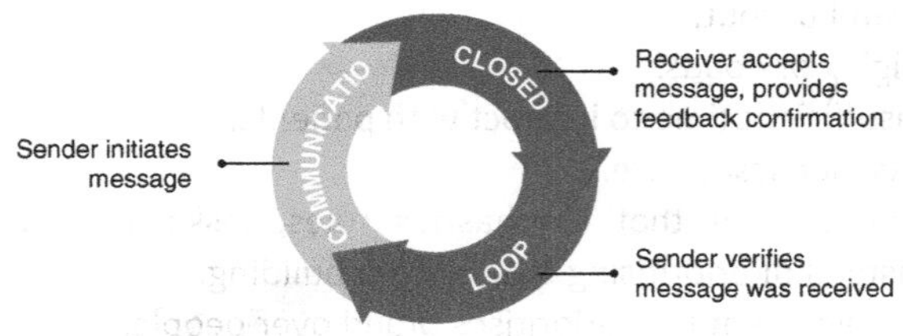
Sender initiates message
COMMUNICATIO
CLOSED
LOOP
Receiver accepts message, provides feedback confirmation
Sender verifies message was received
SLIDEMODEL.COM

FIGURE 7.8 Closed-loop communication. Source: SlideModel / https://slidemodel.com/teamwork-managers-guide/002-closed-loop-communication-diagram-powerpoint-slide/.

TABLE 7.15 Closed-loop communication.

Closed-loop communication	Provider A: '*Name*, we are needing to provide patient X with . . . Because . . .' Provider B: '*Name*, we are going to provide patient X with . . . Because . . .'
	Provider A: '*Name*, the patient (name) presents with . . . let's insert a urinary catheter.' Provider B: '*Name*, you are advocating for urinary catheter insertion because . . .'
	Provider A: '*Name*, can you please prepare ___ mg of Midazolam and ___ of Fentanyl.' Provider B: '*Name*, yes, I am preparing ___ mg of Midazolam and ___ of Fentanyl.'

Clinical handover

Clinical handover refers to the communication exchange that occurs when transferring responsibility for patient care between providers. Human factors and cognitive bias generate ineffective communication during clinical handovers. The cognitive bias of diagnostic momentum, for example, engenders the subconscious tendency for providers to simply accept and pass on a diagnosis between each other, without individually pausing to assure diagnosis validity. This is a common cause of patient under-triage, misdiagnosis, and harm. Including the patients in their transfer of care by maintaining an open dialogue with the patient regarding the process is known to reduce handover miscommunication and patient harm. In addition, there are system-wide communication tools that can be implemented to minimise clinical handovers risks. These communication tools vary depending on setting and allow for flexibility whilst creating common language and expectations amongst all providers.

Ambulance to emergency department: pre-arrival handover

If working as a paramedic for an ambulance service, pre-arrival handovers via radio notification are a form of clinical handover reserved for patients who are significantly unwell, at risk of deterioration, or require specialist resources. Pre-arrival handovers are succinct. The aim is to alert the hospital of the severity or complexities of a patient's presentation, such that the hospital can prepare resources prior to ambulance arrival – i.e. resuscitation cubicle preparation, staff-skill-mix assurance, security if needed, specialist services as required, biohazard preparedness, etc. Pre-arrival handovers may include:

- Ambulance 'crew' identification
- Patient age
- Presenting concern + relevant comorbidities (brief)
- Presenting signs and symptoms (brief)
- Resources required on arrival
- Estimated time of arrival

Ambulance paramedic to triage nurse: clinical handover

If working as a paramedic for an ambulance service, handing over to an emergency department (ED) triage nurse is a requisite for succinctly illustrating how unwell a patient may be so that they can be assigned an appropriate triage category. Ineffective communication at triage can result in delayed patient care secondary to under-triage. This type of handover is not intended to be as comprehensive as a 'bed-side' handover' but it demands provision of 'essential' information. There are several internationally recognised communication tools that can be used to facilitate a clinical handover to a triage nurse. One example is the 'IMIST-AMBO' acronym (see Table 7.16). This can be used to help colleagues communicate patient-related information during a clinical

TABLE 7.16 Description of the IMIST-AMBO tool.

I	Identification (patient)*
M	Mechanism of injury/medical complaint
I	Injuries/information related to the complaint
S	Signs and symptoms, including GCS and vital signs
T	Treatment given and trends noted
A	Allergies
M	Medications (patient's regular medications)
B	Background history (patient's past history)
O	Other information (scene, social, valuables, advanced directives, family informed)

TABLE 7.17 Information shared during clinical handover.

Patient identity + allergies	**Preferred name, gender identity, pronouns, cultural background, patient decision-making capacity, advanced care directives, next-of – kin**
Presenting complaint	Initial patient concerns/signs and symptoms
Prodrome	Patient physical, social, environmental health in the lead up to sign and symptom development
Physical assessment findings	Neurological, cardiovascular, respiratory, gastrointestinal, genitourinary, integumentary, musculoskeletal, neurovascular, blood work, imaging results, etc (dependent on work setting)
Medical history and risk factors	Former diagnoses, genetic risk factors, lifestyle risk factors
Medication	Dose, duration, compliance
Social health	Social resources/link ins, financial risks, safety risks
Environmental health	Housing risks, food/water access, safety risks
Preliminary diagnoses	Differential conditions that have been considered/treated
Care provision	Technical and non-technical healthcare provided

handover in an accurate way that adheres to a specific sequence. This tool guides the practitioner to structure the communication, as well as helping them to remember the necessary data that has to be shared with others when performing an urgent or emergency clinical handover.

Comprehensive paramedic clinical handovers

Globally, paramedics work in a variety of primary, acute, and emergency care settings. Understanding the potential range and comprehensiveness required of a handover is essential. Be it an ED bedside handover or a primary Healthcare Facility Handover, Table 7.17 summarises information that a provider might share when engaging in a comprehensive clinical handover.

Interdisciplinary debriefing

Team debriefing remains an emerging skill for many healthcare providers. It refers to a structured communication approach that unpacks the events of an episode care with all providers involved. A debrief can be 'hot', i.e. occur immediately after an event. Alternatively, a 'debrief' can be 'cold', occurring at a later time or in a

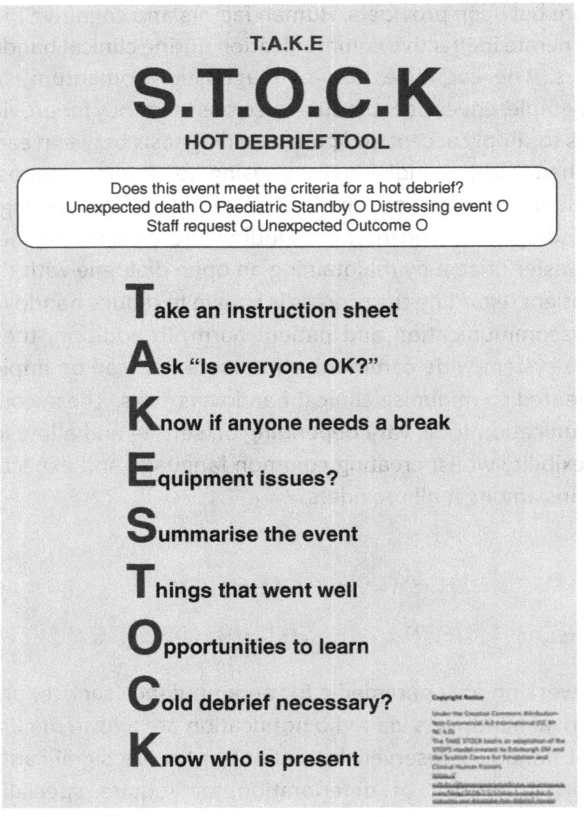

T.A.K.E
S.T.O.C.K
HOT DEBRIEF TOOL
Does this event meet the criteria for a hot debrief?
Unexpected death O Paediatric Standby O Distressing event O
Staff request O Unexpected Outcome O
Take an instruction sheet
Ask "Is everyone OK?"
Know if anyone needs a break
Equipment issues?
Summarise the event
Things that went well
Opportunities to learn
Cold debrief necessary?
Know who is present

FIGURE 7.9 Team debrief: take stock. Source: www.rcem-learning.co.uk.

different environment to where the episode of care took place. Typically, debriefs are conducted such that one person takes the role of 'lead' communicator. The 'lead communicator' will use a designated debrief communication model to facilitate the debrief. All forms of team debriefing are associated with improved team performance (improved interdisciplinary communication, interdisciplinary understanding, improved team reflexivity, improved recognition of patient threats). There remains a need to ensure health providers involved in a debrief, particularly in 'hot debriefs', are in a psychosocially safe place to participate. Debriefs are intended to be safe, respectful, compassionate, and non-judgemental spaces. Team debrief communication frameworks vary. See Figures 7.9, 7.10, and 7.11.

Conclusion

Communication competency, regardless of clinical setting, is a core paramedic capability. When used effectively, interpersonally and interculturally aware communication drives patient safety, resulting in improved health equity and health outcomes.

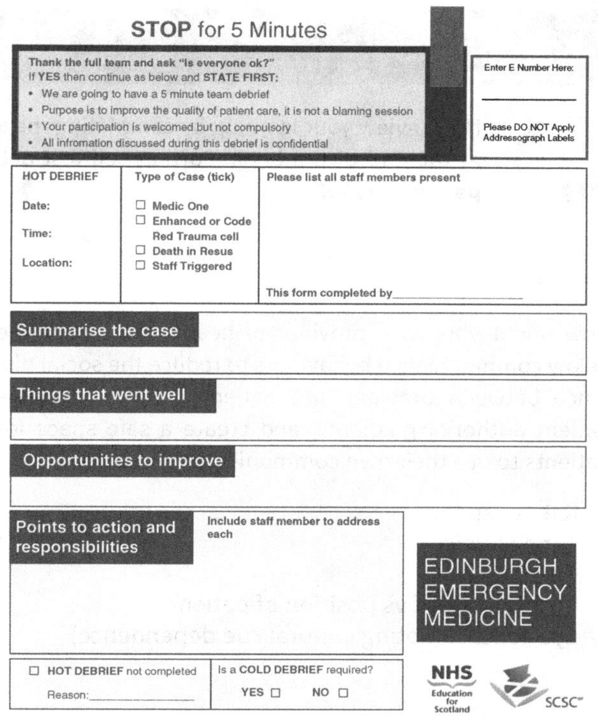

STOP for 5 Minutes

Thank the full team and ask "Is everyone ok?"
If **YES** then continue as below and **STATE FIRST:**

- We are going to have a 5 minute team debrief
- Purpose is to improve the quality of patient care, it is not a blaming session
- Your participation is welcomed but not compulsory
- All infromation discussed during this debrief is confidential

Enter E Number Here: ____

Please DO NOT Apply Addressograph Labels

HOT DEBRIEF	Type of Case (tick)	Please list all staff members present
Date: Time: Location:	☐ Medic One ☐ Enhanced or Code Red Trauma cell ☐ Death in Resus ☐ Staff Triggered	This form completed by____________

Summarise the case

Things that went well

Opportunities to improve

Points to action and responsibilities — Include staff member to address each

☐ HOT DEBRIEF not completed Reason:____________	Is a COLD DEBRIEF required? YES ☐ NO ☐

FIGURE 7.10 Team debrief: stop. Source: https://www.edinburghemergencymedicine.com/blog/2018/11/1/stop-5-stop-for-5-minutes-our-bespoke-hot-debrief-model.

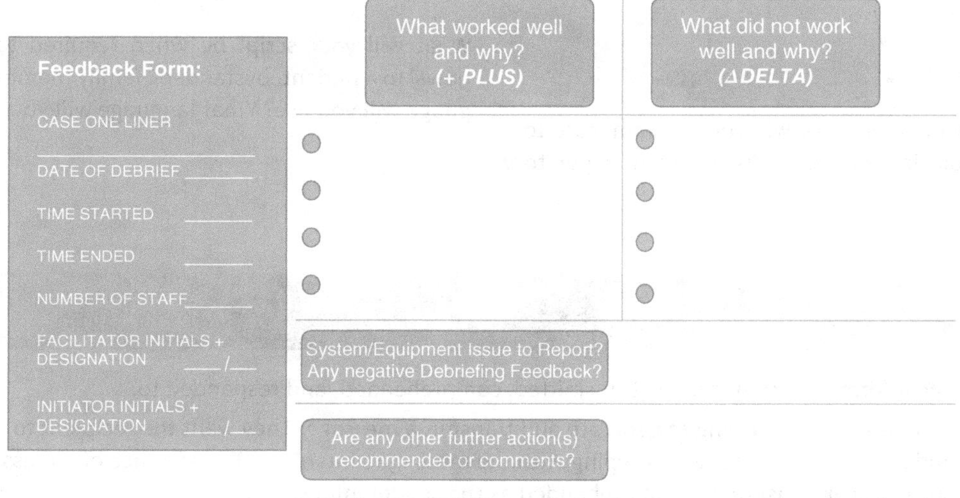

Feedback Form:

CASE ONE LINER ____________

DATE OF DEBRIEF ______

TIME STARTED ______

TIME ENDED ______

NUMBER OF STAFF______

FACILITATOR INITIALS + DESIGNATION ___/___

INITIATOR INITIALS + DESIGNATION ___/___

What worked well and why? *(+ PLUS)*	What did not work well and why? *(ΔDELTA)*
●	●
●	●
●	●
●	●

System/Equipment Issue to Report? Any negative Debriefing Feedback?

Are any other further action(s) recommended or comments?

FIGURE 7.11 Team debrief: generic exemplar. Source: Coggins et al. 2020, p. 3 /Springer Nature / CCBY 4.0 / Public domain.

Activities

Now review your learning by completing the learning activities in this chapter. The answers to these appear at the end of the book. Further self-test activities can be found at **www.wileyfundamentalseries.com/paramedic/3e.**

Activity 7.1

How might you, as a provider of healthcare, adapt the below communicative behaviours to reduce the social distance between provider and patient, flatten provider–patient authority gradients, and create a safe space for patients to use their own communicative cues?

- Rate of speech
- Tone of voice
- Gestures
- Position of self vs position of patient
- Eye contact (noting cultural cue dependence)

Activity 7.2

As a healthcare provider, how will you explicitly acknowledge the presence of private patient information? How will you, together with the patient, establish privacy rules and boundaries?

Activity 7.3

As a healthcare provider, how will you communicate to a patient your role in obligatory disclosure to regulatory bodies or law enforcement? (For instance, communicable diseases in keeping with reporting requirements; child abuse in keeping with legislation.)

Activity 7.4

Can you think of a time when you felt disregarded or unheard by a healthcare provider?

- Describe this experience? (Description)
- How did this experience make you feel? (Feelings)
- How did this affect your healthcare experience? (Evaluation)
- How did this impact your relationship with your healthcare engagement? (Analysis)
- What did this experience teach you? (Conclusion)
- As a healthcare provider, how will you ensure that clients feel heard and validated? (Action Plan)

Activity 7.5

What will your script be when required to deliver 'bad news' to a patient, bystanders, family members? What language will you use? What language will you avoid?

Glossary

Message: The information that is being transmitted, comprehended, and responded to.

Sender: Participant who is trying to generate and transmit a message. They want the recipient to receive and understand the message, in keeping with the message's intention. Transference of a message does not automatically ensure it is comprehended as the sender intended.

Encoding: An internal cognitive process that allows the 'sender' to turn thoughts into communication. Encoding is influenced by numerous variables: language, personal attitudes, knowledge base, social circumstances, stressors, and more.

Channel: The medium through which a message is conveyed, and the sensory route through which an encoded message travels between sender and receiver. Was the message relayed verbally, non-verbally, in writing? How has the episode of communication been heard, seen, smelt?

Receiver: Persons to whom the message is directed.

Decoding: Internal cognitive process through which the receiver turns communication into thoughts/makes meaning of information presented. Receiver message interpretation is influenced by personal attributes, perspectives, knowledge base, attitudes, and motivations. Differences between sender and receiver education, experience and personal circumstances can result in communication cues holding different meanings between parties.

Feedback: The process of determining if and how a message has been received. This involves communication cues from both sender and receiver that indicate how well, accurately, or inaccurately a message has been understood. Feedback can occur verbally or non-verbally. It can incorporate techniques such as paraphrasing, summarising, and inaction reflection. Feedback processes clarify communication intent and prevent miscommunication. In healthcare, this serves as a patient-safety and harm-preventative strategy.

Noise: Any interference that occurs during a communication process is referred to as noise. Noise can be one's internal dialogue, or it can be external distractions. Self-awareness tactics are key to preventing internal noise from interrupting a communication process. External noise, particularly in the setting of healthcare, can be challenging to mitigate. Recognition of external noise placing a patient care episode at risk is an essential healthcare provider skill. Applying structured communication scaffolds and using communication tactics to lessen the potential of distraction is a key patient-safety concept.

Context: The physical and psychological setting in which communication is occurring. Physical context refers to environmental factors that play into a communication encounter. Location, temperature, size of a space, lighting all influence communication. As a healthcare provider, busy, loud, out of hospital care settings with numerous bystanders (as an example) will influence communication. Working in a crowded hospital cubicle with limited room to move will influence communication. The psychological context of a communication encounter leans into human factors such as participant mental load and emotional state, the nature of any previous interaction participants may have had, cultural differences, authority gradients, and more. The way in which the context of a communication interface is managed directly impacts the success of communication transmission and meaning making.

References

ACSQHC. (2020). Communicating for safety: improving clinical communication, collaboration and teamwork in Australian health services. Scoping Paper.

Baliga, K., Coggins, A., Warburton, S. et al. (2022). Pilot study of the DART tool – an objective healthcare simulation debriefing assessment instrument. *BMC Medical Education* **22** (636): 1–9.

Barrier, P.T.J. and Jensen, N. (2003). *Mayo Clin Proc* **78:** 211–214.

Beach, M. and Inui, T., Relationship-centered-care-research-network. (2006). Relationship-centred care: a constructive reframing. *J Gen Intern Med* **21.**

Birkhäuer, J., Gaab, J., Kossowsky, J. et al. (2017). Trust in the health care professional and health outcome: a meta-analysis. *PMC* **12** (2).

Bylund, C., Peterson, E., and Cameron, K. (2012). A practitioner's guide to interpersonal communication theory: an overview and exploration of selected theories. *Patient Education and Counseling* **87** (3): 261–267.

Coggins, A., De Los Santos, A., Zaklama, R. et al. (2020). Interdisciplinary clinical debriefing in the emergency department: an observational study of learning topics and outcomes. *BMC Emergency Medicine* **20** (79): 1–10.

Coiera, E. (2006). Communication systems in healthcare. *Clin Biochem Rev* **27.**

Cox, L. and Best, O. (2022). Clarifying cultural safety: its focus and intent in an Australian context. *Contemporary Nurse* **58** (1): 71–81.

Epstein, R.M., Fiscella, K., Lesser, C.S. et al. (2010). Why the nation needs a policy push on patient-centered health care. *Health Affairs* **29** (8): 1489-1495.

Farzadnia, S. and Giles, H. (2015). Patient-provider health interactions: a communication accommodation theory perspective. *International Journal of Society, Culture & Language*, *3*(2): 17–34.

Foster, C. (2019). The rebirth of medical paternalism: an NHS Trust v Y. *J Med Ethics* **45:** 3–7.

Guttman, O., Lazzara, E., Keebler, J. et al. (2021). Dissecting communication barriers in healthcare: a path to enhancing communication resiliency, reliability, and patient safety. *Journal of Patient Safety* **17** (8): e1465–e1471.

Halbach, A. (2012). Questions about basic interpersonal communication skills and cognitive language proficiency. *Applied linguistics* **33** (5): 608–613. doi: 10.1093/applin/ams058.

Hoeln-Rabbersvik, E., Thygesen, E., Eikebrokk, T. et al. (2018). Barriers to exchanging healthcare information in inter-municipal healthcare services: a qualitative case study. *BMC Medical Informatics and Decision Making* **18** (92): 1–14.

Jahromi, V., Tabatabaee, S., Adbar, Z. et al. (2016). Active listening: the key of successful communication in hospital managers. *PMC* **8** (3): 2123–2128.

Jull, G. (2017). Biopsychosocial model of disease: 40 years on. Which way is the pendulum swinging? *British Journal of Sports Medicine* **51** (16): 1187–1188. doi: 10.1136/bjsports-2016-097362.

Kitson, A., Marshall, A., Bassett, K. et al. (2013). What are the core elements of patient-centred care? A narrative review and synthesis of the literature from health policy, medicine and nursing. Journal of advanced nursing. *Journal of Advanced Nursing* **69** (1): 4–15.

Kolbe, M., Marty, A., Seelandt, J. et al. (2016). How to debrief teamwork interactions: using circular questions to explore and change team interaction patterns. *Advances in Simulation* **1** (29): 1–8.

Krumrey-Fulks, K. (2023). Intercultural communication. In: Nonverbal Communication (ed.K. Krumrey). Open, Oregon: Press Books.

Kuipers, J., Cramm, J., Nieboer, A. (2019). The importance of patient-centred care and co-creation of care for satisfaction with care and physical and social well-being of patients with multi-morbidity in the primary care setting. *BMC Health Services Research* **19** (13): 1–9.

84

Kwame, A. and Petrucka, P. (2021). A literature-based study of patient-centered care and communication in nurse-patient interactions: barriers, facilitators, and the way forward. *BMC Nursing* **20** (158): 1–10.

Lapum, J., St-Amant, O., Hughes, M. et al. (eds.). (2020a). *Introduction to Communication in Nursing*. Open, Oregan: Pressbooks.

Lynøe, N.E. and Juth, N. (2021). How to reveal disguised paternalism: version 2.0. *BMC Medical Ethics* **22, Article 170**.

Merriman, C.D., Stayt, L.C., and Ricketts, B. (2014). Comparing the effectiveness of clinical simulation versus didactic methods to teach undergraduate adult nursing students to recognize and assess the deteriorating patient. *Clinical Simulation in Nursing* **10** (3): e119–e127. doi: 10.1016/j.ecns.2013.09.004.

Minnican, C. and O'Toole, G. (2020). Exploring the incidence of culturally responsive communication in Australian healthcare: the first rapid review on this concept. *BMC Health Services Research* **20** (20): 1–14.

Nancarrow, S., Booth, A., Ariss, S. et al. (2013). Ten Principles of good interdisciplinary team work. *Human Resources for Health* **11** (19): 1–11.

Pearson, J.C. and Nelson, P.E. (2000). *An Introduction to Human Communication: Understanding and Sharing.* McGraw-Hill Higher Education.

Preston, P. (2005). Nonverbal communication: do you really say what you mean? *Journal of Healthcare Management* **50** (2): 83–86. doi: 10.1097/00115514-200503000-00004.

Queensland Health. (2015). Aboriginal and Torres Strait Islander Cultural Capability. Available at: Cultural Capability | Queensland Health (accessed 23 October 2023).

Relman, A.S. (2001). The institute of medicine report on the quality of health care crossing the quality chasm: a new health system for the 21st century. *New England Journal of Medicine* **345:** 702–703.

Rider, E. and Keefer, C. (2006). Communication skills competencies: definitions and a teaching toolbox. *Medical Education* **40:** 624–629.

Ruben, B.D. (2016). Communication theory and health communication practice: the more things change, the more they stay the same. *Health Communication* **31** (1). doi: 10.1080/10410236.2014.923086.

Ruhl, D. and Homan, M. (2020). An example of employing the principles of bioethics to medical decision making in the Covid-19 era. *The Laryngoscope* **130**.

Servotte, J., Welch-Horan, T.B., Mullan, P. et al. (2020). Development and implementation of an end-of-shift clinical debriefing method for emergency departments during Covid-19. *Advances in Simulation* **5** (32): 1–11.

Siewert, B. (2017). Building a new culture of safety. *HealthManagement .org* **17** (5): 388–390.

Tosas, M.R. (2022). Interrupting patients in healthcare settings: what is being interrupted? *Cult Med Psychiatry* **46:** 827–845.

University of Buffalo. (2015). What is Trauma-informed Care. Work.

Uono, S.H. and Hietanen, J.K. (2015). Eye contact perception in the west and east: a cross-cultural study. *PMC* **10** (2).

Wanko Keutchafo, E.L., Kerr, J., and Jarvis, M.A. (2020). Evidence of nonverbal communication between nurses and older adults: a scoping review. *BMC Nurs* **19** (53). doi: 10.1186/s12912-020-00443-9.

WHO. (2007). *People Centred Health Care – A Policy Framework.* World Health Organization.

Yianni, L. and Rodd, I. (2017). G236(P)Pace – 'probe, alert, challenge, escalate' model of graded assertiveness used in paediatric resuscitation. *Archives of Disease in Childhood* **102** (1).

Bibliography

ACSQHC. (2017). National Safety and Quality Health Service Standards. Available at: https://www.safetyandquality.gov.au (accessed February 2023).

ACSQHC. (2022a). Communicating for safety. Available at: https://www.safetyandquality.gov.au (accessed February 2023).

ACSQHC. (2022b). Communicating with patients and colleagues. Available at: https://www.safetyandquality.gov.au/our-work/communicating-safety/communicating-patients-and-colleagues (accessed February 2023).

ACSQHC. (2023a). Clinical Handover. Available at: Available at: https://www.safetyandquality.gov.au/our-work/communicating-safety/clinical-handover (accessed February 2023).

ACSQHC. (2023b). Communicating for safety resource portal. Available at: https://c4sportal.safetyandquality.gov.au/communicating-with-patients-and-colleagues (accessed February 2023).

ACSQHC. (2023c). Communication at clinical handover. Available at: https://www.safetyandquality.gov.au/standards/nsqhs-standards/communicating-safety-standard/communication-clinical-handover (accessed February 2023).

ACSQHC. (2023d). Communication of critical information. Available at: https://www.safetyandquality.gov.au/standards/nsqhs-standards/communicating-safety-standard/communication-critical-information (accessed February 2023).

ACSQHC. (2010). OSSIE guide to clinical handover improvement. Available at: https://www.safetyandquality.gov.au/sites/default/files/2019-12/ossie_guide_to_clinical_handover_improvement.pdf (accessed February 2023).

Dixson, M., Greenwell, M., Rogers-Stacy, C. et al. (2016). *Instructor's Corner: Nonverbal Immediacy Behaviors and Online Student Engagement*. National Communication Association. Available at: https://www.natcom.org/communication-currents/instructor's-corner-nonverbal-immediacy-behaviors-and-online-student (accessed February 2023).

Kumar, A. (2021). types of communication: verbal, non-verbal, written, visual, feedback, mass, group communication. Available at: https://getuplearn.com/blog/types-of-communication (accessed February 2023).

Lapum, J., St-Amant, O., Hughes, M. et al. (2020b). *Types of Interviewing Questions*. Open, Oregan: Pressbooks. Available at: https://pressbooks.library.torontomu.ca/communicationnursing/chapter/types-of-interviewing-questions (accessed February 2023).

Menschner, C. and Maul, A. (2016). Key ingredients for successful trauma – informed care implementation. Available at: https://www.samhsa.gov/sites/default/files/programs_campaigns/childrens_mental_health/atc-whitepaper-040616.pdf (accessed February 2023).

MHCC. (2022). *Recovery Orientated Language Guide – Words Matter*. M.H.C.C. NSW. Available at: https://mhcc.org.au/wp-content/uploads/2022/07/Recovery-Oriented-Language-Guide-Mental-Health-Coordinating-Council-2022.pdf (accessed February 2023).

OpenRN. (2023). *Proxemics*. Open Education Alberta. Available at: https://openeducationalberta.ca/foundationsforsuccessinnursing/chapter/2-2-basic-communication-concepts (accessed February 2023).

Rogers, K. (2023). *Interactive model of communication: definition & application*. Study.com. Available at: https://study.com/academy/lesson/interactive-model-of-communication-definition-application.html (accessed February 2023).

SAHealth. (2013). *The Teach - Back Method*. SA Health Safety and Quality Unit. https://www.sahealth.sa.gov.au/wps/wcm/connect/acb97c004e4552aeac22af8ba24f3db9/HLT-TeachBackMethod-T4-PHCS-SQ-20130118.pdf (accessed February 2023).

Srivastava, S. (n.d.). The patient interview. Available at: https://samples.jbpub.com/9781449652722/9781449645106_ch01_001_036.pdf (accessed February 2023).

SwitzerOnLeadership. (2023). The communication process – seven essential elements. Available at: https://www.switzeronleadership.com/the-communication-process-seven-essential-elements (accessed February 2023).

TraumaVic. (2023). Teamwork and communication. Available at: https://trauma.reach.vic.gov.au/guidelines/teamwork-and-communication/dealing-with-issues (accessed February 2023).

University of Minnesota. (2023). The communication process. Available at: https://open.lib.umn.edu/communication/chapter/1-2-the-communication-process (accessed February 2023).

University of Minnesota. (2023). Communication in the real world. Available at: https://open.lib.umn.edu/communication/chapter/4-2-types-of-nonverbal-communication (accessed February 2023).

WA.gov. (n.d.). *Culturally responsive assessment questions for CBT+ - DCYF*. Available at: https://www.dcyf.wa.gov/sites/default/files/pdf/CulturallyResponsiveQuestions.pdf.

Windle, R. and Warren, S. (2017). Communication Skills. The Centre for Appropriate Dispute Resolution in Special Education. Available at: https://www.cadreworks.org/resources/communication-skills (accessed February 2023).

CHAPTER 8

Practice-based learning

Joe Copson

Lecturer in Paramedic Science, University of East Anglia – PhD student, University of Hertfordshire, UK

Vince Clarke

Principal Lecturer and Programme Leader Paramedic Science, University of Hertfordshire, UK

Contents

LEARNING OUTCOMES

On completion of this chapter the reader will be able to:

- Recognise the importance of practice-based learning in initial paramedic education.
- Understand the role of the student in practice-based learning.
- Understand the role of the practice educator in practice-based learning.
- Identify how learners might seek further support when undertaking practice-based learning.
- Engage in reflective practice.
- Recognise the challenges associated with transition to practice.

Fundamentals of Paramedic Practice: A Systems Approach, Third Edition. Edited by Sam Willis and Ian Peate.

Companion website: www.wiley.com/go/willis/paramedic3e

Case study

Jess and Josh are first-year student paramedics who are about to embark on their first practice placement. They want to learn more about why they are undertaking practice placement, what they are likely to learn, what their responsibilities are, and who will support them through the process.

This chapter will help Jess and Josh to recognise the reasons for undertaking practice placement, as well as providing details about skills they may learn and develop throughout their experience. The chapter will also provide Jess and Josh with considerations to optimise their readiness for practice-based learning, learning opportunities and their enjoyment of their experience in the placement environment.

Introduction: the evolution of UK paramedic practice-based learning

The paramedic role has developed significantly since its inception. In the 1960s the role was often defined as that of an 'ambulance driver', and staff were unqualified and untrained. By the late 1990s, the paramedic role had developed to that of a registered healthcare professional, and paramedic practice utilised fundamental principles from medicine and nursing to inform practice (Clarke 2020).

Nursing philosophy underpinned higher education routes for paramedic training and education, as well as principles, from established healthcare programmes such as occupational therapy, radiography, and physiotherapy (Donaghy 2010; Clarke 2020).

The first UK national paramedic training programme, approved by the Department of Health and Social Security, was piloted in 1986. As part of the paramedic extended skills training, placements in hospitals were introduced, which developed the use of practice-based learning in paramedic education. However, the initial focus of these placements was psycho-motor skill acquisition, linking theory and practice by undertaking skills in a hospital environment, notably different from the reality of practice for the majority of paramedics (Clarke 2020). As a result, it was identified in 2000 that paramedic education and experience needed to be:

> *"broadened and improved for those personnel involved in pre-hospital care and specifically for paramedics . . . [concluding that] . . . paramedic training does not provide the underpinning education for sound clinical judgement to be exercised or indeed expected" (JRCALC 2000, p. 3)*

Critical thinking is a prerequisite for sound clinical judgement in practice, and paramedic education required a greater depth of underpinning theoretical content to facilitate the development of critical thinking skills (Fero et al. 2010). A diverse range of practice experiences was, therefore, required to apply and consolidate theoretical concepts (Clarke 2020). Following the recommendations of JRCALC (2000), the professional regulation of paramedics in 2001, and to facilitate the increased need for theory and practice alignment in paramedic education and practice, paramedic higher education programmes were further developed (Clarke 2020).

Paramedic programmes routinely place learners in the ambulance service setting, most often on a double-crewed ambulance as an additional person, i.e. supernumerary. Such placements can be undertaken in blocks, generally of four to six weeks, or in a more flexible 'day release' approach where learners will attend their education provider for two or three days each week and their placement on the remaining days. Placement providers tend to find block placements easier to facilitate, so these are by far the most common approach.

The development of the paramedic profession, and wider recognition of the diverse skillset of paramedics, has led to an increased diversity of opportunities for paramedic employment in multiple healthcare settings. In addition to the ambulance service, paramedics can now be found working in primary and urgent care, hospital departments, and many other areas of practice (Clarke 2020). This variety of settings has broadened the provision of placements within some educational programmes to give learners a greater breadth of experience within their practice-based learning opportunities.

Learning point: *understanding your history can help with your future* (Clarke 2020, p. 5)
Knowledge of the history of the profession, and the development of paramedic education and training, is important for students and educators. This knowledge aids understanding of the way in which contemporary methods of education were developed.

Apprenticeships

Historically, paramedics were educated through in-service, employed, models. Although not strictly 'apprenticeships', these routes to qualification shared many characteristics with modern day degree apprenticeships for paramedics. Apprenticeships are programmes used in vocational professions to combine employment with education. Student learning through apprenticeship schemes provides a process of observation, with incremental increases in participation in practical elements of the job.

In other disciplines, apprenticeships have been seen to bridge the theory–practice gap (Akkerman and Bakker 2012). Within the paramedic profession, the initial work-based schemes contained limited classroom-based learning and, over time, struggled to adapt educational content alongside the real-world developments in terms of patient presentations, equipment used in practice, and patient care techniques used by paramedics (Clarke 2020).

In recent times in the UK, degree-level apprenticeships have been developed to facilitate training of paramedics to the threshold level required for registration. Degree-level apprenticeship programme facilitation is complex, and flexible programme design is critical (King et al. 2016). Amalgamation of higher education provided by universities, which combines higher-level thinking, with the vocational aspects of on-the-job training is essential for success in this model (Mulkeen et al. 2019).

Learners on apprenticeships face different challenges to those on full-time undergraduate programmes because of the duality of their role, i.e., they are both an employee and a learner. As an employee, the apprentice may be working alongside non-registered support staff and responding to a range of urgent and emergency ambulance calls to deliver care one day, then be working under the supervision of a practice educator and expected to take on the role of the learner and approach cases in a different way the next day. The differing pressures of being an employee and a learner can be challenging for both the learner and the employer to navigate. As such, it often falls to the education provider to ensure that learners undertaking an apprenticeship are fully and appropriately supported by their employer to balance their education needs.

Undergraduate degrees

Increasingly, across the world, completion of an undergraduate degree is necessary to become a paramedic. Undergraduate degrees for paramedics have been developed based on the recognition of the expansion of the paramedic scope of practice. Historically, the paramedic role covered a wide demographic of patients across the lifespan but recently has expanded rapidly in terms of clinical skills, decision-making, equipment usage, and treatment options for individuals at all stages of life.

Degree-level education aims to teach students fundamental principles, which can be applied in a variety of settings, developing students' ability to learn and problem solve in any given situation. Recognising the variety of presentations that paramedics may be faced with, and the inability to solely use rote learning to effectively deal with the complexity of contemporary practice, undergraduate degrees must adequately prepare student paramedics for transition into a complex adaptive system.

Originally, degrees tended to be closely aligned to traditional ambulance service pathways, with extra modules taught in areas such as law and ethics and biosciences. These modules were often adapted from other allied health profession degree courses and delivered by academics from these courses (Clarke 2020). As there are now many suitably qualified paramedic academics, paramedic degrees are currently widely provided by profession-specific academic staff.

Paramedic degree programmes are also increasingly able to develop their own syllabus, aligning with the standards of both regulators and professional bodies. This has allowed for integration of further pedagogical and learning theory within the paramedic curriculum. Developing the pedagogical approach to paramedic education allows teaching of fundamental theoretical elements that can then be applied in a practice placement setting. Taylor (2007) notes that clinical placements allow recognition of theoretical principles in the real world. Undergraduate degrees attempt to instil the congruence of science and art required to be a successful paramedic, the underpinning scientific knowledge, and the art of applying this across varied austere settings. In order to be successful in this endeavour, both academic staff and practice educators must be suitably qualified to provide optimal educational experiences.

> ***Learning point:*** *a graduate profession*
> *"The evolution to a graduate profession does not prevent non-graduate paramedics from supporting learners in practice."* (Clarke 2020 p. 7) There remains a high number of very experienced and capable non-degree educated paramedics in the workforce. The benefits to the learner of the wealth of experience of non-degree paramedic practice educators cannot be understated.

Paramedic students as practice-based learners

Practice-based learning undertaken during practice placements and sometimes known as work integrated learning, provides students with opportunities to increase their knowledge and apply previously gained theoretical understanding in the clinical environment (Kirkpatrick et al. 1991; Wills 1997; Atack et al. 2000).

Additionally, practice-based learning enables students to develop wider, interpersonal attributes like communication and empathy alongside other professional attributes such as professional identity (Clarke 2020).

For practice placements to achieve any of these outcomes they must be carefully planned and the placement setting well prepared for students to attend. This means having practice educators, or similar, available to students for the entirety of their placement experience. This requirement is generally well met in the context of ambulance service placements; however, student paramedics attend a variety of placements in a wide range of health and social care settings. For these placements to be beneficial for the student, the placement provider and the practice educator must be made aware of the purpose and learning outcomes associated with each placement setting (Clarke 2020).

Students rely heavily on their assigned practice educators during practice and socialisation of the paramedic student is often dependent on that single relationship (Lane et al. 2016).

There are three main purposes of practice placements: to allow students to gain professional skills, attitudes and knowledge; to allow the theorising of practice and the practical application of theory (Schön 1983); and, to allow enculturation and professional identity formation, whereby students adopt their professional culture (Waters 2001).

'Situated learning' is a process during which student paramedics on practice placement construct their professional identity through contributing to the practice environment, and social engagements with the community of practice (Lave and Wenger 1991). Students are likely to work with many different practice educators during their clinical placements. All educators will have had varied experiences of practice, and these experiences will shape the way they perform their clinical role and educate students. The student must find a way to optimally utilise the experiences and knowledge of their educators, and their own exposure to novel and diverse experiences, to contextualise and develop their individual practice (Clarke 2020).

Placements in non-ambulance settings also help the student paramedic's development, although the challenges associated with such placements include a lack of understanding of roles and of the purpose of such placements. As such, appropriate preparation of both student and practice educator or mentor – as well as the placement setting itself – is vital to ensure that such placements help the student develop the necessary attributes and their professional identity, rather than limiting the placement to an observational experience.

The supernumerary learner

The term 'supernumerary' is often used when describing practice-based learning, especially in undergraduate programmes. The term simply means 'present in excess of the normal or requisite number'. Within paramedic education, there has been an increase in supernumerary learner numbers within ambulance services as degree programmes have expanded, although apprenticeship schemes sometimes do not give as many opportunities for supernumerary practice placements within ambulance settings. In the majority of cases, practice-based learning undertaken in wider healthcare settings, i.e., not ambulance services, will always be in a supernumerary capacity. In these settings it is important to distinguish between supernumerary and 'observational'. This point will be discussed later.

For the student paramedic, the nature of being truly supernumerary reduces ambiguity around the supernumerary status of a learner, which is often lost to remote supervision and service provision in healthcare settings (Sarre et al. 2018). Supernumerary status has clear benefits for student experience and learning as it allows students to work directly alongside experienced educators throughout their training.

There are, however, some key issues that must be considered in relation to supernumerary learning experiences. The nature of being supernumerary means there are differences in experience when compared to the perceived paramedic role. An example of this would be the dynamics of the practical environment, working as part of a three-person crew, as opposed to a two-person crew, and the different challenges that may be faced in decision-making with fewer individuals involved. In addition, supernumerary learners often rely heavily on their practice educator for socialisation and immersion into communities of practice. Supernumerary status, especially as a student from a different institution, can cause difficulties with role identity, onboarding, and socialisation, leading to students feeling subordinate (Elcock et al. 2007; Garratt 2023).

Educators supporting supernumerary learners should be aware of these potential issues to create an optimal learning environment to support the student; guiding the individual through socialisation and onboarding into communities of practice. Educators must encourage discussion around the differences between experiences and potential effects of changing dynamics. Students should attempt to reflect on the impact of direct supervision and support, and how things might change as a new registrant. Students must also feel empowered to seek support where necessary for issues that arise in practice, irrelevant of their supernumerary status.

In order to maximise learning opportunities, it is of particular importance that practice-based learning in non-ambulance settings is professionally managed. Practice educators/facilitators need to be made fully aware of the role and scope of practice of the student paramedic, as well as why they are attending a placement in what might appear to be a 'non-paramedic' setting. Students who are undertaking placement in non-ambulance settings should have knowledge of the learning outcomes for the placement and a clear knowledge of, and access to, equal support systems within this alternative environment.

> ***Learning point:** supernumerary learning*
> Supernumerary learning has clear benefits, but the potential impacts of supernumerary learning in different environments should be considered at student, educator, and organisational levels.

The benefits of practice-based learning

In many disciplines, students are required to engage in practice placements. Practice placements are considered to enable the application of theoretical principles in the real world (Taylor 2007), and give students the opportunity to gain exposure and experience in their role, and to exhibit relevant competencies in the practice environment (Clarke 2020). The benefits of practice-based learning are numerous, as presented by the College of Paramedics (Clarke 2020 p. 15 & p. 16). For the learner these include the opportunity to:

- Translate theory and underpinning knowledge into practice.
- Gain practical experience of providing direct patient care whilst being fully supported.
- Develop appropriate attitude, behaviour, and professional standards.
- Develop as a reflective practitioner, learning from direct experience.
- Develop an understanding of the importance of 'lifelong learning'.

The benefits of practice-based learning for the practice educator include:

- The ability to maintain clinical practice whilst being recognised for knowledge, skills, experience, and leadership.
- Further development of leadership and management skills/competency.
- Development as a reflective healthcare professional with continuous learning from direct experience and chance to translate theory and latest evidence-based research into practice.
- The opportunity to contribute to a 'community of practice' and develop practice education as a key component of the paramedic profession.

Outside of the learner/practice educator relationship, there are many benefits of practice-based learning for patients and service users, practice-based education providers, employers of paramedics, and commissioners of services (Clarke 2020).

The role of the student

The paramedic student is the only participant who plays a role in all aspects of their educational pathway. They are in the classroom, they undertake simulation, and they experience practice placements. As such, it is the responsibility of the student to bring together all of these aspects and consolidate them during practice. Not all students will have exactly the same experiences in each of the learning settings, and to expect this would be unrealistic. It is vitally important that each individual student knows what they are expected to achieve during practice-based learning, whether this be in ambulance or wider healthcare settings.

Having clear learning objectives, from both a course and an individual perspective, is key in achieving effective practice-based learning. In the majority of cases, these learning objectives are dictated by the education provider. However, individualised learning objectives should be encouraged, and these should be owned by the learner and shared with their practice educator at the beginning of any practice-based learning opportunity. Such initial meetings and discussions are key in all settings but can prove particularly beneficial in wider health and social care placements where the scope of practice of the paramedic may not be fully understood by the placement provider/mentor and there is greater scope for a failed placement experience.

Clarke (2020, p. 26) states that the student is *"the conduit by which theory and practice will both be experienced and integrated into their understanding of their professional role and the development of their own personal professional knowledge."* As such, it is important that they adopt appropriate methods of development and metacognition such as reflective practice. Taking responsibility for one's own learning is a key expectation of students in practice. Students are expected to adhere to policies set by education providers and placements such as uniform dress code, confidentiality, and health and safety. Failure to meet these standards may result in a failed placement experience. Some students find the transition from the education provider to the workplace, where there are sometimes very different expectations in regard to behaviours, to be a particular challenge.

Developing reflective practice

The ability to reflect on one's own professional practise is a fundamental skill for any healthcare practitioner. Reflective practice is essential for maintaining the ability to practice safely within complex and dynamic healthcare contexts and developing as a practitioner. Comprehensive reflection aids systematic and thorough development of oneself as a professional, recognising areas for development as well as areas of strength. As a result, paramedic educational curriculums now widely incorporate reflective practice.

The development of the requisite skills to effectively engage in reflective practice is imperative for the transition to professional practice as a new registrant. Beyond the university setting opportunities to receive structured formal feedback, or for facilitated reflection, may be limited. It is therefore important for student paramedics to utilise practice education experiences to develop and apply reflective techniques.

Reflective practices have developed markedly in recent times, and there is an abundance of theoretically based techniques to deploy whilst engaging in reflection. Multiple models exist to aid in the process of reflection and are widely adopted within education and healthcare. Models, including Kolb's (1984) Experiential Learning Cycle, Gibbs's (1988) Reflective Cycle, Rolfe et al.'s (2001) Reflective Model, and Driscoll's (2007) Model of Reflection, utilise theoretical concepts to provide a structured process for reflective activities. In addition, several paramedic specific approaches to reflective practice have been developed including those of Willis (2010), Smart (2011), Pocock (2013), and Turner (2015).

Traditionally, reflection was seen as a process carried out by individuals on their individual actions, hopefully leading to an individual change or development of practice. Whilst individual reflection still has its merits, there are benefits to reflecting as a team or with peers. It is important to remember as a student or new registrant one may have less of an intuitive ability to be able to reflect effectively; peer reflection can help with this. In addition, there has been a shift from independence to interdependence in reflection, and individuals are encouraged to use their own reflections to recognise issues and inspire change and quality improvement on a wider scale.

In-depth reflection helps people to analyse their previous experiences and preconceptions, and what they, as an individual, bring to a situation. Engaging in reflection is important to recognise how previous experiences are informing and impacting one's current practice, both positively and negatively.

Reflection is fundamental to continuing to develop as a professional and to performing at the highest level possible. Developing strategies for embedding reflection and reflexivity into one's practice is an essential skill for any paramedic. Within paramedic practice, the necessity of engagement with CPD has been demonstrated by the paradigm shift in the paramedic role over recent years. Understandably, professional bodies and regulators often have standards of proficiency directly related to reflective practice. As an autonomous evidence-based practitioner, one must continuously develop contemporaneously with evidence-based changes, modern technologies, and new techniques to continue to practice effectively. Reflection on one's own practice as a way of identifying areas for development is essential for safe clinical practice.

The student's ability to link theory and practice is enhanced through the combination of clinical practice experiences, and theoretical teaching. This amalgamation is key *in "perpetuating a developmental learning cycle of the type proposed by Kolb (1984)."* (Clarke 2020, p.10).

The relationship between the practice educator and the student paramedic can be mutually beneficial, as a successful relationship will empower both individuals to develop their practice (Clarke 2020). This development of practice is formulated through critical discussion and utilisation of the model of professional thinking.

Professional thinking is described by Clarke (2020, p. 28) as *"the ability to clearly analyse decision-making and engage in self and peer reflection. This involves a combination of deliberation and discussion, rational thinking, clinical reasoning, professional knowing, and expertise gained from previous knowledge."*

Professional thinking in the practice environment should be collaboratively developed between the student paramedic and the practice educator, reinforcing the symbiotic relationship that enables reflection and will enhance the practice of both individuals (Clarke 2020).

As a student, feedback from peers and practice educators will be fundamental in supporting an individual's development as a reflective practitioner. As such, it is important that students adopt responsibility for proactively seeking feedback during practice education.

Although the student is central to their own development, external factors can have a significant impact on the student's ability to link theory and practice, including the practice educator. A key role of the practice educator must therefore be to facilitate learning and encourage students to engage in reflective practice whilst congruently reflecting on their own clinical and educational practice.

The role of the practice educator

Practice educators in paramedic practice-based learning are referred to variously as mentors, supervisors, work-based trainers, and clinical tutors. The nomenclature itself is less important than clarity around the definition of the term, and therefore the role. Defining the term 'practice educator' allows delineation of the responsibilities of the role and provides coherence for practice educators and students which enables effective management of expectations and development of successful educator-student relationships (Clarke 2020).

The College of Paramedics (Clarke 2020, p.28) defines a practice educator as follows:

> *"The practice educator (PEd) undertakes a multi-faceted role, including being a Role Model, Leader, Teacher, Coach, Assessor and Mentor. They have a responsibility for ensuring the clinical supervision and development of a learner in the practice-based environment."*

The practice educator role is considered to be that of a paramedic who is directly supporting the development of a student paramedic in practice. Other terms may be adopted for ongoing support of qualified/registered individuals, for example, preceptor or clinical mentor. The remit of these roles, however, is somewhat different to that of the practice educator.

The successful facilitation of practice education involves enabling the practical application of theoretical principles and knowledge, skill acquisition and development, and enhancement of critical thinking and decision-making abilities (Clarke 2020). Roles undertaken by practice educators to facilitate practice education are varied and multiplex, as practice educators are responsible for "*creating, nurturing, and managing an effective learning environment, in partnership with the learner.*" (Clarke 2020 p. 28).

In order to achieve this goal, practice educators should be well prepared for their role, with the College of Paramedics advocating a minimum of a level 6 academic qualification in practice education for any paramedics undertaking the role.

Practice educators are expected to undertake the ongoing support, development, and assessment of their students alongside being clinically responsible for any service users that they attend. On occasion, the service user will take priority over the student and learning is facilitated following an incident rather than during it. This should be a reasonably expected approach to development and the student should be prepared to engage with learning discussions before, during, and after incidents.

It is not the role of the practice educator to teach students the theoretical principles behind their approaches/interventions. This is the role of the education provider and the student.

Learner support: neurodiversity

Some students may be diagnosed with developmental conditions such as autistic spectrum disorders (ASD), dyslexia, or dyspraxia. These conditions are often recognised by legislation (e.g., in the UK as part of the Equality Act 2010), meaning that it is against the law for an education provider or employer to discriminate against such individuals on the basis of their diagnosis (Clarke 2020).

Education providers and employers have a duty to make 'reasonable adjustments' to ensure these learners are not discriminated against. Such adjustments may include providing extra support and aids such as computers or overlays for books and/or screens, as well as additional time for examinations and assessments (Clarke 2020).

"The practice-based learning environment of the paramedic is sometimes not conducive to making the same reasonable adjustments that may be put in place for classroom teaching and assessment. Practice educators who are supporting learners with identified learning differences must be familiar with the potential impact that this will have on the learning experience." (Clarke 2020, p. 92). Working in close partnership with the student and their education provider will help support not only the student but also the practice educator and, as such, tripartite meetings should be encouraged and supported to identify challenges and support mechanisms early in a student's placement experience.

Learner well-being

A learner's experiences during practice placements contribute to the development of their individual approaches to resilience and self-care; elements that can be considered as 'well-being'. Resilience can be defined as the ability to feel better quickly after unpleasant experiences such as shock or injury (OALD 2024), which often involve challenging situations the learner/student paramedic may be encountering for the first time. Resilience can be learned, although it is often tacit learning, which the individual is not necessarily fully aware of (Clarke 2020).

Developing resilience is unique to the individual. By appreciating that experiences will impact on individuals in different ways, both the learner and the practice educator can be open to discussing how incidents have been perceived and how, perhaps by a process of reflection, better understanding of the situation and its impact on the learner can be explored. Such self-awareness, supported by the input of the practice educator, can facilitate development of a learner's resilience over time.

Early identification of any potential challenges, related to either mental or physical health, is key in gaining the most appropriate support. Practice educators may be the first to notice changes in a learner's behaviour. For example, the learner may have become more withdrawn and less communicative over their time in practice. Early communication between the learner and the practice educator is needed so that both parties can access appropriate support and help. Practice educators are not necessarily in the best position to offer specific guidance to learners in relation to their mental well-being; however, they are in a position to seek guidance from the education provider and to work with education providers to determine the best method of support for learners. On occasion, it may be best if a learner is temporarily removed from placement, although the potential impact of such a move on the learner's mental health must be considered.

Learners' self-identification of negative feelings in relation to practice is very important to prevent a negative impact on all aspects of their study and life. Seeking help should be considered a strength and recognition of particular triggers or situations that give rise to negative feelings is key in developing coping strategies over time.

Support structures

It is essential for students to know how to access the support structures available to them whilst immersed in practice education.

Ahead of a first placement, students should ensure that they are aware of how to access support from the education provider, the practice environment organisation, and any other support services that may be relevant to them as an individual. This includes gaining contact details for the individuals who act as the first point of contact when support is required and clarity on the processes in place.

Remember that peer support can be fundamental to thriving as a student. Encouraging development of peer support structures will be of benefit to all students.

Transition to practice (initial)

Every student enters their first practice placement with differing previous life, workplace, and clinical experiences. As a result, ahead of first immersion into clinical practice, individuals have varying preconceptions, which may be influenced by anticipatory socialisation. Anticipatory socialisation is a process by which individuals outside the paramedic profession, who aspire to join it, may attempt to adopt perceived values and standards of the profession. However, lack of exposure to the professional environment may mean these preconceptions are formed by external influences such as social media and television, resulting in a distorted view of the paramedic experience (Devenish et al. 2016).

Managing expectations and preparing individuals for their first experiences of professional practice is challenging due to the dynamic nature of paramedic practice, the challenging environment, and the diversity of potential exposure.

Individuals must be adequately prepared to experience a wide range of clinical scenarios, without any guarantees of specific clinical exposure. Students must not act outside of their scope of practice, and so it is imperative that students and educators understand their scope of practice and what is expected of them during individual placements. As a student, speaking to senior staff, lecturers, and educators prior to a first placement will help to understand one's scope of practice and the realities of placement, limiting the impact of any potential misconceptions.

As an educator it is important to understand the student as an individual and their previous experiences and exposures as much as possible. Alongside this, educators must display adaptability, recognising that during a first placement the student is academically and clinically at a different level to others who may be further into their programme. Knowledge of the individual scope of practice of the student is essential to avoid both unnecessary stress for the student and the potential for students to be asked to act outside of their scope of practice, for example, performing skills they have not been verified as competent to complete.

A thorough induction to the clinical placement is paramount for students during their initial transition to practice and requisite knowledge of the practice environment must be provided to new students. Additionally, it is imperative that students know their own responsibilities and where support is available. Effective inductions are beneficial from multiple perspectives and help students transition to the practice environment from logistical, socialisation, safety, and well-being perspectives.

Conclusion

In a rapidly evolving profession, where individuals' responsibilities are continually expanding, a greater appreciation of the role of practice-based learning in the initial development of paramedics cannot be understated.

Paramedic practice-based learning has many similarities with other professions; however, it also has its own unique challenges. Such challenges need to be understood by learners, practice educators, placement facilitators, and educational establishments in order to ensure that learners remain safe and supported whilst developing their professional skills and identity.

Activities

Now review your learning by completing the learning activities in this chapter. The answers to these appear at the end of the book. Further self-test activities can be found at **www.wileyfundamentalseries.com/paramedic/3e.**

Test your knowledge

1. How might practice-based learning enhance paramedic students' overall competence?
   (a) By relying solely on theoretical knowledge.
   (b) By minimising the importance of practical skills.
   (c) By integrating classroom learning with real-world experiences.
   (d) By reducing exposure to patient care scenarios.
2. What is the primary focus of practice-based learning for paramedic students?
   (a) Academic research and publishing papers.
   (b) Hands-on training in real care settings.
   (c) Observing clinical procedures from a distance.
   (d) Memorisation of details in textbooks.
3. Practice-based learning enables paramedic students to:
   (a) Avoid the application of theoretical knowledge in real-life situations.
   (b) Develop expertise without practical experiences.
   (c) Apply classroom knowledge to clinical scenarios.
   (d) Rely solely on textbooks for patient care.
4. What role does reflection play in practice-based learning for paramedic students?
   (a) It is not necessary for the learning process.
   (b) It helps in memorising medical terminology.
   (c) It allows students to analyse their experiences and learn from them.
   (d) It only focuses on theoretical concepts.
5. Which approach is often used in practice-based learning for paramedic students to enhance clinical skills?
   (a) Participating in real world patient scenarios.
   (b) Watching instructional videos only.
   (c) Reading health and care journals and articles.
   (d) Attending lectures without hands-on training.

Activity 8.1

Set yourself some targets for what you would like to achieve in your next placement and how you can demonstrate these. Share them with your practice educator.

Activity 8.2

How would you measure these achievements? How would you ensure you have met your intended outcomes?

Activity 8.3

Using a reflective model of your choice, reflect on some experiences that led you to this point. For example, the reasons you wanted to be a paramedic.

Activity 8.4

Speak to your lecturers about the support processes in place for students in university and on placement and make sure you have a record of the relevant contact details.

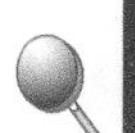

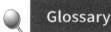

Glossary

Learner: Used to describe any individual who is undertaking learning in the practice setting. This will include students on formal educational pathways and those who have achieved qualification and are being supported in their transition to practice period.

Practice placements: Any formally arranged periods in which a learner is placed in a clinical area where they have direct contact with service users.

Practice-based learning: Also referred to as 'work integrated learning', this is the process by which a learner develops in the practice setting, more often than not under the guidance and support of a practice educator. In some settings, the terms 'practice placements', 'work integrated learning', and 'clinical placements' are used synonymously with practice-based learning.

Practice educator: The individual who directly supports a learner who is undertaking practice-based learning during a practice placement. In the ambulance service setting, the practice educator is usually expected to be the person with whom the learner is working on a daily basis. A practice educator is generally assigned to learners who have not yet achieved their qualification/registration and who are on a programme of study.

Mentor: The term 'mentor' is more generally used to describe individuals who support peers, i.e. those who have gained qualification/registration but are new to their work role. It is, however, sometimes also used to describe a practice educator. The term 'preceptor' is sometimes used when there is a formal preceptorship period a learner is required to undertake.

References

Akkerman, S.F. and Bakker, A. (2012) Crossing boundaries between school and work during apprenticeships. *Vocations and Learning* **5:** 153–173. doi: 10.1007/s12186-011-9073-6.

Atack, L., Comacu, M., Kenny, R. et al. (2000). Student and staff relationships in a clinical practice model: impact on learning. *Journal of Nursing Education* **39** (9): 387–400.

Clarke, V. (ed.) (2020). *Paramedic Practice-Based Learning: A Handbook for Practice Educators and Facilitators*. Bridgewater: College of Paramedics.

Devenish, A., Clark, M. and Fleming, M. (2016). Experiences in becoming a paramedic: the professional socialization of university qualified paramedics. *Creative Education* **7** (6): 786–801.

Donaghy, J. (2010). Equipping the student for workplace changes in paramedic education. *Journal of Paramedic Practice* **2** (11): 524–528.

Driscoll, J. (2007). *Practising Clinical Supervision: a Reflective Approach for Healthcare Professionals*. 2e. Edinburgh: Baillière Tindall Elsevier.

Elcock, K.S., Curtis, P., and Sharples, K. (2007). Supernumerary status–an unrealised ideal. *Nurse Education in Practice* **7** (1): 4–10.

Fero, L.J., O'Donnell, J.M., Zullo, T.G. et al. (2010). Critical thinking skills in nursing students: comparison of simulation-based performance with metrics. *Journal of Advanced Nursing* **66** (10): 2182–2193.

Garratt, M. (2023). For when you just can't talk to 'normal' people... exploring the use of informal support structures by supernumerary university paramedic students: findings from a phenomenological study. *British Paramedic Journal* **7** (4): 1–7.

Gibbs, G. (1988). *Learning by Doing: A Guide to Teaching and Learning Methods*. Oxford: Oxford Further Education Unit.

Joint Royal Colleges Ambulance Liaison Committee. (2000). *The Future Role and Education of Paramedic Ambulance Service Personnel*. London: JRCALC.

King, M., Waters, M., Widdowson, J. et al. (2016). Higher technical skills: learning from the experiences of English FE colleges and Australian technical and further education institutes. *Higher Education, Skills and Work-Based Learning* **6** (4): 329–344. doi: 10.1108/HESWBL-06-2016-0039.

Kirkpatrick, H., Byrne, C., Martin, M. et al. (1991). A collaborative model for the clinical education of baccalaureate nursing students. *Journal of Advanced Nursing* **16** (1): 101–107.

Kolb, D. (1984). *Experiential Learning: Experience as the Source of Learning and Development*. Englewood Cliffs, NJ: Prentice-Hall.

Lane, M., Rouse, J. and Docking, R.E. (2016). Mentorship within the paramedic profession: a practice educator's perspective. *British Paramedic Journal* **1** (1): 2–8.

Lave, J., and Wenger, E. (1991). *Situated Learning: Legitimate Peripheral Participation*. Cambridge: Cambridge University Press.

Mulkeen, J., Abdou, H., Leigh, J. et al. (2019). Degree and higher level apprenticeships: an empirical investigation of stakeholder perceptions of challenges and opportunities. *Studies in Higher Education* **44** (2): 333–346. doi: 10.1080/03075079.2017.1365357.

Oxford Advanced Learners Dictionary (2024). *Definition of Resilience*. Available at: http://www.oxfordlearnersdictionaries.com/definition/english/resilience

Pocock, H. (2013). SQIFED: A new reflective model for action learning. *Journal of Paramedic Practice* **5** (3):146–151.

Rolfe, G., Freshwater, D., and Jasper, M. (2001). *Critical Reflection in Nursing and the Helping Professions: A User's Guide*. Basingstoke: Palgrave Macmillan.

Sarre, S., Maben, J., Aldus, C. et al. (2018). The challenges of training, support and assessment of healthcare support workers: a qualitative study of experiences in three English acute hospitals. *International Journal of Nursing Studies* **79:** 145–153.

Schön, D.A. (1983). *The Reflective Practitioner*. London: Temple Smith.

Smart, G. (2011). I.F.E.A.R reflection: an easy to use, adaptable template for paramedics. *Journal of Paramedic Practice* **3** (5): 255–257.

Taylor, C.A. (2007). Collaborative approach to developing 'learning synergy' in primary health care. *Nurse Education in Practice* **7** (1): 18–25.

Turner, H. (2015). Reflective practice for paramedics: a new approach. *Journal of Paramedic Practice* **7** (3): 138–141.

Waters, B. (2001). Radical action for radical plans. *The British Journal of Occupational Therapy* **64** (2): 577–578.

Willis, S. (2010). Becoming a reflective practitioner: frameworks for the prehospital professional. *Journal of Paramedic Practice* **2** (5): 212–216.

Wills, M. (1997). Link teacher behaviours: student nurses' perceptions. *Nurse Education Today* **17** (3): 232–246.

CHAPTER 9

Well-being for paramedics

Emma Geis

Lecturer, Award Lead MSci Paramedic Science, Keele University, UK

Katie Pavoni

Associate Professor, BSc Paramedic Science
Course Director & Pastoral Lead,
St George's, University of London, UK

Contents

LEARNING OUTCOMES

On completion of this chapter, the reader will be able to:

- Understand the context of paramedic well-being and associated stigma.
- Discuss the factors within paramedic practice that can have an adverse impact on well-being.
- Recognise signs of distress and personal vulnerability.
- Understand the importance of looking after one's emotional health and well-being as a health care professional, along with adopting self-care strategies and accessing support as required.

Fundamentals of Paramedic Practice: A Systems Approach, Third Edition. Edited by Sam Willis and Ian Peate.

Companion website: www.wiley.com/go/willis/paramedic3e

Case study 1

Kori is a student paramedic currently on ambulance practice placement. Kori recently experienced the breakdown of their long-term relationship and has since been working overtime at their job in a local restaurant to pay their rent, often meaning that with placement hours they are working multiple days and nights in a row.

Kori has recently been more irritable than usual with patients and appears to be more on edge. They mention to you that they have a reduced appetite, and that they have been withdrawing from their family and friends as they 'don't feel in the mood' for socialising. They also tell you they feel they are falling behind with university work and are 'losing motivation' for their study.

Consider:

1. What signs are there that Kori may be struggling with their well-being?
2. What factors may be impacting how Kori is feeling?
3. How would you respond to Kori and offer a supportive conversation?
4. What support strategies may be helpful for Kori?

Introduction

Mental health and well-being, just like physical health, affects us all. It is often described as a continuum (WHO 2022) and can change depending upon our health, life experiences, challenges, and individual circumstances. As human beings we are all vulnerable to times in our lives where we may experience difficulty, and we all experience mental health differently. No one is exempt from it; it is a human part of our existence and should be recognised as such, with the importance, equality, and compassion it deserves.

Although it is estimated that at any given time 25% of the population will experience a mental health problem (WHO 2023) there is still substantial stigma and negative, often discriminatory, attitudes and perceptions remain. This can create a barrier for individuals to seek help and prolongs their distress.

Mind (2020) identifies mental well-being as the state of a person who can contribute to their community, work productively and cope with normal stressors of life. Absence of a mental health condition does not naturally mean a person has a good well-being and caring for oneself by eating healthily, exercising, and sleeping well, for example, can promote healthy well-being (Mental Health Foundation 2021a).

The National Union of Students (NUS) (2023) states that the number of students in higher education experiencing mental health problems has doubled since 2014/2015. This may be as a result of a range of complex factors; however, it is recognised that higher education represents a significant period of transition and change, which can be intensified by distance from social support, financial pressures, and the evolution of personal identity (HEPI 2019).

This applies to all students at university; however, for healthcare students these risks can be amplified due to the unique challenges, pressures, and stressors of the healthcare environment and exposure to difficult and emotive situations whilst undertaking clinical placement (Van der Riet et al. 2015).

According to Kushal et al. (2018), 62% of healthcare professionals show stress associated symptoms. Johnson et al. (2018) affirm that mental well-being and burnout are considered to be an international concern for healthcare professionals. Further evidence from Shanafelt et al. (2017) highlights that alongside an impact on the individual, burnout and poor mental well-being can also reduce the quality of care given to patients. Recent research has also highlighted that in addition to facing well-being challenges, healthcare workers are at a greater risk of developing mental health conditions such as depressive disorders and post-traumatic stress disorder (PTSD) as a result of occupational factors.

The context of paramedic practice further exacerbates this risk, as individuals working within the profession often experience frequent exposure to traumatic situations, social isolation, operational demands, and emotional labour (Ramey et al. 2018). Therefore, awareness of these complex factors and of looking after our mental health and well-being early on in our career is essential. It will in turn support us as the future workforce.

Within the healthcare environment we often hear the expression 'You need to take care of yourself before you take care of others', or similar analogies that express the importance of self-care but often lack authentic enactment for a variety of reasons explored in this chapter. For paramedics, it is reported that individuals frequently fear disclosure due to preconceptions and stereotypes, and often feel that in some way, as the helpers, they are 'invincible' or heroes without problems or health needs of their own (Mind 2019a).

As students and paramedics, it is vital that we challenge these perceptions and acknowledge individual factors and the risks related to our profession that can impact our mental health and well-being. We need to recognise our own vulnerabilities, be mindful of our emotional responses and the signs that we may be struggling, and take steps to practice self-care, prevention, and self-compassion and proactively access support when needed.

This awareness of our mental health and well-being is at the heart of being a healthcare professional and is supported by professional and regulatory bodies such as the Health Care Professions Council (HCPC 2023). However, despite the importance and relevance to our patients, we must not forget that taking care of our mental health has humanitarian value, as it is what we all deserve.

This chapter will explore the context of well-being both as student paramedics and in the transition to paramedic practice. It will promote strategies for self-awareness and individual coping and resilience, and explore the importance of person-centred support.

Definitions

Understanding the range of terminology and language associated with mental health is important, not only in terms of recognition of our own emotional states and responses but also when accessing support.

Often terms such as 'mental health', 'mental illness', and 'mental well-being' are discussed interchangeably, but these have frequently subtle but important differences. For the purposes of this chapter, the following definitions will be used (WHO 2022):

- **Well-being:** a dynamic state that incorporates positive mental, physical, and social health. It includes individual prosperity, quality of life, and personal fulfilment.
- **Mental health:** 'a state of wellbeing in which the individual realises his or her abilities, can cope with the normal stresses of life, work productively and fruitfully, and is able to make a contribution to his or her community' (WHO 2022).
- **Mental health condition:** the presence of diagnosable or classified mental illness.

As mentioned earlier, the absence of a mental health condition does not naturally mean a person has a good well-being. Taking steps to care of oneself such as eating healthily, exercising, and sleeping well can promote a healthy well-being (Mental Health Foundation 2021a).

Similarly, recognition that the presence of a mental health issue or condition does not necessarily result in poor mental health and well-being is essential. With support and adaptive coping strategies, an individual's health can thrive in the way that it does with physical health. Conversely, experiencing challenges with our well-being does not mean that we have a mental health condition. This distinction is vital in terms of challenging stigma and acknowledging times of personal distress and difficulty.

Resilience

Resilience is a common term when discussing well-being and has a range of diverse interpretations within the literature. Despite this lack of firm definition, there is a consensus that personal resilience encompasses our ability to cope and 'keep going' in times of difficulty and to adapt and respond to challenging life experiences (Bennett 2015; British Red Cross 2023a). This can often be referred to as 'bouncing back'. However, rather than being static or fixed, the development of individual resilience is an ongoing and dynamic process, shaped and influenced by our unique circumstances.

Although our life challenges and resilience are unique to us all, it is vital to recognise that some people experience greater difficulty. This can be because of issues such as discrimination, including racism, transphobia, and homophobia, socio-economic deprivation, health challenges, and lack of access to support (Mind 2023a). Many individuals may experience multiple barriers, which can have a substantial impact upon well-being and resilience. Being mindful of this is essential when considering ourselves and supporting others.

For student paramedics, recognising that one is an individual and will have a unique journey when it comes to personal resilience is essential. It is important to also be aware that to be resilient does not mean the absence of difficulty, nor does it mean that we are not permitted to have emotional responses to emotive or challenging situations. Being resilient means being able to recognise difficult times, having the tools to cope, and knowing when to seek support.

Resilience can therefore be enhanced and evolved by being self-aware and identifying personal vulnerabilities, by adopting and developing adaptive coping strategies and support networks, and by looking after and nurturing our well-being.

Stigma

Although we can all experience challenges with our mental health and well-being, significant stigma is still associated with our psychological health (Mind 2023b). Furthermore, people experiencing mental health problems often face unacceptable discrimination, along with negative attitudes and perceptions that can have a detrimental impact upon engagement with support and recovery (Mental Health Foundation 2021b). Stigma is a complex entity with several subdivisions. For the context of this chapter, this has been streamlined and the core aspects of social stigma (or public stigma), self-stigma (or internalised stigma), and professional stigma (Subu et al. 2021) will be explored.

Social stigma

Social stigma is the negative public attitudes and stereotypes regarding mental health (Subu et al. 2021). Literature suggests that people experiencing mental health challenges are more likely to experience social stigma than people with physical illnesses. These thoughts and beliefs are often based upon media misrepresentation, which has created a sense of fear and a lack of compassion and understanding as a result of the damaging misconception that mental health problems are a 'choice' (Kowalski and Peipert 2019). Therefore, not only do people have to manage the impact of their condition but also often demeaning and detrimental public attitudes alongside it.

Often social stigma can lead to direct discrimination, with individuals being treated differently as a result of their mental health diagnosis or well-being challenges (Haddad and Haddad 2015). For example, a person may be excluded being from social events, or have different requirements because of mental health medication. This often results in unnecessary delays in the disclosure of difficulty and accessing support, with people suffering for longer in silence. This discrimination, alongside being morally and ethically unjust, is illegal in the UK. The Equality Act (2010) safeguards the rights of individuals with protected characteristics such as health challenges and states that no one should be discriminated against or treated unfairly as a result.

Self-stigma

Self-stigma relates to negative attitudes and perceptions that are internalised, leading to guilt, blame, low self-esteem, and hopelessness (Haddad and Haddad 2015). These cognitive processes can often result in social isolation, withdrawal, and concealment of emotional distress (Stolzenburg et al. 2017; Gartner et al. 2022). This can again lead to a delay in accessing help.

Professional stigma

Professional stigma relates to the negative attitudes and perceptions of healthcare professionals regarding people with mental health problems and well-being challenges (Gartner et al. 2022). This is particularly concerning, as several studies have highlighted inequitable care and treatment within a variety of healthcare services, to which unfortunately paramedics have been no exception (Rees et al. 2015; Knaack et al. 2017; Gartner et al. 2022).

Stigma in paramedic practice

For paramedics, the culture surrounding our well-being has been historically far from positive (Melow 2017). It is reported that paramedics are the most likely to experience mental health challenges but the least likely of all emergency services staff to access help and support (Mind 2019b). Many studies have highlighted that this may be due to paramedics perceiving themselves to be invincible (Mendes 2019) and believing that the admission of distress may show 'weakness' or lack of personal resilience (Mind 2016; Jones 2017) and directly opposes the 'hero' notion held by the general public (Rees et al. 2022). For paramedic students, this can often be enhanced by a desire to prove professional capability, perceived hierarchy such as fear of disclosing the information to a practice educator, and masking of emotional responses in order to 'fit in'. Furthermore, paramedic students can often face compounded stigma and multiple intersected demands such as academic work, navigating practice and university life, and personal challenges, which can all take a cumulative toll on well-being and impact confidence to disclose and willingness to reach out for support.

Challenging stigma

Challenging the culture of stigma at individual, cultural, and practice levels is therefore vital if we are to ensure the compassionate care that people in distress deserve. There are some helpful ways to challenge stigma (social, self, and professional):

- Be mindful of our language. Is it compassionate? Is it kind? Would we utilise the same words when discussing physical health?
- Gently challenge an idea or opinion if we feel safe to do so or raise concerns where appropriate (particularly within paramedic working contexts).
- Reach out to people in distress and offer support. This can make a real difference to feelings of shame and isolation.
- Check in on your peers and help normalise the conversation around well-being.
- Avoid assumptions and stereotypes and engage in conscious reflection. Call out our own stereotypes, perceptions, and attitudes.
- If we are finding things difficult, remember we deserve self-compassion and support. There is no shame in struggling.

Intersectionality

It is important to note that factors such as culture, race, ethnicity, sexuality, gender identity, disability, socio-economic status, and neurodiversity create a variety of lived experiences and can cumulatively compound stigma, discrimination, and inequality with regards to mental health, resilience, and well-being. It is therefore essential to take a person-centred approach, and to be mindful of the importance of our unique community and individual contexts.

'The stress bucket': what factors can affect your well-being?

Our well-being is dynamic, and is influenced by our interactions, personal circumstances, life experiences, and life events. Some of the factors that can affect our well-being may include:

- Health concerns
- Life events, e.g. bereavements/relationship breakdowns
- Caring responsibilities
- Work/academic pressures
- Socio-economic challenges
- Change

Responses to and impact of these factors will be unique to each person, but they can either individually or cumulatively result in significant distress and difficulty. A way of exploring cumulative stress is through the 'stress bucket' (Brabban and Turkington 2002), adapted and shown in Figure 9.1. This explores how when a person, represented by a bucket, experiences multiple difficult or stressful situations, represented by water, this causes their internal water or stress levels to rise. At the time where this reaches the top of the bucket, or when a person is struggling to manage, we will often see signs that a person's bucket is overflowing, in the form of physical, emotional, cognitive, and/or behavioural changes. This stress, or distress, can be managed through individual coping strategies

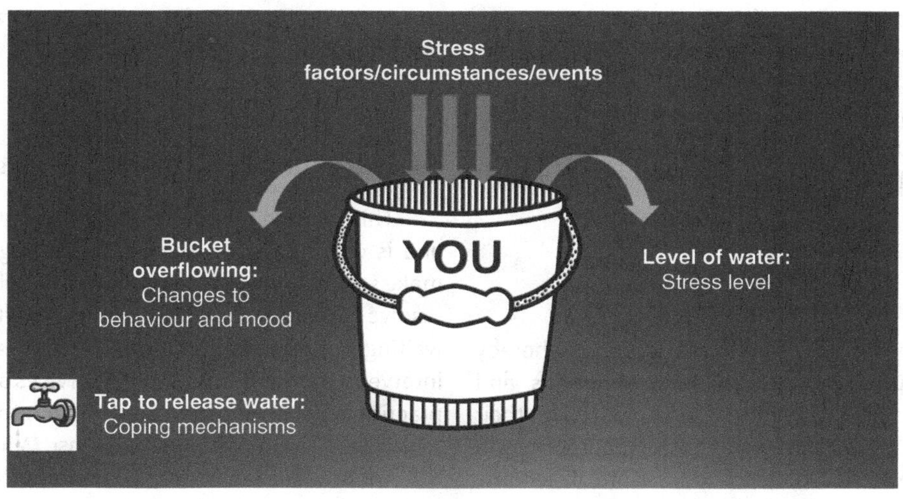

FIGURE 9.1 Stress bucket. Source: Adapted by Pavoni 2023, based on the original concept from Brabban and Turkington 2002.

such as self-care or formal support, represented by the tap, which releases the internal pressure.

It is important to note that our you're andividual resilience, e.g. the size and strength of our metaphorical bucket, will be shaped by complex biopsychosocial factors, including our past experiences, genetics, and social-cultural contexts.

Context of paramedic mental health and well-being

Paramedics are first and foremost human beings, who unfortunately are not exempt from the life experiences described above. However, in addition to these generic factors, there are specific factors that apply to our community of practice, which leads to an increased risk in vulnerability to experiencing poor mental health and well-being. These factors include:

- Exposure to emotional labour and traumatic incidents.
- Shift work.
- Lone working.
- Working in complex and often unpredictable environments.

Emotional labour

Emotional labour is the way in which we manage our emotional responses to fulfil our professional roles and in a way that is deemed socially acceptable. Within healthcare, it is used to supress or regulate emotions when attending patients, for example, with a significant injury (Aung et al. 2019). Fouquereau et al. (2019) suggest that there are two types of emotional labour: 'surface acting' and 'deep acting'.

Surface acting

Surface acting, the first type of emotional labour, is whereby an individual supresses their authentic emotions and instead opts to act in a manner that does not reflect their true feelings. This can in turn lead to stress, burnout, and cognitive weariness, due to the suppression of genuine feelings (Sousan et al. 2022).

Deep acting

In contrast, the second type of emotional labour is deep acting, which is the ability to manage our feelings to be more appropriate to the audience, to show a genuine outward emotion (Johnson et al. 2007). Theodosius (2008) suggests that deep acting can benefit well-being by encompassing a positive attitude.

Some research such as Jennings (2017) highlights that student paramedics often supress their emotions whilst on placement. This could be due to students not having the confidence to discuss their feelings outwardly with practice educators in clinical practice. Developing a positive learning environment that encourages students to speak freely about their feelings and utilising reflection to debrief after incidents can help manage emotions and hopefully reduce the risk of cognitive weariness and burnout.

Although paramedics are at undeniably greater risk than the general population, being mindful of our personal vulnerabilities and the risks associated with our role can lead to greater self-awareness, the development of individual coping skills and resilience, and early access to help and support in times of adversity.

Exposure to traumatic incidents

The incidents that the ambulance service is exposed to can have a significant impact upon our psychological health. Traumatic incidents can be cumulative in nature or related to a singular event.

In the immediacy after exposure to traumatic event, a person may:

- Replay the incident.
- Experience anxiety and low mood.
- Sleep badly due to intrusive memories and flashbacks.

This is often referred to as an 'acute stress reaction' and is common when the brain is trying to process and make sense of an adverse incident. This will usually fade or resolve within a few days or weeks. Often a 'watchful waiting' approach is advocated during this time but further intervention from formal health services such as a general practitioner (GP) is advocated if symptoms persist over four weeks or are particularly intense (Mind 2022).

For student paramedics, it is important to recognise that any incident can be challenging or resonate with an individual personally due to our unique life contexts. For example, a patient may be reminiscent of a loved one, or a situation we have personally encountered. Furthermore, one may be seeing these incidents for the first time, and simultaneously trying to process the emotive nature of the environment, alongside practice educators' clinical actions and responses. Remembering to practice self-care and reaching out to support networks is essential to help individuals process the challenging situations being encountered, make sense of them, and develop personal resilience.

Moral injury

Moral injury can be defined as the feelings or emotions a person experiences when they are exposed to situations or actions that may go against their beliefs and values (Mind 2022). This can be associated with difficult decision-making in clinical situations or operational pressures.

Practice insight

What situations do paramedics face that could cause a risk of moral injury?

It is important to seek support if one is feeling distressed, frustrated, or angry or is experiencing guilt or self-blame about a particular incident. Support can be accessed through the university or external counselling services, peers, practice educators, or specific ambulance service charities. Allowing space and time to process and talk through how we are feeling may prevent any continuation and worsening of these11ffing11sssing symptoms and future mental health challenges. It will also nurture one's overall health. This approach will also enable individuals to have the cognitive and emotional energy and capacity to continue to care for others.

The extra challenge

The NUS (2023) states that the number of students in higher education experiencing mental health problems has doubled since 2014/2015. This can be due to a range of complex factors, and for paramedic students, alongside the awareness of our professional context, it is important to understand how academic pressures can also influence well-being.

The learning environment

When moving from college or school to university there is a significant transition to an often-new learning environment. This is due to the higher level of academic ability that is needed, as well as the organisational and managerial complexity (Cabras et al. 2018). Tharani et al. (2017) suggest that within the nursing discipline the learning environment is a main contributor to students' stress and, worryingly, Bamuhair et al. (2015) state that a high level of stress due to a poor learning environment can impact on academic ability. Recognising the impact of this transition is important, along with using helpful coping strategies during times of difficulty.

Academic demands

A further large contributor to stress for undergraduate students is the academic demands and understandably, as Lotz and Sparfeldt (2017) indicate, the increased anxiety levels around the pinch point of university assessments. Not only are there academic assessments within university but whilst on clinical placement there is also an expectation to be successful at the clinical elements of the course. Although the learning environment will change at university, being able to manage time effectively and plan and organise assignments can significantly help with a reduction in this stress. Consider the best time of day to do work – when there is the least distraction and the most motivation – and plan your university work around this time.

Signs your bucket is overflowing: recognition of distress

Mood, cognition, and emotional states will be affected by our individual circumstances, interactions, and life events and can be transitory. However, being mindful of changes and persistency is an important step in either initiating

TABLE 9.1 Potential indicators of distress.

Physical	Emotional	Cognitive	Behavioural
Changes to sleep	Persistent sadness	Low self-esteem	Isolation and/or avoidance
Changes to appetite	Irritability/frustration/anger	Helplessness/hopelessness	Withdrawal
Feeling panicked or 'on edge'/hypervigilance	Feeling 'numb'	Ruminating and/or intrusive thoughts (including flashbacks)	Risk-taking behaviour (e.g. alcohol, substances)
Fatigue	Feeling tearful	Persistent worry	Difficulty with decision-making
Palpitations	Feeling overwhelmed	Difficulty concentrating and remembering things	Changes to routine
Gastrointestinal problems, including nausea and stomach aches	Lack of joy in activities that usually bring happiness or pleasure	Lack of motivation	Difficulties in looking after oneself, e.g. personal hygiene
Headaches	Exhaustion	Increased negative thinking	'Out of character' behaviour
Panic attacks	Feeling disconnected	Suicidal thoughts	Self-harm

self-care or having a supportive conversation with a person who may be struggling.

Signs of distress will be unique to everyone and it is important when reflecting on our own emotions, and those of people around us, not to make assumptions but to consider any changes to what is normal for a person. For example, has it been difficult to sleep recently? Is a friend or colleague who is usually calm and measured becoming more easily irritable? Perhaps a person who is known for their humour is now quiet and withdrawn?

Some potential signs of distress are outlined in Table 9.1.

Recognition of distress in ourselves and colleagues can be the first step to ensuring help and support.

Attaching the tap to the bucket: adaptive coping strategies

There are a number of different strategies that have been identified within research that can help promote positive well-being. One of the most well-known is the 'Five ways to well-being', shown in Figure 9.2. This was defined by the New Economics Foundation in 2008 and has since had a number of adaptations across different disciplines and sectors. This section will explore some healthy, or 'adaptive' coping strategies for paramedic students, which aim to put a tap on the 'stress bucket'.

Take notice

One of the first and most important steps in maintaining well-being is to recognise how we are feeling and acknowledge that our emotions are valid. It may be helpful to write down how we are feeling, to consider what is in our control, and to identify areas where further help and support to manage these challenges may be required (British Red Cross 2023b). Understanding what is in our personal 'buckets' can then lead to considering what type of support may be most helpful.

Self-compassion

Practising self-compassion as healthcare workers is essential. It involves recognising our thoughts and emotional responses,

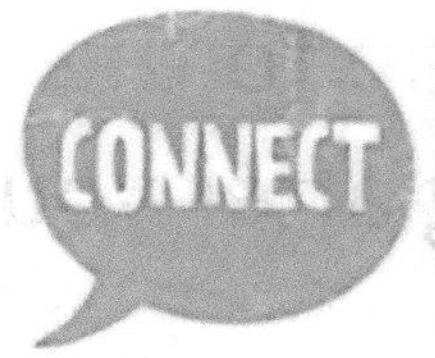
CONNECT
TALK & LISTEN,
BE THERE,
FEEL CONNECTED
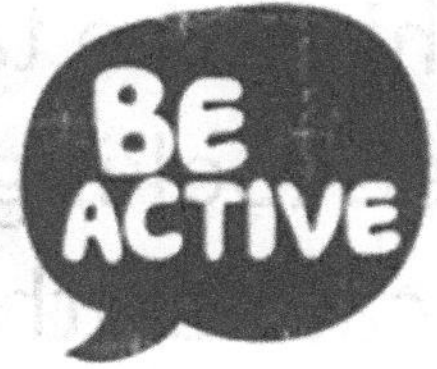
BE ACTIVE
DO WHAT YOU CAN.
ENJOY WHAT YOU DO.
MOVE YOUR MOOD

TAKE NOTICE
REMEMBER
THE SIMPLE
THINGS THAT
GIVE YOU JOY
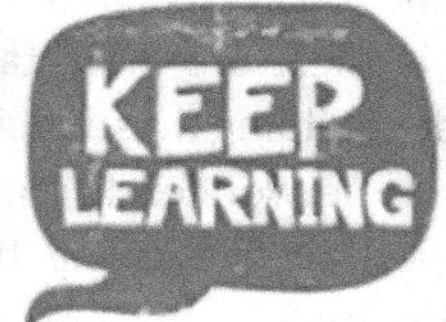
KEEP LEARNING
EMBRACE NEW
EXPERIENCES.
SEE OPPORTUNITIES.
SURPRISE YOURSELF

Give
Your time,
your words,
your presence

FIGURE 9.2 Five ways to well-being. Source: Adapted from New Economics Foundation 2008.

taking a non-judgemental approach to our feelings and difficulties, avoiding unhelpful self-criticism, and being aware of the need to apply the same kindness and empathy to ourselves as we do to others (Hashem and Zeinoun 2020). This approach also recognises that struggling is a natural part of our human existence and nothing to be ashamed of. Being self-compassionate can reduce the risk of burnout and poor well-being, develop our personal resilience, and allow us to continue to give compassionate care to our patients (Kotera et al. 2021).

Take time for you to be you

Sometimes, when juggling the intense demands of being a student paramedic or paramedic, it can be easy to lose track of what we enjoy, and other aspects of our identity. Try to create space to undertake activities and personal interests such as hobbies. These can feel challenging during times of significant academic pressure and shift work but building in even small amounts of time within the day to go for a walk, listen to music, or read is a really important aspect of self-care, which promotes positive well-being (Mind 2023).

Relaxation techniques such as yoga and mindfulness can be very helpful, particularly in situations that feel overwhelming. It allows space to take notice how one is feeling within the moment and can make times of stress feel manageable (MIND 2023). Although it is important to find the right approach, as we may all have different ways of relaxing such as being in nature or reading.

Connections

Similarly, connecting with people can be a helpful way of boosting our well-being (British Red Cross 2023). Spending time with family, friends, and those that matter to us can increase our self-esteem, allow space to discuss how we are feeling, and provide an opportunity for support (NHS 2023). For paramedic students and paramedics connecting with people in our support network, and people who make one feel 'like oneself' is essential to developing resilience.

Social support

Alsubaie et al. (2019) suggest that sources of social support are key for mental well-being and research such as Sun et al. (2019) highlights the significant impact that both conversational and relational aspects of social interaction have on a person's mental well-being, especially for introverts. One of the complex factors of moving to university is loneliness due to leaving all usual social support behind and needing to create new social circles (Vasileiou et al. 2019). Worryingly, Peltzer and Pengpid (2017) found that students who self-reported loneliness also reported sleeping problems, tobacco use, aggressive behaviour, and risk-taking behaviour. Interestingly Apostolou and Keramari (2020) state the main reason why making new friends and creating new social circles can be difficult is due to a lack of trust. Combined with moving into university halls and having to live with new people, this can understandably cause interpersonal stress. An increase in interpersonal stress can cause depression, anxiety, and a reduction in engagement for students (Coiro et al. 2017). It is therefore important when moving to university to consider building those social circles and developing a social support network early on.

The value of peer support in well-being has been widely documented (Mental Health Foundation 2022a). For paramedic students, this sense of connection with others with shared experiences and insight can be a helpful way of processing the unique challenges of the profession. However, some paramedic students may find interactions with friends outside of practice more useful. It is advocated that a combination may be most beneficial, to help nurture the different aspects of a student's life and personal connections.

Reflection

Reflection is introduced early within academic study for healthcare professionals, usually as a core assessment technique. The HCPC (2021) states that reflection is a positive technique to identify ways that you can improve service delivery and your practice. Reflection enables professionals to develop knowledge, question, clarify, and improve performance (Turner 2015). In addition to its being an important technique for improving practice, it is essential to recognise the benefits that reflection can have on well-being. Williams (2013) suggests that reflection and sharing experiences can support students in the ongoing emotional workload that is required to be a paramedic. A study within nurses also recommends that providing opportunities for reflection is crucial for developing a workforce that is able to face health crisis (Martin-Delgado et al. 2021). There are multiple ways to reflect, for an assessment, on your own during placement and as a group to share experiences. These reflections can be in any format. Considering different learning styles, it may be easier to write the reflection down or to record it as a voice note (HCPC 2021). Reflection can also help us identify patterns or trends where we may need support, for example, certain calls and circumstances that you may find more personally challenging. It is important to remember that reflection is not just an assessment technique and learning how to reflect early within your studies can be a positive support mechanism for maintaining a healthy well-being and developing resilience as a student, and as you embark upon your future paramedic career.

Attaching the tap to the bucket: looking after your physical health

The relationship between food and mood

The result of unhealthy eating on well-being and mental health is worrying, with studies revealing high depression and stress scores associated with a low fruit and vegetable intake and not maintaining the Mediterranean diet. The Mediterranean diet according to Castro-Quezada et al. (2014) is a way of eating based on traditional cuisine of countries surrounding the Mediterranean Sea and consists of high levels of fruit, vegetables, grains, beans, nuts, and seeds. This is seen as the healthiest diet. Although most people understand the requirement of eating healthy foods and can see the relationship between food and mood, it can become difficult to maintain a healthy lifestyle when working shift work within healthcare. Healthcare shift workers often may not have access to cooking appliances for cooking or heating up pre prepared food, which can encourage collection of fast food for ease and convenience. During night shifts, healthcare workers are also more likely to have cravings for sugary snacks and drink less fluids, which contributes to a poor diet (Gifkins et al. 2018).

When considering students, Antonopoulou et al. (2020) highlight that students living away from home have a significantly low Mediterranean diet and tend to focus on unhealthy foods. One reason for this is the increase in fast food restaurant attendance, which Scott et al. (2020) suggest could be due to either bad time management or an increase in social activities involving groups of students eating out together. Therefore, healthcare students need to be mindful of the difficulties these complex issues present and consider ways to manage this. Some tips from the NHS (2022) on how to maintain a healthy diet include basing meals on higher fibre starchy carbohydrates, eating lots of vegetables and fruit, consuming lots of fish, cutting down on sugar and fats, and eating no more than 6g of salt a day. Specifically for shift work, preparing healthy meals to have at work, ensuring lots of healthy snacks are available, and trying to maintain mealtimes – e.g. not skipping breakfast – can also help maintain a healthy diet.

Sleep

Schlarb et al. (2017) suggest up to 60% of university students experience poor sleep quality with Sivertsen et al. (2019) claiming that sleep problems among university students rose from 22.6% in 2010 to 30.5% in 2018. Stress reduces sleep and could be one reason for students lacking the sleep required at university due to increased academic stress. Another reason is the lack of knowledge around sleep hygiene, specifically for medical students (Campbell et al. 2018).

Cherry (2023) states that the lack of sleep can cause significant mental health issues and, worryingly, insomnia can cause depression. Mind (2020) highlight one of the potential issues of struggling to sleep as being increased loneliness due to the lack of energy to meet up with friends.

The impact that shift work alone can have on mental health is staggering, this is due to the circadian misalignment and sleep displacement that is caused through working different hours (Savarese and Di Perri 2020). Owens (2017) suggested that a staggering 95.65% of nurses stated they are fatigued and that the job is mentally and physically draining. As paramedics and nurses work similar shift patterns, we can assume this would be a comparable statistic for paramedics. In addition, Pryce (2016) suggests that sleep deprivation can reduce an individual's psychomotor skills as much as drinking alcohol; therefore reducing the quality of care being provided to patients. With a reduction in sleep being proven to affect clinical care, this can then cause more stress and unfortunately end in a cycle of reduced sleep and increased mental health illness (Merill 2022).

An undergraduate paramedic student will typically spend 50% of their degree in a clinical placement setting. Therefore, it is important to consider the impact that shift work can have right from the start of university. Mind (2021) identify some tips for healthy sleep, including:

- Creating a dark, quiet, cool environment to provide a restful sleeping area. Confronting sleepiness –if you have tried to fall asleep but feel like you are lying awake then do not force it.
- Writing down worries, this can be especially important as a healthcare professional, potentially journalling or debriefing after clinical incidents attended.
- Cutting out alcohol and caffeine before sleeping.
- Exercising and moving more.

Exercise

A final complex factor that affects well-being is lack of exercise. As Mikkelsen et al. (2017) suggest, exercise can alleviate anxiety, depression, and stress. Berk et al. (2013) state that depression is an inflammatory disease. They identify a range of factors that can increase the risk of systematic inflammation and are therefore associated with depression such as poor diet, obesity, and lack of physical activity. Over an eleven-year period, a study of 33,908 adults found that 12% of new cases of depression may be prevented if individuals do one hour of physical activity a week (Harvey et al. 2018).

Healthcare students may struggle to exercise regularly due to the continuous changing of shift patterns and lack of structure within the timetable at university. This can cause students to struggle to find a regular routine, potentially demotivating them to keep up with regular exercise. Sleep deprivation associated with shift work can also demotivate people to take part in certain activities, one of these being exercise. Exercise as defined by the NHS (2021) can be a range of moderate, vigorous, and very vigorous activity. The recommendation for adults aged nineteen to sixty-four is at least 150 minutes of moderate intensity exercise a week, which could include brisk walking, riding a bike, and dancing. Seventy-five minutes of vigorous exercise such as netball, football, running, and swimming can have similar health benefits as 150 minutes of moderate activity.

Supportive conversations

The ways in which we respond to individuals who are struggling can have a significant impact on their health and overall recovery. It is important to be mindful that due to the stigma surrounding mental health, and in particular within paramedic practice, you may be the first person an individual speaks to about how they are feeling. Therefore, a compassionate, empathetic, and supportive approach can make a real difference and provide hope in times of distress. Box 9.1 offers tips that can enhance supportive conversations.

BOX 9.1 Tips for supportive conversations

- Consider the environment: is it suitable and confidential?
- At first, a person may respond with 'I'm fine'. Consider asking twice, as you may be the first person they have spoken to.
- Demonstrate active listening – think about your non-verbal communication, including body language and tone of voice.
- Utilise silences and allow space for responses.
- Use open questions and do not be afraid to ask difficult questions particularly around thoughts of suicide and self-harm.
- Validate feelings and recognise a person's emotions, e.g. 'I can't imagine how hard that is', 'It sounds like you have been through a lot'.
- Be kind and reassuring.
- Avoid relaying your own experience wherever possible, as although usually this is well intended it can sometimes be counterproductive.
- Remember it is not your role to diagnose a person but rather to empower them to think about support options and next steps.
- Be honest if you feel you may need to inform a trusted person or contact emergency help if you are concerned there may be an imminent risk of harm.

Accessing external support

Along with self-care and positive coping strategies, we may need additional support to manage our mental health and well-being. This will depend upon the nature of our distress, any specific causing factors (for example, witnessing a traumatic incident or experiencing a bereavement, financial stressors, relationship problems, or academic pressures), social support, and the degree to which it is impacting our day-to-day lives.

Examples of support will be different in each geographical area; however, you may wish to consider:

- Self-referral to counselling services.
- GP appointments.
- Employer or university support services.
- Listening support lines and paramedic specific mental health helplines.
- Mental health crisis support lines if you are feeling unsafe or experiencing thoughts of harm.
- Emergency department if you are feeling at imminent risk of harm (NHS 2022).

It is vital as healthcare professionals that we take steps to keep ourselves well and there is no shame in doing so.

Conclusion

When starting university life and shift work, it is important to consider the change of lifestyle and new challenges that are ahead. Utilise the stress bucket and spend some time thinking about how these changes may impact you and how you can maintain a healthy well-being to reduce your risk of developing any mental and physical ill health during your studies.

Maintaining a healthy well-being, understanding how to recognise stress within yourself, and identifying how to seek support will help you build resilience moving into full time healthcare. It is also imperative in building a healthy future workforce.

Case study 2

Ava is a first-year student on her last week of placement. She has been an eager and engaged student throughout her first placement but has recently seemed tired, withdrawn, and at times disinterested. This has culminated in missing days of placement, decrease in performance, and an overall lower mood.

Recently she has often been just on time or slightly late for shifts and has been appearing unkempt at times.

On these occasions she states she is 'sorry' for being late with minimal explanations, often citing her commute or poor sleep but rarely providing any reason at all.

Consider:

1. What is your initial response to this change in Ava's behaviour and what questions may you want to ask her?
2. What factors may be affecting Ava?
3. What ongoing strategies could you suggest to support Ava?

Activities

Now review your learning by completing the learning activities in this chapter. The answers to these appear at the end of the book. Further self-test activities can be found at **www.wileyfundamentalseries.com/paramedic/3e.**

Test your knowledge

1. What do you understand by the term mindfulness?
2. What coping mechanism might people use as they try to cope with workplace stress?
3. When faced with stress, the body undergoes a series of physiological changes as part of the 'fight or flight' response. Discuss the psychological and psychological responses that can be experience during the fight or flight response.
4. What is the role of the stress hormone cortisol?
5. Depression can vary in its severity; it is a complex condition with both biological and environmental factors playing a role. Discuss this.

Activity 9.1

Creating a personalised well-being plan is an effective way to outline specific goals and strategies for improving your overall physical, mental, and emotional health. Here are some headings that you might use in creating that plan. Take some time to create your own personalised well-being plan using these headings:

Step 1: Self-assessment
(Here you need to reflect on your current well-being.)

Step 2: Set specific well-being goals
(Define clear and achievable well-being goals.)

Step 3: Prioritize your goals
(Determine which goals are most important to you and which ones you would like to focus.)

Step 4: Identify strategies
(For each well-being goal, brainstorm specific strategies and actions you can take to work toward that goal.)

Step 5: Create an action plan
(Develop a detailed action plan for each goal, outlining what you need to do daily, weekly, or monthly to make progress.)

Step 6: Gather resources and support
(Identify the resources and support you may need to achieve your well-being goals.)

Step 7: Implement and monitor
(Begin implementing your action plan and regularly monitor your progress.)

Step 8: Practice self-care

Step 9: Evaluate and adjust
(Periodically assess your progress and evaluate.)

Step 10: Celebrate achievements
(Acknowledge and celebrate your achievements along the way.)

Glossary

Burnout: A state of physical, emotional, and mental exhaustion resulting from chronic work-related stress, potentially leading to a decrease in well-being.

Cultural competence: The ability to understand, appreciate, and effectively interact with individuals from diverse cultural backgrounds, promoting well-being for all.

Depression Mental health condition characterised by persistent and profound feelings of sadness, hopelessness, and a lack of interest or pleasure in activities that were once enjoyable.

Emotional resilience The ability to bounce back and adapt positively to challenging or stressful situations, promoting mental well-being.

Mental health: Refers to emotional and psychological well-being, encompassing factors such as mood, stress, and coping mechanisms.

Self-care Activities and practices individuals engage in to maintain and improve their own physical, mental, and emotional well-being.

Stress	A natural and common response that our bodies and minds experience when we encounter challenges, demands, or threats.
Stress management	Strategies and techniques used to cope with and reduce the impact of stress on mental and physical health.
Well-being	The overall state of being healthy, happy, and content in various aspects of life, including physical, mental, and emotional health.

References

Alkhateeb, S.A., Alkhameesi, N.F., Lamfon, G.N. et al. (2019). Pattern of physical exercise practice among university students in the Kingdom of Saudi Arabia (before beginning and during college): a cross-sectional study. *BMC Public Health* **19** (1): 1–7.

Alsubaie, M.M., Stain, H.J., Webster, L.A. et al. (2019). The role of sources of social support on depression and quality of life for university students. *International Journal of Adolescence and Youth* [e-journal] **24** (4): 484–496.

Antonopoulou, M., Mantzorou, M., Serdari, A. et al. (2020). Evaluating Mediterranean diet adherence in university student populations: does this dietary pattern affect students' academic performance and mental health? *The International Journal of Health Planning and Management* [e-journal] **35** (1): 5–21.

Apostolou, M. and Keramari, D. (2020). What prevents people from making friends: A taxonomy of reasons. *Personality and Individual Differences* [e-journal] **163:** 110043.

Aung, N. and Tewogbola, P. (2019). The impact of emotional labor on the health in the workplace: a narrative review of literature from 2013–2018. *AIMS Public Health* **6** (3): 268.

Bamuhair, S.S., Farhan, A., Althubaiti, A.et al. (2015). Sources of stress and coping strategies among undergraduate medical students enrolled in a problem-based learning curriculum. *Depression* **20:** 33.

Bani-Issa, W., Radwan, H., Al Marzooq, F. et al. (2020). Salivary cortisol, subjective stress and quality of sleep among female healthcare professionals. *Journal of Multidisciplinary Healthcare* **13:** 125–140.

Bennett, K. (2015). Emotional and personal resilience through life. Available at: https://assets.publishing.service.gov.uk/media/5a808fd8ed915d74e622f2b2/gs-15-19-future-ageing-emotional-personal-resilience-er04.pdf (accessed 18 July 2023).

Berk, M., Williams, L.J., Jacka, F.N. et al. (2013). So depression is an inflammatory disease, but where does the inflammation come from? *BMC Medicine* **11** (1): 1–16.

Brabban, A. and Turkington, D. (2002). The search for meaning: detecting congruence between life events, underlying schema and psychotic symptoms. In: *A Casebook of Cognitive Therapy for Psychosis* (ed. Morrison, A.P.). New York: Brunner Routledge.

British Red Cross. (2023a). Resilience building activities to improve your wellbeing. Available at: https://www.redcross.org.uk/get-help/get-help-with-loneliness/wellbeing-support/resilience-building-activities (accessed 18 July 2023).

British Red Cross. (2023b). Five ways to improve your wellbeing: tips and ideas for people to build resilience to cope with stress and support wellbeing. Available at: https://www.redcross.org.uk/get-help/get-help-with-loneliness/wellbeing-support/five-ways-improve-wellbeing (accessed 12 July 2023).

Cabras, C. and Mondo, M. (2018). Coping strategies, optimism, and life satisfaction among first-year university students in Italy: Gender and age differences. *Higher Education* [e-journal] **75** (4): 643–654.

Campbell, R., Soenens, B., Beyers, W. et al. (2018). University students' sleep during an exam period: the role of basic psychological needs and stress. *Motivation and Emotion* [e-journal] **42** (5): 671–681.

Castro-Quezada, I., Román-Viñas, B., and Serra-Majem, L. (2014). The Mediterranean diet and nutritional adequacy: a review. *Nutrients* **6** (1): 231–248.

Cherry, K. (2023). How does sleep affect mental health. Available at: How Sleep Affects Mental Health (verywellmind.com*)* (accessed 17 March 2023).

Coiro, M.J., Bettis, A.H., and Compas, B.E. (2017). College students coping with interpersonal stress: examining a control-based model of coping. *Journal of American College Health* [e-journal] **65** (3): 177–186.

Fouquereau, E., Morin, A.J., Lapointe, É. Et al. (2019). Emotional labour profiles: associations with key predictors and outcomes. *Work & Stress* [e-journal] **33** (3): 268–294.

Gärtner, L., Asbrock, F., and Salzmann, S. (2022). Self-stigma amongst people with mental health problems in terms of warmth and competence. *Frontiers in Psychology* **14** (13): 877491. doi: 10.3389/fpsyg.2022.877491.

Gifkins, J., Johnston, A., and Loudoun, R., 2018. The impact of shift work on eating patterns and self-care strategies utilised by experienced and inexperienced nurses. *Chronobiology International* **35** (6): 811–820.

Haddad, P. and Haddad, I. (2015). Mental health stigma. British Association of Psychopharmacology. Available at: https://www.bap.org.uk/articles/mental-health-stigma/ (accessed 18 July 2023).

Harvey, S.B., Øverland, S., Hatch, S.L. et al. (2018). Exercise and the prevention of depression: results of the HUNT Cohort Study. *Am J Psychiatry* **175** (1): 28–36.

Hashem, Z. and Zeinoun, P. (2020). Self-compassion explains less burnout amongst healthcare professionals. *Mindfullness (NY)* **11** (11): 2542-2551. doi: 10.1007/s12671-020-01469-5.

HCPC (Health & Care Professionals Council). (2021). What is reflection? Available at: What is reflection? | (hcpc-uk.org) (accessed 4 October 2022).

HCPC. (2023). Standards of conduct, performance and ethics. Available at: https://www.hcpc-uk.org/standards/standards-of-conduct-performance-and-ethics/ (accessed 18 October 2023).

HEPI (Higher Education Policy Institute). (2019). Measuring well-being in higher education. Available at: https://www.hepi.ac.uk/wp-content/uploads/2019/05/Policy-Note-13-Paper-May-2019-Measuring-well-being-in-higher-education-8-Pages-5.pdf (accessed 10 June 2023).

Jennings, K. (2017). Emotional labour in paramedic practice: Student awareness of professional demands. *Journal of Paramedic Practice* **9** (7): 288–294.

Johnson, H.M. and Spector, P.E. (2007). Service with a smile: do emotional intelligence, gender and autonomy moderate the emotional labor process? *Journal of Occupational Health Psychology* **12:** 319–333.

Johnson, J., Hall, L.H., Berzins, K. et al. (2018). Mental healthcare staff well-being and burnout: a narrative review of trends, causes, implications, and recommendations for future interventions. *International Journal of Mental Health Nursing* [e-journal] **27** (1): 20–32.

Jones, S. (2017). Describing the mental health profile of first responders: a systematic review. *Journal of the American Psychiatric Nurses Association* **23** (3): 200–214. doi: 10.1177%2F1078390317695266.

Kandola, A., Ashdown-Franks, G., Hendrikse, J. et al. (2019). Physical activity and depression: towards understanding the antidepressant mechanisms of physical activity. *Neuroscience & Biobehavioral Reviews* **107:** 525–539.

Kotera, Y., Jackson, J.E., Kirkman, A. et al. (2023). Comparing the mental health of healthcare students: mental health shame and self-compassion in counselling, occupational therapy, nursing and social work students. *Int J Ment Health Addict.* **13:** 1–18. doi: 10.1007/s11469-023-01018-w.

Kowalski, R.M. and Peipert, A. (2019). Public- and self-stigma attached to physical versus psychological disabilities. *Stigma and Health* **4** (2): 136–142. doi: 10.1037/sah0000123.

Kushal, A., Gupta, S., Mehta, M. et al. (2018). Study of stress among health care professionals: a systemic review. *Int J Res Foundation Hosp Healthcare Adm* **6** (1): 6–11.

Lotz, C. and Sparfeldt, J.R. (2017). Does test anxiety increase as the exam draws near? Students' state test anxiety recorded over the course of one semester. *Personality and Individual Differences* **104:** 397–400.

Martin-Delgado, L., Goni-Fuste, B., Alfonso-Arias, C. et al. (2021). Nursing students on the frontline: impact and personal and professional gains of joining the health care workforce during the COVID-19 pandemic in Spain. *Journal of Professional Nursing* **37** (3): 588–597.

Mellow, R. (2017). Groundbreaking data collected on mental health of first responders. *Journal of Emergency Medical Services* **11** (42). Available at: https://www.jems.com/2017/11/01/groundbreaking-data-collected-on-mental-health-of-first-responders/ (accessed 11 May 2023).

Mental Health Foundation. (2021a). What is good mental health? Available at: What is good mental health? | Mental Health Foundation (accessed 6 January 2023).

Mental Health Foundation (2021b) Stigma and discrimination. Available at: https://www.mentalhealth.org.uk/explore-mental-health/a-z-topics/stigma-and-discrimination (accessed 23 October 2023).

Merrill, R.M. (2022). Mental health conditions according to stress and sleep disorders. *International Journal of Environmental Research and Public Health* **19** (13): 7957.

Mikkelsen, K., Stojanovska, L., Polenakovic, M. et al. (2017). Exercise and mental health. *Maturitas*, **106:** 48–56.

Mind. (2016). Wellbeing and mental health support in the emergency services. Available at: https://www.mind.org.uk/media/34555691/20046_mind-blue-light-programme-legacy-report-v12_online.pdf (accessed 20 April 2023).

Mind. (2019a). Wellbeing and mental health in the emergency services. Available at: https://www.mind.org.uk/media-a/4525/blue-light-programme-legacy-report_english-summary.pdf (accessed 18 May 2023).

Mind. (2019b). Post traumatic stress disorder (PTSD). Available at: https://www.mind.org.uk/information-support/types-of-mental-health-problems/post-traumatic-stress-disorder-ptsd-and-complex-ptsd/about-ptsd/ (accessed 12 July 2023).

Mind. (2020). How to cope with sleep problems. Available at: Sleep and mental health | Mind, the mental health charity - help for mental health problems (accessed 17 March 2023).

Mind. (2021). How to cope with sleep problems. Available at: Tips to improve your sleep - Mind (accessed 11 March 2023).

Mind. (2022). Coping with what you experience in the ambulance service. Available at: https://www.mind.org.uk/news-campaigns/campaigns/blue-light-programme/blue-light-information/coping-with-what-you-experience-in-the-ambulance-service/ (accessed 12 July 2023)

Mind. (2023a). Managing stress and building resilience. Available at: https://www.mind.org.uk/information-support/types-of-mental-health-problems/stress/managing-stress-and-building-resilience/ (accessed 23 October 2023).

Mind. (2023b). How to improve your mental wellbeing. Available at: https://www.mind.org.uk/information-support/tips-for-everyday-living/wellbeing/ (accessed 6 February 2023).

New Economics Foundation. (2008). Five ways to wellbeing. Available at: https://neweconomics.org/2008/10/five-ways-to-wellbeing (accessed 23 October 2023).

NHS (National Health Service). (2021). Physical activity guidelines for adults aged 19 to 64. Available at: Physical activity guidelines for adults aged 19 to 64 - NHS (www.nhs.uk) (accessed 14 March 2023).

NHS. (2022). Mental health services. Available at: https://www.nhs.uk/nhs-services/mental-health-services/ (accessed 18 July 2023).

NHS. (2023). Five steps to mental wellbeing. Available at: https://www.nhs.uk/mental-health/self-help/guides-tools-and-activities/five-steps-to-mental-wellbeing/ (accessed 12 July 2023).

NUS (National Union of Students). (2023). Mental health policy. Available at: Mental Health- NUS UK (accessed 15 February 2023).

Owens, B. (2017). The impact of shift work on nurses' quality of sleep. *ABNF Journal* **28** (3).

Peltzer, K. and Pengpid, S. (2017). Loneliness: its correlates and associations with health risk behaviours among university students in 25 countries. *Journal of Psychology in Africa* [e-journal] **27** (3): 247–255.

Pryce, C. (2016). Impact of shift work on critical care nurses. *Canadian Journal of Critical Care Nursing* **27** (4).

Ramey, S., MacQuarrie, A., Cochrane, A. et al. (2019). Drowsy and dangerous? Fatigue in paramedics: an overview. *Irish Journal of Paramedicine* **4** (1). doi: 10.32378/ijp.v4i1.175.

Rees, N., Rapport, F., Snooks, H. John, A., Patel, C. (2017) 'How Do Emergency Ambulance Paramedics View the Care They Provide to People Who Self Harm?: Ways and Means' *International Journal of Law and Psychiatry,* **50**, pp. 61-67, DOI: 10.1016/j.ijlp.2016.05.010

Rees, N., Williams, J., Hogan, C., Smyth, L. Archer, T. (2022) 'Heroism and paramedic practice: a constructivist metasynthesis of qualitative research' *Front. Psychol.* **13**, https://doi.org/10.3389/fpsyg.2022.1016841

Schlarb, A.A., Friedrich, A., and Claßen, M. (2017). *Sleep problems in university students – an intervention. Neuropsychiatric Disease and Treatment* [e-journal] **13:** *1989.*

Scott, S., Muir, C., Stead, M. et al. (2020). Exploring the links between unhealthy eating behaviour and heavy alcohol use in the social, emotional and cultural lives of young adults (aged 18–25): a qualitative research study. *Appetite* [e-journal] **144:** 104449.

Savarese, M. and Di Perri, M.C. (2020). Excessive sleepiness in shift work disorder: a narrative review of the last 5 years. *Sleep and Breathing* **24:** 297–310.

Shanafelt, T.D. and Noseworthy, J.H. (2017). Executive leadership and physician well-being: nine organizational strategies to promote engagement and reduce burnout. In: *Mayo Clinic Proceedings* (Vol. 92, No. 1), pp. 129–146. London: Elsevier.

Sivertsen, B., Vedaa, Ø., Harvey, A.G. et al. (2019). Sleep patterns and insomnia in young adults: a national survey of Norwegian university students. *Journal of Sleep Research* [e-journal] **28** (2): e12790.

Sousan, A., Farmanesh, P., and Zargar, P. (2022). The effect of surface acting on job stress and cognitive weariness among healthcare workers during the COVID-19 pandemic: exploring the role of sense of community. *Front Psychol* **13:** 826156.

Stolzenburg, S., Freitag, S., Evans-Lacko, S. et al. (2017). The stigma of mental illness as a barrier to self labelling as having a mental illness. *J Nerv Ment Dis* **205** (12). doi: 10.1097/NMD.0000000000000756.

Subu, M.A., Wati, D.F., Netrida, N. et al. (2021). Types of stigma experienced by patients with mental illness and mental health nurses in Indonesia: a qualitative content analysis. *International Mental Health Syst* **15** (1). doi: 10.1186/s13033-021-00502-x.

Sun, J., Harris, K., and Vazire, S. (2020). Is well-being associated with the quantity and quality of social interactions? *Journal of Personality and Social Psychology* **119** (6): 1478–1496. doi: 10.1037/pspp0000272.

Tharani, A., Husain, Y., and Warwick, I. (2017). Learning environment and emotional well-being: a qualitative study of undergraduate nursing students. *Nurse Education Today* [e-journal] **59:** 82–87.

Theodosius, C. (2008). *Emotional Labour in Health Care: The Unmanaged Heart of Nursing*. London: Routledge.

Turner, H. (2015). Reflective practice for paramedics: a new approach. *Journal of Paramedic Practice* **7** (3): 138–144.

Van de Riet, P., Rossieter, R., Kirby, D. et al. (2015) Piloting a stress management and mindfulness program for undergraduate nursing students: student feedback and lessons learned. *Nurse Education Today* **31** (1): 44–49. doi: 10.1016/j.nedt.2014.05.003.

WHO (World Health Organization). (2022). World mental health report: transforming mental health for all. Available at: https://www.who.int/publications/i/item/9789240049338 (accessed 25 October 2023).

WHO. (2023). Mental health. Available at: https://www.who.int/health-topics/mental-health#tab=tab_1 (accessed 25 October 2023).

Williams, A. (2013). A study of emotion work in student paramedic practice. *Nurse Education Today* **33** (5): 512–517.

Van de Riet, P., Rossieter, R., Kirby, D. et al. (2015). Piloting a stress management and mindfulness program for undergraduate nursing students: student feedback and lessons learned. *Nurse Education Today* **31** (1). doi: 10.1016/j.nedt.2014.05.003.

Vasileiou, K., Barnett, J., Barreto, M. et al. (2019). Coping with loneliness at University: a qualitative interview study with students in the UK. *Mental Health & Prevention* [e-journal] **13:** 21–30.

Zhai, K., Gao, X., and Wang, G., 2018. The role of sleep quality in the psychological well-being of final year undergraduate students in China. *International Journal of Environmental Research and Public Health* [e-journal] **15** (12): 2881.

CHAPTER 10

Mental health for paramedics

Renate Taylor

Senior Lecturer in Mental Health Nursing and Nurse Education, University of Roehampton, UK

Jade Speed

London Ambulance Service Safeguarding Specialist and Paramedic

Contents

LEARNING OUTCOMES

On completion of this chapter, the reader will be able to:

- Define mental health.
- Identify personal risk factors.
- Reflect on demands of the job in relation to self-awareness and emotional and physical well-being.
- Actively engage in promoting and maintaining good mental and physical health for self and colleagues (others).
- Know where to ask for help.
- Become part of a workforce protecting and contributing to improving mental health outcomes for paramedics.

Case Study

Rob was called out on a job. His colleague on the ambulance is a newly qualified paramedic. Rob sighs deeply, he is feeling anxious of the unknown in relation to the call out for a road traffic collision. His newly qualified colleague Dean observes this. To break the ice in the silence of moving off, Dean states 'I am nervous, but I know we can always ask for help.' Rob remains silent and responds eventually with 'You just get on with the job – seventeen years in and nobody has ever offered me any help.'

Fundamentals of Paramedic Practice: A Systems Approach, Third Edition. Edited by Sam Willis and Ian Peate.

Companion website: www.wiley.com/go/willis/paramedic3e

Introduction

Welcome to 'Mental health for the paramedic'. This chapter will complement all the chapters related to your learning and development in this book. It will explore and highlight the state of paramedics' mental health and well-being. The information and data in the chapter will present a universal overview of how paramedics, student paramedics, and Retired paramedics report on work, working in learning, and post-work maintenance of their mental and physical health and well-being. This chapter will work on a fundamental term of engagement to develop interest and self-awareness to promote and understand how critical incidents and getting on with the job can result in emotional suppression. There will be opportunity to embrace, through the discussion of their effect on mental health and physical health, the protective and coping mechanisms used in the challenging work, including personal satisfaction and building resilience. Your active participation through reflection and learning can assist to move from reported feelings of isolation and withdrawal to support and open disclosure by asking for help. This in turn will highlight occupational input and educational support for student paramedics. The intended audience for this chapter is global and for clarity it is acknowledged that the term paramedic also refers to first responders, emergency medical technicians, emergency medical personnel, and call takers (Lawn et al. 2020).

What is mental health?

Good question. How do we define mental health? The World Health Organization (WHO) is often turned to for the global generic definition of mental health. 'Mental Health is a state of mental well-being that enables people to cope with the stresses of life, realize their abilities, learn well and work well, and contribute to their community' (WHO 2022, p. 1). The above concept of mental health is an encapsulation of a much broader and conscious paradigm that sets out to offer inclusivity and acknowledgement of fluidity in striving for and maintaining good mental health whilst living with a mental health diagnosis, disability, or poor physical health. WHO state that 'Mental Health is a basic human right' (WHO 2022, p.1). The King's Fund in their Prioritising Mental Health Report (2015) further elaborate on this with a statement that enhances the understanding of good mental health, embracing the notion that it is not only based on the absence of mental illness. Good mental health is inclusive of 'how we cope with our lives, handle situations, relate to others and make choices. Fundamentally that mental health cannot be separated from physical health' (The King's Fund 2015, p. 1).

When exploring the nature of mental health and what is good or developing coping strategies to maintain good well-being, it is important to bear in mind the intrinsic link between mental and physical health. The principle of this so-called 'parity of esteem' is ensuring that mental and physical health are given equal importance (Department of Health 2012). It is important to remember that whilst this chapter will focus mainly on the challenges of the paramedic workforce in relation to psychological impact, physical pain is equally evident. Work-related injuries, for example, back pain, can lead to poor mental health such as depression and psychological therapy is recommended alongside a physical health treatment package (National Institute for Health and Care Excellence (NICE) 2016) where required.

What are the factors affecting mental health on the job?

There are many factors associated with mental distress on the job and the reported associated physical effects, described as psychological injury, experienced by ambulance personnel (Lawn et al. 2020). In a systematic review of qualitative research, Lawn et al. (2020) explored thirty-nine areas of study. A significant finding was that the management of how the organisation responds to and acknowledges incidents or mental distress has an impact on the well-being of paramedics. The organisational input will be further discussed in this chapter.

Factors affecting mental health on the job as highlighted in Table 10.1 are inclusive but not entirely representative of all factors. When exploring the literature, it is important to note that the information is vast and additional supported reading is recommended. It is, however, encouraging that there is a continuing developmental strategy for the mental health of paramedics to help define healthier outcomes and improve organisational support. Harris (2017) provides a real-life account of action when a job of unpredictable environment starts with the alarm being raised – one hour before the end of the shift. The psychological pressure starts with the call: 'Patient is trapped under the transport truck, but speaking' (Harris 2017,

TABLE 10.1 Factors affecting mental health on the job.

Factors	Global	Paramedic workforce
Unpredictable environments	Australia, New Zealand, UK, USA, Sweden	Paramedics, students, call handler
Everyday experience of trauma	Australia, New Zealand, UK, USA, Sweden, Canada	Paramedics, students
Levels of stress	Australia, New Zealand, UK, South Africa, Canada, Sweden	Paramedics, students, retired personnel
Dysfunctional peer support	Australia, USA, UK	Paramedics, students
Violence and aggression	Australia, USA, UK	Paramedics, students
Negative attitudes to emotional expression	Australia, UK, New Zealand, Canada	Paramedics, students
Shift patterns and target expectations	Australia, UK, USA	Paramedics, students
Not knowing how to answer family concerns	UK	Students.
Lack of control	UK	Paramedic
Family concerns	Australia, New Zealand, UK	Paramedics, students
Us and them culture	UK	Call handlers
Organisational support/lack of support	Australia, UK	Paramedics, students, retired personnel

Source: Lawn et al. 2020; Warren-James et al. 2021.

p. 1). Already physiologically tired nearing the end of a shift, the attendance, organisation of support to the scene i.e. air ambulance crew, handing over of the patient, and then return to complete the extensive paperwork, clean up, decontamination, and replacement of equipment result in long hours of overtime (Harris 2017). It is evident that the job itself has impact on the physical and mental well-being of the paramedic. Harris (2017) provides tips on self-care and mental health management explored later in this chapter.

Psychological preparedness has been described as the physical visibility of a paramedic to the public. This visual element includes, as noted by Rolfe et al., (2019) the costume, the (military style) protective uniform of durable green material and heavy boots, which signifies the role and profession and differentiates the paramedic from all others. In addition to the uniform's protective qualities it is also one way of establishing professional boundaries. Although presenting as strong and in control when others need them, the paramedic is a human being and the uniform is not an impermeable shield that can prevent the emotional strain of responsibility in the provision of providing care in unpredictable environments.

Global assessment of the well-being of paramedics

Between 2015 and 2019, the UK mental health charity Mind developed the Blue Light Programme, aimed at reducing stigma and improving mental health support for emergency services such as police, ambulance, and fire and rescue services. An initial survey was conducted in 2015 (3,600 respondents) relating to mental health triggers, the support available, and what the participants thought about that organisational support. The study found a clear need for mental health support. This was followed up with a 2019 survey (5,081 respondents). The findings report that 78.5% of ambulance staff, including volunteers, had experienced personal mental health problems (Mind 2019). Exploring emergency response, including correctional workers, a Canadian study found paramedic anxiety rates as high as 22%, depression 10%, and suicidal ideation at 10% (Carleton et al. 2018). Similarly, a prevalence of Post Traumatic Stress Disorder (PTSD) of 15–20%, is reported in Australia (Khan 2020). Larsson (2016) argues that whilst the focus of these studies highlights PTSD, there is a notion that other types of stress-related factors are not included or risk being neglected in PTSD such as, 'wear and tear stress reactions', (Larsson 2016). So, how does this look in relation to what is affecting the mental well-being of paramedics?

From a physiological perspective sleep is crucial to mental and physical well-being. For paramedics, who are working often extended shifts, dealing with the unexpected, being relied upon in the face of adversity for reassurance and life-saving care, lack of sleep is reported to be one of the most common contributing factors affecting mental and physical well-being. Good sleep hygiene is wholly established in health promotion (NICE 2022). Job-related factors that interrupt good sleep can be thinking about the day's events, struggling with guilt, and feeling helpless, which is most commonly reported with the loss of a child. This can result in symptoms of irritability, mood changes, lethargy, anxiety, and worry about the next day. In turn this will become an interrelated cycle, as can be seen in Figure 10.1. Diet will also affect how one is feeling. Missing breaks, dehydration, and often eating quick snacks or fast food on the go, or no meal at all, will exacerbate the same irritability and poor functionality on the job itself.

There are also the effects on relationships with family and colleagues. With shift work often leaving little time for recovery, rest, and social activity, this can lead to a sense of isolation and feeling withdrawn, less compassionate, and projecting blame (Lawn et al. 2020).

Thoughts can linger, keep presenting themselves, and take away one's attention from the present moment. This is unproductive but not at all uncommon. Paramedics attending scenes involving physical risk such as fire, violence, and accidents also have the psychological impact of dealing with that. Rumination, focusing on negative aspects or disturbing thoughts and beliefs of self-blame or questioning, can result. The emotions that arise from those thoughts can lead to a sense of failure, guilt, or blame. These emotions can become suppressed and carried around indefinitely. A challenging but achievable concept of acceptance is having the ability to reflect on and accept these thoughts and emotions without trying to evaluate them (Gartner et al. 2019). In light of this there is also the requirement for paramedics to remain professional despite the potential for both physical and verbal abuse, and the perceived lack of organisational support.

Focusing on the student paramedic, evidence suggests that feelings of anxiety are due to uncertain outcomes, answering questions from family members, and the risk of clinical mistakes, including experiencing a person's death (Warren-James et al. 2021).

Paramedic training has moved from work-based learning, i.e. learning on the job, to university degree courses that include work-integrated learning (WIL) (placement settings) and incorporate classroom focus on teamwork, leadership, and critical thinking. Evidence shows that this training itself can be a compounding contributing factor to suppressed emotion. One of the benefits of on-the-job

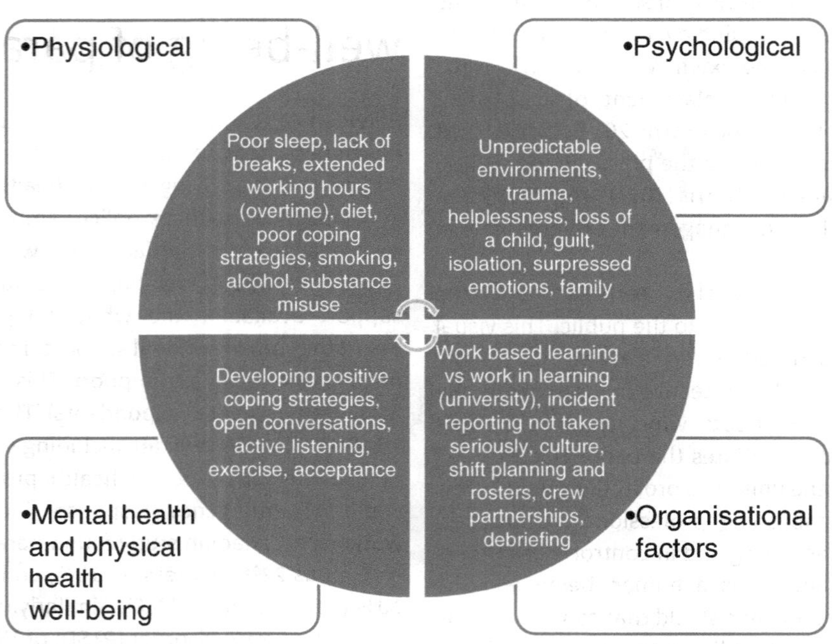

FIGURE 10.1 Overview of contributing factors on physical and mental well-being.

training was the substantial clinical experience gained. A reported prediction of students developing PTSD was the identification of critical incidents exposure, dysfunctional peer support, and negative attitudes towards emotional expression. This was found to account for a 30% variance in the symptomology of trauma-related events (Fjeldheim et al. 2014).

Emotional suppression and workplace culture

Paramedics often describe their work as being highly demanding with little control and low levels of support (Lawn et al. 2020; Warren-James et al. 2021). The demands of the job lead to – but are not restricted to – an emotional, excessive, and exhausting workload. The limited control a paramedic has over situations reflects their lack of opportunity for decision-making and lack of support from managers. Keeping the paramedic student in mind, in a UK study, Jennings (2017) found that 78% of respondents identified that there was a covering up of emotions or feelings in relation to the emotional demands of the role. The paramedic students reported that they became more aware of their emotions in their placement, developing from early on an unspoken need to cover them up. When this was explored further by Holmes et al. (2017), paramedic students and university course coordinators in Australia and New Zealand reported that challenges relating to mental health within the profession were not appropriately covered in courses. A parallel insight is that student nurses find WIL placements equally challenging mentally, and this is particularly noted for third year final students, where expectations of demonstrating knowledge, skills, and clinical competence are increased and often critical decision-making is vital (Edwards et al. 2017). This is compounded by limited time and workplace culture expectations that are more stressful as the student progresses in the course.

Currently paramedicine is generally being offered as a university course, with professional status on completion. It could be argued that within the university culture students are encouraged to seek help and support. This could be concerning their academic work, mental health and well-being, counselling, and supportive physical hobbies and activities. Alzahrani et al. (2023) found in a small cross-cultural study that students sought and received support from academics for their mental health and well-being. However, isolated students who did not ask for help were sometimes the ones most in need of it. Nevertheless, universities do offer academic tutor support and access to mental health and well-being support. This is encouraging, as students recognise that there is an outlet for their thoughts and feelings and that suppressing emotions or the unspoken need to cover them up will promote anxiety and stress rather than reduce them. Reflective practice (Jasper 2013), a valuable developing skill for students, is now embedded in healthcare courses, and the expectation is that the workplace offers the same. For newly qualified paramedics there is evidence that the support of continuing reflection in the workplace is limited or rarely available (Howlett 2019). The strength of reflective practice is that it enables students to consider their actions, delivers care, and makes a link between theory and practice, including organisational policy and management. Reflective practice and the support and learning it provides encourages the student paramedic to be open and honest, and feelings are a central part of it. It will be stressful therefore to experience a closed and challenging mindset of 'just get on with the job'. It is understandable that stresses, traumatic experiences, and physiological outcomes can result in stress, symptoms of depression, and anxiety (Khan 2018). Student and qualified paramedics continue to learn and develop what the dominant group has constructed and found to be acceptable. Suppressing emotions becomes the normal way of thinking and working, despite, as evidenced, causing more harm when behaviours are modelled in order to fit in (Avraham et al. 2014).

Building resilience in the workplace is something that paramedics develop through the sociocultural aspects of the job and also on a personal level. Paramedics enter the profession for a number of reasons, including caring about people, the excitement of variety, childhood and/or life experience, or wanting a change of career. Workload pressures as discussed include the impact of healthcare reforms, which are challenging and demanding. Health and social care systems are measured against key performance indicators and have targets to meet, which are there in the background when attending a job. There are moments where the job is meaningful, when it provokes emotion on a personal level and human connections are made (Clompus et al. 2016). Coping strategies can be informal such as using a form of humour, acceptance and detachment, family and friends, banter with work colleagues. There are also formal coping and resilience strategies, including management, appraisal, debriefing, and external referrals (Clompus et al. 2016; Lawn et al. 2020). Positively for paramedic mental health, there is also a sense of camaraderie, status, identity, and sense of belonging offered through routine and structure for the complex and challenging work (Lawn et al. 2020).

Six distinct stages of critical incidents

Critical incidents can have an impact on mental health for the paramedic and student paramedic. These are what can be known as traumatising events – i.e. events that may cause psychological distress. A common feature of a critical incident is when it becomes overwhelming, bringing to the surface unusual emotional reactions that are strong and may interfere with their functioning. This can be before, during, or post event. These emotions and disturbances differ from the normal stressors of workplace settings. Prehospital care rates the highest in screening for mental disorders such as PTSD (Loef et al. 2021). For a full overview of mental illnesses, please see Chapter 11 of this volume, 'Mental health and out-of-hospital care. There are a number of stages in the response to traumatic events:

- Anticipation stage – preparation for the unknown. Feelings of responsibility with some anxiety and fear of making mistakes. Progression of the event can lead to paramedics feeling worthless and insufficient – despite having done all they could do. This demonstrates how the tough, reliable exterior (uniform) and professional face can camouflage the internal tension and turmoil. Post event, the paramedic may be physiologically exhausted and psychologically confused. Underlying emotions may include anger, sense of rejection from family, loss of control, feeling trapped and helpless (Lawn et al. 2020).
- Effects of relationships with others in the workplace. Interactions with others and lack of compassion causes social withdrawal, isolation and blaming others, especially those close to the paramedic. This is a way of releasing built-up stress and distancing themselves from their own negative feelings. In relation to family, this is a hyper alertness of being protective of their family and friends. It relates to the experience of witnessing worst-case scenarios.
- Organisational observations and operational features – due to the nature of the job, precedence of sick leave, high levels of exposure, and excessive occupational demands. Targets, key performance indicators, and monitored response times all have an impact on paramedics' physical and mental health. Call takers report being on edge because the recording of calls gives them a feeling of being watched. Paramedics also felt that due to previous responses violent and aggressive events often went under-reported, as the culture suggests that is part of the job.
- Perceived control, real control, and nature of critical incident. As previously mentioned, significant stress occurs when a child/baby is involved. Other stressful situations include abuse, harm, suicide, and harm to colleagues. Personal significance can also amplify feelings, for example, when there are triggers such as personal recognition of an event or knowing a patient who has died, this is considered perceived control. Lack of control – either real or perceived – is seen as lack of control over the work environment and knowledge of the outcomes of the event, plus the lack of clinically received feedback after the event. Loss of control relates to workplace safety, bullying, and physical and verbal threats, leading to isolation and withdrawal.

  Protective and coping strategies – compartmentalising. This can help in the short term but could be detrimental in the longer term. This can lead to paramedics distancing themselves from the patient; to avoidance and searching for information (Lawn et al. 2020).

Loef et al. (2021) focused on newly qualified (up to two years in practice) paramedics in the Netherlands. The paramedic course differs somewhat where the students undertake a full nursing course first or a minimum two years of nursing followed by paramedic training. The study found that the paramedics described de-personification of the patient as a coping mechanism – approaching each patient as a medical case rather than a person. When events become critical, to actively avoid getting to know the patient, paramedics tend to not look at the face or personal belongings such as photographs. The paramedics report that when personal identification is made with the patient they see family or their own living environment – they identify with the patient and a strong emotional connection is felt. Examples of this could include someone of the same age, from their neighbourhood, or personally known to them. Tougher times are reported to be when the patient's family is present and they begin to get to know the patient, or tragic cases such as where a young man dies and his baby is due the next day.

As a coping mechanism, paramedics reported that once a call is received, they focus on their medical skills in preparation and discuss an action plan with their crew partner. Checking protocols and staying distanced emotionally helps. On arrival at the scene, all participants depersonify the patient and focus on their clinical and medical skills. After the event, the paramedics describe sharing their feelings with the nearest on-the-scene colleague. They utilise ambulance care professionals – mostly over coffee, and on occasions by actively contacting management. Interestingly, the participants (paramedics) in this study say that the workplace culture is to essentially share their feelings relating to a critical incident:

> *I really need confirmation, from my driver, from my other colleagues I worked with. Did we see the same things? Did we feel the same things? Did we do it well? . . . It reassures me. (participant 12) (Loef et al. 2021)*

For a difficult, challenging, and most rewarding job, the support given and received by colleagues can build confidence, teamwork, and trust, and in turn begin to disperse a culture of unspoken emotions.

Changing the stigma and finding support

What is stigma?

> *A stigma is a negative attitude or idea about a mental, physical, or social feature of a person or group of people. This implies that there is social disapproval. Stigmas are a major concern because they can lead to negative effects such as discrimination. (Olivine 2022)*

To know if we are subject to stigma, it is pivotal that we understand how we can recognise stigma and in what form we may experience or witness it. Some signs of stigma may be noticeable and obvious; however, they can also be subtle and hence sometimes go unrecognised. The mental health stigma experienced by paramedics is often a negative attitude that will prevent the individual from sharing their thoughts and feelings and often inhibits them from seeking the correct support they both want and need.

When considering different generations of paramedics, it can be seen that the level of stigma has transformed throughout the years to now be at a lower level. This might be believed to be due to a reduction in the stigma surrounding mental health itself, mental health training within organisations, and the encouragement to be open, talk, be honest, and seek support. Support comes in many ways, shapes, and forms and can be accessed by everyone from student paramedics to fully qualified paramedics. It is really important to seek advice and know where support opportunities are in one's university or service.

Support can also come through conversation with your colleagues, friends, or family and it is important that you do not let stigma interfere with receiving the support you need. You may often find yourself working with different colleagues on a regular basis, which can minimise opportunities to build a rapport for emotional support and hinder your honesty and openness due to fears around stigma and judgement. However, the chances are that your colleague has either previously experienced or will experience in the future similar feelings to those you are facing at that moment in time. Box 10.1 outlines some top tips for combating stigma.

Self-care and well-being of a paramedic

Throughout our lives, things that happen within our personal life (for example, relationship challenges, sickness, a change in circumstances, or bereavement) or at work that can all influence our mental health and well-being. There will be times where you may be flourishing, thriving, and doing well and then periods where you might be struggling to cope, feeling down, or even in crisis. Research by the mental health charity Mind (2021) found that emergency medical services employees were twice as likely as the general population to identify problems at work as the main cause of their mental ill health. As a paramedic, it is vital that your own self-care and well-being is taken seriously and at the forefront of your daily routine. Everyone is individual and self-care can come in many ways, shapes, and forms depending on the paramedic's needs at that current time.

BOX 10.1 Top tips for combating stigma

- Seek treatment for mental health conditions.
- Reach out and seek support from your university, workplace, and other health service resources.
- Pick up on signs of stigma such as withdrawal and reach out to people who may be experiencing this.
- Educate others in order to destigmatise mental health.
- Be mindful of your choice of words in order to remain sensitive to others.
- Bring awareness to the language and actions around stigma to make a change.
- Demonstrate and show your fellow students and/or colleagues that stigmas are not accurate or acceptable.

Self-care for paramedics can include:

- Getting enough quality sleep.
- Maintaining a well-balanced diet.
- Taking exercise.
- Reaching out to others.
- Setting realistic expectations.
- Practising self-awareness and self-management.
- Committing to a healthy work–life balance.
- Practising wellness through relaxation techniques and mindfulness.
- Keeping a positive attitude.

Since 2020 there has been added extra pressure and strain on the paramedic professional with the impact from the Covid-19 global pandemic. The pandemic placed substantial demands on an already understaffed, overstretched, and under-resourced health system and it stretched practitioners to the limits of their competence causing a considerable impact on their health and well-being. According to a survey conducted by Mind (2021), ambulance staff were the most likely (77 %) to say their mental health has worsened since the start of this pandemic, compared to police (66 %) or fire (65 %). One in four (25 %) 999 staff and volunteers surveyed rated their current mental health as poor or very poor.

Many clinicians had to balance their professional and personal values and commitments alongside the risks that were posed to themselves and their families and their duty to care for patients. Paramedics who had to self-isolate and stay away from their support networks suffered a negative effect on their mental health on top of their professional stress and pressure. The College of Paramedics conducted a survey in 2021 and found that 89% of paramedics reported their jobs were taking a toll on their mental health and 69% agreed that the toll on their mental health had intensified since the start of the Covid-19 pandemic (College of Paramedics 2021).

Whilst all emergency services personnel are faced with tragic and highly stressful events during their career, paramedics are often exposed to these types of dealings on a daily basis. For the majority of the time, most paramedics are resilient, however, traumatic events still take their toll, particularly when considering the cumulative effect of repeated exposure.

> *Paramedics are well-trained to deal with medical emergencies and the horrific aftermath of accidents and disaster scenes. Focusing on the job at hand is an effective way of coping and keeping an emotional distance from the event.*
> *(Phelps 2018)*

What we need to be extremely aware of is that there will be cases that will slip behind the professional guard and become personal. This could be due to being confronted by a scene or patient that strikes a personal chord for some reason. In this case, paramedics are expected to put on a brave face and deal with the challenge ahead. However, this will severely impact the paramedic's own well-being and is something that needs to be addressed by seeking support from available resources.

Burnout is something that many student paramedics and paramedics experience throughout their carer and this often affects the quality of care that patients then receive. Burnout can be caused by long shifts without an appropriate break, shifts over running, staff shortages, and even queuing for hours outside a hospital whilst waiting to hand over the care of their patient. If a paramedic is experiencing burnout it may lead to them making bad decisions and therefore poor patient care. Despite experiencing this, paramedics often feel a personal pressure to carry on and deliver care to more patients due to service pressures. However, it is vital that at this time we acknowledge that we are experiencing symptoms of burnout, talk to the university lead or manager and receive the support that is require for our well-being.

In March 2022, the Association of Ambulance Chief Executives and the College of Paramedics requested that the new tailored mental health continuum for the sector was used by all UK NHS ambulance service employees and volunteers.

Take a moment for yourself and STOPP

STOPP

TAKE A BREATH

OBSERVE: What am I thinking? What am I reacting too? What am I feeling?

PULL BACK: Put in some perspective. See the bigger picture. Is this fact or opinion?

PRACTISE WHAT WORKS: What is the best thing to do for me, for others and for the situation?

Source: getselfhelp 2023. https://www.getselfhelp.co.uk/docs/STOPP.

What is the mental health continuum?

The mental health continuum is a tool which helps us to think about our wellbeing and what actions we can take to improve it. The mental health continuum helps us to identify where our mental health is low. (Association of Ambulance Chief Executives 2023)

The mental health continuum can be used by anyone and recognises that mental health exists on a spectrum anywhere between the two extremes of mental health and mental illness. It also recognises that mental health can be fluctuating: it is not all or nothing and there are a multitude of factors that affect our mental health on a daily basis. The continuum helps us to identify when our mental health is low and what actions and steps can be taken to improve it. Seeing mental health as a visual spectrum allows us to be more forgiving to ourselves and others as well as understanding and acknowledging when it is time for us to seek help from professionals in the hope of preventing a long-term impact that can push us to an extreme.

Conclusion

Throughout the chapter the importance of the mental health of paramedics has been explored in thorough detail and hopefully you now feel more confident around this topic. In order to ensure an understanding of what mental health is and how this can be implemented within your paramedic practice it was imperative to recognise the factors are that affect mental health on the job, the global assessment of the well-being of paramedics, the emotional suppression and workplace culture and the six distinct stages of critical incidents. This will therefore enable you to feel confident to challenge and change the stigma around mental health for paramedics and the process of finding support as well as understanding the importance of self-care and the well-being of a paramedic. Throughout this chapter and along with further reading, all the above will have become clearer and you may now have a deeper and clearer understanding of mental health for paramedics.

It is recommendation that you take care of yourself and others and remember to seek help whenever you feel it is necessary and do not delay this process. It is wholly recommended that you open up conversations with friends, family, and colleagues as it is healthy to discuss changes in your mental health and this will allow the correct pathway to assist you in the best capacity. 'We as paramedics need to remember that we are just as human as our patients. We bleed, cry, and hurt, and that's OK.' (Harris, 2017).

Activities

Now review your learning by completing the learning activities in this chapter. The answers to these appear at the end of the book. Further self-test activities can be found at **www.wileyfundamentalseries.com/paramedic/3e.**

Activity 10.1

- Visit https://www.who.int/news-room/fact-sheets/detail/mental-health-strengthening-our-response#SnippetTab.
- Read the determinants of mental health.
- Make some notes of what stands out to you. What relates to your current work experience?
- Activity time thirty minutes to one hour.

Activity 10.2

Go back to the Case study at the start of this chapter. Read it again and make a few notes. It is a short case study.

Now, using the Rolfe et al. (2001) Model of Reflection, reflect on:

What? What is happening? Who are the individuals in the case study?

So what? What are the feelings of the individuals? What are they saying? What do you think each one is thinking.

Now what? What are you feeling? What are your thoughts? Reflect on how you engage/listen/offer support/open conversation.

Activity 10.3

Access and read the mental health continuum chart. Complete the below next time you are on a shift:

Start of shift check in:

Where are you on the continuum?

Is there anything that you can consciously do to change where you are on the continuum?

End of shift check in:

Where are you on the continuum?

Are you in a different place now than you were at the start of your shift?

If so, what has contributed?

For further reading on paramedic mental health and well-being see https://collegeofparamedics.co.uk/COP/Member_/Paramedic_Mental_Health_and_Wellbeing.aspxeofparamedics.co.uk.

Glossary

Compassion: Often regarded as being sensitive to the emotional aspects of the suffering of others.

Competence: The ability to do something successfully or efficiently.

Critical incident: An event that occurs out of the range of normal experience; one that is sudden and unexpected, involves the perception of a threat to life, and may include elements of physical and emotional loss.

Key performance indicators: Used by many organisations including healthcare providers to see if they are meeting their objectives.

Post-traumatic stress disorder: A mental health condition caused by a traumatic experience.

Resilience: The ability to cope mentally or emotionally with a crisis or to return to pre-crisis status quickly.

Sleep hygiene: This encompasses both environment and habits, it can pave the way for higher-quality sleep and better overall health.

Stigma: *A* negative and often unfair social attitude that is attached to a person or group, this can often place shame on them for a perceived deficiency or difference.

Suicidal ideation: Often called suicidal thoughts or ideas, this is a broad term that is used to describe a range of contemplations, wishes, and preoccupations with death and suicide.

Workplace culture: The shared values, belief systems, attitudes, and set of assumptions that people in a workplace share.

References

Alzahrani, A., Keyworth, C., Wilson, C. et al. (2023). Causes of stress and poor wellbeing among paramedic students in Saudi Arabia and the United Kingdom: a cross-cultural qualitative study. *BMC Health Serv Res* **23** (1): 444. doi: 10.1186/s12913-023-09374-y. PMID: 37147658; PMCID: PMC10163716.

Association of Ambulance Chief Executives. (2023). The mental health continuum. Available at: https://aace.org.uk/mental-health-continuum/ (accessed 1 June 2023).

Avraham, N., Goldblatt, H., and Yafe, E. (2014). Paramedics' experiences and coping strategies when encountering critical incidents.

Qual Health Res **24** (2): 194–208. doi: 10.1177/1049732313519867. PMID: 24495988.

Centre for Mental Health. (2023). Parity of esteem. Available at: "Parity of esteem" | Centre for Mental Health (accessed 20 June 2023).

Carleton, R., Afifi, TQ., Turner, S. et al. (2018). Mental disorder symptoms among public safety personnel in Canada. *Can Journal of Psychiatry* **68** (1): 54–56. Available at: Mental Disorder Symptoms among Public Safety Personnel in Canada - PubMed (nih.gov) (accessed 25 June 2023).

Clompus, S.R. and Albarran, J.W. (2016). Exploring the nature of resilience in paramedic practice: A psycho-social study. *International Emergency Nursing* **28**: 1–7. doi: 10.1016/j.ienj.2015.11.006.

College of Paramedics. (2021). Paramedic mental health and wellbeing. Available at: https://collegeofparamedics.co.uk/COP/News/college_of_paramedics_survey_results_2021.aspx (accessed 1 June 2023).

Department of Health. (2012). Compassion in practice. Available at: Microsoft Word - 121203_Compassion in practice_FULL DW (england.nhs.uk) (accessed 23 October 2023).

Edwards, M.J., Bassett, G., Sinden, L., and Fothergill, R.T. (2015). Frequent callers to ambulance service: patient profiling and impact of case management on patient utilisation of the ambulance service. *Journal of Emergency Medicine* **32** (5): 392–396.

Fjeldheim, C.B., Nöthling, J., Pretorius, K. et al. (2014). Trauma exposure, posttraumatic stress disorder and the effect of explanatory variables in paramedic trainees. *BMC Emerg Med* **14**: 11. doi: 10.1186/1471-227X-14-11.

Gärtner, A., Behnke, A., Conrad, D. et al. (2019). Emotion regulation in rescue workers: differential relationship with perceived work-related stress and stress-related symptoms. *Front Psychol* **9**: 2744. doi: 10.3389/fpsyg.2018.02744. PMID: 30687192; PMCID: PMC6335291.

Harris, N. (2017). Equipping paramedics to look after their mental health and wellbeing. *Journal of Paramedic Practice.* Available at: Equipping paramedics to look after their mental health and wellbeing | Journal Of Paramedic Practice (accessed 19 June 2023).

Health and Social Care Act. (2012). Available at: Health and Social Care Act 2012 (legislation.gov.uk) (accessed 19 June 2023).

Holmes, L., Jones, R., Brightwell, R. et al. (2017). Student paramedic anticipation, confidence and fears: do undergraduate courses prepare student paramedics for the mental health challenges of the profession? *Australasian Journal of Paramedicine* **14:** 1–12. Doi: 10.33151/ajp.14.4.545.

Howlett, G. (2019). Nearly qualified student paramedics perceptions of reflection and use in practice. *Journal of Paramedic Practice* **11** (6): 258–263.

Jasper, M. (2013). *Beginning Reflective Practice*. Australia: Cengage Learning, EMEA.

Jones, J. (2020). As a paramedic in England, I'm shocked at assaults on ambulance staff during Covid. *The Guardian.* Available at: As a paramedic in England, I'm shocked at assaults on ambulance staff during Covid | Jake Jones | The Guardian (accessed 26 June 2023).

Jennings, K. (2017). Emotional labour in paramedic practice: student awareness of professional demands. *Journal of Paramedic Practice* **9** (7): 288–294. doi: 10.12968/jpar.2017.9.7.288.

Khan, W.A.A., Conduit, R., Kennedy, G.A. et al. (2020). Sleep and mental health among paramedics from Australia and Saudi Arabia: a comparison study. *Clocks Sleep* **2** (2): 246–257. doi: 10.3390/clockssleep2020019. PMID: 33089203; PMCID: PMC7445850.

Larsson, G., Berglund, A.K., and Ohlsson, A. (2016). Daily hassles, their antecedents and outcomes among professional first responders: a systematic literature review. *Sc and J Psychol* **57** (4): 359–367. doi: 10.1111/sjop.12303. PMID: 27291300.

Lawn et al. (2020). The effects of emergency medical service work on the psychological, physical, and social well-being of ambulance personnel: a systemic review of qualitative research. *BMC Psychiatry* **20** (1): 348. doi: 10.1186/s12888-020-02752-4.

Loef, J., Vloet, L.C.M., Vierhoven, PH. et al. (2021). Starting ambulance care professionals and critical incidents: a qualitative study on experiences, consequences and coping strategies. *BMC Emerg Med* **21:** 110. doi: 10.1186/s12873-021-00500-9.

Mind. (2019). Mental health in the emergency services: our 2019 survey results – Ambulance Service. London: Mind.

Mind. (2021). Mind survey reveals toll of pandemic on ambulance workers' mental health. Available at: https://www.mind.org.uk/news-campaigns/news/mind-survey-reveals-toll-of-pandemic-on-ambulance-workers-mental-health/ (accessed 1 June 2023).

National Institute for Health and Care Excellence (NICE). (2016). Lower back pain and sciatica in over 16s: assessment and management. Available at: Overview | Low back pain and sciatica in over 16s: assessment and management | Guidance | NICE (accessed 19 June 2023).

National Institute for Health and Care Excellence (NICE). (2022). Sleep hygiene. Available at: Sleep to treat insomnia and insom nia symptoms (nice.org.uk) (accessed 25 June 2023).

Olivine, A. (2022). What is stigma? Available at: Stigma: Definition, Signs, Impact, and Coping (verywellhealth.com) (accessed 16 June 2023).

Phelps, A. (2018). Paramedics need more support to deal with daily trauma. The University of Melbourne. Available at: Paramedics need more support to deal with daily trauma (theconversation.com) (accessed 23 October 2023).

Rolfe, G., Freshwater, D., and Jasper, M. (2001). *Critical Reflection in Nursing and the Helping Professions: A User's Guide*. Basingstoke: Palgrave Macmillan.

The King's Fund. (2015). Prioritising mental health. Available at: Prioritising mental health | The King's Fund (kingsfund.org.uk) (accessed 15 June 2023).

Warren-James, M. et al. (2021). Paramedic students' experiences of stress whilst undertaking ambulance placements – An integrative review. *Australasian Emergency Care* **24** (2021): 296–301.

World Health Organization (WHO). (2022). *Mental Health*. Available at: https://www.who.int/newsroom/factsheets/detail/mental-health-strengths-our-response (accessed 15 June 2023).

CHAPTER 11

Responding to mental health in the community

Marie Boulianne

Clinical Nurse Manager Bethesda Clinic, Western Australia, Australia

Contents

LEARNING OUTCOMES

On completion of this chapter, the reader will be able to:

- Define positive mental health and mental illness.
- Understand the general intent of the mental health legislation in Australia.
- List the common symptoms of dementia, affective disorders, anxiety disorders, post-traumatic stress disorder, schizophrenia, and psychotic disorders.
- Explain the primary considerations in conducting a risk assessment.
- Identify often confused physical conditions or medication side effects for mental health symptoms.
- Describe simple strategies to care for someone experiencing a mental health crisis and for oneself.

Fundamentals of Paramedic Practice: A Systems Approach, Third Edition. Edited by Sam Willis and Ian Peate.

Companion website: www.wiley.com/go/willis/paramedic3e

Case study

An ambulance is called to a private residence to attend to a forty-seven-year-old man with chest pain and shortness of breath. The paramedics assess for cardiac difficulties whilst also considering symptoms of anxiety. How would they identify and evaluate each of these? What would be the inclusion and exclusion criteria?

Introduction

Everyone goes through life's ups and downs, which are often caused by everyday events. These events usually have their own timeline, and the person will eventually return to a state of well-being.

We each deal with life's challenges and pressures in various ways, often implementing healthy or unhealthy **coping mechanisms**. For example, physical exercise is regarded as a healthy coping mechanism, whereas consuming large amounts of alcohol is not. Excessive use of unhealthy coping mechanisms can create their own problems such as alcohol dependence and exacerbate the original issue.

However, some problems may persist longer, leading to mental health conditions that may affect the individual on a range of severity from mild anxiety to psychosis.

Mental health challenges can be difficult to identify. Psychiatric symptoms may be hard to assess objectively and vary significantly between individuals. What we feel inside is not always easily visible on the outside and can often be difficult to describe to someone else. It can be highly subjective and provoke a strong personal response from those around us.

This chapter will present the reader with an introduction to the concepts of mental health and will provide a concise overview of the leading mental health conditions encountered on the road. The chapter offers strategies to assist paramedics called to attend to adult patients with a variety of mental health concerns.

Positive mental health and mental illness

Mental illness is usually understood in the context of a person experiencing mental health symptoms (e.g. persistent feelings of sadness, insomnia) and **psychopathology** (e.g. major depressive disorder, schizophrenia, anxiety disorder). **Positive mental health** refers to a person's overall subjective psychological well-being (Ryff 1989) and their ability to function optimally (Huppert 2005). Various personal resources are conducive to this full functioning, including one's character strengths (Peterson and Seligman 2004), flourishing (Keyes 2002), resilience (Bonanno 2004), life satisfaction (Diener et al. 1985), quality of interpersonal relationships (Reis and Gable 2003), and purpose and meaning in life (Steger et al. 2006).

Mental health is often described on a bipolar continuum from positive mental health to mental illness (Figure 11.1) (Trent 1992).

However, there is growing evidence suggesting that these concepts exist independently yet are intricately influenced by one another and overlap in several ways (Iasiello and van Agteren 2020). It is possible to be experiencing highly positive mental health resources despite a diagnosis of a mental illness (Heiervang et al. 2008). And reversely, the absence of mental illness does not guarantee positive mental health (Jahoda 1958). Mental health is therefore better understood in subgroups that account for the presence or absence of mental illness and the presence of high or low positive mental health (Keyes 2005; Iasiello and van Agteren 2020). These four subgroups are:

1. Complete mental health
2. Symptomatic
3. Struggling
4. Vulnerable

Stigma

People experiencing mental health conditions are often subject to stigma. Stigma in mental health relates to the validation of negative stereotypes and the labelling of an individual who is experiencing mental health challenges (Corrigan and Wassel 2008). The individuals are also subject to labelling themselves, which is referred to as **internalised stigma** or **self-stigma** (Lyon and Mortimer-Jones 2020). This personal judgement can negatively affect concordance with treatment and recovery and increase symptomology. In attending to persons in the community, paramedics need

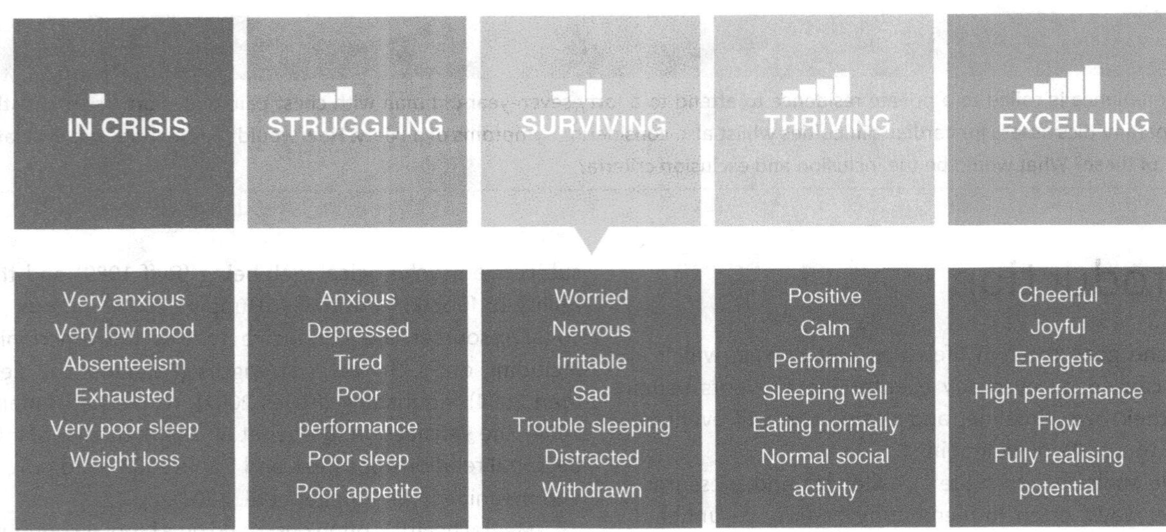

IN CRISIS
STRUGGLING
SURVIVING
THRIVING
EXCELLING
Very anxious
Very low mood
Absenteeism
Exhausted
Very poor sleep
Weight loss
Anxious
Depressed
Tired
Poor performance
Poor sleep
Poor appetite
Worried
Nervous
Irritable
Sad
Trouble sleeping
Distracted
Withdrawn
Positive
Calm
Performing
Sleeping well
Eating normally
Normal social activity
Cheerful
Joyful
Energetic
High performance
Flow
Fully realising potential

FIGURE 11.1 Mental health continuum. Source: Delphis. https://delphis.org.uk/mental-health/continuum-mental-health/.

to be aware of the role played by stigma. For instance, the person in need of care may not have reached out for help by fear, or past experience, of being stigmatised (see section below on Borderline Personality Disorder). Bystanders may negatively label the person or their behaviour ('acting like a crazy person', 'loony'), or the paramedic may themselves approach the person or the behaviour undesirably, responding to their own negative feelings. Self-reflection plays a significant role in identifying and dealing with these harmful cognitive and emotional responses (O'Connor and O'Hara 2018).

Mental health legislation

Within Australia, mental health legislation was developed to protect the rights and dignity of people experiencing mental health difficulties affecting their capacity to make sound decisions. In Australia, the Mental Health Act (MHA) differs between states and territories, though the essence of the legislation is shared across the country. It covers voluntary and involuntary admissions in mental health facilities, stipulating the boundaries of involuntary detention, transfer to another facility, and treatment (including the provision of electroconvulsive therapy) in the community or facilities. It details restrictive practices such as physical, chemical, and mechanical restraint within authorised hospitals. For a quick reference guide, visit the RANZCP (2017) Mental Health Acts - comparative tables (ranzcp.org).

Additionally, the MHAs promote a recovery-oriented practice that provides the person with the right to joint decision-making in their care and the involvement of the person/s caring for them. Paramedics called to attend to a person who is experiencing mental health distress can transport them to an authorised mental health facility or emergency department (alternative place) if they have reasonable grounds to believe that the person is mentally ill or disturbed. Paramedics can also request police assistance if they have serious concerns for their safety or that of the person/s they are attending. It is estimated that prehospital mental health emergencies account for 11% of calls received (Morisson-Rees et al. 2015; Duncan et al. 2019).

Overview of common mental health conditions and illnesses

Dementia

Dementia is an umbrella term that comprises several symptoms relating to progressive neurological conditions affecting the brain. There are several types of dementia, and they have different causes and symptoms. These are presented in Table 11.1. The risk of developing dementia increases with age, and symptoms become apparent in

TABLE 11.1 Types of dementia and their causes and symptoms.

Type of dementia	Causes	Symptoms
Alzheimer's disease Most frequent form of dementia	Mostly unknown though general health risk factors may contribute to its development (e.g. lack of mental exercise, obesity, alcohol, high blood pressure, smoking, and physical inactivity).	Frequent, ongoing, and persistent memory loss, disorientation to time, place, and person. Difficulty with thinking, planning, solving problems and executive functions. Language and comprehension difficulties. Reduced motivation. Changes in personality and mood. Symptoms can be variable throughout the day, change between days, and be negatively affected by fatigue, stress, and ill-health.
Vascular dementia	Single or multiple strokes. Untreated hypertension or diabetes causing vascular damage to the small blood vessels in the brain. Brain functions will be affected according to the size and location of the damage in the brain.	Reasoning and thinking skills deterioration. Mild memory issues. Walking and movement difficulties. Behavioural changes. Incontinence.
Lewy Body disease	Term that includes Parkinson's disease and dementia with Lewy bodies (microscopic structures of abnormal protein deposits in brain cells).	Alterations of movements, thinking abilities, and behaviour. Apathy, anxiety, depression, fatigue, constipation, urinary incontinence, excessive sleepiness, poor sense of smell, and delusions.
Frontotemporal dementia	Progressive damage to either/or/both the frontal and temporal brain lobes. Most common in people under the age of sixty-five. There are several subtypes of frontotemporal dementia with varying signs and symptoms.	Alterations of movements, thinking abilities, and behaviour. Fixed mood and behaviour, appearance of selfishness and inflexibility, apathy and amotivation. Loss of empathy and/or emotional warmth. Easily distracted and impulsive. Changes in eating preferences. Decline in self-care and personal hygiene. Lack of insight. Repetitive motor behaviours (e.g. counting, collecting, tapping). *Note: memory often remains unaffected, particularly in early stages. In addition to behaviour changes, symptoms for some subtypes can include progressive aphasia (loss of language) and semantic (ability to assign words).
Alcohol syndrome dementia	People with excessive alcohol consumption over several years (though not all will develop the condition). Diet and lifestyle factors are believed to play a role. Men over forty-five years of age are most commonly affected.	Impaired cognitive abilities. Personality changes Issues with decreased initiative, spontaneity, memory. Difficulty maintaining clear and logical cognitive tasks requiring planning, organising, common sense judgement, and social skills. Difficulty with equilibrium.

Source: Dementia Australia 2022.

those over sixty-five years. However, people in their forties and fifties have also been diagnosed with dementia.

Affective disorders

Depression

Depression is a widespread condition that ranges in severity from mild to severe and life-threatening. More females than males (8.5% vs 6.2%) are diagnosed with depression (ABS 2022). There are different types of depression, including postnatal depression (PND), seasonal affective disorder (SAD), and bipolar disorder (see below).

Depression with symptoms lasting over twelve months is known as major depressive disorder or clinical depression. It is a common and severe disorder affecting one in sixteen Australians (ABS 2022).

Symptoms can include low mood, tearfulness, changes (increase or decrease) in appetite and sleep patterns, social isolation or withdrawal, loss of libido and interest in previously enjoyable activities, low self-esteem, reduced confidence, and hopelessness. Some people, but not all, may experience suicidal thoughts and engage in self-harm behaviour (see below). However, people with depression are not 'down, sad, and depressed' all of the time. Some may still be able to engage in humour, smile, or exhibit traits that could appear inconsistent with popular expectation of depression.

Bipolar

Bipolar disorder is characterised by extreme shifts in moods, from mania ('high') to severe depression ('low') that can persist for weeks. However, there may be long periods of stable mental health (weeks or even years) between episodes.

There are two predominant types of bipolar disorder: Bipolar I and Bipolar II. The main difference between the two lay in the severity of the manic episode. People with Bipolar I will experience a full episode of mania, whilst someone with Bipolar II will experience hypomania, which is less severe or long-lasting than mania.

Mania can be experienced as feeling intensely upbeat, jumpy, or wired, with a marked increase in energy, activity, or agitation. Some people experience an exaggerated sense of self or self-confidence (grandiosity), excitement or happiness (euphoria). Periods of mania tend to precede periods of depression. However, despite common extreme mood shifts, symptoms will vary between individuals.

During manic phases, there is often an increase in risk-taking behaviours. Paramedics may be called to attend to consequences of intrusive and disinhibited behaviour, road accidents from dangerous driving, or casualty from perilous behaviour (e.g. setting themselves on fire to remove parasites on skin as a result of tactile hallucinations, jumping from high altitude thinking they can fly, etc.).

Anxiety disorders

Humans (as well as animals) experience a state of **anxiety** when their well-being or survival is under perceived or actual threat. Experiencing anxiety is normal and necessary to remain alive. Anxiety increases arousal, activates the autonomic and neuroendocrine systems and vigilance, moving us into action to deal with a potential threat.

An **anxiety attack** is characterised by the experience of persistent irrational fears or thoughts whilst a **panic attack** also includes physiological symptoms (see below).

Generalised anxiety disorder (GAD) is when anxiety symptoms emerge in the absence of threat. The person additionally finds it difficult to control their worry more often than not and symptoms occur over several months, impacting their normal functioning.

Physiological symptoms can include feeling dizzy/faint/lightheaded or unsteady, shortness of breath, tachycardia, chest pain, nausea, abdominal upset, sweating, shaking, chills or heat sensations, and paraesthesia. The person may also experience a fear of dying or losing control, **dissociation** such as **derealisation** (feeling removed from reality, as if in a movie), or **depersonalisation** (feeling detached from, or outside of, own self/body).

Obsessive-compulsive disorder (OCD) relates to when an individual is experiencing obsessions, compulsions, or both. **Obsessions** are experienced as unwanted or intrusive, persistent, and recurring urges, thoughts, or images that cause significant anxiety or distress. The person cannot ignore, suppress, or neutralise (by performing a compulsion) these urges, thoughts, or images. **Compulsions** are repetitive behaviours (e.g. checking, ordering, hand-washing, etc.) or mental acts (e.g. counting, silently repeating words, praying) that a person feels urged to perform because of the obsessions, or in accordance with an inflexible set of rules that must be applied. These are aimed at preventing or reducing distress experienced by the obsession, a dreaded event, or situation. These behaviours or acts may or may not be logically connected with what they aim to neutralise and can be overly excessive. The obsessions and compulsions account for more than one hour per day and cause significant distress or impairment in daily functioning, work, or socialisation. There are several misconceptions about OCD; the disorder is often reduced to being 'a clean freak' or said of someone ordering their pencils by colour and there are often misrepresentations in public culture (Kim 2021).

Personality disorders

Some people with mental health disorders can present with challenging behaviours. **Emotional Unstable Personality Disorder (EUPD)** and **Borderline Personality Disorder (BPD)** are often encountered. They can be particularly exigent when the person is emotionally dysregulated and/or affected by substances. Their behaviours can affect personal relationships, amplified by an increase in mood lability, risky and impulsive actions, self-harming, and their often-extreme reactions to abandonment (perceived or real), chronic feelings of emptiness, and shame (Perrotta 2020). BPD has been linked to childhood adversity (Porter et al. 2019). Stigma around these diagnostic terms, particularly from health care providers, is prevalent (Papathanasiou and Stylianidis 2022). Some people even express they avoid seeking help when they are in crisis due to past adverse experiences that increased their distress rather reduce it (Ng et al. 2019). Self-harm is a common presentation to paramedics in those who present with personality disorders, usually in the form of cutting of the skin.

Post-traumatic stress disorder

Post-traumatic stress disorder (PTSD) is when acute stress from a traumatic event remains unresolved and symptoms are still present after one month from exposure and are causing distress and functional impairment (such as affecting work or socialisation). A person may have experienced a traumatic event such as exposure to actual or threat of death, serious injury, or sexual violence. This exposure may have been:

Direct: person directly affected by the trauma.
Vicarious: as a witness to the traumatic event.
Indirect: learning that a relative/friend/close person was exposed to a trauma, or being exposed to the details of trauma, often through work duties (first responders, crime scene investigators, medics).

Symptoms can include:

Intrusions: nightmares, flashbacks, unwanted upsetting memories, emotional distress, physical reactivity.
Avoidance: person may avoid any trauma-related thoughts, feelings, or external reminders.
Negative cognitive alterations: negative thoughts or feelings at the onset or following the trauma, e.g. inability to recall details of the trauma, feeling isolated, negative affect and difficulty experiencing a positive one, exaggerated blame towards self or others for causing the trauma.
Arousal and reactivity alterations: changes in arousal and reactivity at the onset or following the trauma, e.g. irritability or aggression, risky or destructive behaviour, hypervigilance, easily startled, difficulty with concentration or sleep.
Dissociation: depersonalisation or derealisation.

Schizophrenia and psychotic disorders

Psychosis is a condition whereby a person loses touch with reality. It includes a combination of symptoms affecting thinking patterns, behaviour, and perceptions.

These symptoms are classed as either 'positive' or 'negative'. This does not refer to the quality (as in 'good' or 'bad') but as to whether the symptoms are 'added on' (**positive**) or 'take something away' or express a reduction in normal functioning or affect (**negative**).

Hallucinations are erroneous alterations of sensory perceptions that the person believes to be true but others around them cannot experience the same. They can involve any of the five senses. See Table 11.2 for more details and examples.

TABLE 11.2 **Positive and negative psychotic symptoms.**

Symptoms		Description	Example
Positive			
Hallucinations	Visual	Seeing things (people, objects, or images) that others cannot see.	Faces, flashes, particular shapes.
	Auditory	Hearing specific voices that are not their own and are coming from an external point (not a person's own inner voice). These can also be specific noises.	Hearing voices from either known or unknown people; content can be complementary, derogatory, or commanding. Hearing music, laughing, humming, tapping, etc.
	Olfactory	A smell that only the person can smell and is most frequently unpleasant.	Excrement, rotten fish, or eggs, oil.
	Gustatory	Tasting of unpleasant food that others cannot.	Taste of spoiled food.
	Tactile	Feeling something on the skin that is not there.	Bugs crawling up on their skin.
Delusions	Ideas of grandeur, or Grandiosity	Believing they are 'bigger' than they are or have special powers.	Being God or the prime minister; ability to control the weather with their thoughts.
	Paranoia	Being watched, monitored, followed.	There is a camera in the licence plate in the car in front of them; their phone is being tapped and others are listening in on their conversations.
	Reference	Specific sounds or sights are directed at them with a hidden message; or normal daily events have a special meaning that only they know about.	The person reading the news on the television is talking about them; numbers printed on the newspaper add up to the formula to cure cancer.
	Influence	Other people are manipulating or controlling them.	Medication being prescribed is to poison or control them.
	Persecutory	Believing that some life events happen to punish past wrongdoings.	A bushfire or car pile-up on the freeway is their fault.
	Religious	Believing they have a special connection with God or a deity.	God is speaking to them directly or sending special messages.
Thought	Insertion	Others are putting thoughts into their head, or they are experiencing own thoughts as that of someone else's.	
	Withdrawal	Someone is taking away their thoughts or there is an interruption in the flow of thoughts as if 'someone took them out'.	
	Broadcasting	Believing others can hear their thoughts or know what they are thinking about.	
Disorganised thought or speech	Tangential	Digressing or being off topic.	Talking about cars, electric cars, then hydroelectricity and hydrogen.
	Derailment	Ideas are semi- or non-related.	Talking about cars, to mice, to cereals.

TABLE 11.2 *(Continued)*

Symptoms		Description	Example
Positive			
	Neologism	Creating new words.	
	Flight of ideas	Multiple ideas spoken very fast and erratically.	
	Blocking/mutism	Stop talking mid-sentence and resume several seconds or minutes later often changing the topic.	
	Circumstantiality	Going around in circles and adding too many irrelevant or unnecessary details.	
	Word salad	Mostly incoherent collection of words.	
Negative			
Reduced/flat affect		Monotone voice, reduced/lack of variability in facial expression.	
Reduced/lack of enjoyment		Reduced/lack of ability to find pleasure in daily life.	
Reduced/lack of speech		Only speaks when forced to interact.	
Personal hygiene		Neglecting personal hygiene – not showering, wearing the same clothes for several days.	
Activities of daily living		Needing help to complete everyday activities; may appear to be 'lazy' and unmotivated.	
Social withdrawal		Avoiding going outside of their house and being afraid to do so.	

Schizophrenia is a mental illness that includes psychosis but to a more severe extent. To reach a diagnosis of schizophrenia, some of the symptoms must last continuously for at least six months. A person with schizophrenia may have one or multiple episodes of psychosis or of being unwell throughout their life; however, symptoms can often be managed with a combination of medication, psychotherapy, and support.

There are several misconceptions about schizophrenia. The illness is erroneously associated with a 'split personality', and the stigma that people with schizophrenia are 'dangerous' is also false (Goodwin 2014). Most of them tend to be more afraid of others due to their symptoms. If they exhibit violent behaviour, it is generally due to reacting out of fear rather than being overly aggressive. However, individuals with a diagnosis of schizophrenia who have comorbid substance misuse, a history of antisocial conduct, or a trauma history are at increased risk of violence (Fazel et al. 2009; De Girolamo et al. 2021). Additionally, the person can have prolonged periods of remission and can resume normal functioning.

Self-harm and suicide

A person who **self-harms** may engage in the behaviour to reduce emotional pain and distress or due to overwhelming feelings. They may also seek to regain a sense of control over their life, to 'feel something' to counteract feelings of numbness or 'being dead inside', to feel pleasure or to inflict self-punishment. However, self-harm does not have the primary intention of causing death. This is also termed **non-suicidal self-injury** (NSSI).

Self-harm can be performed in a variety of ways. A person may cut, scrape, pierce, bite, burn, or pick their skin; hit or punch themselves or bang their head; eat glass; pull their hair or eyebrows; swallow batteries; insert foreign objects in skin or body cavities; poison or misuse drugs, medication, or alcohol; misuse food (not eating or overeating); exercise to the point of exhaustion; engage in fights that they are likely to get hurt in; or have unsafe sex.

Suicide refers to a direct personal attempt at ending one's life. It is also possible for a person to engage in NSSI and to accidentally die by suicide.

Family and intimate partner violence and assaults

Intimate partner violence refers to aggression and abuse committed in the context of a current or former romantic relationship. Other family members may also inflict abuse

TABLE 11.3 Risk assessment factors

	Possible risks to self or others, or by others
Historical / background	Previous history of an attempt of own life or self-harm behaviour Major physical disability or illness Family history of suicide History of abuse or trauma
Current	Current attempt on own life (or expressing distress, intent, or plan) Medical condition (e.g. terminal illness) Psychiatric condition (paranoid ideations, command hallucinations) Current abuse or trauma Misuse of alcohol and other drugs Weapons or firearms (knives, ropes, guns) Behavioural: reduced self-control, impulsivity, anger, frustration
Circumstantial factors	Recently separated/widowed/divorced Loss of job Homelessness Significant life event
Protective factors	**Any factors that may reduce the risk of suicidality or violence, increase reasons to seek help or personal strengths** e.g.: Having a child/grandchild, pet Support from a partner/significant other, family member, carer, or social network Religious faith

Note: being male, LGBTQIA+, and under the age of thirty-five also significantly increase the risk of suicidality.

or commit violent acts towards others in the household. The violence or abuse perpetrated may be physical, verbal, sexual, emotional, financial, or social. The purpose of this is to instil fear in the partner or family member to maintain, or gain, control over them.

Within Australia in 2021, more than one in two recorded assaults involved domestic or family violence. Almost one in four women (23%) and one in seven men (7.8%) have experienced sexual and/or physical violence by an intimate partner at least once since the age of fifteen (AIHW 2022).

Risk assessment

A **risk assessment** is an important tool that aims to identify potential dangers and predict the likelihood and level of harm that could occur (Ayhan and Üstün 2021). This risk assessment allows the creation of a risk management plan that identifies interventions and actions that can reduce the threat or harm level.

A person may be at risk from their own behaviour or suicidality (**risk to self**), from someone else (**risk by others**), or to someone else (**risk to others**). Risk can also be increased by historical or current factors or lessened by protective factors (Wu et al. 2011; Ayhan and Üstün 2021). Table 11.3 provides explanations and examples.

Differential diagnosis

Some symptoms that appear a priori to be related to a mental health condition may be due to a physical cause. It is crucial for health professionals to remain objective and consider the differential diagnosis. Table 11.4 lists psychiatric symptoms with possible physiological causes.

Similarly, some medications can cause side effects that could be mistaken for mental health symptoms (Table 11.5).

Several homeless and vulnerable people with confusion due to organic factors (e.g. diabetic ketoacidosis, sepsis, intracranial bleeding) have been neglected to near or actual death in emergency departments and police lock ups because they were thought to be just drunk, stoned, or fabricating. People experiencing homelessness often have multi-morbidities (Vallesi et al. 2021) and the chance of misdiagnosis is high. It is therefore appropriate for paramedics to have a high index of suspicion because they can colour the diagnostic leanings during assessment.

Practice considerations

In addition to attending to acute deterioration, there are several practical considerations that you will need to take whilst caring for a person in mental distress.

Priorities as a first responder

As a paramedic several considerations will impact attending a person with, or affected by, a mental health condition. The first priorities will be the dispatch considerations – how many paramedics are needed to attend, is reinforcement needed, e.g. other paramedics, police, fire brigade – the

TABLE 11.4 Common psychiatric symptoms with possible physiological causes.

Symptom	Possible physiological causes
Anxiety	Anaemia Endocrine disorders (e.g. hyperthyroidism) Hypoglycaemia Neurological disorders Pheochromocytoma Dyspnoea (e.g. secondary to other disease including anaemia, lung disease such as asthma, COPD, interstitial lung disease, etc.) Substance withdrawal (sudden cessation of alcohol, benzodiazepines, narcotics, including commencement of naltrexone)
Depression	Autoimmune disease (e.g. lupus, rheumatoid arthritis, et al.) Cancer (incl. paraneoplastic syndromes) Diabetes mellitus Endocrine disorders (hypothyroidism, Addison's disease, parathyroid gland disease) Electrolyte imbalance (e.g. hyponatraemia) Infection Neurological disorders (e.g. dementia, epilepsy, Parkinson's disease, stroke)
Fatigue	Anaemia Cancer Chronic infection Endocrine disorders (e.g. hypothyroidism, Addison's disease, Cushing's syndrome) Radio/chemotherapy Electrolyte imbalances – hyponatraemia, hypokalaemia, hypocalcaemia, hypomagnesaemia
Headache	Brain tumour Migraine Temporal arteritis Subarachnoid haemorrhage
Weakness	Autoimmune disease (e.g. myasthenia gravis, rheumatoid arthritis) Neurological disorders (e.g. Parkinson's disease) Peripheral neuropathy
Confusion/ Psychosis	Sepsis Intracranial neoplasm Metabolic disturbances (incl. hypercalcaemia, hypophosphatasaemia, Diabetic ketoacidosis) Creutzfeldt-Jakob disease

assessment of the scene and the first impressions. To do so, the paramedic will heavily rely on their ability to effectively engage and build rapport with the patient, often requiring using de-escalation techniques. This will help them complete their assessment, manage possible intoxication, reduce risk level, and initiate appropriate interventions.

Engagement and de-escalation

The first resource available is how we engage with the person. Our body language (as well as theirs!) will quickly signal our attitude toward another person. It is essential to allow sufficient space for self and others (to react in a dangerous situation or to avoid creating fear in the other), maintaining a low, calming, and reassuring voice and conveying genuine interest in the person. Acknowledge their distress, maintain eye contact, and have an open body posture. Try to offer realistic options. Small gestures like providing them with a blanket and ensuring they are warm may serve to protect, calm, and reassure.

Fear and unpredictability

A person experiencing symptoms of psychosis may be fearful of the attending paramedic (review symptoms of psychosis above). They may be experiencing hallucinations or delusions that make it difficult for them to feel safe around first responders. This could increase the risk of unpredictable behaviour.

Intoxication

Another element to consider that may impact a person's presentation is whether they are intoxicated. This can negatively affect their judgement and their unpredictability. Depending on the substance, this may increase risks such as vomiting and obstructing airways, overdose, respiratory distress, or cardiac arrest.

Reducing risk – dos and don'ts

It is crucial to assess whether there is a risk of suicidality. First, ask direct questions: Do they want to kill or harm themselves? Do they have means (such as medication or weapons)? Have they thought of a plan or where they would do this? Have they already taken a substance?

TABLE 11.5 Medication side effects causing possible mental health symptoms.

Side effects	Medication
Acute confusion and delirium	Antimuscarinics (e.g. procyclidine) Beta-blockers Central nervous system depressants (e.g. hypnotics, sedatives, antidepressants, antihistamines) Cimetidine Digoxin
Behavioural disturbance	Anaesthetic agents Antipsychotics Benzodiazepines Lithium toxicity
Depression	Amphetamines Anticonvulsants Antihypertensives Antipsychotics Benzodiazepines Corticosteroids Opioids Oral contraceptives Levodopa
Elated mood	Antidepressants (including selective serotonin reuptake inhibitors (SSRIs) given to a person with Bipolar Affective Disorder) Antimuscarinics (e.g. benzhexol) Corticosteroids
Psychotic symptoms	Appetite suppressants Barbiturates Beta-blockers Corticosteroids Methamphetamines Opioids Narcotics Non-steroidal anti-inflammatory drug (NSAIDs) – including indomethacin and celecoxib via inhibition of prostaglandin synthesis and Akt signalling Levodopa
Immunotherapy agents	Interferon alpha: long-term fatigue, insomnia, anxiety, and depression Monoclonal antibody immunotherapy: depression, psychosis (though agent specific and rare) Cytokine based immunotherapy: a range of neuropsychiatric adverse events including psychosis

You may need to remove means to avoid further danger (if appropriate), attend to a physical condition (bleeding, vomiting, choking, deterioration), or provide emergency treatment such as opioid overdose reversal, and first cardiopulmonary resuscitation.

It is important that you do not dismiss or invalidate the patient's reason for their distress, verbalise your frustration, or express criticism or judgement such as saying that they are selfish, seeking attention, or not requiring emergency care. Do not make promises you cannot keep.

Humour can be helpful to engage and defuse tension (Rolfe et al. 2020) but there is also a danger it could be misinterpreted. Be careful to use it purposely and respectfully.

Communication and documentation

It is vital to obtain collateral when available from carers or next of kin at the scene. Ensure that accurate records are taken and handed over to treating teams when transferring patients to hospitals or other settings to reduce miscommunication and ensure appropriate patient care and treatment planning is established.

Importance of language

The words we use are compelling and have the potential to offend, create a power imbalance, or disempower someone.

Also, in considering gender and cultural diversity, remember to ask the person how they want to be addressed, e.g. which pronoun they want to be addressed as (he, she, they) or what name (e.g. an Aboriginal person who prefers to be called 'Bill' though their registered name is Roger).

Apply the person-first approach. This means to refer to the person first before their condition. In the context of a mental health condition, ask yourself if the label is necessary.

Don't say	Instead say
Committed/completed/ successful suicide	Died by suicide
Unsuccessful suicide	Attempted suicide
Patient is non-compliant with . . .	Person does not adhere to . . .

Don't say	Instead say
Schizo Bill	Bill who lives with schizophrenia
She's crazy!	She is unusual, or distressed
Trauma/domestic violence victim	Survivor of trauma/ domestic violence
They are an addict!	A person who lives with substance use condition

Collaboration and innovations

Collaborative practice between disciplines such as paramedicine, nursing, and medicine has led to great innovations. For instance, some hospitals now use virtual emergency medicine during ambulance transport to accelerate assessment, triage, or rerouting (SMHS 2021).

Responders' mental health

Paramedics, as first responders, are at a higher risk of developing PTSD due to the nature of their work. Kyron et al. (2022) surveyed nearly 15,000 ambulance, police, emergency, and first responders. They found that most paramedics reported low well-being (26.7%), high to very high psychological distress (28.6%), and 64.8% had a current diagnosis of either anxiety, depression, or PTSD. Ten per cent of them also either had had suicidal thoughts or behaviour in the previous twelve months. Alcohol consumption was a concern for over 60%, whilst over 27.4% binged drank, and 9.3% reported using illicit drugs.

Despite these high figures, very few identified as needing of psychological help and reported receiving adequate mental health support. The near majority (56%) failed to identify they had a problem, needed help, or reported seeking help. Only 15.9% stated they were receiving adequate help (Kyron et al. 2022).

Several positive coping strategies are offered to paramedics to address or maintain their mental health. Paramedics often resort to black humour as a coping strategy to distance themselves from difficult and emotional situations and value peer support (Risson et al. 2022). Additionally, most employers offer free counselling support sessions through Employee's Assistance Program (EAP). Alternatively, there is access to psychological services funded by Medicare or reimbursed through private health. There are also dedicated and specialised veterans and first responder's trauma response psychiatric care groups usually offered in private hospitals.

Conclusion

A person's mental health is as integral to their well-being as their physical condition. Several factors can affect a person's mental health, and several overlaps can impact paramedics called to attend to a person in distress. Attending and caring for people in an emergency can accumulate and take a toll on the paramedic's own well-being. Being able to recognise the signs and symptoms of mental health challenges can help paramedics attend to patients on the road and benefit attending to their own self-care.

Activities

Now review your learning by completing the learning activities in this chapter. The answers to these appear at the end of the book. Further self-test activities can be found at **www.wileyfundamentalseries.com/paramedic/3e.**

Test your knowledge

1. What is the primary intention and function of the mental health legislation in Australia?
2. What is the difference between mental illness, psychopathology, and positive mental health?
3. Discuss the difference between positive and negative symptoms and provide examples.
4. Identify and discuss physiological symptoms that could present as psychosis.

5. Discuss the main practical steps in attending to a person who presents in mental distress.
6. Describe the common symptoms of depression, bipolar disorder, schizophrenia, and dementia.
7. Identify and discuss factors considered in conducting a risk assessment.
8. What constitutes intimate partner violence?
9. What type of exposure could lead to PTSD?
10. What could be the advantages and disadvantages of using humour in paramedicine?

Glossary

Anxiety: A state of increased arousal, activated autonomic and neuroendocrine systems, and vigilance to help deal with a potential or actual threat.

Anxiety attack: Persistent irrational fears or thoughts in the absence of threat.

Bipolar: A mental health disorder characterised by extreme mood shifts from mania to depression.

Compulsions: Repetitive behaviours or mental acts that a person feels urged to perform to prevent or reduce distress caused by obsessions.

Coping mechanisms: Means used to deal with life's challenges and pressures. They can be regarded as healthy or positive, e.g. appropriate amount of physical exercise; or unhealthy or negative e.g. alcohol dependence.

Dementia: Umbrella term comprising several symptoms relating to progressive neurological conditions affecting the brain.

Depersonalisation: Feeling detached from or outside of one self/body.

Depression: Widespread condition that ranges in severity from mild, to severe and life-threatening. Individuals can experience a variety of physical, psychological, and social symptoms.

Derealisation: Feeling removed from reality.

Dissociation: Process of disconnecting from own thoughts, feelings, memories, or sense of self.

Emotional Unstable Personality Disorder (EUPD) and Borderline Personality Disorder (BPD): Mental health disorders characterised by emotional dysregulation, difficult behaviours that affect interpersonal relationships, and often extreme reactions to abandonment and persistent feelings of emptiness.

Generalised Anxiety Disorder (GAD): When a person experiences anxiety symptoms in the absence of threat that are difficult to control more often than not, over several months and which affect their normal functioning.

Internalised stigma: When an individual is labelling themselves. Also called self-stigma.

Intimate partner violence: Aggression or abuse committed by a current or former romantic partner.

Mania: A marked increase in energy, activity or agitation that can be experienced by feeling intensely happy, excited, upbeat, jumpy, wired, or an exaggerated sense of self.

Mental illness: The experience of mental health symptoms, e.g. insomnia, persistent feelings of sadness.

Negative symptoms: Reduction in normal functioning or affect.

Non-suicidal self-injury (NSSI): Self-harm that is not intended to cause death.

Obsessive-compulsive disorder (OCD): The experience of obsessions, compulsions, or both.

Obsessions: Unwanted or intrusive, persistent, and recurring urges, thoughts or images causing significant anxiety or distress.

Panic attack: Anxiety attack accompanied with physiological symptoms such as shortness of breath, sweating, shaking, tachycardia.

Positive mental health: A person's overall subjective psychological well-being and optimal functioning.

Positive symptoms: Experience of new symptoms such as hallucinations and delusions.

Post-traumatic stress disorder (PTSD): Unresolved episode of acute stress following an event causing distress and functional impairment. The event may have been direct, vicarious, or indirect.

Psychopathology: A mental health disorder, e.g. major depressive disorder, bipolar disorder, and schizophrenia.

Psychosis: Mental health condition characterised by loss of contact with reality.

Risk assessment: Identification of potential dangers, the prediction of its likelihood and potential level of harm.

Self-harm: Hurtful acts performed to oneself to reduce emotional pain or distress or due to overwhelming feelings.

Schizophrenia: Severe mental health illness that includes psychosis to a severe extent.

Stigma: Negative stereotypes and labelling of an individual who is experiencing mental health challenges.

Suicide: A direct attempt at ending one's life.

References

Australian Institute of Health and Welfare. (2022). Family, domestic and sexual violence data in Australia. AIHW, Australian Government. Available at: https://www.aihw.gov.au/getmedia/348b5559-ad3b-48a7-8e79-cea0a6c11076/Family-domestic-and-sexual-violence-data-in-Australia.pdf.aspx?inline=true (accessed 24 January 2023).

Australian Bureau of Statistics (ABS). (2022). National study of mental health and wellbeing. Available at: https://www.abs.gov.au/statistics/health/mental-health/national-study-mental-health-and-wellbeing/latest-release#key-statistics (accessed 19 February 2023).

Australian Capital Territory. (2021). Mental Health Act 2015. Available at: www.legislation.act.gov.au (accessed 19 February 2023).

Ayhan, F. and Üstün, B. (2021). Examination of risk assessment tools developed to evaluate risks in mental health areas: A systematic review. *Nursing Forum* **56** (2): 330–340. doi: 10.1111/nuf.12557.

Bonanno, G.A. (2008). Loss, trauma, and human resilience: have we underestimated the human capacity to thrive after extremely aversive events? *Psychological Trauma: Theory, Research, Practice, and Policy* **S** (1): 101–113. doi: 10.1037/1942-9681.S.1.101

Papathanasiou, C. and Stylianidis, S. (2022). Mental health professionals' attitudes towards patients with borderline personality disorder: the role of disgust. *International Journal of Psychiatry Research* **5** (1): 1–13.

Corrigan, P.W. and Wassel, A. (2008). Understanding and influencing the stigma of mental illness. *Journal of Psychosocial Nursing and Mental Health Services* **46** (1): 42–48. doi: 10.3928/02793695-20080101-04.

De Girolamo, G., Iozzino, L., Ferrari, C. et al. (2021). A multinational case–control study comparing forensic and non-forensic patients with schizophrenia spectrum disorders: the EU-VIORMED project. *Psychological Medicine* **53** (5): 1–11. doi:10.1017/S0033291721003433.

Dementia Australian. (2022). About dementia. Available at: www.dementia.org.au (accessed 19 February 2023).

Diener, E., Emmons, R.A., Larsen, R.J. et al. (1985). The satisfaction with life scale. *Journal of Personality Assessment* **49** (1): 71–75. doi: 10.1207/s15327752jpa4901_13.

Duncan, E.A., Best, C., Dougall, N. et al. (2019). Epidemiology of emergency ambulance service calls related to mental health problems and self harm: a national record linkage study. *Scandinavian Journal of Trauma, Resuscitation and Emergency Medicine* **27** (1): 1–8. doi: 10.1186/s13049-019-0611-9.

Fazel, S., Gulati, G., Linsell, L. et al. (2009). Schizophrenia and violence: systematic review and meta-analysis. *PLOS MED* **6** (8): e1000120. doi: 10.1371/journal.pmed.1000120. PMID: 19668362; PMCID: PMC2718581.

Goodwin, J. (2014). The horror of stigma: psychosis and mental health care environments in twenty-first-century horror film (part II). *Perspectives in Psychiatric Care* **50** (4): 224–234.

Heiervang, E., Goodman, A., and Goodman, R. (2008). The Nordic advantage in child mental health: separating health differences from reporting style in a cross-cultural comparison of psychopathology. *Journal of Child Psychology and Psychiatry* **49** (6): 678–685. doi: 10.1111/j.1469-7610.2008.01882.x.

Huppert, F.A. (2005). Positive mental health in individuals and populations. In: *The Science of Well-being* (ed. F.A. Huppert, N. Baylis, and B. Keverne), pp. 307–340. Oxford: Oxford University Press.

Iasiello, M., and van Agteren, J. (2020). Mental health and/or mental illness: A scoping review of the evidence and implications of the dual-continua model of mental health. *Evidence Base: A Journal of Evidence Reviews in Key Policy Areas* (1): 1–45. doi: 10.3316/informit.261420605378998.

Jahoda, M. (1958). *Current Concepts of Positive Mental Health.* London: Basic Books.

Keyes, C.L.M. (2005). Mental illness and/or mental health? Investigating axioms of the complete state model of health. *Journal of Consulting and Clinical Psychology* **73** (3): 539–548. doi: 10.1037/0022-006X.73.3.539.

Keyes, C.L. (2002). The mental health continuum: From languishing to flourishing in life. *Journal of Health and Social Behavior* **43** (2): 207–222. doi: 10.2307/3090197.

Kim, A.J. (2021). The metanarrative of OCD. Deconstructing positive stereotypes in media and popular nomenclature. In: *Metanarratives of Disability* (ed. D. Bolt), pp. 61–76. London: Routledge.

Kyron, M.J., Rikkers, W., Bartlett, J. et al. (2002). Mental health and wellbeing of Australian police and emergency services employees. *Archives of Environmental and Occupational Health* **77** (4): 282–292. doi: 10.1080/19338244.2021.189363.

Lubman, D.I., Heilbronn, C., Ogeil, R.P. et al. (2020). National Ambulance surveillance system: a novel method using coded Australian ambulance clinical records to monitor self-harm and mental health-related morbidity. *PLOS ONE* **15** (7): e0236344. doi: 10.1371/journal.pone.0236344.

Lyon, A.S. and Mortimer-Jones, S.M. (2021). The relationship between terminology preferences, empowerment and internalised stigma in mental health. *Issues in Mental Health Nursing* **42** (2): 183–195. doi: 10.1080/01612840.2020.1756013.

Morisson-Rees, S., Whitfield, R., Evans, S. et al. (2015). Investigating the volume of mental health emergency calls in the Welsh ambulance service trust (WAST) and developing a pre-hospital mental health model of care for application and testing. *Emergency Medicine Journal* **32** (5): e3-e3.

New South Wales Government. (2007). Mental Health Act 2007. Available at: http://www.legacy.legistation.nsw.gov.au (accessed 19 February 2023).

Ng, F.Y.Y., Townsend, M.L., Miller, C.E. et al. (2019). The lived experience of recovery in borderline personality disorder: a qualitative study. *Borderline Personality Disorder Emotional Dysregulation* **6**, 10: 1–9. doi: 10.1186/s40479-019-0107-2.

Northern Territory Government. (1998). Mental Health and Related Services Act 1998. Available at: http://www.legislation.nt.gov.au (accessed 19 February 2023).

O'Connor, C. and O'Hara, J. (2018). Reflections on reflective practice among pre-hospital emergency care practitioners in Ireland. *Irish Journal of Paramedicine* **3** (2). doi: 10.32378/ijp.v3i2.155.

Perrotta, G. (2020). Borderline personality disorder: definition, differential diagnosis, clinical contexts and therapeutic approaches. *Annals of Psychiatry and Treatment* **4** (1): 43–56. doi: 10.17352/apt.

Peterson, C. and Seligman, M.E. (2004). *Character Strengths and Virtues: A Handbook and Classification* (Vol. 1). Oxford: Oxford University Press.

Porter, C., Palmier-Claus, J., Branitsky, A. et al.(2020). Childhood adversity and borderline personality disorder: a meta-analysis. *Acta Psychiatrica Scandinavica* **141** (1): 6–20. doi: 10.1111/acps.13118.

Queensland Government. (2016). Mental Health Act 2016. Available at: http://www.legislation.qld.gov.au (accessed 19 February 2023).

Reis, H.T., and Gable, S.L. (2003). Toward a positive psychology of relationships. In: *Flourishing: Positive Psychology and the Life Well-lived* (ed. C.L.M. Keyes and J. Haidt), pp. 129–159. Washington, DC: American Psychological Association.

Risson, H., Beovich, B., and Bowles, K.A. (2022). Paramedic interactions with significant others during and after resuscitation and death of a patient. *Australasian Emergency Care* **26** (2): 113–118. doi: 10.1016/j.auec.2022.08.007.

Rolfe, U., Pope, C., and Crouch, R. (2020). Paramedic performance when managing patients experiencing mental health issues–exploring paramedics' presentation of self. *International Emergency Nursing* **49**: 100828. doi: 10.1016/j.ienj.2019.100828.

Royal Australian and New Zealand College of Psychiatrists (RANZCP). (2017). RANZCP Mental health legislation – comparative tables. Available at: https://www.ranzcp.org/files/resources/college_statements/mental-health-legislation-tables/mental-health-acts-comparative-tables.aspx (accessed 19 February 2023).

Ryff, C.D. (1989). Happiness is everything, or is it? Explorations on the meaning of psychological well-being. *Journal of Personality and Social Psychology* (**6**): 1069–1081. doi: 10.1037/0022-3514.57.6.1069.

Steger, M.F., Frazier, P., Oishi, S. et al. (2006). The meaning in life questionnaire: assessing the presence of and search for meaning in life. *Journal of Counselling Psychology* **53** (1): 80–93. doi: 10.1037/0022-0167.53.1.80.

South Metropolitan Health Service (SMHS). (2021). SMHS virtual emergency medicine service set to expand. Available at: https://smhs.health.wa.gov.au/News/2021/08/12/SMHS-Virtual-Emergency-Medicine-service-set-to-expand (accessed 19 February 2023).

Trent, D.R. (1992) The promotion of mental health: fallacies of current thinking. In: *Promoting Mental Health (2)* (ed. D.R. Trent and C. Reed), pp. 561–568. Aldershot: Avebury.

Vallesi, S., Tuson, M., Davies, A. et al. (2021). Multimorbidity among people experiencing homelessness – insights from primary care data. *International Journal of Environmental Research and Public Health* **18** (12): 6498. doi: 10.3390/ijerph18126498.

Wu, C., Chang, C., Hayes, R. et al. (2012). Clinical risk assessment rating and all-cause mortality in secondary mental healthcare: the South London and Maudsley NHS Foundation Trust Biomedical Research Centre (SLAM BRC) case register. *Psychological Medicine* **42** (8): 1581–1590. doi: 10.1017/S0033291711002698.

CHAPTER 12

De-escalation

Simon Menz

Clinical Support Paramedic, St John Ambulance, Western Australia, Australia

Contents

LEARNING OUTCOMES

On completion of this chapter the reader will be able to:

- Define the term de-escalation.
- Identify the importance of de-escalation.
- Understand a variety of techniques to be utilised for effective de-escalation.
- Recognise the flexible adaptive nature of de-escalation.

Case study

You are working with a senior paramedic in your first week when you're tasked to a priority 2 case for a twenty-two-year-old female who has self-harmed by cutting her wrists with a razor blade. The patient's family are on scene and have advised that the bleeding is now controlled, and the razor blade has been removed from the patient. However, she has now locked herself in the bedroom and is yelling at her family about not wanting to go to hospital.

When you arrive, police are out the front of the house talking with the family and they inform you that the patient has a history of self harm and depression. She is currently refusing to engage with the police.

Fundamentals of Paramedic Practice: A Systems Approach, Third Edition. Edited by Sam Willis and Ian Peate.

Companion website: www.wiley.com/go/willis/paramedic3e

Introduction

De-escalation is considered an essential skill for paramedics. This skill can come naturally to some, whilst others are able to develop it over time. When presented with an agitated patient, the art of de-escalation can have several benefits, from reducing harm to patients though to creating a safe working environment for the paramedics and other professional agencies involved. By having well established de-escalation skills, paramedics are often able to prevent people from becoming aggressive. Throughout this chapter, a variety of different techniques will be investigated to assist with improving overall knowledge regarding the safe and effective de-escalation of agitated and aggressive patients, including an individualised patient approach, spatial awareness, verbal and non-verbal communication, remaining calm, altering stimuli, agreeing to disagree, empowering patients, informing patients, utilising common interests, and setting boundaries. De-escalation techniques discussed in this chapter are generalised and can be tailored for different groups of people with specific needs, including but not limited to the elderly, children, people with disabilities, and drug affected persons. Topics discussed in this chapter will be beneficial in assisting people to re-stabilise from an agitated state; however, they can also be used more frequently to prevent a patient becoming agitated (Goodman et al. 2020). To assist with recalling the recommendations from the chapter, the acronym 'C-I-LISTEN-AS-I-C' is proposed:

C – Calm
I – Inform
L – Language
I – Individual approach
S – Spatial awareness
T – Tone
E – Empower
N – Non-verbal/body language
A – Agree to disagree
S – Stimuli
I – Identify
C – Common interests

Background

De-escalation can be defined as a collaborative process that involves a range of verbal and non-verbal interventions to reduce agitation or violence (Patel et al. 2018). The World Health Organization (WHO) estimates that 8–38% of all healthcare workers globally are physically assaulted at some stage in their career, with many more experiencing patient aggression (WHO 2022). Ambulance Victoria reports an unacceptably high level of violence and aggression experienced by their paramedics, citing an average of one paramedic being assaulted every fifty hours (Ambulance Victoria 2022). An American study found that 69% of emergency medical services (EMS) workers were exposed to violence or aggression in the past twelve months (Gormley et al. 2016). These findings are supported by a Switzerland study reporting an 84% exposure of violence and aggression towards paramedics (Savoy et al. 2021). With such high rates of occupational violence and aggression exposure, the need for all paramedics to be knowledgeable in the area of de-escalation is clear. Healthcare workplace violence is known to have significant impacts on both the physiological and psychological wellness of the practitioners involved (Ali Abozaid et al. 2022). De-escalation training that equips health care workers with practical training results in an increase in confidence when addressing a potentially aggressive patient (Ali Abozaid et al. 2022). A study that asked individuals who have recently been assaulted what could be done to reduce assaults, de-escalation training was a strong recommendation (Maguire et al. 2018). Physical restraint of an individual is likely to have a negative effect on the patient's aggressive behaviour (Bailey 2022), hence the importance of having individuals skilled in de-escalation with the patient as soon as possible.

Identify

Building rapport with an individual is an essential aspect of being able to de-escalate situations. The fundamental building block of rapport building is understanding who each other are. Early introductions including name and job title will take the paramedic from being an anonymous paramedic to a paramedic who is seen as a fellow human with a name and a purpose. An agitated individual is less likely to want to harm someone they can bond with in a meaningful way.

Another benefit of early introductions is that you can correctly pronounce the person's name and refer to them by their name. Simply using a person's name instead of generic terms such as 'mate' or 'darling' creates an environment of respect, facilitating a more well-balanced and considered conversation (Michigan University 2017). An individual is also more attentive when their name is used (Tamura et al. 2016). When making introductions be sure not to forget to introduce your colleague or anyone else who has arrived with you. An example of this would be:

> *'Hi, my name is Chris, I'm a paramedic and this is my partner, Beth. What is your name?'*

Introductions may be difficult in the first instance depending on how agitated and aggressive the patient is but should be made as soon as reasonably practicable. Early introductions can create an environment of familiarity, strengthening the rapport you're going to be building with them. This strategy will be one that becomes 'second nature' to the experienced paramedic, likely resulting in a decreased incidence of patients becoming escalated and agitated in the first place.

Making assumptions about a person's name, pronoun, or relationship status with the patient can prevent rapport building. An effective way around this is to respectfully enquire about the relationship to the patient or by asking for their preferred name. For example, some people will provide their legal name to the operations centre when calling for an ambulance but are commonly known by a 'nickname' or use their middle name as their primary name. Listening to bystanders on scene to understand what name they are using for the patient can be helpful here. If the patient's name is not one that you're comfortable pronouncing, confirm with them or a family member for the correct pronunciation. This will show the patient that you're interested in them as an individual and are willing to tailor your care to their specific needs.

TABLE 12.1 AHPRA and national board code of conduct.

Principle 1	Put patients first – safe, effective, and collaborative practice
Principle 2	Aboriginal and Torres Strait Islander health and cultural safety
Principle 3	Respectful and culturally safe practice for all
Principle 4	Working with patients
Principle 5	Working with other practitioners
Principle 6	Working within the healthcare system
Principle 7	Minimising risk to patients
Principle 8	Professional behaviour
Principle 9	Maintaining practitioner health and well-being
Principle 10	Teaching, supervising, and assessing
Principle 11	Ethical research

Source: AHPRA and national boards 2022.

Individual approach

A patient-centred approach is a focus across all health professions, and paramedicine is no exception to this. The Australian Health Practitioner Regulation Agency's (APHRA) national code of conduct for registered paramedics in Australia highlights this patient-centred approach with four of the eleven principles being focused on an individually tailored patient-centred approach to all patient interactions (see Table 12.1 for AHPRA code of conduct standards). New Zealand and the UK have similar underpinnings in their paramedic codes of conduct – for example, the standards of proficiency for paramedics (HCPC 2018) and the Kaunihera Manapou Paramedic Council Code of Conduct (Kaunihera Manapou Paramedic Council 2020) – further supporting the notion of focused patient-centred care. A paramedic will see many patients across a single shift, and each one of these patients should be treated as an individual to optimise their care. It can sometimes be easy for paramedics to become complacent and lose empathy for their patients, especially if that's not the first time seeing a similar presentation that shift. Paramedics must always remember that whilst that patient's presentation may be routine and common for them, for the patient, it could be the most significant life-altering event they will experience all year.

When it comes to implementing effective de-escalation techniques, it must be understood that not every technique will work for every patient. As paramedics become more experienced, they develop an understanding for what techniques will be more beneficial for different demographics of patients, however, this is not a guarantee and the paramedic must be willing to rapidly adapt and amend their approach based on the response from the patient or the bystanders involved.

The ability to adapt and adjust the approach may require the 'attending' or 'treating' officer to swap out with their partner to facilitate this individual approach. The key here is not to take this personally and understand that some people will be able to connect with and relate to the patient more than others. Being flexible in this way also shows the patient that your team is willing to adjust to put the patent's interests first, increasing the likelihood of building rapport with them. By establishing rapport with the patient, de-escalation is more likely to be effective (Johnston et al. 2022).

Spatial awareness

Spatial awareness is a skill that comes naturally to some but needs to be learnt and reinforced for others. Being aware of an individual's physical comfort zone is important in the process of de-escalation (Richmond et al. 2012). Not only will a good sense of spatial awareness aid in building rapport it will also keep you safe in the event the patient becomes violent.

Each individual will make you aware of their level of comfort with how close you get through their body language (and sometimes verbal language). If you are comfortable with deeming it safe to get close to the patient, getting down to their level will help to break down any perceived power gradients. Standing up whilst the patient is sitting can be perceived as being intimidating towards the patient. To assist in making the patient feel comfortable with your presence, getting to their level by kneeling down next to them, or pulling up a chair near them will have a noticeable difference in building a positive relationship. Most people will naturally do this when interacting with children, it's important to continue these good habits with all patients where safe to do so.

Your position within a room can also have an impact on the overall de-escalation of the patient. Whilst it may be considered ideal to position yourself close to the patient, it might not always be safe, in which case you have to communicate with the patient from a distance. In these circumstances, it's important to note your position in the room to prevent a feeling of being 'trapped'. In a room with only one exit, the paramedic will often place themselves close to the exit. This is generally a good idea as it will allow a rapid exit in the event the patient becomes violent. If, however, you position yourself between the patient and the exit, the patient may feel as though their exit is blocked, resulting in a potential increase in their anxiety and agitation. The way around this is to find a position that is safe and off to the side of the line between the patient and the exit. If the patient then decides they wish to exit, they don't feel as though they have to 'get past' a paramedic. In the event the patient makes a violent outburst directed towards the paramedic, there is still a close route to the exit for the paramedic.

Non-verbal and verbal communication

Verbal and non-verbal communication have been studied with varying estimates on the role each plays in communication. It's been estimated that non-verbal communication accounts for 60–90% of all communication (Argyle, 1988; Wanko Keutchafo et al. 2020). These differences may come about with some authors considering environmental factors, some considering tone of voice, and others looking only at non-oral communication.

The key to de-escalation with non-verbal communication is to ensure one's overall demeanour is warm, welcoming, non-threatening, and open to input from others (Egan 2002; Fulde and Preisz 2011). Whilst this will need to be tailored to each individual situation, some overarching concepts of positive non-verbal communication are:

- Maintain a calm and reassuring tone.
- Adjust your speed of language to be slightly slower.
- Remain even toned.
- Keep hands out of pockets.
- Avoid a splayed stance.
- Avoid crossing arms.
- Open stance.
- Open hands (avoid closed fists).
- Face towards the patient.
- Carry a smile.
- Use eye contact, avoid prolonged eye contact.

The generic concepts listed above are helpful in maintaining self-awareness, however, the complexities of non-verbal communication have been suggested to be subtle and not assessable in studies attempting to differentiate between verbal and non-verbal communication. Non-verbal de-escalation has more emphasis placed on it in situations where verbal communication is limited, for example, with a deaf patient (Jeffery and Austen 2005).

Altering stimuli

Excessive stimuli are common triggers for agitated individuals (Fulde and Preisz 2011;Iroku-Malize and Grissom 2018), especially those with dementia (Janzen et al. 2013). Many skilled paramedics will develop a habit of switching off the TV and asking for music to be dimmed upon entry into any premises. Not only does this enhance the ability to communicate with the patient and their family but it can also reduce stimuli input for the individual, reducing agitation. There are no guarantees around this, however, as gentle music has been found to have calming effects (Hung Hsu et al. 2015). An individual's agitation may be exacerbated by something as simple as feeling claustrophobic, so opening the blinds may be what is required to reduce the agitation. Removing excess people from the room can also aid in the reduction of unnecessary stimuli. This approach to altering stimuli has to be considered in the context of the situation and be an individual approach. It would be wise to involve family, carers, or support workers when deciding which stimuli to reduce and which stimuli would enhance the de-escalation process.

Frustration is considered a common cause for agitation, especially in those with dementia (Dementia Australia 2020). Some easy to implement strategies to reduce frustration are to improve vision or hearing through the return of glasses, hearing aids, or even false teeth. Altering light levels in the room or rear of the ambulance can also have a positive impact on the level of agitation being experienced by the patient.

Consider this example:

You have successfully managed to build some rapport with your patient, and they are calm and compliant during transport to hospital. During transport, you have dimmed the lights, adopted a calm, quiet tone, and promoted a sense of relaxation in a one-on-one environment. Upon arrival at hospital, you take the patient into triage where you leave them to wait with your partner whilst you discuss the case with the triage nurse. The patient is now in a loud, busy environment, surrounded by lots of unfamiliar people, and the fluorescent lights are bright. How would you expect the patient to feel and react to this sudden change of environment?

Remain calm

Paramedics are often described as being akin to a duck, appearing calm on the outside whilst paddling quickly below the surface. The concept behind this is that the emotions that we exhibit will be mimicked by those around us (Fischer and Hess 2017). By remaining calm and having a calm presence on scene, the patient and bystanders will begin to reduce their level of agitation and aggression (Iroku-Malize and Grissom 2018; Todak and James 2018; Johnston et al. 2022). This concept is not going to have immediate effect and it will take some time for emotions to slowly come down from a heightened state. If a paramedic finds themselves becoming frustrated, angry, or annoyed with an individual, the result will be two or more people with heightened emotions and no one to bring the emotions back down again.

Let's relate this to the Case study at the beginning of the chapter. If the agitated patient is yelling and arguing with others on scene, the goal would be to reduce this level of agitation and yelling so a meaningful conversation can be had with the patient. If the paramedics on scene approach this situation by yelling back at the patient, she will presume this level of emotion and type of behaviour is acceptable and continue yelling and being generally agitated, potentially even increasing her agitation.

This skill of remaining calm in the face of agitation can be difficult. Student paramedics may not have faced many of these situations before. A conscious effort to be aware of your emotions, body language, verbal language, and tone of voice is crucial in maintaining a calm presence whilst with the patient (Robins 2019). This calm presence can also have the effect of preventing a patient from becoming agitated in the first place, and in the case of an agitated or aggressive person, prevention is always better than a cure.

Language

Breaking bad news to a patient regarding mortality requires excellent communication skills on behalf of the practitioner as this increases the recipient's ability to process the associated negative emotions (Ptacek and Ptacek 2001). Poor communication when breaking bad news has been shown to result in pathologic grief reactions (Park et al. 2010).Whilst research in this area primarily relates to advising of mortality, research is lacking when it comes to breaking bad news to a patient who is being transported to hospital as an involuntary patient. The confidence level and knowledge base of paramedics in the field of breaking bad news is described as being insufficient, with recommendations for more training in the delivery of bad news to be implemented (Rasmus et al. 2020).

Understanding that paramedics have some improvement to make regarding communication in breaking bad news, this may also be the case for de-escalation communication strategies, as quite often in these situations bad news will be broken to the patient, especially if they are going to be transported as an involuntary mental health patient. When it comes to breaking bad news to an agitated patient, where appropriate, it may be best to wait until the patient has been de-escalated before advising them of the bad news, to optimise their ability to process it. On the other hand, it may be the delivery of the bad news that leads to the patient or bystander becoming aggressive. The importance of being open and honest with the individual also needs to be considered. Being transparent in communication also has a significant impact on the development of rapport with the individual.

The language or words used can have a significant impact on the trajectory of the interaction moving forward, with non-threatening words being optimum for de-escalation (Robins 2019). The most important underlying concept that a paramedic can adopt is:

Have a helping attitude, not a telling attitude.

By approaching conversations with a helping attitude, the individuals involved are more likely to sympathise with the paramedic, rapidly strengthening the rapport-building process. A telling attitude can be considered to be when the paramedic has an authoritarian approach. This is evident when the paramedic perceives themselves to hold all the power in the relationship and believes that people will do as they're told. The telling attitude can cause feelings of resentment towards the paramedic, making it difficult to ascertain information or gain compliance from the patient. Consider the following statements:

'Sit down whilst I assess you'.
'Can I help you sit down so I can assess you?'

The language used in both statements is trying to achieve the same outcome, with a simple change, however, one is telling the patient what to do, whilst the other is asking if the paramedic can help the patient whilst suggesting to them what they would like to be done. This helping attitude also often results in the patient feeling more involved and more empowered in the decisions relation to their ongoing care. Some agitated patients may only be directing their anger towards certain individuals. For example, if the police are on scene and you hear the phrase, 'I like you ambos, it's the police I have a problem with', it becomes obvious who the anger is directed towards. This attitude has most likely come from previous experiences and interactions where the paramedics are perceived as being there to help, whilst the police are perceived as being there to enforce the law and act in an authoritative manner. This scenario may be a misperception held by the patient prior to the police and paramedics arriving, so it's important to recognise this and show that patient that the police are also there to help.

Another example of the helping vs telling attitude is:

'You need to calm down'.
'I would like to help you to calm down'.

Again, a small change in the wording yet a powerful impact on the relationship with the patient. Recall being in an argument with someone and the words, 'You just need to calm down' were said. What was the impact of this? Did the person spontaneously calm down? Generally this would result in further escalation of the argument, something we are actively trying to avoid in these situations. It must also be remembered that we will inevitably make mistakes in these situations and saying the wrong thing isn't always going to be *catastrophic* , it may just make it a little more challenging getting to the end goal of a calm and compliant patient.

The phrase 'I understand' also has the potential to negatively impact the rapport-building process if used inappropriately. Paramedics have likely at some stage in their career used the phrase 'I understand' and been met with a response similar to 'You don't understand'. The 'I understand' statement can have benefits if the paramedic is able to demonstrate to the individual that they have been through or experienced similar life events that are currently causing their emotional distress and are willing to explain this to them. In situations where we cannot relate to their situation, saying to them 'Can you help me understand' demonstrates interest on our behalf. This is also an invitation for the patient to explain what they are currently experiencing, allowing them to offload their frustration of feeling isolated and not listened to.

Common interests

This may seem like common sense for some, yet the idea of finding common interests can easily be lost in the moment as the clinical priorities begin to sink in. It's well known that when an individual is new to learning a task, their cognitive workload is great, with small details of the task requiring more cognitive processing effort. For student paramedics, the focus is generally on the clinical assessment of the patient and beginning to think of a clinical management plan for the patient. With this taking up a significant amount of cognitive power, the interpersonal skill of ensuring a rapport is built with the patient can be lost. It's important to remember that if a paramedic is able to build rapport with the patient early, they will be more successful in obtaining pertinent information that may alter clinical decisions moving forwards.

In the context of the agitated and aggressive patient, taking the time to find some common interests will strengthen the rapport-building process. Finding common interests can be done in multiple ways. One way to is suggest common themes that the majority of society may have an interest in such as sport. This is especially effective for the intellectually disabled cohort as these individuals often have a passion for being passionate about certain sports. This has an impact on the de-escalation of the patient as it distracts them from their emotions. On top of this, it allows the patient to see us as more than paramedics, as another person with whom a connection can be made. An individual is less likely to want to harm or argue with a person they have a rapport with and is more likely to be compliant with that person's requests for assessment and transport.

Agree to disagree

Another crucial tool in the kit to aid in de-escalation is the concept of agreeing to disagree with the patient (Richmond et al. 2012). In most instances, being able to agree with the patient is an effective, rapid pathway to building rapport, however, some statements made by patients are not wise to agree with. Having some boundaries as to what is suitable to agree with and what is not can take some time to develop. By agreeing to disagree with the individual, we're showing the patient that we have boundaries and cannot be manipulated by them. It also instils a level of trust and respect from the patient as agreeing to disagree shows that we have actively listened to what they have said and given it our full attention. By agreeing to disagree with the patient the paramedic is also avoiding an argument with them. If the paramedic was to tell the patient that they don't agree with what they are saying without acknowledging that their opinion is valid, they may try and argue until the paramedic agrees with them. This may result in further escalation from the patient.

Defer authority

The concept of deferring authority aims to show the patient that the reason for the paramedic's attendance is to help them and look out for their best interests. Deferring authority is when one suggests that someone else is responsible for a decision, protocol, or intervention. If the patient tries to blame the paramedic for something they don't agree with, it can be beneficial to pass that blame onto a faceless organisation or someone who is not on scene. They will find it more difficult to be angry with an organisation or faceless individual than the people on scene with them.

An example of this relating back to the Case study example would be:

Patient: 'Why can't you take my friend in the ambulance with me to hospital?'

Paramedic: 'I would really like to help you out here and get your friend to hospital, however, it's the policy of the ambulance service that we cannot transport anyone other than the patient'.

Or

Patient: 'Why are the police here with you?'

Paramedic: 'I didn't call the police, however, it's standard policy to have them come along to assist every now and again'.

Empower with choices

When interacting with an agitated patient, their agitation and frustration can be enhanced by the feeling that they have lost control of the situation and the right to make decisions about their treatment. Therefore, an effective tool in being able to de-escalate an individual is to provide them with options and choices (Richmond et al. 2012). This empowers and provides them with a sense of control over the situation. This isn't always as easy as it seems with it not being possible to give some choices to the patient. For example, in the Case study at the beginning of the chapter, the patient may be managed as involuntary under the mental health act and has lost the ability to decide if they are transported to hospital or not. The paramedic can re-empower her by offering other choices such as sitting in the chair in the ambulance or being transported on the stretcher. The paramedic may even be in a position where they offer her a choice of having observations being assessed or not. These choices may be as benign as a choice of what shoes to wear to walk to the ambulance.

Boundaries and social contracts

Along with understanding the importance of empowering patients with choices, there comes a balance with setting boundaries (Fulde and Preisz 2011; Richmond et al. 2012; Robins 2019). Some patients might try to get away with certain behaviours that may be unsafe for themselves or the paramedics attending to them (Goodman et al. 2020). By setting boundaries early, as paramedics we are able to establish with the patient a level of respect that shows them we are willing to help them but not to do anything at all just to make them happy. Setting boundaries for patients can sometimes be seen as a social contract, as a breach of the boundaries will carry a consequence that needs to be verbalised to the patient. An example of setting a boundary may be:

> *'We can take your bag with your belongings but we can't take your suitcase as we cannot secure it in the ambulance'.*
>
> Or
>
> *'You can have a cigarette before we leave for the hospital but you can't have several cigarettes'.*

These boundaries show the patient that their wishes and needs are respected without letting them take advantage of the situation. In these situations, it's important to remember to say less to anger the patient (Richmond et al. 2012) by establishing what some triggers for them might be.

Inform the patient

Knowledge is a powerful asset. The more knowledge the patient has, the more comfortable they're going to be with a situation (Fulde and Preisz 2011). A fear of the unknown can cause anxiety and agitation for some patients, as there are countless options or scenarios that the patient may be concerned about. With timely information being provided to the patient, these fears can be diminished, allowing the anxiety and agitation to fade away. Sometimes it may be important to inform the patient of their rights to refuse certain assessments and/or interventions, as the fear of a needle when having a blood glucose test may be the trigger causing their agitation.

Informing the patient of the anticipated upcoming management for them will also allow them to prepare for what is ahead. Consider the following ongoing situation from the Case study at the beginning of the chapter:

> *You have successfully managed to build rapport with your patient, and they have agreed to calmly be transported to hospital for a mental health assessment. On the way to hospital you are speaking in a calm, quiet manner, the lights are dimmed, and it's just yourself and the patient in the back of the ambulance. You have agreed to let the patient listen to her favourite music. When you arrive at the hospital, you take the patient into the emergency department triage area where there are multiple other patients, paramedics, and nurses, all talking among themselves making lots of noise. The fluorescent lights are bright and there is a lack of privacy for the patient. You, the paramedic who has built rapport with them leave them to discuss their personal details with the triage nurse. After a few minutes a triage nurse comes over to the patient, grabs her wrist to feel her pulse whilst asking why she is here. The triage nurse asks her to take her headphones out and stop listening to her music.*

Now imagine yourself in the patient's position. Would it be surprising when the patient suddenly becomes agitated and starts trying to abscond?

By 'pre-briefing' the patient, the paramedic informs them of what is to be expected upon arrival at the emergency department. This creates an opportunity to discuss and identify any potential triggers for the patient and should trigger the paramedic to work on a plan to prevent escalation of the patient in the triage area. The skill of 'pre-briefing' can also be used for other patients who have not displayed signs of violence or aggression. This allows the practice of 'pre-briefing' to become a standard aspect of patient care, coming more naturally when needed with patients where de-escalation has been achieved.

Conclusion

Throughout this chapter, multiple different tips and techniques have been investigated to assist with improving the effectiveness of on-scene de-escalation of violent and aggressive patients. It's important to remember that these tips are not always going to work for every patient and should be tailored to the needs of each specific patient.

The techniques of de-escalation discussed here are not all inclusive, further reading is encouraged to increase knowledge in this area. As a paramedic student, the art of de-escalation requires practice and experience with feedback of what works in different situations helping to evolve the skill as time goes on. Being able to safely de-escalate situations will result in improved outcomes for patients. Unsuccessful attempts of de-escalation often result in chemical sedation or physical restraint, both of which will cause a negative experience and association with paramedics or police, potentially making any future efforts of de-escalation more difficult. Chemical and physical restraint should be used as an absolute last resort (Iroku-Malize and Grissom 2018) with a primary focus on achieving safe and more patient focused outcomes through the use of a variety of de-escalation techniques.

Activities

Now review your learning by completing the learning activities in this chapter. The answers to these appear at the end of the book. Further self-test activities can be found at **www.wileyfundamentalseries.com/paramedic/3e.**

Activity 12.1

Read and review the following case study.

Irene is a seventy-eight-year-old lady who lives in an aged-care facility. Carl, a paramedic, has been called to assess Irene for displaying some aggressive behaviour towards the care facility staff and other residents.

As Carl arrives, he finds Irene sitting on her bed yelling at a staff member who is standing next to her. Carl approaches Irene, introduces himself, his partner and states his qualifications. He has his hands on his hips as he stands next to the other staff member already in front of Irene and away from the door. Carl begins to question Irene about why he has been called. Carl askes Irene if she has any pain or is feeling unwell. Irene's attention is split between Carl and the other staff member. Irene continues to yell at the staff member, now becoming agitated that Carl is asking her a lot of questions that she cannot understand. The staff member explains that Irene has recently lost her hearing aids and is having trouble hearing people. Carl is able to remain calm as he attempts to talk to Irene from a closer distance so she can hear him. Carl slows his speech and uses non-medical language in an effort to assist Irene to understand him.

Activity 12.2

List three de-escalation techniques that were implemented by the paramedic in the case study.

Activity 12.3

List three de-escalation techniques that were not implemented by the paramedic in the case study.

Glossary

Chemical sedation: The administration of a drug/medication to restrain an individual with the goal of reducing agitation, consciousness, and/or physical movement or strength

Cognitive workload: The level of mental effort required to complete one or multiple tasks at a time.

De-escalation: A collaborative process that involves a range of verbal and non-verbal interventions to reduce agitation or violence.

Empathy: The process of understanding the emotions and feelings of others.

Open stance: A body position where the feet are side by side approximately shoulder width apart with the torso facing forward and the arms out by the side.

Patient-centred approach: The medical approach to patient assessment and management that considers the patient first, taking into consideration all aspects of the patients wants, needs, and preferences.

Rapport: The harmonious relationship developed between two or more individuals based on mutual respect and understanding of each other's feelings, emotions, and needs.

Spatial awareness: A complex cognitive skill involving receiving and interpreting information about one's surroundings. It involves being aware of your own position in an environment as well as the impact of other persons or objects within the same environment.

Splayed stance: A standing body position where one foot is in front of the other with the torso rotated slightly to the side. This is a common stance seen in combat situations.

References

Ali Abozaid, A., Momen, M., Fawzy Abou El Exx, N. et al. (2022). Patient and visitor aggression de-escalation training for nurses in a teaching hospital in Cairo, Egypt. *BMC Nursing* **21** (1): 63. doi: 10.1186/s12912-022-00828-y.

Ambulance Victoria. (2022). Violence against paramedics is never ok. Available at: https://www.ambulance.vic.gov.au/campaigns/violence-against-paramedics-is-never-ok (accessed 4 July 2022).

Argyle, M. (1988). *Bodily Communication*. 2e. London: Routledge.

Bailey, H.E. (2022). *Violence against Nurses and Patient Behavior Management in the Emergency Department*. Phoenix, AZ: Grand Canyon University ProQuest Dissertations Publishing.

AHPRA and national boards. (2022). Code of conduct. Available at: https://www.paramedicineboard.gov.au/ (accessed 4 July 2022).

Dementia Australia. (2020). *Changed behaviours*. Available at: https://www.dementia.org.au/ (accessed 22 July 2022).

Egan, G. (2002). *The Skilled Helper: A Problem-Management and Opportunity-Development Approach to Helping*. 7e. Pacific Grove, CA: Brooks/Cole.

Fischer, A. and Hess, U. (2017). Mimicking emotions. *Current Opinions in Psychology* **17:** 151–155. doi: 10.1016/j.copsyc.2017.07.008.

Fulde, G. and Preisz, P. (2011). Managing aggressive and violent patients. *Aust Prescr* **34:** 166–168. doi: 10.18773/austprescr.2011.061.

Goodman, H., Brooks, C., Price, O. et al. (2020). Barriers and facilitators to the effective de-escalation of conflict behaviours in forensic high-secure settings: a qualitative study. *Int J Mental Health Systems* **14** (1): 59. doi: 10.1186/s13033-020-00392-5.

Gormley, M.A., Crowe, R.P., Bentley, M.A. et al. (2016). A national description of violence towards emergency medical services personnel. *Prehosp Emerg Care* **20** (4): 439–447. doi: 10.3109/10903127.2015.1128029.

Hung Hsu, M., Flowerdew, R., Parker, M. et al. (2015). Individual music therapy for managing neuropsychiatric symptoms for people with dementia and their carers: a cluster randomised controlled feasibility study. *BMC Geriatrics* **15** (1): 84 doi: 10.1186/s12877-015-0082-4.

Iroku-Malize, T. and Grissom, M. (2018). The agitated patient: steps to take, how to stay safe. *J Family Pract* **67** (3): 136–147.

Janzen, S., Zecevic, A.A., Klosek, M. et al. (2013). Managing agitation using nonpharmacological interventions for seniors with dementia. *Am J Alzheimer's Disease & Other Dementias* **28** (5): 524–532. doi: 0.1177/1533317513494444.

Jeffery, D. and Austen, S. (2005). Adapting de-escalation techniques with deaf service users. *Nursing Standard* **19** (49): 41–47.

Johnston, I., Price, O., McPherson, P. et al.(2022). De-escalation of conflict in forensic mental health inpatient settings: a Theoretical Domains Framework-informed qualitative investigation of staff and patient perspectives. *BMC Psychology* **10** (1): 30 doi: 10.1186/s40359-022-00735-6.

Maguire, B.J., O'Neill, B.J., O'Meara, P. et al. (2018). Preventing EMS workplace violence: a mixed-method analysis of insights from assaulted medics. Injury, **49** (7): 1258–1265. doi: 10.1016/j.injury.2018.05.007.

Michigan University. (2017). Using a person's name in conversation. Michigan: Michigan State University. Available at: https://www.canr.msu.edu/ (accessed 6 July 2022).

Patel, M.X., Sethi, F.N., Barnes, T.R.E. et al. (2018). Joint BAP NAPICU evidence-based consensus guidelines for the clinical management of acute disturbance: de-escalation and rapid tranquillisation. *J Psychopharmacology* **32** (6): 601–640. doi: 10.1177/0269881118776738.

Park, I., Gupta, A., Mandani, K. et al. (2010). Breaking bad news education for emergency medicine residents: a novel training module using simulation with the SPIKES protocol. *J Emerg Trauma Shock* **3** (4): 385–388.

Ptacek, J.T. and Ptacek, J.J. (2001). Patients' perceptions of receiving bad news about cancer. *J Clin Oncol* **19** (21): 4160–4164. doi: 10.1200/JCO.2001.19.21.4160.

Rasmus, P., Kozlowska, E., Robaczynska, K. et al. (2020). Evaluation of emergency medical services staff knowledge in breaking bad news to patients. *J International Medical Research* **48** (6). doi: 10.1177/0300060520918699.

Richmond, J.S., Berlin, J.S., Fishkind, A.B. et al. (2012). Verbal de-escalation of the agitated patient: consensus statement of the American Association of Emergency Psychiatry project beta de-escalation workgroup. *Western J Emerg Med: Integrating Emerg Care with Primary Health* **13** (1): 17–25 doi: 10.5811/westjem.2011.9.6864

Robins, K.C. (2019). De-escalation in healthcare. *Nephrology Nursing Journal* **46** (3): 345–346.

Savoy, S., Carron, P.N., Romain-Glassey, N. et al. (2021). Self-reported violence experienced by Swiss prehospital emergency care providers. *Emerg Med International* **17** (2021). **doi**: 10.1155/2021/9966950.

Tamura, K., Mizuba, T., and Iramina, K. (2016). Hearing subject's own name induces the late positive component of event-related potential and beta power suppression. *Brain Research* **1635:** 130–142. doi: 10.1016/j.brainres.2016.01.032.

Kaunihera Manapou Paramedic Council. (2020). The Kaunihera Manapou Paramedic Council Code of Conduct. Available at: https://www.paramediccouncil.org.nz/ (accessed 4 July 2022).

Health and Care Professionals Council (HCPC). 2018). The standards of proficiency for paramedics. Available at: https://www.hcpc-uk.org/standards/standards-of-proficiency/paramedics (accessed 6 July 2022).

Todak, N. and James, L. (2018). A systematic social observation study of police de-escalation tactics. *Police Quarterly* **21** (4): 509–543. doi: 10.1177/1098611118784007.

Wanko Keutchafo, E.L., Kerr, J., and Jarvis, M.A. (2020) Evidence of nonverbal communication between nurses and older adults: a scoping review. *BMC Nurs* **19** (1): 1–13. doi: 10.1186/s12912-020-00443-9.

World Health Organization (WHO). (2022). Preventing violence against health workers. Available at: Preventing violence against health workers (who.int) (accessed 23 July 2022).

CHAPTER 13

Public health and health promotion

Michael Fanner
Department of Social Policy and Intervention, University of Oxford, UK

Contents

LEARNING OUTCOMES

On completion of this chapter the reader will be able to:

1. Understand the public health model in the promotion, management, and protection of health in populations, especially public health priorities.
2. Become aware of the changing nature of local and national demography and how these impact upon population health and well-being, integrated care, and the role of paramedics.
3. Recognise the value of health promotion in episodic care within paramedic practice in the context of modifying health behaviours.

Introduction

Public health and health promotion are both significant within paramedic practice, not least because they are far-ranging concepts that are universally understood throughout the multidisciplinary team, and more distantly, by the public. In 1988, Sir Donald Acheson, the Chief Medical Officer at the time, defined public health as 'the science and art of preventing disease, prolonging life and preventing disability through the organised efforts of society' (Acheson 1988, p. 1). The emphasis Acheson makes between 'science' and 'art' is a

Fundamentals of Paramedic Practice: A Systems Approach, Third Edition. Edited by Sam Willis and Ian Peate.

Companion website: www.wiley.com/go/willis/paramedic3e

seminal and distinct feature of all public health definitions. For example, the science of the Covid-19 pandemic could relate to the accelerated vaccine design and investment to prevent or lessen the pathogenesis of SAR-CoV-19 on the general population (Fanner 2022a). Yet, the art could relate to the UK government's public information strategy outlining Covid-19 lay-friendly preventative measures, with memorable slogans such as 'Hands. Face. Space.', which urged the public to wash their hands, cover their face, and make space in an attempt to control infection rates (Department of Health and Social Care 2020). Public health and health promotion is not down to one professional group to 'own' but requires multidisciplinary and multi-agency coordination and working, including the paramedic profession. This chapter is not exhaustive in covering all ground in public health and health promotion and is positioned as an introduction to the essential concepts – so further reading is strongly encouraged.

The importance of social determinants of health

The relationship between the 'health' of populations and how individuals perceive, negotiate and navigate their health throughout their lives (particularly their sense of well-being) becomes a fundamental juncture in public health and health promotion. This juncture creates the need for public health (and resulting health promotion practice) to be best understood as a more non-linear, complex system, and to explicitly consider the socio-economic status and psychological well-being of individuals, groups, and communities within the population. Public health as a 'system' and the need for greater integration of care will be discussed in this chapter.

Whilst public health efforts (and indeed, interventions) have become more obvious, ubiquitous features of everyday life since the Covid pandemic, public health should always consider the social and environmental factors of health, best conceptualised through the social determinants of health. Social factors of health can include individuals being able to feel connected in their local communities and being able to enjoy recreational activities. Environmental factors of health can include individuals being able to afford basic living amenities (such as food, heating, and rent or mortgage payments) or how governments calculate any increases in state welfare benefits in each fiscal budget. To support this wider consideration of the social determinants of health, Marmot et al. (2020) have observed a decade-long marked decline in England's population health, across the social gradient, correlative to the lack of government attention and investment to public health and well-being. They highlighted that at the start of the twentieth century, England had made uninterrupted progress in life expectancy increases, but from 2011, these improvements had practically stopped, and had in fact fallen in the most socially excluded and deprived communities. Marmot et al. (2020) evidenced these claims through strong statistical inferences demonstrating the interdependence between socio-economic vulnerabilities (social inequalities) and poorer health (health disparities).

Practice insight: social determinants of health

The social determinants of health are the social and environmental factors that influence health outcomes. Social and environment factors can include income, poverty, education, food insecurity, housing, early childhood development, and social inclusion, as a few examples. These factors create the daily living conditions and pressures that individuals are born into, grow, work, and retire within. The more negative social determinants of health an individual is subject to, the greater the adversity on their health and life chances. Social determinants of health are often measured comparatively through the exposure to, and experience of, social inequalities and health disparities across the population.

There is a lack of comparable international equivalents to Marmot et al.'s (2020) work within the literature, but it is highly likely other countries (with similar or poorer fiscal policy history) have similar population health and well-being statuses since the 2007–2008 global financial crisis and the Covid-19 pandemic. Developing countries, by contrast, will have far greater public health needs, which will often mean vaster and disproportionate mortality and morbidity rates across populations, especially during the perinatal period and in childhood. Marmot et al.'s statistical observations raise academic and professional concern, especially in the context of continuous claims making by governments of 'record investments' into national health and social care services; illustrating that public health spending is generally underestimated and under-conceptualised (i.e. the impact of non-health related fiscal policy affecting the social and economic mobility of individuals to improve their own health and well-being). The European Public Health Alliance (2020) strongly argue for the need for comprehensive policy, starting from early childhood and addressing the significant factors resulting in health inequalities throughout adulthood, are needed to achieve health equity and social fairness, and sustainable and equitable economics and societies. Paramedics indeed work with all age groups and communities within the population so gain unique insight to a diversity of individuals' livelihoods, including becoming acutely aware of emerging and long-standing socio-economic issues that impact upon health such as increasing fuel poverty.

The public health movement

Public health has evolved throughout human history, largely driven by the 'trial and error' of intergenerational expansion of scientific and medical knowledge and as part of the continued and increasing civilisation and socialisation of communities (e.g. urbanisation) (Tulchinsky and Varavikova 2014). Tulchinsky and Varavikova (2014) believe both parallel events have created the need for concerted efforts for organised health protection within populations. The shaping of public health throughout history has needed both public acceptance for disease control and public confidence with the medical and public health professions' ability to respond to diseases, advancing their knowledge of the basic science, causes, diagnosis, and treatments of diseases. Public engagement and acceptance are vital for effective public health policy and practice in order to demonstrate maximised achievement of positive health experience and outcomes (Sharp et al. 2020), and each health professional group has a role to play within this. In 1978, an international conference on primary healthcare (where the Alma-Ata Declaration was adopted) led to a new integrative approach to global health in the name of 'New Public Health', which ambitiously wanted a system-wide awareness and application of many dimensions and parts of society to be involved in achieving an acceptable level of Health for All by the year 2000 (Joomun 2023). The Declaration of Alma-Ata explicitly underlined the paramountcy of primary healthcare provision as a key to attainment in achieving the Health for All goal. The Declaration of Alma-Ata celebrated its fortieth anniversary at the Global Conference on Primary Health Care in Astana in October 2018, reaffirming that robust primary healthcare is crucial to achieve universal health coverage. These conferences are historically pertinent milestones for paramedic practice to reflect upon in its expanding roles in primary care services and systems.

The New Public Health approach relies upon contemporary and comprehensive evidence-based scientific, technological, and management system implementation to monitor and measure the health of individuals and populations, which includes system learning (Tulchinsky and Varavikova 2010). System learning entails the political will and subsequent (and rapid) policy generation from lessons learned from past success and failures in public health measures in combatting existing, evolving, or re-emerging health or social concerns, conditions, threats, or risks (Platt et al. 2020). Whilst the New Public Health approach is still in existence, since 2015, all United Nations members adopted the 2030 Agenda for Sustainable Development, made up of 17 Goals and 169 targets, to transform the world by ending poverty and inequality as well as protecting the planet. However, without sounding cynical, previous global health commitments by governments have yet to be fully achieved, so the 2030 commitment is unlikely unless international progress is increased and maintained (Caballero 2019). It is important to note that eleven of the seventeen Sustainable Development Goals relate to health (Marmot et al. 2020), which means the paramedic profession should make all attempts to contribute as critically and as practically as possible for the sake of local, national, and global health.

The (in)visibility of paramedics in public health

Paramedics have evolved from 'ambulance drivers' with basic first aid qualifications to registered out-of-hospital (OOH) care professionals (McCann et al. 2013), holding expertise in responding to known emergency health needs such as cardiac arrests (Weiss et al. 2018) as well as unknown emergency health needs such as critical illness caused by Covid-19 (Fanner 2022b). Paramedicine continues to evolve in its contribution to health and public health, in both similar and distinct ways from other professional groups. Dissecting Williams et al.'s (2021) proposed international definition of paramedicine in relation to public health, paramedics contribute a significant role to healthcare systems, primarily as the first responders to emergency, urgent and unplanned health needs of populations through their possession of 'complex knowledge and skills, a broad scope of practice . . . and . . . practic[ing] under medical direction or independently, often in unscheduled, unpredictable or dynamic settings' (Williams et al. 2021, pp. 3561–3562). Together with this increased professionalisation and definitional consensus of the paramedic profession, there has also been a year-on-year accelerated surge in ambulance demand from the public, which potentially dilutes the visible progression of the paramedic profession contributions to public health, more generally.

To add to this, there is no clearly defined model of public health approaches within the ambulance sector (Crabtree and James 2021), leading to varied and different use of paramedics in ambulance services and wider health and care systems. This heterogenous and widespread use, without a clearly defined public health approach within the ambulance service, means paramedics become lost in plain sight in public health systems but the profession's evolutionary history may offer some explanation to this (further reading on the brief history of paramedic education/professionalisation can be found in Fanner 2022b). So, paramedics should not only consider their knowledge to be limited to individual emergency health responses to public health threats/issues but also consider how the data and evidence they use in practice on a day-to-day basis is informed by the public health model, thus operationalising public health concepts in very 'real-world' ways. Paramedics need to be cognisant of the particular groups and communities who are more vulnerable to social inequalities and health disparities than others in their local geographies; this leads to a professional stimulation of awareness of specific public health issues (through local data and evidence) that may affect these groups or communities more than others. In such instances, paramedics can apply specific health promotion advice in each clinical contact with specific groups or communities. For example, in the case of people with intellectual disabilities, bespoke advice can be offered on increasing oral hydration during heatwaves, or encouraging seasonal immunisation offers during winter periods.

Practice insight: unwarranted variations in NHS ambulance trusts

Following Lord Carter of Cole's successful review into the operational productivity of acute non-specialist trusts in England in 2016, a similar review was requested by the ambulance sector. In 2018, Carter's review entitled 'Operational productivity and performance in NHS Ambulance Trusts: unwarranted variations' (NHS England 2018) was published, which centred on the varying hospital conveyance rates across all ten ambulance services in England. Carter identified that reducing avoidable conveyance to hospital would make savings of £300 million a year, which would in turn make more money available for reinvesting in services.

Carter proposed three structural problems were causal to the high variation of conveyance across England and included: access to GP and community services, the need for urgent treatment centres, and the reduction in ambulance handover delays. Carter recommended a move towards a common operating model across ambulance services in the country, with productivity opportunity in three main areas: staff engagement, better use of technology, and improved fleet management.

The public health model

The public health model builds upon other models of health such as the biomedical and biopsychosocial models but addresses health (and social) problems through a population-based and comprehensive approach in the promotion, management, and protection of health through epidemiologic surveillance, health promotion, disease prevention, and the accessibility and availability of universal healthcare services. As an example, the UK's NHS is the only comprehensive health system in the industrialised nations that does not determine accessibility of healthcare according to wealth, so the NHS is in itself a public health strategy (Naidoo and Wills 2016). To put it simply, the public health model largely adopts a preventative approach to population health by targeting state-level interventions at the known risk factors of a health or social concern, condition, threat, or risk (hereafter, health concern), identifying and responding to the concerns as they arise as quickly as possible to ensure that their long-term impact is minimised. For example, NHS ambulance services are essentially the state-funded interventions that are responsible for responding to patients who require emergency assessment and interventions, as they are the best and quickest public health resource to ultimately save lives and lessen the longer-term health impacts from an injury or illness, i.e. reducing unnecessary mortality and morbidity within the population.

As part of the identification and response to health concerns, risk and protective factors are considered as components of the development and testing of novel or established interventions or strategies, which are then subsequently evaluated for effectiveness. In 2004, the World Health Organization (WHO) proposed three different types of public health interventions (within a mental health context – but it is also equally applicable to physical health): universal, indicated, and selective prevention (WHO 2004), defined as:

- Universal prevention is designed to target the entire general public, in an indiscriminate way, not targeting specific groups on the basis of increased risk/low protective factors. For example, the 999 emergency telephone service, or the legal requirement for seat belt use in vehicles.
- Indicated prevention is designed to target groups within the general population who may be at heightened risk of a health concern, evidenced by their biopsychosocial risk and protective factors. For example, individuals who smoke heavily are at increased risk of respiratory health problems, or a mental health car within an ambulance service.
- Selective prevention is designed to target high-risk individuals who may already be showing signs of a particular health concern but do not yet meet diagnostic criteria. For example, individuals who live in poor housing conditions with excessive damp and mould and are showing signs of respiratory problems, or a dedicated 'frequent caller' team within an ambulance service, focusing specifically on patients who have a high call volume.

In other texts, public health prevention can be defined as primary, secondary, and tertiary prevention and hold similar definitions to the above.

In order to ensure that public health interventions or strategies are 'fit for purpose', public health professionals study health concerns through three essential public health concepts: demography, epidemiology, and health inequalities. These concepts are also used when little is known about or something new evolves in a previously understood health concern, or in other words, when previously 'known knowns', 'known unknowns', or 'unknown unknowns' come to light (Pawson et al. 2011). Each concept will now be briefly discussed.

Demography

Demography is the study of populations, including their size, structure, density, distribution, and growth. As the demographics of any given population change, the requirement to evolve how we measure population also changes. Model-based demography (Burch 2018) exists to as accurately as possible respond to these changes in how population numbers are measured and indeed 'categorised', for example, with straightforward categories like age, or less straightforward categories like future public health adherence. Model-based demography allows dynamic inferences to aid policymakers, researchers, and clinicians in developing appropriate and contemporary health and social care systems, strategies, and interventions. For example, developing a palliative and end-of-life care specialist paramedic team in local geographies with dense communities of older people.

Epidemiology

Epidemiology is the study of disease (or health concern) pattern occurrence within whole, and subgroups of the population (Coggon et al. 2009). Epidemiology utilises different types of data collection methods and statistical measurement tools to determine how populations are affected by the outcomes of disease, as well as how populations are exposed to disease (Celentano and Szklo 2019). Epidemiological data can be either descriptive, i.e. everyone's counted, or analytical, i.e. making inferences from a sample of the population, and offers greater insight to disease for policymakers, researchers, and clinicians through:

- New or continued learning about the **natural history of diseases,** meaning how a disease behaves within or affects the human body over time, with and without medical intervention. For example, there is an average 90% mortality between eight to ten years after initial HIV infection without anti-retroviral therapy but near-normal life expectancy and no onward transmission with optimised anti-retroviral therapy.
- Development of **case definitions,** meaning how diseases are defined and qualify as a clinical diagnosis, using different types of criteria, made of:
  - Laboratory criteria, e.g. test findings of a biological sample (a clinical criteria as defined below would often indicate the need for a laboratory test);
  - clinical criteria e.g. whereby a clinician observes a symptom or set of symptoms; and

  - epidemiological criteria, e.g. population-level symptom reporting, such as Office for National Statistics self-report surveys on particular health concern symptoms in different parts of the population.
  - Clinical and epidemiological criteria are often solely used as part of a clinical diagnosis in paramedic practice. For example, two to three symptoms of influenza may be considered clinically equal to 'laboratory-confirmed' influenza, without the need for testing and can be offered best practice treatment advice.
- **Disease causation and association** such as crowded environments and respiratory viruses (often causation) or observed increases in both the sale of ice creams and the rate of intentional fatality injuries/homicide during hot weather periods (association!).
- **Disease surveillance** such as statutory duties for clinicians to notify certain infectious diseases to local health protection teams, for example, suspected food poisoning.
- **Disease screening and testing development or improvement and data** such as the development of home rapid lateral flow test kits for Covid-19 or the need for improving screening in unexpected increases in Tuberculous positivity rates in homeless or incarcerated communities.
- **Intervention development** such as novel antimicrobial therapy for bacterial infections or more technologically sophisticated OOH equipment such as hand-held ultrasound devices.
- **Measurement of outcomes or intervention responses** such as observing a reduction or eradication of vaccinatable diseases, or measuring survival rates of patients who arrived by ambulance compared to those who self-presented at an emergency department.

Health inequalities

Health inequalities are important considerations and influencing factors in public health, as they denote differences in (often negative) health experience and outcomes between individuals, groups, and communities within populations. Health inequalities often present or situate individuals or groups within the population in conditions that ultimately influence their opportunities for good health by shaping how individuals think, feel, and act within their health and well-being. Health inequalities can be righted through health, social, and economic interventions, e.g. increasing the access to culturally safe healthcare or government action on improving the social determinants of health. More recently, health inequalities are now better understood as health inequities (focusing on individual/subgroup access and support needs for achieving optimal health rather than standardisation/equal access of services) and are more likely to be achieved through social justice approaches as described in the health visiting/public health nursing literature (Fanner et al. 2022).

Paramedic practice, public health, and integrative care systems

As populations grower older with increasing complex care needs, the health and social care service requirements and professions have to also evolve, including ambulance services and the paramedic profession. Many people with

Case study: carrying out your own transect walk

In order to become familiar with your local area (and indeed develop a local case study), a transect walk (or, simply put, a systematic walk) is a very effective way of identifying the health and social assets and vulnerabilities that may impact upon local public health. You can search online for different transect walk questions, but four simple questions could be:

1. What does it feel like to live in the local area?
2. What social or environmental factors within the local area may lead to poorer health?
3. What access to healthcare is available in the local area, particularly out of hours and beyond emergency health services?
4. What might it be like for at-risk socially excluded groups such as people of colour, people from Gypsy, Roma, and Travellers of Irish Heritage communities, or non-English speaking asylum seekers to navigate the above three questions?

Please always consider your and others' health and safety when carrying out a transect walk.

multiple long-term conditions are living longer, requiring more than one health and/or social care service to support their holistic needs, leading to fragmented care (The King's Fund 2022). As a result, healthcare systems across the globe now seek to respond to this demand through integrated models of service delivery, encompassing diverse ways of improving integration of care within and across services (Baxter et al. 2018). In England, the Health and Care Act 2022 formally created integrated care systems, as legal entities, managed by integrated care boards, with four key aims:

- *improving outcomes in local population health and health care*
- *tackling inequalities in outcomes, experience and access*
- *enhancing productivity and value for money*
- *helping the NHS to support broader social and economic development.*
(The King's Fund 2022)

This official policy move to integrated care works extremely well within the public health model to truly ascertain the local population health needs and appropriate system-level response. However, Rutter et al. (2017) propose advancing the public health model by arguing for the need for a complex system model of evidence for public health. They rightly assert that many health concern are often measured through simple, short-term, individual-level health outcomes, failing to contextualise and consider the complex, multiple, and upstream population-level actions. Rutter et al. (2017) go on to suggest that this data issue in the published evidence leads policymakers to prioritise individual-level interventions over system-wide and system-level responses. An example is given in the paragraph below.

During the recent Covid-19 pandemic, government rules and regulations (and indeed legislation) evolved as the pandemic continued from weeks to months, from an initial focus on individuals 'washing their hands' and working from home to system-wide responses such as flight restrictions and temporary flight bans. During the Covid-19 pandemic, there became great exacerbation of the issue of hospital discharge delay caused by long-standing lack of social care provision in the community, which had a knock-on effect on ambulance handover delays, emergency department overcrowding, and hospital bed capacity.

A complex systems model of public health evidence ensures that when a health concern is measured it is theorised as an outcome of an assembly of interdependent elements, whether obvious or subtle, that come together as a whole (Rutter et al. 2017). For instance, whilst health services may declare full equality, diversity, and inclusion commitments, wider structural oppression may still undermine the health experience of minoritised groups. Bohensky et al. (2010) have previously commented that policymakers, researchers, and clinicians are increasingly interested in using different and multiple sources of data to aid the measurement of clinical performance and health outcomes of patients, which wholly adopts a public health approach in its conception and employment as a research method.

Practice insight: data linkage studies

Data linkage is an important tool in observational research methods. In health research, data linkage studies essentially follow the same individual patients through their healthcare journeys, combining multiple and different data sources from the same or different health services, to create a more enhanced data resource. This then allows researchers to be able to fully understand the potential issues and successes in health experience and outcomes from a systems-level to improve healthcare services. Data linkage studies are extremely valuable research methods in ambulance service and paramedic research.

To apply this complex systems model to OOH care, Crabtree and James (2021) have helpfully proposed a consistent public health approach to the ambulance sector, especially with regard to a call for more unified population health management. Population health management is an increasingly used term to describe the way in which historical and current data can be utilised to better understand what factors influence health and well-being of communities and how (Crabtree and James 2021). For example, ambulance dispatch data has been used, albeit small-scale and inconsistently, as an early indicator of endemic influenza-like illnesses (Mostashari et al. 2003), to establish relationships between temperature and heat-related illnesses (Bassil et al. 2009) and even monitor violent crime (Sutherland et al. 2021). Excitingly, since the successful implementation of the new Ambulance Response Programme in England in 2017, following the largest clinical ambulance trials in the world (Turner and Jacques 2018), there has been official recognition for the need to understand how and why individuals use ambulance services to improve their experience and outcome of OOH care. This recognition has led to a new national development of the

Ambulance Data Set (ADS) in England, to consistently collect data on the following:

- *Patient demographics (gender, ethnicity, age at activity date);*
- *Episode information (including arrival and conclusion dates and times, source of referral and attendance category type);*
- *Clinical information (chief complaint, acuity, diagnosis, investigations and treatments);*
- *Injury information (data/time of injury, place type, activity and mechanism);*
- *Referred services and discharge information (onward referral for treatment, treatment complete, streaming, follow-up treatment and safeguarding concerns). (NHS Digital 2022)*

Not only will this ADS inform future paramedic/public health practice, in wholesale and holistic ways, in integrative care systems, it will also ensure paramedics and ambulance services are recognised in their current (under-recognised) roles in the health and social care landscape. In a scoping review of the literature on integrative care, Allana et al. (2022) observed that paramedics often 'bridge' the gaps that fall between existing health and social care partnerships such as primary care, hospitals, and social care by offering reactive and preventative care. Although it may not be planned as such, this new data makes a good case for the significance of paramedics within public health systems, i.e. integrated care systems.

Practice insight: Ambulance Response Programme

Since 2017, the NHS offers a national ambulance response standard across England to ensure the sickest patients get the fastest response and that all patients get the right response first time – meeting the acutest needs of high public health priorities. The Ambulance Response Programme was developed to improve patient outcomes and increase the operational efficiency of ambulance service provision. This new system replaced a decades-old system of localised telephone OOH triage protocols to a more comprehensive electronic clinical decision support service to support more effective remote assessment of callers to emergency services. Each category is defined in Table 13.1.

TABLE 13.1 Ambulance Response Programme categories.

Category	Response	Response time to 90% of all incidents
Category 1	Life threatening An immediate intervention or resuscitation to a life-threatening condition such as cardiac arrest	15 minutes
Category 2	Emergency A serious condition such as stroke, which may require rapid on-scene assessment and intervention, and urgent transport	40 minutes
Category 3	Urgent An urgent problem that is not life threatening such as a psychotic episode, which requires referral/transport to an acute setting in order to receive onward treatment	2 hours
Category 4	Less urgent A less urgent problem, such as recent moderate symptom continuation in an older adult, which requires transportation to an acute or primary care setting	3 hours
Category 5	Non-urgent A non-urgent problem such as a small cut to a finger, which requires home first aid management and self-monitoring for signs of infection	Self-care/home management only

Health promotion

The WHO (1998) defines health promotion as 'the process of enabling people to increase control over, and to improve their health'. In 1986, the Ottawa Charter for Health Promotion (WHO 1986) was presented at the first international conference on health promotion (mainly but not exclusively focused on the needs of industrialised countries) and built on the progress of the Alma-Ata Declaration to achieve Health for All by the year 2000 and beyond (discussed earlier in the chapter). The Ottawa Charter, still relevant today, incorporates five key action areas, through three basic health promotion strategies (enable, mediate, and advocate) including:

- *Build healthy public policy*
- *Create supportive environments for health*
- *Strengthen community action for health*
- *Develop personal skills*
- *Re-orient health services*
  (Joomun 2023)

As previously discussed in this chapter, the 2030 Agenda for Sustainable Development now drives government efforts in public health, and this also includes the continued expectation of health promotion as framed by the Ottawa Charter. Health promotion is still in its early days in paramedicine, with limited research to support its place, but the health-promoting role of the paramedic is starting to gain traction within wider health policy (Schofield and McClean 2022). However, the role of the paramedic in health promotion is unique, as Fanner (2022a) has previously pointed out, in respect of immunisation advice and information as one example. All paramedics are likely to meet patients who have had a varied health services experience; therefore it is vital to include health promotion advice at each clinical interaction, especially if the patient's presenting complaint relates to a health promotion opportunity. So, for this reason, paramedics should not completely rely upon other health professionals to offer the necessary health promotion advice and information.

In current clinical practice, paramedics utilise different health promotion approaches within their work, but many rely upon the Making Every Contact Count (MECC) initiative. The evidence-based MECC approach aims to improve the health and well-being of an individual by helping them change their health behaviours through the use of conversations on the risk factors that lead to poorer health such as physical inactivity, smoking, and alcohol intake (NICE 2023). Other approaches contextualised by health promotion theories also exist and are outlined further in this chapter.

Health behaviours

Health behaviours can be defined as the actions taken by individuals that impact upon their health and well-being, whether intentional or unintentional, dependent upon their ability to control their lives. For many health concerns, health behaviours can often be a causal factor, an action (or series of actions) in the management of a health concern, as well as an exacerbating factor of progression. However, the amount of 'control' an individual has on the ability to change a health behaviour depends upon their unique social determinants of health. A consistent change in health behaviours can be slow, or even reverse a health condition altogether (such as Type 2 Diabetes Mellitus). Paramedics should note that not all health concerns (and outcomes) are entirely behaviourally based, and constitutional factors including age, biological sex, and genetics can mean an individual has a higher propensity of developing certain diseases (Benton 2012). Individuals with known family histories of certain diseases such as hypertension or particular cancers should still be afforded the same attention to their health behaviours, as the continuation of poor health behaviours may increase the risk of development of these diseases.

It is important to consider that health behaviours change over time and intergenerationally, for example, compared with previous generations, people spend more time in environments that not only restricts physical activity but also necessitates prolonged sitting, risking new health risks due to sedentary behaviour (Owen et al. 2010). Not only does sedentary behaviour affect physical health but meta-analysis of longitudinal research suggests that a lack of physical activity is also associated with poorer mental health (Schuch et al. 2018), meaning that paramedics should always consider the impact of health behaviours through both physical health as well as mental health paradigms.

Health behaviours can be influenced by paramedics utilising different health promotion theories and models and approaches as outlined in the remaining sections of this chapter.

Health promotion theories

There are different theories and models that can both contextualise health behaviours and help to facilitate and guide effective paramedic practice. Many theories and models have been applied to different health settings and not all are applicable to every situation.

- **The Health Belief Model** theorises that an individual's decisions or actions are mostly dependent on their perceived susceptibility, severity, benefits, barriers, cue to action (the need to change), and self-efficacy (their confidence to change) relating to a health behaviour.
- **Stages of Change Model (also known as the Transtheoretical Model)** theorises the process in which an individual decides to change a health behaviour through six stages:
  - Precontemplation (does not recognise the need to change a health behaviour).
  - Contemplation (recognises the need to a health behaviour but is not ready, is ambivalent, or lacks confidence to make the change)
  - Preparation or determination (begins to make small changes in healthier health behaviours with full belief that it is a better option).
  - Action or willpower (the change or modification in a health behaviour is in motion and intend to adhere to this change or modification).
  - Maintenance (maintains the change or modification in a health behaviour to remain healthier, with a focus on relapse prevention).
  - Termination (no desire to return to a previous health behaviour, without the risk of relapse).
- **Theory of Reasoned Action/Planned Behaviour** theorises an individual's health behaviour is shaped by their behavioural intentions that are guided by both their own attitude and subjective (or social) norms/acceptability. For example, alcohol consumption within a home environment may hold different social norms and acceptability than in a public place.
- **Ecological Model of Health Behaviour** illustrates individual's health behaviours to be determined by the multiple levels or influence of their social, cultural, and physical environments on their knowledge, attitudes, and beliefs.
- **Social Cognitive Theory** theorises an individual's health behaviours to be influenced by how they socially learn, cognitively decide, and take actions within their social environment. For example, a child or young person will need to become aware of the importance of 'consent' when accessing and engaging with health services, in preparation for adulthood. So, in order for this social learning to occur, a paramedic can influence a child's health behaviours, by taking the same steps used within the normative 'consent' process when assenting them for a clinical assessment (providing there is also parental consent).

Each theory or model guides health promotion practice for policymakers, researchers, and clinicians in their hypotheses to improve health promotion outcome effectiveness. More pertinently, each theory or model can also help inform paramedics in their offer of different health promotion approaches.

Health promotion approaches

There are different ways of approaching health promotion, some of which may not be appropriate and therefore should be applied to practice with professional discretion. However, it is entirely possible for paramedics to incorporate health promotion approaches in all episodic care.

- **Prevention:** the aim of a preventative approach, also known as the behaviour-change or behaviourist approach, is for the health-promoting paramedic to encourage an individual to adopt a healthier lifestyle through changing their current beliefs and attitude to health.
- **Empowerment:** the aim of the empowerment approach, also known as the client-centred approach, is for the health-promoting paramedic to offer evidence-based information to individuals to facilitate well-informed decisions about their health. This approach requires the paramedic to see the individual as an equal partner in the changes required in their health behaviour, in need of support to make the right decision for them whilst bearing in mind they have ultimate control of their own lives.
- **Educational:** the aim of the educational approach, also known as the informative approach, is for the health-promoting paramedic to raise and inform individuals of evidence-based information about health issues to allow them to make decisions but is not dependent on any kind of facilitative support from the health-promoting paramedic.
- **Use of fear:** the aim of the fear approach, also known as the approach to frighten individuals into rapid health behaviour change, is for the health promoting paramedic to create scenarios (often exaggerated or actual worst case) as a method of explaining facts about continued health behaviours. Television advertisements on road safety often use fatality of others to promote speed awareness, for example.
- **Use of disgust:** the aim of the use of disgust approach, also known as the regret approach, is for the health-promoting paramedic to explain the consequences of health behaviours with unpleasant and graphic details to an individual to invoke an emotionally primed risk aversion to a health behaviour. For example, detailing the necrotic complications of uncontrolled Diabetes Mellitus.

- **Medical:** the aim of the medical approach, also known as the interventionist approach, is to relieve an individual of pain and suffering, the promotion of health and the prevention of disease, the forestalling of death and the promoting of a peaceful death, and the cure of disease when possible and the care of those who cannot self-care through medical interventions. This approach is likely to be very familiar with paramedics as this is a de facto response often expected by members of the public!

Conclusion

This chapter has explored the essential knowledge of public health and health promotion that paramedics need on a day-to-day basis. In order to address complexity in population health and well-being and the service provision landscape, the enactment of public health and health promotion practice ultimately sits within two parts, part science-based and part art-based, echoing Acheson's (1998) public health definition. People are complex beings, with their own (genetic) individual variation, destined by health behaviours (whether they are in control of them or not), thus requiring paramedics (and indeed, all health professionals) to offer person-centred and unique responses as informed by the evidence base.

Whilst there is great attention on the needs of public health and health promotion practice towards individuals, paramedics must consider the system-wide issues and politics that ultimately make the bigger changes in population health. Global commitments to improving everyone's health through more person-centred as well as environmentally friendly policy may seem somewhat impossible to achieve, but with countries, including England, now with laws to improve care through integrative care systems, there is hope for improved population health status across the world.

Though public health and health promotion may be somewhat novel concepts within paramedic practice, there is strong momentum to change this within the profession, especially with the future impact of the ADS and the desire within the ambulance sector to standardise its approach towards public health. Paramedics should absolutely contextualise their practice to go beyond the individual emergency health needs of patients and incorporate wider public health learning and knowledge to improve, consolidate, and make visible the paramedic contributions to public health and integrative care systems.

Activities

Now review your learning by completing the learning activities in this chapter. The answers to these appear at the end of the book. Further self-test activities can be found at **www.wileyfundamentalseries.com/paramedic/3e.**

Test your knowledge

1. Is public health defined as art-based practice, science-based practice, or both?
2. Why is public acceptance and confidence required in public health policy?
3. How many UN Sustainable Development Goals relate to health?
4. Why might paramedics not be considered as traditional public health professionals?
5. Why is a 'complex systems model of public health evidence' more effective in assessing population health?
6. How many key action areas does the Ottawa Charter for Health Promotion incorporate?
7. What health promotion initiative is commonly relied upon in paramedic practice?
8. What is sedentary behaviour?
9. What factors are individuals unable to change in relation to health concerns?
10. What is a social determinant of health?
11. How many health promotion approaches can paramedic potentially utilise in their practice?

Glossary

Demography: The study of populations, including their size, structure, density, distribution, and growth.

Epidemiology: The study of disease (or health condition) pattern occurrence within whole and sub-parts of the population.

Health behaviours: Actions taken by individuals that impact upon their health and well-being, whether intentional or unintentional, dependent upon their ability to control their lives.

Health disparities: Preventative differences in the burden of illness, injury, and violence or health-enhancing/recreational opportunities to achieve optimal health (often socially disadvantaged populations are more affected).

Health inequalities: Avoidable differences in health outcomes between groups or populations.

Integrated care: The organised partnership(s) of health and social care services to plan and deliver joined up services for the benefit of those receiving care in the least fragmented way.

Public health model: A population-based and comprehensive approach in the promotion, management, and protection of health through epidemiologic surveillance, health promotion, disease prevention, and the accessibility and availability of universal healthcare services.

Social gradient (of health): A term used to describe the relationship between socio-economic position and health status (for example, people with less socio-economic advantage tend to have worse health and shorter lives).

Further reading

Fanner, M. (2022). Immunisations. In: *Fundamentals of Pharmacology for Paramedics* (ed. Peate, I. Clegg, L., and Evans, S.), pp. 299–318. Chichester: Wiley.

Celentano, D.D. and Szklo, M. (2019). *Gordis Epidemiology.* 6e. Canada: Elsevier.

References

Acheson, D. (1988). *Public Health in England: The Report of the Committee of Inquiry into the Future Development to the Public Health Function.* 1e. London: Stationery Office Books.

Allana, A., Tarvares, W., Pinto, A.D. et al. (2022). Designing and governing responsive local care systems – insights from a local scoping review of paramedics in integrated models of care. *International Journal of Integrated Care* **22** (2): 1–19.

Bassil, K.L., Cole, D.C., Moineddin, R. et al (2009). The relationship between temperature and ambulance response calls for heat-related illness in Toronto, Ontario, 2005. *Journal of Epidemiology & Community Health* **65** (9): 829–831.

Baxter, S., Johnson, M., Chambers, D. et al. (2018). The effects of integrated care: a systematic review of UK and international evidence. *BMC Health Services Research* **18:** 1–13.

Benton, T.G. (2012). Individual variation and population dynamics: lessons from a simple system. *Philosophical Transactions of the Royal Society of London. Biological Sciences* **367** (1586): 200–210.

Bohensky, M.A., Jolley, D., Sundararajan, V. et al. (2010). Data linkage: a powerful research tool with potential problems. *BMC Health Serv Res* **10:** 346. doi: 10.1186/1472-6963-10-346.

Burch, T. (2018). *Model-Based Demography. Essays on Integrating Data, Technique and Theory.* Cham: Springer Open.

Caballero, P. (2019). The SDGs. Changing how development is understood. *Global Policy* **10** (1): 138–140.

Celentano, D.D. and Szklo, M. (2019). *Gordis Epidemiology.* 6e. Canada: Elsevier.

Coggon, D., Rose, D., and Barker, G. (2009). *Epidemiology for the Uninitiated.* 5e. London: BMJ Books.

College of Paramedics. (2019). *Paramedic Curriculum Guidance.* 5e. College of Paramedics.

Crabtree, R. and James, S. (2021). Developing a public health approach within the ambulance sector. Discussion Paper. Public Health England and Association of Ambulance Chief Executives.

Department of Health and Social Care. (2020). New campaign to prevent spread of coronavirus indoors this winter. Press Release. Available at: https://www.gov.uk/government/news/new-campaign-to-prevent-spread-of-coronavirus-indoors-this-winter (accessed 2 January 2023).

Eaton, G., Wong, G., Williams, V. et al. (2020). Contribution of paramedics in primary and urgent care: a systematic review. *British Journal of General Practice* **70** (695): e421–e426.

European Public Health Alliance. (2020). The Marmot Review 10 years on and its implications for a healthy Europe. Position Paper. European Public Health Alliance.

Fanner, M. (2022a). Immunisations. In: Fundamentals of Pharmacology for Paramedics (ed. Peate, I. Clegg, L. and Evans, S.), pp. 299–318. Chichester: Wiley.

Fanner, M. (2022b). Reflecting on population health learning in pre-registration paramedic education during a global pandemic. In *Digital Connections in Health and Social Work: Perspectives from Covid-19* (ed. Turner, D. and Fanner, M.), pp. 23–36. St Albans: Critical Publishing Limited.

Fanner, M., Whittaker, K., and Cowley S. (2022). Being oriented towards social justice: Learning for health visitor practice. *Nurse Education Today* **116:** 105386.

Fenn, K. and Byrne, M. (2013). The key principles of cognitive behavioural therapy. *InnovAiT* **6** (9): 579–585.

Joomun, L. (2023). Health Promotion. In: *Fundamentals of Public Health Practice* (ed. Holland, A. et al.), pp. 28–39. London: Sage.

Marmot, M., Allen, J., Boyce, T. et al. (2020). Health equity in England: The Marmot Review 10 years on. Institute of Health Equity. Available at: https://www.health.org.uk/publications/reports/the-marmot-review-10-years-on (accessed 10 January 2023).

McCann, L., Granter, E., Hyde, P. et al. (2013). Still blue-collar after all these years? An ethnography of the professionalisation of emergency ambulance work. *Journal of Management Studies* **50** (5): 750–776.

Mostashari, F., Fine, A., Das, D. et al. (2003). Use of ambulance dispatch data as an early warning system for communitywide influenzalike illness, New York City. *Journal of Urban Health* **80** (2) (Supplement 1): i43–i49.

Naidoo, J. and Wills, J. (2016). *Foundations for Health Promotion.* 4e. London: Elsevier.

National Institute for Health and Social Care Excellence (NICE). (2023). Making Every Contact Count. Available at: https://stpsupport.nice.org.uk/mecc/index.html (accessed 15 January 2023).

NHS Digital. (2022). Ambulance Data Set (ADS). Available at: https://digital.nhs.uk/data-and-information/data-collections-and-data-sets/data-sets/ambulance-data-set/about-the-ads (accessed 14 January 2023).

NHS England. (2018). Operational productivity and performance in England NHS Ambulance Trusts. Unwarranted variations. Available at: https://www.england.nhs.uk/publication/lord-carters-review-into-unwarranted-variation-in-nhs-ambulance-trusts/ (accessed 12 January 2023).

Owen, N., Sparling, P.B., Healy, G.N. et al. (2010). Sedentary behaviour: emerging evidence for a new health risk. *Mayo Clinical Proceedings* **85** (12): 1138–1141.

Pawson, R., Owen, L., and Wong. G. (2011). Known knowns, known unknowns, unknown unknowns: the predicament of evidence-based policy. *American Journal of Evaluation* **32** (4): 518–546.

Platt, J.E., Raj, M., and Wienroth, M. (2020). An analysis of the learning health system in its first decade in practice: scoping review. *Journal of Medical Internet Research* **22** (3): e17026.

Rutter, H., Savona, N., Glonti, K. et al. (2017). The need for a complex systems model of evidence for public health. *The Lancet* **390** (10112): 2602–2604.

Schofield, B. and McClean, S. (2022). Paramedics and health promotion. *Perspectives in Public Health* **142** (3): 135–136.

Schuch, F.B., Vancampfort, D., Firth, J. et al. (2018). Physical activity and incident depression: a meta-analysis of prospective cohort studies. *American Journal of Psychiatry* **175** (7): 631–648.

Sharp, C.A., Bellis, M.A., Hughes, K. et al. (2020). Public acceptability of public health policy to improve population health: a population-based survey. *Health Expectations* **23** (4): 802–812.

Sutherland, A., Strang, L., Stepanek, M. et al. (2021). Tracking violent crime with ambulance data: how much crime goes uncounted? *Cambridge Journal of Evidence-Based Policing* **5**: 20–39.

The King's Fund. (2022). Integrated care systems explained: making sense of systems, places and neighbourhoods. Available at: https://www.kingsfund.org.uk/publications/integrated-care-systems-explained#:~:text=Where%20next%3F-,What%20are%20integrated%20care%20systems%3F,reducing%20inequalities%20across%20geographical%20areas (accessed 17 January 2023).

Tulchinsky, T. and Varavikova, E.A. (2014). A history of public health. In: *The New Public Health* (ed. Tulchinsky, T. and Varavikova, E.A.), pp. 1–42. London: Elsevier.

Tulchinsky, T. and Varavikova, E.A. (2010). What is the "New Public Health"? *Public Health Reviews* **32**: 25–53.

Turner, J. and Jacques, R. (2018). Ambulance Response Programme Review. University of Sheffield. Available at: ambulance-response-programme-review.pdf (england.nhs.uk) (accessed 12 October 2023).

Weiss, N., Ross, E., Cooley, C. et al. (2018). Does experience matter? Paramedic cardiac resuscitation experience effect on out-of-hospital cardiac arrest outcomes. *Prehospital Emergency Care* **22** (3): 332–337.

Williams, B., Beovich, B., and Olaussen, A. (2021). The definition of paramedicine: an international Delphi study. *Journal of Multidisciplinary Healthcare* **14**: 3561–3570.

WHO (World Health Organization). (1986). Ottawa Charter for Health Promotion. Available at: Ottawa Charter for Health Promotion (who.int) (accessed 25 October 2023).

WHO. (1998). Health promotion glossary. Available at: Health promotion (who.int) (accessed 25 October 2023).

WHO. (2004). *Prevention of Mental Disorders: Effective Interventions and Policy Options*. Available at: Prevention of mental disorders: effective interventions and policy options (who.int) (accessed 12 October 2023).

CHAPTER 14

Leadership in paramedic practice

Jack Howard

Intensive Care Paramedic, Ambulance Victoria, Melbourne, Australia

Contents

LEARNING OUTCOMES

On completion of this chapter the reader will be able to:

- Recognise how all roles in paramedic practice involve aspects of mentorship and leadership in terms of influencing and engaging others.
- Identify leadership behaviours.
- Recognise the value of leadership theory in enhancing practice for the out-of-hospital care professional.
- Discuss leadership styles and approaches.
- Apply theories and principles of leadership theory to develop practice at an individual level, when supervising others and when working with teams.

Fundamentals of Paramedic Practice: A Systems Approach, Third Edition. Edited by Sam Willis and Ian Peate.

Companion website: www.wiley.com/go/willis/paramedic3e

Case study

You are a local single responder paramedic who has arrived on scene at a high speed, motor vehicle accident. A car has swerved off the road and into a tree. There is a single patient, mechanically trapped with critical injuries. The job has triggered a multi-agency response with firefighters, police, and a dual paramedic crew in attendance. The scene is chaotic, emotive, and highly charged. There is a great deal of commotion but little progress in extricating the patient and moving towards hospital. The multiple agencies on scene do not appear to be working together. The other paramedic crew are junior in their experience levels, you are the senior paramedic on scene.

Introduction

Leadership in paramedic practice permeates all facets of everyday work life. From the coal face of emergency operations, like the scenes represented by the Case study above, to the offices of upper management, leadership is not only required it is essential.

Paramedicine is a rapidly growing and changing profession steadily being influenced and shaped by out-of-hospital (OOH) research and from the benefits of cross pollination with medical bodies. Strong leadership is required not only in the traditional clinical management front but also in education, research, and culture (van Diggele et al. 2022).

In general, leadership is defined as: whereby an individual influences a group of individuals to achieve a common goal (Northouse, 2019). Whilst this is an adequate definition to cover the broad strokes of leadership theory, to define leadership in paramedicine is far more complex and multifaceted. The reason for this is influence in paramedicine can be actioned on multiple levels from a personal scale to organisation wide. The face of leadership in this context has numerous formats or styles and can be tailored to suit the individual needs of the target audience, indeed a paramedic can switch between multiple styles of leadership all within a single patient care episode depending on the needs of the patient, peers, bystanders, or situation. If all the above was not enough, leadership undergoes constant evolution through a paramedic's career, influenced from self-experience and increasing research surrounding the subject, and as such, demands continual revision (Mercer et al. 2018). Clearly the subject of leadership is of real importance in the field of paramedicine.

This chapter will provide a blueprint you can use to revise and enhance your own leadership skills. You will be challenged to think and address common leadership problems that are often faced by paramedics in the workplace, such as:

- How do I manage myself and maximise my own performance and professional contribution?
- How effectively do I work with other individuals, especially where I hold a mentoring or supervisory role relative to that person?
- How effectively do I work with teams and, where I encounter challenge and conflict in teamwork, what models and processes do I draw upon in order to find a way forward?
- Finally, how do I see my own paramedic practice fitting into the wider picture of my organisation and how does my contribution help to shape that wider picture?

The need to develop and expand leadership skills is vital for all paramedics. Quality patient care and advocacy in the uncontrolled, unscheduled, and unplanned OOH environment demands robust leadership. Recent research demonstrates that high-quality patient care is achieved through collaborative leadership approaches, a style well suited to the team-based approach paramedics work in (Turner 2019).

Every chapter in this book is important, however, there are not many other OOH subjects that have such far-reaching and significant influence upon every aspect of your practice as this one does. Your attention to the learning in this chapter will guide the way you practice, educate, and lead as a paramedic.

Whilst it is true not everyone possesses natural leadership qualities; it is also true to say this does not mean that one cannot learn to be a better leader. Everyone has individual strengths of character, those strengths naturally lend themselves to certain aspects of leadership, empathetic individuals have an increased ability to form connections with others, conscientious personas tend to shoulder more responsibility and accept more accountability. In addition to our natural leadership strengths, there is no reason we cannot expand, develop, and strengthen leadership in other areas, in fact research strongly supports this. Whether you are a university student about to take your first step into the emergency service workforce or a manager with decades of experience, this chapter is relevant to you.

Theories of leadership: a brief overview

The importance of leadership has been greatly emphasised regarding patient outcomes and team building in recent years by health care professions. Literature and research into the topic of leadership has increased exponentially and hence so has our understanding and awareness. Out of hospital bodies are dedicating resources to developing leadership from within their own workforces (Barr and Dowding 2022; Gopee and Galloway 2017).

Leadership comes in many forms and styles, differing situations or personnel on scene can dictate how you communicate and lead. Therefore, it is important to understand that leadership theories are most helpful when used pragmatically to provide a framework for looking constructively at a situation, or identifying a way forward when a challenge, dilemma, or problem has arisen. With this practical orientation in mind, let us briefly review some of the key leadership styles and approaches, as defined in the current research. The discussion is organised in three key sections: definitions, leaders and leadership behaviours, and leadership styles and approaches.

Definitions of leadership

The Old English etymology of the verb *to lead* can be traced back to the word *lædan,* which means 'to show the way' (*Oxford English Dictionary* (Online) 2000). Clearly, the general meaning behind the word leader has not changed in over a thousand years. Leadership is fundamentally related to the idea of setting direction and guiding oneself or others. Modern day leadership has expanded on its Old English origins, identifying a set of skills, traits, and behaviours that allow individuals to lead and motivate a team to a specific goal. For paramedics this can look like a team synergistically providing high-quality patient care, through implementing organisational clinical or cultural change. Whatever the end goal may be, we can be certain that leadership is an everyday requirement of a paramedic.

Effective leadership requires specific characteristics and skills. Traits such as strong communication skills, empathy, decisiveness, integrity, and confidence have been identified as key contributors to effective leadership. However, the application of leadership does not require the same character traits and skills every time (Price-Dowd 2020). Adaptability is especially relevant in the OOH world, where the unexpected and unanticipated are common encounters (Johnson et al. 2018). Leadership is articulating the vision or goal and instilling a sense of ownership in the team to motivate, direct, and support leading to achievement; how the leader accomplishes this can vary from situation to situation.

Although leaders may possess the required characteristics or skills, a large portion of effective leadership is about building and maintaining, the ability to build relationships features heavily in successful teams. Good leaders inspire, foster trust, and encourage collaboration amongst their team. The most effective leaders promote an environment where individuals feel safe to voice opinion and share new ideas. When this leadership model is applied, there are benefits to patient outcomes (Sfantou et al. 2017).

From leaders to leadership behaviours

Contemporary discussions of leadership have gradually but consistently shifted from discussing leadership in terms of individual *leaders* to considering the topic in relation to leadership *behaviours* (Barr and Dowding 2019). It is natural to look towards great leaders from history such as Nelson Mandela or Mahatma Gandhi and try to define leadership from their examples. Using these individual exemplars, the exploration of their leadership would then work backwards to try to establish their leadership characteristics of a good leader – the assumption being that if we can work out what these great leaders have in common, we can seek to imitate it.

There are obvious limitations to such an approach. First, there is the issue of transferability: is the effective leadership of Nelson Mandela, to lead his people through such oppression, transferable to leading an OOH team to strive for a positive patient outcome?

Second, to start with examples of great leaders and then look for underlying principles of great leadership is challenging when it comes to less tangible and fluid leadership qualities involving personality and style. For example, the eminent leaders mentioned were much noted for their 'charisma' or 'charm' – a personal quality that is not generally viewed as something that can be imitated, developed, or adopted.

This method of deriving leadership principles from famous examples can lead to the perpetuation of the view that great leaders are 'born, not made', arriving in the world with in-built traits that naturally set them apart. Whilst the above examples undoubtedly possessed natural personality traits advantageous to inspirational leadership, recent research into the study of personality traits to enhance our own leadership skills known as **trait theory of leadership** have found inconsistent relationships between individual traits and leadership effectiveness.

Practice insight

Next time you are at station, ramped at hospital, or on standby, discuss the subject of leadership with your crew mate or colleagues. Ask them do they think leaders are born or developed? Also ask them what they think are the essential characteristics of a leader?

Thus, it has been recognised as more helpful to move away from focusing on individual leader traits and instead focus on leadership *behaviours* (Turner 2019). Although most personality 'traits' tend to be innate and cannot be easily adopted, leadership behaviours can be. Recent research into leadership effectiveness shows there is far more practical value studying and improving upon leadership behaviours. It is an obligation to current or aspiring leaders to actively develop leadership behaviours and styles that combine with our natural personal traits and values. This will result in an effective and flexible approach to leadership. It is now time to consider what some of those styles and behaviours might involve.

Leadership styles and approaches

There is no current evidence suggesting a leader must adopt a singular style to become an effective leader. Each leader works in their own particular way to suit their own leadership style, an extremely effective leader can even suit this approach to the situation at hand. The ability of a team leader in paramedicine to stay flexible and adaptable is of great importance in the field. Supporting this statement are the theories of **situational leadership** (Hersey and Blanchard 1969, 1993) and **contingency theory** (Fiedler 1969). The most effective leaders in paramedicine are flexible and adaptable according to context.

TABLE 14.1 Classical styles of leadership.

Autocratic leadership	A leader adopting an autocratic approach would make unilateral decisions without team consultation or input.
Democratic leadership	A leader adopting this approach would be highly consultative and would seek guidance, input, and sometimes formal voting on leadership decisions and actions.
Laissez-faire leadership	A leader adopting this approach is 'hands off' in dealings with colleagues; they are trusted to get on with the task in hand and are left room for individual judgement and for making mistakes.
Distributed leadership	This model develops further the idea of democratic leadership: in this co-leadership model decision-making and responsibility are shared.

Some of the most distinctive and classical leadership styles are set out in Table 14.1.

Tragedies in healthcare are unfortunately commonplace thus the need to throw the spotlight on leadership and its impact upon patient outcomes. Research recently has heavily focused on leadership styles and new models are being developed and expanded constantly as we become more aware of how leadership can affect patient outcome. Tragic healthcare cases throw into stark reality the importance of a team-based and collaborative leadership style, and how input from all within the team ensures we achieve high-quality clinical care.

With this in mind, we will now look at a small sample of various contemporary leadership styles that are being increasingly championed by healthcare organisations due to their success in team building, individual development, and improved patient outcomes.

Transformational leadership is associated with increased employee satisfaction, a reduction in episodes of burnout and improved patient outcomes (Steinmann et al. 2018). Transformational leaders motivate and inspire teams to achieve excellence by showing followers what they might get out of doing a task, how they might learn and develop whilst doing it, and how they might want to use their own initiative and skill set in accomplishing the task. Transformational leadership involves a more coaching orientation to working with others and has been shown to bring positive results to an organisation in terms

Reflection point: mind that label!

Whilst it may sometimes be helpful to label different leadership behaviours and approaches to discuss practice, it is crucial that we remain critically aware and do not use labels in an unexamined or casual manner. It would be a mistake, for example, to label an individual leader 'a transactional leader' based on only one or two interactions or decisions. Likewise, it would be simplistic to suggest 'I am a transformational leader' based on only a snapshot of practice; the truth is always more complex and fluid than this.

Indeed, it is far better to avoid labelling any individual an 'X' or 'Y' kind of leader (this is inevitably a simplistic approach). Instead, think in terms of a continuum between different leadership behaviours and approaches and consider where *individual leadership decisions or actions* fall on that continuum. Despite being quite contrasting styles, transformational and transactional leadership styles have been proven to combine into an extremely effective leadership approach. Ensure your leadership style stays fluid to the situation you find yourself in.

of developing more motivated, engaged, and confident employees.

In contrast, **transactional leadership** is based on the relationship between leaders and followers. The leader dictates a clear set of expectations, oversees the performance of their followers, and provides rewards or punitive actions accordingly. In transactional leadership engagement, expectations are clear, and results are predictable (van Diggele et al. 2020).

However, healthcare systems are moving away from these downward-style power gradient leadership models (Rahbi et al. 2017; Leclerc et al. 2021) and favouring styles such as **servant leadership**, a style that emphasises a leader's duty to the well-being of the patient and empowerment of their healthcare team. It involves leaders prioritising the needs of others, instituting a supportive and collaborative environment that encourages team members to achieve their full potential.

Another leadership style with an emphasis on team building is **authentic leadership**, a style that promotes transparency and ethical behaviour in its leaders. Authentic leadership is focused on building trust, openly collaborating, and advocating for the well-being of both team members and patients. Authentic leadership has been linked with happier and more productive workplaces, increased collaboration between team members, and reduction in adverse patient outcomes (Lyubovnikova et al. 2017).

The spectre of Covid-19 has impacted global healthcare agencies in many ways, one such way being a forced rethink into effective leadership strategies (Kumar 2022). Given the positive influence certain modern leadership styles encourage there is almost a universal emphasis being placed into team building, empowerment, and collaboration in an attempt to reduce burnout and inspire happy teams. It has been widely proven empowered and collaborative teams produce stronger outcomes for their patients (Sfantou et al. 2017; van Diggele et al. 2020).

Leadership at the individual level

What does all this theory mean for us at a personal level? The process by which we learn to regulate ourselves as professionals, monitor our own performance, and find ways to improve that performance is itself a leadership process. Thinking about our individual development in relation to the concept of leadership can be a helpful way to gain self-knowledge and to learn more about not only how we perceive ourselves but also how we are perceived by others. The ability to inspire and motivate others does not require an official rank or seniority, leadership first starts within oneself before it can be extended to those around you.

Practice insight

In order to keep up to date with service developments, including new roles that emerge over time, be sure you read all e-mails and in-house communications placed on noticeboards sent from the service. Engage in discussions regarding developments with paramedic colleagues and be sure to attend as many ambulance service study days and events as possible. This includes events held by the professional body. Go one step further and become a student ambassador with the professional body and be active in raising standards. Drive the culture of your station and inspire others around you to do the same.

Leadership and the mentoring or supervisory role

Of all the leadership roles within the field of paramedicine, it can be argued that one of the most important is that of a mentor or supervisor. The importance of guiding an inexperienced student through the challenges of becoming a paramedic cannot be understated. The mentor is not just influencing this singular individual, they are shaping the desired culture and expected professional standards of the organisation for years to come (Hodge et al. 2018).

The performance of this leadership role has no minimum attendance, you can be guiding large teams of paramedics or supervising the learning and development of a singular trainee. The requirements of leadership are equal to both scenarios and of equal importance.

The Covid-19 pandemic placed a significant burden on ambulance response times (Andrew et al. 2022), paramedic organisations around the world are finding themselves hiring increasing numbers of students and trainees. The role of leadership in the mentoring role has been thrown into sharp relief, and it is well known that OOH organisational culture and clinical skills rely heavily on trainers and mentors (Bell and Whitfield 2021).

Effective leadership of someone's learning and development also benefits from acquaintance with a certain amount of educational theory. You may have heard of theories such as learning styles or multiple intelligences, which contend that individuals may prefer to learn or process information via a certain format such as a visual, auditory, or kinaesthetic (active) emphasis. These theories suggest students learn best when teaching aligns with their preferred learning style. It is important to note that these traditionally well-accepted theories have been widely questioned in recent years due to a lack of supporting evidence promoting their effectiveness.

Individual differences in learning preferences still exist. Some students prefer certain learning styles. Unfortunately, there is a lack of evidence existing that points to the effectiveness of these well-known theories in predicting and improving learning outcomes. Concentrating on one aspect of learning also tends to limit student learning opportunities by pigeonholing them into a narrow category instead of encouraging the development of a balanced set of learning and problem-solving skills.

It is good practice to be aware of such theories, to personalise the learning journey of the mentee as much as possible, but also to be aware that good communication (the key to all forms of leadership) and a better approach to education is about making **multiple representations** of the same idea: conveying the same message in different ways, providing different examples, and expressing the idea in different registers or forms of words. Multiple representations have been proven to be an effective tool in education, as they can cater to learning preferences, improve accessibility, and promote a deeper understanding, whilst engaging and motivating students.

Reflection point

Think of a situation where an instructor or senior colleague was teaching you a principle or procedure and it took some time for you to grasp the point they were making. Can you remember that feeling of 'the penny dropping' when you finally wrapped your head around it? Did the point finally hit home when a different representation of the same idea was made?

Leadership and teamwork

One of the most exhilarating experiences as a paramedic is coming together as a productive team to rescue a critically ill patient. This exemplifies the role of paramedics and when the team is working at peak efficiency, solving every problem that arises, achieving the desired patient outcome drives home why we do what we do.

However, the art of collaboration and teamwork can be a double-edged sword, it can also provide one of the biggest challenges paramedics face in the field. Just the slightest amount of desynchrony in a paramedic team has the ability to destabilise patient outcomes and deflate the team.

Effective teamwork has been shown to improve patient outcomes, operational efficiency, and overall job satisfaction: whilst the problems arising from a dysfunctional team can create disproportionate stresses, tensions, and inefficiencies in the workplace (Schmutz et al. 2019).

Somewhat unique to paramedicine is the variability in coming together of teams. Commonly, two paramedics function as a two up crew and perform the bulk of paramedic function. However, as the complexity in patient presentation or the number of patients escalates so does the need for increased members and diversity of skill. This may involve the need for intensive care paramedics, manual handling specialists, in-field managers, and health commanders often in combination with personnel from other disciplines such as fire and rescue or police. A good leader will adapt their leadership style and communication between these different groups, often multiple times in a job.

To help you lead in these challenging events it can be helpful to know a little about the differences of personality, working style, and team role preference that can sometimes lead to conflict in a team. Dr Meredith Belbin's seminal work on **team roles** is widely consulted and well respected (Belbin 2010). Belbin's work suggests that there are several pronounced and distinctive roles that an individual might adopt when working in a team, outlined in Table 14.2.

TABLE 14.2 Belbin's team roles.

Plant	The team member most associated with creativity, with 'blue skies' thinking, and with identifying innovative solutions to tasks and challenges.
Monitor-evaluator	The team member most consistently focused on monitoring team performance and measuring this against desired goals and outcomes.
Co-ordinator	The team member most comfortable with taking a directive role and marshalling the other team members once the team goals and direction have been settled upon.
Resource investigator	The team member best placed to help locate and draw upon the resources required for the team to complete the task.
Implementer	The team member best equipped or most motivated to see through the different phases of the team's tasks.
Team worker	Perhaps the most flexible and adaptable member of the team, who will adapt readily to others and work collaboratively without any overriding preference or particular model of working.
Shaper	The team member most likely to want to shape or influence an existing idea and to attempt to shape how the team achieves its goal.
Completer-finisher	The team member most focused on seeing all constituent steps of a task through to completion.
Specialist	Added as a development of Belbin's original research, the specialist is the member of a team most likely to contribute key or specialised knowledge relevant to a given task.

As with the previous discussion of leadership approaches and styles, it is likewise important to avoid using Belbin's team roles as absolute labels for oneself or members of your team. Make sure to keep a balanced approach between theory and real-world application.

The different roles are helpful only as a frame of reference, to be used judiciously when analysing a team, specifically looking at what works well or what might be going wrong within a group.

Do not pigeonhole members of your team into certain roles. No well-rounded professional could be described as only a 'completer-finisher' or solely a 'plant'; each of us occupies a number of roles according to the team we are working in or the task we are dealing with. Thus, for Belbin's team roles (Belbin 2010) to be helpful to us, we need to apply them sparingly and with the knowledge that they will shift and overlap when applied to any given group of people.

Your leadership as a paramedic is vital to the efficacy of a team working together. Your ability to stay calm and in control will stabilise the team at any scene. The importance of clear communication from leaders cannot be understated. Constant updates to the team on what is happening and where the job is heading are vital to the team understanding their roles and responsibilities. As a leader you are responsible for every team member understanding their role and understanding what is required from them at any case.

Think of your team as a machine of cogs and wheels, dedicated to producing positive patient outcomes. Your team members are represented by the cogs. No matter how effectively the cogs turn, all it takes is one cog working out of synch and your previously well-oiled machine will seize up and cease to operate effectively. Every cog that makes up the machine is of vital importance to its operation. Contemporary healthcare leadership represents this to a fault, and it is the leader's responsibility to ensure the entire team are working together to advocate for the most important person, the patient.

Ongoing leadership development

In the course of your career in paramedic practice, you may well wish to progress into a specialist paramedic role with particular responsibility for mentoring, supervision, or leadership; the prevalence of roles of this kind is increasing

Reflection point

Think back to an incident where conflict arose in a team in which you have worked. If you were to think about the team members in terms of Belbin's team roles, was there a clear distribution of roles between members? Might any conflicts within the team be explained in terms of a clash between roles? Or by the fact that there were too many individuals vying for the same role? How might airing the problem and using the language of team roles have helped to resolve the situation and move things forward?

with the development of the profession (Paramedics Australasia 2016; College of Paramedics 2023). Regardless of whether you adopt a specialist role, there is value for all paramedics in undertaking ongoing leadership development and in accessing professional development related to teamwork, personal resilience and well-being, and personal development. Development opportunities of this kind will be extended to you throughout the course of your career, and it is recommended that you embrace these with a reflective, enquiring, and constructive approach.

Conclusion

In this chapter we have explored the value of leadership theory as a framework for thinking about how a paramedic perceives their own professional role, their interactions with those they are supervising or mentoring, and their collaborations with wider teams of professionals. We have seen how leadership influence and initiative can be shown at all organisational levels, rank and seniority are not a requirement to possess and exhibit leadership. We have also discussed how a good working knowledge of leadership theory can help the OOH professional to map their own learning and development across the span of their career. Leadership is a subject that permeates every facet of daily life for a paramedic. The uncontrolled and dynamic arena that is our workplace demands strong and adaptable leadership. Studying the theories and concepts detailed in this chapter will help with your readiness and resilience in the face of these challenges. All that is required for lasting change is a willingness to apply yourself and a passion to advocate for your patients and co-workers.

Activities

Now review your learning by completing the learning activities in this chapter. The answers to these appear at the end of the book. Further self-test activities can be found at **www.wileyfundamentalseries.com/paramedic/3e.**

Test your knowledge

1. What did the word 'leader' originally mean?
2. What does 'situational' or 'contingency' leadership involve?
3. Identify three distinct leadership styles.
4. Name five of Dr Belbin's team roles.

Activity 14.1

Consider the many different leader–follower engagements that make up paramedic practice. How often and in what contexts do junior colleagues and senior colleagues meet? Who sets direction and gives instructions, and in what style of engagement do they do this? How much scope is there for adopting a 'transformational' approach to some of these engagements (involving colleagues in decision-making, communicating a vision, helping them to identify a stake in the goals to be achieved, helping them to learn and grow as a result of undertaking the task)? What examples can you think of where a transformational approach would be inappropriate, and a transactional approach is absolutely required?

Activity 14.2

Look back at the Case study at the start of this chapter. How would you approach this scene? What are some of the leadership styles that may help at a difficult case such as this? Do you think there is room for the implementation of several styles? Which would you use?

Glossary

Authentic leadership: A leadership approach that emphasises self-awareness, transparency, and ethical behaviour to inspire and empower team members.

Leadership: The process of motivating, engaging, influencing, and persuading others towards the achievement of a common goal.

Multiple intelligences theory: The notion that in addition to a traditional 'intelligence' measured by IQ, there are significantly different ways in which we process, experience, and understand the world, encompassing musical–rhythmic, visual–spatial, verbal–linguistic, logical–mathematical, bodily–kinaesthetic, interpersonal, intrapersonal, and naturalistic intelligences.

Multiple representations: Conveying the same idea in different ways such as suggesting the circulatory system is like a series of connecting rivers and streams, or like a car engine, or like a road network of A roads and B roads.

Servant leadership: Prioritising the well-being and development of followers, with a focus on emphasising service, humility, and meeting their needs.

Situational leadership: Adapting one's leadership style or approach according to the needs of each follower and the specific situation at hand.

Team roles: The behaviours we typically adopt and the roles we typically fulfil when working in a team.

Trait theory of leadership: The attempt to derive leadership principles from examples of eminent leaders in history – and thus a theory that implies that leaders are 'born not made'.

Transactional leadership: A leadership style that concentrates on the exchange of rewards and punishments to motivate and manage individuals towards achieving a goal.

Transformational leadership: A widely espoused style of leadership that involves winning the hearts and minds of followers and engages with colleagues on a person-focused rather than task-focused level.

References

Andrew, E., Nehme, Z., Stephenson, M. et al. (2022). The impact of the COVID-19 pandemic on demand for emergency ambulances in Victoria, *Australia. Prehospital Emergency Care* **26** (1): 23–29. doi: 10.1080/10903127.2021.1944409.

Barr, J., and Dowding, L. (2022). *Leadership in Health Care.* 5e London: SAGE Publications.

Belbin, R.M. (2010). *Management Teams Why They Succeed or Fail.* 3e. London: Butterworth-Heinemann.

Bell, A. and Whitfield, S. (2021). Mentor or tormentor? A commentary on the fractured role of mentoring in paramedicine. *Australasian Journal of Paramedicine* **18:** 1–3. doi: 10.33151/ajp.18.984.

Bennett, R., Mehmed, N., and Williams, B. (2021). Non-technical skills in paramedicine: A scoping review. *Nursing & Health Sciences* **23** (1): 40–52. doi: 10.1111/nhs.12765.

College of Paramedics. (2023). *Paramedic Career Framework.* London: College of Paramedics.

Fiedler, F.E. (1969). Leadership: a new model. In: *Leadership* (ed. C.A. Gibb), pp. 230–241. Harmondsworth: Penguin.

Gopee, N. and Galloway, J. (2017). *Leadership and Management in Healthcare.* 3e. Thousand Oaks: SAGE Publications.

Hodge, A., Swift, S., and Wilson, J.P. (2018). Maintaining competency: a qualitative study of clinical supervision and mentorship as a framework for specialist paramedics. *British Paramedic Journal* **3** (3): 10–15. doi: 10.29045/14784726.2018.12.3.3.10.

Hersey, P. and Blanchard, K.H. (1969). The life cycle theory of leadership. *Training and Development Journal* **23** (5): 26–34.

Hersey, P. and Blanchard, K.H. (1993). *Management of Organizational Behavior: Utilizing Human Resources.* 6e. Englewood Cliffs, NJ: Prentice Hall.

Johnson, D., Bainbridge, P., and Hazard, W. (2018). Understanding an alternative approach to paramedic leadership. *Journal of Paramedic Practice: The Clinical Monthly for Emergency Care Professionals* **10** (8): 1–6. /doi: 10.12968/jpar.2018.10.8.CPD2.

Kumar, R.D.C. (2022). Leadership in healthcare. *Clinics in Integrated Care* **10:** 100080. doi: 10.1016/j.intcar.2021.100080.

Leclerc, L., Kennedy, K., and Campis, S. (2021). Human-centred leadership in health care: A contemporary nursing leadership theory generated via constructivist grounded theory. *Journal of Nursing Management* **29** (2): 294–306. doi: 10.1111/jonm.13154.

Lyubovnikova, J., Legood, A., Turner, N. et al. (2017). How authentic leadership influences team performance: the mediating role of team reflexivity. *Journal of Business Ethics* **141** (1): 59–70. /doi: 10.1007/s10551-015-2692-3.

Mercer, D., Haddon, A., and Loughlin, C. (2018). Leading on the edge: the nature of paramedic leadership at the front line of care. *Health Care Management Review* **43** (1): 12–20. doi: 10.1097/HMR.0000000000000125.

Northouse, P.G. (2019). *Leadership: Theory & Practice*. 8e Thousand Oaks: SAGE Publications.

Oxford English Dictionary (Online). (2000). Oxford: Oxford University Press.

Paramedics Australasia (2016). Paramedicine role descriptions. Paramedics Australasia.

Price-Dowd, C.F.J. (2020). Your leadership style: why understanding yourself matters. *BMJ Leader* **4** (4): 165–167. doi: 10.1136/leader-2020-000218.

Rahbi, D.A., Khalid, K., and Khan, M. (2017). The effects of leadership styles on team motivation. *Academy of Strategic Management Journal* **16** (3): 1–14.

Schmutz, J.B., Meier, L.L., and Manser, T. (2019). How effective is teamwork really? The relationship between teamwork and performance in healthcare teams: a systematic review and meta-analysis. *BMJ Open* **9** (9): e028280–e028280. doi: 10.1136/bmjopen-2018-028280.

Sfantou, D.F., Laliotis, A., Patelarou, A.E. et al. (2017). Importance of leadership style towards quality of care measures in healthcare settings: A systematic review. *Healthcare (Basel)* **5** (4): 73–90. doi: 10.3390/healthcare5040073.

Steinmann, B., Klug, H.J.P., and Maier, G.W. (2018). The path is the goal: How transformational leaders enhance followers' job attitudes and proactive behavior. *Frontiers in Psychology* **9**: 2338–2338. doi: 10.3389/fpsyg.2018.02338.

Turner, P. (2019). *Leadership in Healthcare Delivering Organisational Transformation and Operational Excellence*. 1e. London: Springer International Publishing.

van Diggele, C., Burgess, A., Roberts, C. et al. (2020). Leadership in healthcare education. *BMC Medical Education* **20** (Suppl 2): 456–456. doi: 10.1186/s12909-020-02288-x.

van Diggele, C., Roberts, C., and Lane, S. (2022). Leadership behaviours in interprofessional student teamwork. *BMC Medical Education* **22** (1): 834–834. doi: 10.1186/s12909-022-03923-5.

CHAPTER 15

The foundations of research in paramedic practice

Elicia Austin

School of Health and Social Work, University of Hertfordshire, UK

Contents

LEARNING OUTCOMES

On completion of this chapter the reader will be able to:

- Understand the basis of the theories that underpin research projects.
- Identify the differences between the three opposing research methodologies.
- Recognise the various study designs that will influence the research process.
- Identify some of the most common data-collection methods available.

Introduction

Research is critically important to paramedics, as it is a reliable source of evidence that underpins all of our practice; it increases the evidence available to practitioners through systematic investigation and scientific evaluation. Research is fundamental to the evolution of paramedic practice, as it provides a rationale for challenging our existing guidelines, or forming innovate and original guidelines, based on the result of new valid information.

This chapter is written with the beginner or intermediate paramedic researcher in mind. It offers simplified yet fundamental explanations of the theories underpinning healthcare research, helping you to understand the most common research designs and processes utilised within the paramedic profession. The aim is to develop your skills

Fundamentals of Paramedic Practice: A Systems Approach, Third Edition. Edited by Sam Willis and Ian Peate.

Companion website: www.wiley.com/go/willis/paramedic3e

of interpreting research and to grow your confidence, so you can use research to support your clinical judgement.

It should be noted that the healthcare research community has over time developed its own terms, outlined later in this chapter. You may think that these terms sound complicated, and this can sometimes make the novice researcher apprehensive about reading research. Do not panic, with a little perseverance recognising these concepts becomes easier over time.

Research paradigms

In the early stages of any healthcare research project, the researcher will need to determine which overarching research ideology will fit the theme or idea for their project.

A paradigm itself can be thought of as a set of beliefs and practices that will be used to regulate or standardise a method of research inquiry. These values will be shared by communities of researchers within paramedic science or healthcare research. In other words, this is the idea that there are different systems, which can be used to examine a research topic from very different perspectives (Levers 2013; Brown and Dueñas 2020). This concept of looking at the world (and research) from viewpoints, as well as the theories that underpin this, can be a more challenging concept in paramedic research education. There are various other paradigms not discussed in this text, however, the ones discussed here highlight the polarity for some of the approaches to beginning a research project. It is important to remember that each paramedic research project will utilise a different paradigm specific to the topic being investigated and that the researchers own beliefs will often have a large impact on the paradigamatic route selected (Wilson et al. 2021; Wilson et al. 2022).

Here is a summary of the three most common and distinct routes that currently exist for a healthcare researcher to select on the start of their journey; each will take the research project in a completely different direction.

1. **Positivism** can be explained as an objective view to a answering a problem. It looks to measure testable metrics in order to generate absolute facts, which are undisputable. This is because the researcher would hold the assumption that there is only one clear verifiable reality. The researcher is acting as a 'realist' in this type of project.
2. **'Constructivism' or 'interpretivism'** are words that may be used interchangeably with **'post-positivism'** in the very novice research community. **Post-positivism** is a diverging view away from positivism, where the researcher views the topic area as a buildable living theory where one absolute truth cannot be achieved, but it follows the idea that the research problem should try to be approached in a critical and objective manor (Levers 2013; Ray 2016).

   Interpretivism is an even more polarised approach away from positivism where the researcher believes the subject topic is relative to the circumstances or environment and will have to be subjectively measured. **'Constructivism' or 'constructionism'** both have some homogenous philosophical principles to the other paradigms mentioned (Levers 2013; Turyahikayo 2014). However, there are subtle nuances between how these research paradigms view the social world in which research will be conducted (Brown and Dueñas 2020). All of these approaches have a similar overall outlook, which is to investigate the social reality of the research question (Holloway and Galvin 2016).
3. **Pragmatism** is a practical approach, which is focused around problem solving whilst understanding an environment's current clinical context. There is an assumption that our knowledge can only be constructed based on interactions between people and their environments. Consequently, it seeks to simultaneously test a problem using a scientific method of inquiry and understand the complexities of the social problems affecting this. This often means the research will be 'patient orientated' and look to pursue the maintenance of social justice. This viewpoint can be extremely valuable in identifying the specific opportunities and barriers to changing clinical care (Allemang et al. 2022).

Paradigms have developed with the philosophical, technological, and economic growth of society, resulting in various ideological shifts with regard to our perception of healthcare and medicine, over the past 150 years (Ho 2019). Consequently, there are speculations that there could be the emergence of a separate fourth paradigm, which would seek to understand the 'real world' in a more purposeful way. Similar shifts in paradigms from other research areas, such as Life Science research (Li et al. 2021), may impact this.

Some newer methodological approaches have already been developed in healthcare research, which rely on more modern types of data sources. For example, 'Netnography', which focuses on studying the impact of social media (Salzmann-Erikson and Eriksson 2021). In the future, further technological breakthroughs in robotics, artificial intelligence (AI), and genomics will likely influence the development of a 'big-data-driven' fourth research paradigm (Schlicher et al. 2021). This will allow new research methods to grow 'in the moment' with our rapidly modernising societal norms. It may focus on drawing information continuously from the current environment, concentrating on the right mix of data, rather than the type of data itself. Theoretically, this paradigm might focus on the use of real-time streams of data collection or processing, from less traditional methods, and utilise more unconventional avenues to do this such as apps, social media, or the information on medical devices (Rapport and Braithwaite 2018).

Research methodologies

After the appropriate paradigm has been identified to fit the idea and outcomes of the research project, an appropriate methodology will be decided.

The methodology itself is a way to underpin the research with another theoretical framework – similar to an algorithm in clinical practice. It is a generalised theoretical guide for the project, which will follow the same paradigmatic assumptions and will generally dictate the research data to be collected. The principle that the paradigm and methodology are linked and will consequently direct the project in a specific way is known as paradigmatic rigidity (Mesel 2013). Thus, the use of three divergent methodologies (see Box 15.1).

1. **A quantitative methodology** will produce only numerical data for the purpose of measurement. It seeks to predict and provide explanations using the data collected in a mathematical and logical way (Jolley 2020). This can help in understanding how commonly something occurs in the data set. The data can also be used to determine a correlation, i.e. when two instances tend to occur together. This kind of research is suitable for testing a hypothesis, i.e. a possible explanation that the researcher has previously developed from theory.
2. **In contrast to this, a qualitative methodology** is about investigating a phenomenon – therefore words or observations form the data, rather than numbers. Often qualitative research projects aim for a much deeper understanding of 'why' or 'how' events occur, and the data will be formed by studying human behaviour, opinions, and emotions. Qualitative investigations can also be used to lay the groundwork for the design of a quantitative project or may seek to explain the real-world limitations of clinical interventions (Pope and Mays 2020).
3. **A mixed methods methodology** is a hybrid of both research methodologies, which blends and integrates both qualitative and quantitative data. It aims to collect numerical and narrative information, with both sets of data ultimately informing the overall interpretation of the results. This follows the concept of methodological eclecticism (Hammersley 1996) – meaning that the methods are chosen and mixed because of their ability to answer the research questions raised. This approach is sometimes called triangulation (Wisdom et al. 2012).

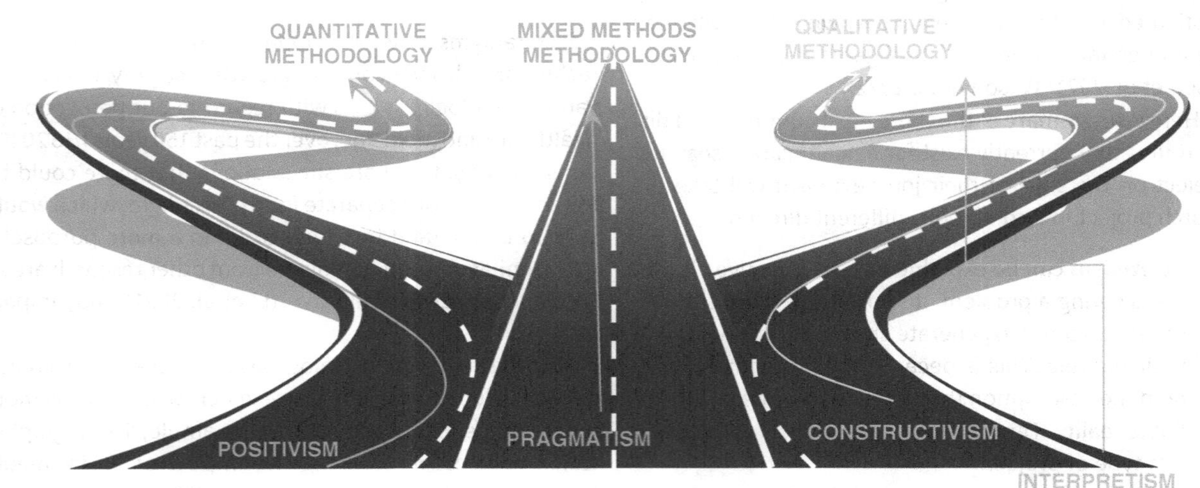

FIGURE 15.1 The different journeys through the theories of research.

BOX 15.1 Three divergent methodologies

As an example, let's explore a 'cardiac arrest' as a basis for a research project whilst looking through the lenses of the three differing paradigms.

A researcher using a positivist paradigm would see a cardiac arrest as a measurable circumstance, as the patient is either dead or alive, and there are no other eventualities or outcomes in this situation. They may argue that this is undisputable, as the absence of breathing and a pulse determines a cardiac arrest. The research project may look to analyse other objective parameters such as length of basic life support (BLS) administration, length of advanced life support (ALS) administration, and number of times a return of spontaneous circulation (ROSC) was achieved.

A researcher using a paradigm based on constructivism or interpretivism may see a cardiac arrest as an opportunity to interpret the family's or bystanders' lived experience. They may argue that every individual would have a different perspective and therefore there is not 'one truth' that can be found to represent all these people's opinions. The research project may look to analyse other subjective parameters such as perceptions of healthcare staff during the event, interpreting bad news, and understanding grief.

A researcher using a pragmatic paradigm may see a cardiac arrest as an opportunity to understand the paramedic's actions in cardiac arrest and their experience of this. They might argue that they would need to collect all data to allow the researcher to holistically interpret the event. Neither type of data on its own would give a comprehensive review of the topic. The research project may look at facts and figures such as compliance of compression depth and rate but may also look to understand the paramedic's thoughts around the human factors preventing these from occurring correctly. This project would be concerned not just with the 'what' happens in a cardiac arrest scenario but also the 'why'.

The research process

Most published research studies have similar formats or layouts, this is because each project follows a similar process and structure of six simple stages when in development:

1. Questions, background, and rationale.
2. Aims and objectives.
3. Study design and research methods.
4. Ethics.
5. Data collection methods and data analysis.
6. Summary, discussion, and limitations.

Question, background, and rationale

Most research projects start with a question. It is good practice to develop a question that is specific and that can realistically be answered with the methods and resources available. The easiest way to develop a question is to read other research: this will help to identify whether the idea is based on clear scientific rationale and whether it will provide new information. There will also be consideration for which paradigm aligns with the research question asked.

Aims and objectives

This is what the researcher is hoping to achieve through carrying out the research. There may be more than one aim described and the researcher may also identify the primary and secondary aims for the project. The researcher will use their aims to measure their question. For some kinds of research (often in quantitative experimental research) the question is written as a hypothesis, or prediction, that will be tested out by the research.

Study design and research methods

This is a categorisation and summary of the specific methods or techniques to be employed in the project. Common phrases will be used to depict exactly how the information will be measured, this may incorporate the type of data that will be collected (primary or secondary), the relation in time (retrospective or prospective), and the output (how the intervention or concept will be measured) (Ranganathan and Aggarwal 2018; Swinscow and Campbell 2021). (See Box 15.2 for common terms used).

Ethics

Ethics is an essential consideration in the research process: the same ethical principles of beneficence, confidentiality, capacity of the participants, informed consent, and non-malfeasance govern research as well as clinical practice (Siriwardena and Whitley 2022). Under an international voluntary code called the Declaration of Helsinki, researchers must weigh the benefits of research against likely harms to participants (Townsend and Luck 2012). Before the project can begin, the researcher must apply for ethical

BOX 15.2 Common terms used to describe the study design

Retrospective study:	A project looking back at something that has already occurred, for example, by asking patients to remember a disease outbreak or by looking at routinely collected operating information.
Prospective study:	A project that plans to observe something in the future, such as participants' response to being given a substance in a drug trial.
Primary data collection:	Information which is collected directly from research participants by the researcher as part of the project.
Secondary data collection:	Information gathering that relies on other research projects as a resource, this will take information from pre-existing published primary research.
Cross-sectional study:	A study collecting data at one point in time (or over a short period), providing a snapshot of the moment.
Longitudinal study:	A study collecting data over a longer period of time with repeated data collection/measurements.
Experimental study:	An experiment by nature where there is the introduction of an intervention actively performed on participants. This will also involve random allocation of the intervention and a comparison to a control group. Examples may be cluster, parallel group or cross over designs.
Quasi-experimental:	An experiment by nature where there is the introduction of an intervention, and a control group, but randomisation will be missing. Examples may be before-and-after studies, time-series, and propensity-matched scoring analyses.
Observational/ non Experimental study:	The formation of data without any manipulation or intervention. Looks to observe or examine relationships.
Descriptive study:	Only look to report the data on one or more characteristics of a group of individuals. These cannot establish relationships between variables or definitively answer questions.
Analytical study:	Establishing causal relationships between variables by testing a hypothesis. The researcher will study the effect of an exposure or intervention, on an outcome.
Forward direction:	The researcher starts with identifying the exposure to a risk factor and then evaluates whether in the future the outcome occurs.
Backward direction:	The researcher starts by recognising whether an outcome is present in the participants and then looks back for the presence of prior exposure to a risk factor.

approval. This is usually done by gaining authorisation from a research ethics committee (REC), where the researcher must justify and manage the risk involved, as well as considering the patient and public involvement in the project (Health Research Authority 2022).

Data collection methods and data analysis

There will be subsequent information provided on the methods that will be utilised in the project. The data collection section will include a detailed description, which enables the reader to fully understand, or visualise, the process used to generate the new data. This may include information on the data collection procedure or tool, the study setting, recruitment of participants, the randomisation process, the sampling process, how the patients were followed up etc. The design and implementation of these sections can affect the overall quality of the research paper. Similarly, the handling and analysis of the data produced is key to obtaining valid results; therefore there may be an explanation for how the data will be analysed and what technology may be utilised to undertake this – for example, ENIVO or SIGMA (Greenhalgh 2014; Jolley 2020).

Summary, discussion, and limitations

In any research paper there must be a clear statement of findings or conclusion, where the researcher should attempt to answer the research question or aims of the study. There has to then be an adequate discussion of the evidence both for and against the researcher's arguments. This can be compared and contrasted to other existing data in order to relate back to the wider context of prehospital or paramedic practice. The researcher should then be critical regarding their own faults or restraints of the project, this may be with regard to any aspect of their research, starting from the question and philosophical underpinnings and finishing at the data analysis (Aveyard 2023). The overall findings from this project should then be published, viewed by other members of the research community, and considered to help towards implementing new future change (Siriwardena and Whitley 2022).

Study designs

This chapter predominately focuses on research designs that follow a quantitative methodology. This seems sensible for the novice paramedic researcher for two reasons. The first is that quantitative-based studies largely generate and apply the majority of the knowledge in evidence-based healthcare (EBHC), so are likely to be available more commonly. Secondly, within this chapter, some ideological assumptions have been simplified. Qualitative research designs require accurate and thorough explanations of the theoretical processes behind them, which would go beyond the breadth of this text. To learn more about this, the recommendation would be to select a text that focuses solely on those nuances.

The study design, data collection, and data analysis methods all have the potential to influence the reliability, validity, trustworthiness, and rigour of the results. Therefore, it is important to understand more about the different types of study designs and how this will influence the evolution of the research project (Cypress 2017).

Case reports

A case report or case study is a concise report of a single patient's or small group of patients' problems, symptoms, or thoughts – it can investigate many different aspects of the patient journey – similar to that of a documentary. As case reports often focus on unusual or new diseases or injuries, they can mirror social changes or foretell epidemiological developments (Patterson et al. 2010). As these only focus on a small number of patients, they generally should not be used to determine the 'cause and effect' or 'prove' something (Pope and Mays 2020) but, rather, should be utilised to generate ideas for the basis of subsequent research projects

(see Table 15.1 for more information).

Cross-sectional studies

A cross-sectional study will normally use a survey as the data collection technique at one point in time but may refer retrospectively to health experiences in the past. These studies aim to predict or find a correlation between identified variables and can also review the relationships between them, but this will only specifically focus on a single time point. Often they may be used to investigate how prevalent or common a disease is within a group or community. Participants will be selected only based on the inclusion and exclusion criteria set for the study, not due to a risk factor or exposure to a disease. A cross-sectional study takes a representative sample of participants and studies them in order to gain answers to a specific clinical question (Greenhalgh 2014) (see Table 15.1 for more information).

Case control studies

A case control study is a development of a case report. This a type of backward-direction study is where the researcher begins by taking cases of ill or injured patients to study a particular condition of interest and compares them to 'healthy' individuals, called controls. The purpose is usually to identify a possible cause (exposure) of the illness, injury, or disease (Siriwardena and Whitley 2022). If there is a systematic difference between patient and healthy person, this difference might have either been caused by or contributed to the illness. Even if the difference is not as clear as if it is affecting all patients or all controls, statistical trends can be sufficient indicators to warrant further investigation. This is the same principle by which the role of smoking in lung cancer was detected: it could be shown that patients with lung cancer were proportionally more likely to be smokers than other members of the population (Ranganathan and Aggarwal 2018) (see Table 15.1 for more information).

Cohort and panel studies

In a cohort study, the participants involved will all be people who share similar characteristics, except for the particular exposure being investigated such as the treatment, therapy, medicine, vaccine, or surgical procedure (see Box 15.3). The participants will be grouped by their relation to the exposure

BOX 15.3 Example cohort study – comparing contraception

Ninety 18-year-old female participants are recruited from a large rural town in the UK. Thirty of these individuals are currently already taking the combined oral contraceptive pill (progesterone and estrogen), 30 currently take the progesterone only oral contraceptive pill, and 30 take no form of contraception. They are interviewed every 2 years, over a 20-year period in total and are questioned regarding the development of breast cancer, ovarian cancer, and pulmonary embolism during this time frame. This helps to understand the relative 'risk' of taking this medication (see Table 15.1 for more information).

and these groups will be compared and followed up to see how many in each group develop a particular disease, complication, or other outcome. This allows an examination of the effects of time and of long-term factors contributing to ill-health – it has a forward direction to the study design. The most typical arrangement is that cohort studies follow a group or cohort of people born within a year in one area. By contrast, a longitudinal panel study will follow a smaller sample of the group. Methods used in these type of longitudinal studies may vary, and often include questionnaires and physical measurements of health. However, by the same token, longitudinal studies take a long time to complete, experience a high dropout rate due to the need for follow-up over time, and are accordingly extremely expensive.

Randomised controlled trials

Randomised controlled trials (RCTs) are used to estimate the impact and effects of an intervention and consequently will provide insight into the effectiveness of treatments.

RCTs compare outcomes for patients receiving a new treatment with outcomes for those receiving either an ineffective 'dummy' treatment, called a placebo, or standard care. If administering a placebo is considered unethical due to the seriousness of patients' conditions, RCTs will administer standard care to the control group instead of a placebo.

One of the hallmarks of RCTs is the allocation to treatment groups by chance, which is called randomisation. Each participant should have the same chance of being allocated to a treatment group. Randomisation is the best safeguard against systematic differences between the treatment and the control group.

Health improvement in response to a medically ineffectual 'dummy' treatment is called the placebo effect (Kaptchuk 1998). As the group receiving the new treatment may have or experience this effect, it is compared against a control group that must also receive a placebo. The patient is kept unaware whether they were assigned to the control or the intervention group, this process is called blinding. Similarly, there is a risk that the assessor – typically the research paramedic –will be biased by their expectations. Hence, some studies are designed so that the researcher is also unaware which group the patient belongs to, this is called double blinding.

RCTs have an intervention, control, and randomisation and therefore have a purely experimental study design. It should be noted that a controlled clinical trial study design is not the same as an RCT. A controlled clinical trial is a type of quasi-experimental comparative study where the participants will be allocated in a non-random manner to either the intervention or control groups (Greenhalgh 2014).

The analysis of RCTs will always be statistical in nature and will use an experienced statistician who calculates an appropriate sample size and interprets whether there is statistical significance of the results (see Table 15.1 for more information).

Critical literature reviews, scoping reviews, systematic reviews, and meta-analyses

These are all forms of secondary research, which compare and synthesise existing research. When beginning any type of research project, the study will be informed by an initial review of the literature, or 'literature review' – which acts as a critical survey of all the authoritative material currently published on a topic, and an evaluation of how far this literature provides a full and robust account of that topic, or leaves gaps for further investigation and collection of new data (Griffiths and Mooney 2011; Aveyard 2023). This is important, as the more comprehensive a literature review is, the less likely it is that a research project will unnecessarily repeat existing work. A scoping review is extremely similar and aims to create a synopsis of the existing evidence; it often will also act as a precursor to a systematic review, as it draws information from a very broad range of studies from a general topic area but will not focus on the quality of those studies specifically. It provides a generic overview or narration of an area of research and therefore will inadvertently identify a gap in the knowledge base (Munn et al. 2022). A systematic review will follow a more structured method than a scoping review and its focus will be on answering a specific question. The conclusion will be drawn by critically appraising the studies and therefore assessing their quality in answering the question (Munn et al. 2018). A meta-analysis has a very similar method but adds on an additional step to the systematic review process, by analysing and combining the individual

TABLE 15.1 Common research study designs and their classifying characteristics.

Study design	Methodology	Relation to time	Data collection	Purpose	Direction	Intervention based
Scoping reviews	Qualitative or quantitative or both	Retrospective	Secondary	Descriptive (Analyses a gap in knowledge/ evidence base)	N/A	No
Literature reviews, systematic reviews, and meta-analysis	Qualitative or quantitative or both	Retrospective	Secondary	Analytical	N/A	No
Case reports	Qualitative or quantitative	Retrospective	Primary	Descriptive	Backward direction	No – observational
Case control studies	Quantitative	Retrospective	Primary	Analytical	Backward direction	No – observational
RCTs	Quantitative	Prospective	Primary	Analytical	Forward directional	Yes – Experimental
Cohort or panel studies	Usually quantitative	Usually prospective (but can be retrospective)	Usually primary	Analytical	Forward directional, and Longitudinal	No – observational
Cross-sectional study	Usually quantitative	Retrospective	Primary	Analytical or descriptive (correlational)	Single point in time	No – observational

results from multiple similar studies. With quantitative data this is a relatively straightforward process, as the appropriate statistical methods can be applied to measure what the overall effect of the individual studies are. A qualitative study of the same kind may be called a 'meta-synthesis' and will use different methods of analysis (Aromataris and Pearson 2014) (see Table 15.1 for more information).

Data collection tools

Questionnaire-based studies

To ensure the quality and reporting is substantial, there are various considerations if creating a questionnaire- or survey-based tool for a research project (O'Connor 2022).

A census is a questionnaire study sent to every individual in a population, whilst a survey is targeted at a sample of the population. As it is rarely possible to contact all members of a population, a sample has to be selected instead. For a quantitative study, this would involve a sample size calculation by a statistician. It is best if the sample is as representative of the overall population as possible, so that wider conclusions can be drawn from the study (Ponto 2015). This is normally most likely to be the case when the sample is selected randomly – this is when every person in the population has an equal likelihood of being selected for inclusion.

A questionnaire may have open-ended (qualitative) questions that allow the participants to write in any answer they wish, this can be contrasted with closed-ended questions that only allow a limited number of answers such as yes/no or multiple-choice selection. However, if large amounts of very descriptive or in-depth information is required then conducting interviews may be considered more appropriate (Boynton and Greenhalgh 2004; Patten 2014). A popular matrix format is called a Likert scale, where the participant will rank a number of statements on a five-point scale (usually these are 'strongly agree', 'agree', 'undecided/don't know', 'disagree', 'strongly disagree'), although this can have up to seven choices in total. Closed-ended questions or rating to a numerical value allow for quantitative data to be collected, whilst open-ended questions normally do not.

It is important for the researcher to arrange questions in a logical order, as a previous question can shape how they think about questions to come. Not only will grouping questions make matters easier for participants but it can also prevent 'leading' them to one or the other statement. The phrasing of questions must also be considered and should not lead the participant, i.e. favour a particular answer. If the question is closed, the researcher must make sure that all possible answers are available. The researcher will also need to avoid double-barrelled questions, ambiguous terms, or negative phrasing (O'Connor 2022).

The delivery or application of the surveys is also important, they can be delivered by post, telephone, the internet, or in person. Telephone or face-to-face surveys tend to be very time-consuming for the researcher but have good response rates. Postal surveys can be sent to large groups of people but suffer from a very low response rate (typically below half). The internet is able to reach a large number of people but response rates to online surveys are also not particularly high. Where the survey is advertised on a website or via mass emails, there will be some selection bias: only people with a relatively strong interest in the topic will respond, whilst a silent majority with different views will desist (Haddad et al. 2022).

The site or setting in which the application of a questionnaire will take place must also be considered. For example, in an ambulance, a patient realistically may not be able to consent, concentrate, or physically complete a survey. However, if a participant took the survey to hospital and home, with the intention to post it back, this would likely yield a low response rate.

Interview-based studies

In-depth individual interviews aim to generate personal narratives, opinions, and beliefs from individuals, through one-to-one questioning (Guest et al. 2020). The most commonly used interview technique within healthcare research is the semi-structured interview. This involves the preparation of a list of topics and some specific questions to take to the interview but also some open conversation with the participant. It allows for more exploration through its flexibility (Kallio et al. 2016). A structured interview may also be used, however, this only involves pre-prepared questions, whilst an unstructured interview is an open invitation to the participant to talk freely about a topic and any aspect of it that they wish to address.

It is the interviewer's job to keep the conversation focused on the topics of interest, sometimes asking the pre-prepared questions. As long as the participant is speaking on topic, it is best not to interrupt unnecessarily. If statements are unclear, a follow-up question can be asked, even if it is not on the original list.

The most common selection strategy for participants to interview is a purposive approach, where participants are invited who are most likely to have valuable insights into a topic. Random selection is unusual because of the small numbers recruited to most interview studies (Sadler et al. 2010; Pope and Mays 2020). It is most effective to send potential participants an explanatory invitation letter before telephoning them about possible participation. Ideally, a study will keep recruiting participants until no significantly new themes emerge in new interviews – a state of affairs that is called data saturation.

It is common practice to audio record an interview, for which written consent must be obtained from the participant before commencing the interview. These will often be transcribed and coded, then a complete thematic analysis of the content will be undertaken.

Focus-group-based studies

Focus groups involve inviting several participants to engage in the data collection at the same time and asking them to discuss a topic. By doing this the participants can agree on their perceptions through discussion, which will highlight the issues on which they openly disagree and can help to stimulate a larger range of ideas overall (Guest et al. 2020). Although it can result in a loss of detail – and has been suggested to discourage those participants who do not enjoy speaking from engaging – or may deter participants from speaking about views or practices that embarrass them (Tausch and Menold 2016).

The overall procedure is similar to interview: a researcher will be present and act as a facilitator utilising open-ended questions and a moderator to the discussion, directing the conversation where necessary (Krueger and Casey 2015). The most straightforward recruitment approach is purposive. It is best to semi-structure the discussion with pre-prepared topics and some questions; this should be audio- or video-recorded and the information then transcribed and analysed from the information on the recording.

Observational and participatory studies

An observational study involves watching participants in action, whilst a participatory design involves taking part in the human activity under study. An observational study of community first responders might involve following such a person for several hours a day like a 'fly on the wall' and noting observations (Fitzpatrick and Boulton 1994). A participatory study of the same would involve volunteering/working as a community first responder for a while, and then writing about this. The longer that is spent with a research participant, the less likely they will be to change behaviour due to the researcher's presence, especially when observing actions that form part of daily routines (O'Reilly 2012). There is also the possibility of observing behaviour in simulated settings. This may be advantageous when there are ethical issues with exposing the participants to certain risks or real life scenarios are rare and occur infrequently. This allows the researcher to create a tailored reproduction of specific conditions and circumstances of clinical practice, which may help enable the participants to practice in a safer or more controlled environment (Lamé and Dixon-Woods 2020).

Review of routinely collected data and chart review

This data collection method involves extracting data from records rather than from individual participants directly. Routinely collected health data will be data that already exists and was originally collected and collated for purposes other than research. This may be data from electronic or paper-based health records, administrative information, and disease databases or registries (Nicholls et al. 2017). This should not be confused with secondary research. The existing data will not have been extracted or analysed and therefore no conclusions can be drawn from this. The researcher will create a project and perform a chart review to first abstract only the relevant data for the topic and then analyse this appropriately, the study design of these projects will often be a retrospective cohort study (Siriwardena and Whitley 2022).

Conclusion

This chapter should provide a foundation of understanding for some of the more complex terminologies and theories that may be found when exploring evidence-based paramedic practice. It has introduced some of the most common structures and methods utilised in healthcare research. A paramedic's research activity will be a journey of personal development – it is advisable to start by attempting to read, interpret, and appraise studies on topics you enjoy. This chapter can help unlock the door to exploring an innovative world of research and practice development.

Activities

Now review your learning by completing the learning activities in this chapter. The answers to these appear at the end of the book. Further self-test activities can be found at **www.wileyfundamentalseries.com/paramedic/3e.**

Test your knowledge

1. What is a paradigm?
2. What are the three different methodologies?
3. Is an RCT the same as a control trial?

Activity 15.1

Try listing the main differences between positivism and post-positivism.

Activity 15.2

In order to practise identifying different research study designs, explore your university's databases and search for a subject of interest to you within the prehospital environment. See if you can find an RCT, case study, and cohort study. Compare the format and content of the articles.

Glossary

Case control study:	A development on a case report. It takes cases of ill or injured patients and compares them to 'healthy' individuals, called controls.
Case report:	A thorough but concise report of a single patient's or small group of patients' problems.
Literature review:	A systematic method for analysing a phenomenon using published research.
Randomised controlled trial (RCT):	An experiment that compares outcomes for patients receiving a new treatment with outcomes for those receiving either an ineffective treatment, called a placebo, or standard care. Participants in the trial are assigned to treatments by chance, i.e. randomly, and then outcomes are compared.
Qualitative research:	Finding out about a phenomenon through word or observation data.
Quantitative research:	Research that produces numerical data for the purpose of measurement.
Research ethics committee (REC):	A committee of research experts who approve or deny research applications.

References

Allemang, B., Sitter, K., and Dimitropoulos, G. (2022). Pragmatism as a paradigm for patient-oriented research. *Health Expectations* **25** (1): 38–47.

Aromataris, E. and Pearson, A. (2014). The systematic review: an overview. *American Journal of Nursing* **114** (3): 47–55.

Aveyard, H. (2023). *Doing a Literature Review in Health and Social Care: A Practical Guide.* 5e. Open University Press.

Boynton, P.M. and Greenhalgh, T. (2004). Selecting, designing, and developing your questionnaire. *British Medical Journal* **328** (328): 1312–1315.

Brown, M.E. and Dueñas, A.N. (2020). A medical science educator's guide to selecting a research paradigm: building a basis for better research. *Med Sci Educ* **30** (2): 545–553.

Cypress, B. (2017) Rigor or reliability and validity in qualitative research: perspectives, strategies, reconceptualization, and recommendations. *Dimensions of Critical Care Nursing* **36** (4): 253–263.

Fitzpatrick, R. and Boulton, M. (1994). Qualitative methods for assessing health care. *Quality in Health Care* **3** (2): 107–113.

Greenhalgh, T. (2014). *How to Read a Paper: The Basics of Evidence-Based Medicine*. John Wiley & Sons, Inc.

Griffiths, P. and Mooney, G.P. (eds.) (2011). *The Paramedic's Guide to Research*. London: McGraw-Hill.

Guest, G., Namey, E., O'Regan, A. et al. (2020). *Comparing Interview and Focus Group Data Collected in Person and Online*. Washington (DC): Patient-Centered Outcomes Research Institute (PCORI).

Haddad, C., Sacre, H., Zeenny, R.M. et al. (2022). Should samples be weighted to decrease selection bias in online surveys during the COVID-19 pandemic? Data from seven datasets. *BMC Med Res Methodol* **22** (1): 63–65.

Hammersley, M. (1996). The relationship between qualitative and quantitative research: paradigm loyalty versus methodological eclecticism. In: *Handbook of Qualitative Research Methods for Psychology and the Social Sciences* (ed. J. Richardson), pp. 159–174. Leicester: British Psychological Society.

Health Research Authority. (2022). Research Ethics Committee – Standard Operating Procedures**.** Available at: https://www.hra.nhs.uk/about-us/committees-and-services/res-and-recs/research-ethics-committee-standard-operating-procedures (accessed 27 October 2023).

Ho, D. (2019). *A Philosopher Goes to the Doctor. A Critical Look at Philosophical Assumptions in Medicine*. New York: Routledge.

Holloway, I. and Galvin, K. (2016). *Qualitative Research in Nursing and Healthcare*. John Wiley & Sons, Inc.

Jolley, J. (2020). *Introducing Research and Evidence-Based Practice for Nursing and Healthcare Professionals.* 3e. Taylor & Francis Group.

Kallio, H., Pietilä, A.M., Johnson, M. (2016). Systematic methodological review: developing a framework for a qualitative semi-structured interview guide. *J Adv Nurs* **72** (12): 2954–2965.

Kaptchuk, T.J. (1998). Intentional ignorance: a history of blind assessment and placebo controls in medicine. *Bulletin of the History of Medicine* **72** (3): 389–433.

Krueger, R.A. and Casey, M.A. (eds.) (2015). *Focus Groups: A Practical Guide for Applied Research.* 5e. Thousand Oaks: Sage.

Lamé, G, and Dixon-Woods, M. (2020). Using clinical simulation to study how to improve quality and safety in healthcare. *BMJ Simulation & Technology Enhanced Learning* **6** (2): 87–94.

Levers, M.-J. D. (2013). Philosophical paradigms, grounded theory, and perspectives on emergence. SAGE Open **3** (4). doi: 10.1177/2158244013517243.

Li, S., Jinwei, B., Jiao, W. et al. (2021). The fourth scientific discovery paradigm for precision medicine and healthcare: challenges ahead. *Precision Clinical Medicine* **4** (2): 80–84.

Mesel, T. (2013). The necessary distinction between methodology and philosophical assumptions in healthcare research. *Scandinavian Journal of Caring Sciences* **27** (3): 750–756.

Munn, Z., Peters, M.D.J., Stern, C. et al. (2018). Systematic review or scoping review? Guidance for authors when choosing between a systematic or scoping review approach. *BMC Med Res Methodol* **18** (1): 143–144.

Munn, Z., Pollock, D., Khalil, H. et al. (2022). What are scoping reviews? Providing a formal definition of scoping reviews as a type of evidence synthesis. *JBI Evidence Synthesis* **20** (4): 950–952.

Nicholls, S.G., Langan, S.M., and Benchimol, E.I. (2017). Routinely collected data: the importance of high-quality diagnostic coding to research. *Canadian Medical Association Journal [journal de l'Association medicale Canadienne]* **189** (33): 1054–1055.

O'Connor, S. (2022). Designing and using surveys in nursing research: a contemporary discussion. *Clinical Nursing Research* **31** (4): 567–570.

O'Reilly, K. (2012). *Ethnographic Methods.* 2e. Oxford: Routledge.

Patten, M.L. (2014). *Questionnaire Research: A Practical Guide.* 4e. Taylor & Francis Group.

Patterson, D., Weaver, M., Clark, S. et al. (2010). Case reports and case series in prehospital emergency care research. *Emergency Medicine Journal* **27** (11): 807–809.

Ponto, J. (2015). Understanding and evaluating survey research. *Journal of the Advanced Practitioner in Oncology* **6** (2): 168–171.

Pope, C. and Mays, N. (2020). *Qualitative Research in Health Care.* 4e. John Wiley & Sons, Inc.

Ranganathan, P. and Aggarwal, R. (2018). Study designs: part 1 – an overview and classification. *Perspectives in Clinical Research* **9** (4): 184–186.

Rapport, F. and Braithwaite, J. (2018). Are we on the cusp of a fourth research paradigm? Predicting the future for a new approach to methods-use in medical and health services research. *BMC Medical Research Methodology* **18** (1): 143–144.

Ray, S. (2016). *Oxford Handbook of Clinical and Healthcare Research. 1e*. Oxford Medical Handbooks.

Ryan, G. (2019). Postpositivist, critical realism: philosophy, methodology and method for nursing research. *Nurse Researcher* **27** (3): 20–26.

Sadler, G.R., Lee, H.-C., Lim, R.S.-H. et al. (2010). Recruitment of hard-to-reach population subgroups via adaptations of the snowball sampling strategy. *Nursing and Health Sciences* **12** (3): 369–374.

Salzmann-Erikson, M. and Eriksson, H. (2021). Netnography in the healthcare and nursing sector. In: *Netnography Unlimited: Understanding Technoculture Using Qualitative Social Media Research* (ed. R.V. Kozinets and R. Gambetti), pp. 71–82. London: Routledge.

Schlicher, J., Metsker, M.T., Shah, H. et al. (2021). From NASA to healthcare: real-time data analytics (mission control) is reshaping healthcare services. *Perspectives in Health Information Management* **18** (4): 1g.

Siriwardena, A.N. and Whitley, G.A. (2022). *Prehospital Research Methods and Practice*. Class Professional Publishing.

Swinscow, T. and Campbell, M. (2021). *Statistics at Square One. 12e*. London: BMJ.

Tausch, A.P. and Menold, N. (2016). Methodological aspects of focus groups in health research: results of qualitative interviews with focus group moderators. *Global Qualitative Nursing Research* **3** (1) 1–12.

Townsend, R. and Luck, M. (2012). *Applied Paramedic Law and Ethics: Australia and New Zealand*. London: Elsevier.

Turyahikayo, E. (2014). Resolving the qualitative-quantitative debate in healthcare research. *Medical Practice and Reviews* **5** (1): 6–15.

Wilson, A., Howitt, S., Holloway, A. et al. (2021). Factors affecting paramedicine students' learning about evidence-based practice: a phenomenographic study. *BMC Med Educ* **21** (1): 45–52.

Wilson, C., Janes, G., and Williams, J. (2022). Identity, positionality and reflexivity: relevance and application to research paramedics. *British Paramedic Journal* **7** (2): 43–49.

Wisdom, J.P., Cavaleri, M.A., Onwuegbuzie, A.J. et al. (2012). Methodological reporting in qualitative, quantitative, and mixed methods health services research articles. *Health Services Research* **47** (2): 721–745.

CHAPTER **16**

Medical terminology

Samantha Sweet

Paramedic, London Ambulance Service, London, UK

Contents

LEARNING OUTCOMES

On completion of this chapter the reader will be able to:

- Recognise the importance of medical terminology in relation to paramedic practice.
- Identify how to break down medical terms to understand them.
- Analyse, recognise, and define medical terms and medical acronyms.
- Pronounce key medical terms.
- Interpret and apply both written and verbal medical terminology.

Case study

You are called to an elderly lady that has had a fall, and she is unsure what has happened. You notice the patient has a cast on her arm and bruising to the right temple. The patient had a fall a week earlier, and her notes are summarised below.

Notes: pt found lying supine on floor post TLOC, deformity to right distal radius/ulna. Pt assisted to sit, however, noted hypotension upon sitting. ECG showing bradycardia. PMHx anaemia and Alzheimer's. Tx – intravenous access, pain relief and transport to hospital.

What does this mean? How did the patient fall? Did the patient get injured on this fall?

Fundamentals of Paramedic Practice: A Systems Approach, Third Edition. Edited by Sam Willis and Ian Peate.

Companion website: www.wiley.com/go/willis/paramedic3e

Introduction

Healthcare professionals including paramedics, are required to document all cases they attend using patient report forms (PRFs), or an alternative electronic version (different countries will have similar reporting systems). PRFs assist to provide the understanding of the assessments and treatments that a person has undergone in any stage of their care journey, and they are a legal documentation into that person's care. As such, PRFs should be complete; both detailing the assessment and treatment that the patient received and any pertinent negatives that have led you to rule out other conditions. Often we use the phrase 'if it is not written down, it did not happen'.

A PRF not only acts as a report for the ambulance service (which can then be used to change practice and influence service provision), and for use by other health professionals in the patient's treatment, but it can also be called on to prove or disprove action that was taken. Therefore, it is vital that the PRF is accurate and consistent, and that there are no 'grey areas' in your report writing.

Medical terminology helps achieve this level of consistency and accuracy and leaves no room for confusion by anybody else who may be reading your report, facilitating communication in the medical field (Walker et al. 2013). Medical terminology is the standardised means of communication in the healthcare industry, allowing understanding across multiple disciplines. Medical terminology is also recognised legally, so in the event that you must recall your information subsequently, there will be no room for misinterpretation of your document.

If you ask a person from a non-medical background if terminology healthcare professionals use is difficult to comprehend, often the answer is yes. Most non-medical people will question why medical terminology is used in the industry when simple English would suffice (Koch-Weser et al. 2009). The rationale for employing medical language is important, as it provides a precise method for the following:

- Accurately locating anatomical landmarks
- Describing medical conditions
- Describing prescribed treatments and interventions

Although there is not a governing body to regulate the professional use of medical terminology, being able to use medical terminology accurately is advocated. Historically, medical terminology was principally used by doctors, specialists, and academics. However, it is now equally vital for paramedics, nurses, and most allied health professions to be proficient in medical language for consistent patient care across all healthcare professionals. Equally, the evolution of primary and secondary healthcare has caused many medical/health support staff such as medical assistants and administration staff to become proficient in medical terminology. Using consistent terminology streamlines reporting, billing, and patient care pathways. With these advances, it is now commonplace for all health professionals to understand medical language and allows for this to be understood worldwide. It is important, however, to remember that patient's and relatives will not be averse to medical terminology, and so language should be appropriately adapted.

This chapter introduces medical terminology, and provides a discussion of medical acronyms, medical abbreviations, and a brief 'Hx' of the development of medical terminology (our first abbreviation = Hx, meaning history), showing the respective influences of Greek, Latin, Arabic, and finally English vocabulary.

A brief history (Hx) of medical terminology

Greek influence

The origins of modern Western medicine are often traced to Hippocrates (460–377 BCE), a Greek physician widely accepted as the founder of medicine in the fourth century BCE. Named the 'father of Western medicine', Hippocrates is attributed as the founder of many influences in medicine. The *Hippocratic Corpus,* a series of sixty texts with many foundational features in medicine, are associated with Hippocrates (Craik 2015). These writings were written in Greek, which is where the beginning of the Greek influence arises. Hippocrates was followed by another two doctors, Galen and Aristotle, both of whom continued the influence that Greek has in the modern medical world. Words arising from Greek include diarrhoea (through flow) and dyspnoea (difficulty breathing), however, you will find more examples through the chapter.

Latin influence

Modern medical terminology owes an equal debt to Latin vocabulary and to the first-century text *De Medicina,* attributed to Roman aristocrat Aulus Cornelius Celsus (Wulff 2004). *De Medicina,* the first surviving attempt at a medical encyclopaedia, shows the extensive influence of Hippocrates and Greek terminology. Celsus translated many Greek terms into Latin but had to import Greek medical terms directly where no Latin equivalent was available (Stephenson 2022). Celsus also adopted the Greek process of likening and describing the shape of anatomical structures to objects of comparable shape, for example, musical instruments (e.g. tuba = trumpet, tibia = flute) or plants (glans = acorn).

Arabic influence

Between 750 and 900 CE, many of the classical Greek medical texts were translated into Arabic throughout the modern-day Middle East (Stephenson 2022). Arabic scholars contributed to the prevailing medical literature and although their influence was relatively small, some Arabic terms found their way into Western medicine (e.g. nucha).

These three influences on medical terminology were cemented in the Renaissance of the sixteenth century when a renewed emphasis on Latin learning and culture saw the retranslation into Latin of the foundational medical texts and the establishment of 'medical Latin' as a body of vocabulary that is still used to this day.

Contemporary English dominance

The final phase in the brief history of the development of medical terminology is the dominance of English terms in the medical lexicon, a dominance that can be directly attributed to the post-war settlement following the Second World War. Although during the twentieth century medical science still used three languages equally (German, English, and French), in the post-war years English established itself as the preferred language at international conferences; just as medical Latin had formed a common language for Renaissance scholars. So, today medical doctors have increasingly chosen English as the single language for international communication. The ongoing impact of this development can be seen in the proliferation of English clinical terms in other languages. For example, the term 'bypass' has been adopted in Italian, German, Dutch, and Romanian. Whereas the Polish and French retain their own terms of *pomostowanie* and *pontage* (Wulff 2004). The importance of English in medical terminology is also reflected in research. Most articles in journals with significant importance to the medical world are often written in English, and so this demonstrates the importance of the English language in medicine.

Medical terminology and word structure

Whilst medical terminology can sound complex, there are some general rules relating to basic word structure that can help us to understand and remember its meaning. In the English language, most words have three possible components (see Table 16.1):

- Root words
- Affixes (prefix and suffix)
- Combining vowel

Root words

Root words contain the main meaning of the sentence. They can be individual words that have their own meaning, or they can be combined with affixes to create more complicated word structures. It is this part of the word that is often linked to words obtained from other languages, often either Greek or Latin. It is important to note, however, some words have both Greek and Latin origins and are used in different settings. Take the kidneys: some terms refer to Latin origin of the word *ren* ('renal failure', meaning kidney failure) whilst others take the Greek origin of the word *nephr* (nephrology, meaning study of kidneys).

Often root words must change form slightly if adding additional components to the word. Many of the examples in

TABLE 16.1 **Description of basic word structure.**

Word root	Fundamental meaning of a medical term, for example, to describe a body part or condition.
Affix	Attached to the beginning (prefix) or end (suffix) of the medical term to modify its meaning.
Combining vowel	Used to allow ease of pronunciation where suffixation has taken place; usually an 'o'.

Table 16.2 end with '/o'. This suggests that in some forms the word adds an 'o' and in others it does not. Whilst many words follow the same rules, there are some exceptions to this. These exceptions are often picked up whilst using the terminology or seen in medical dictionaries. One key change to note is words ending in 'x'. When adding suffixes to these words (see next section for affixes), the 'x' changes to either a 'g' or a 'c' depending on what the preceding letter is; specifically it changes to a 'g' if the preceding letter is a consonant or a 'c' if the preceding letter is a vowel.

Some words are made up of two route words, with no additional prefix or suffix. An example of this would be *cardiovascular*. This term, made up of two route words, relates to both the heart ('cardi' meaning heart) and vessels ('vascul' meaning blood vessels). As such, *cardiovascular* relates to both the heart and blood vessels, describing the network of blood vessels that blood pumps through, supplied by the heart.

TABLE 16.2 **Root words and meanings.**

Medical root words	Meaning
Angi/o	Blood vessel
Cardi	Heart
Cepahl/o	Head
Cerebr/o	Brain
Chrom/o	Colour
Enter/o	Intestine
Derm/o	Skin
Gastr/o	Stomach
Haem/o	Blood
Lapar	Abdomen
Laryng	Lower throat
Myo	Muscle
Neur/o	Nerve
Onych/o	Nail
Oro	Mouth
Osteo	Bone
Phag/o	Eat/swallow
Pharyng	Upper throat
Phleb/o	Vein
Pulmon/o	Lungs
Uria	Urine
Vascul	Blood vessel

Affixes

Affixes only have meaning when they are attached to a root word. A prefix is attached to the start of a root word, a suffix to the end. In medical terminology, a further difference can be observed: here, a prefix at the start of a word often specifies the location, time, or number, whereas a suffix at the end of the word reflects the condition, disorder, disease, or procedure (Walker et al. 2013). Some examples of prefixes and suffixes are listed in Tables 16.3, 16.4, and 16.5.

Familiar examples of terms using a prefix include 'hypertension' (meaning 'high blood pressure'), where the prefix 'hyper-' (meaning 'above' or 'more than normal') is added to the root word 'tension', which in medical terminology means blood pressure. Likewise, the word 'bradycardia' means 'slow heart', a meaning generated by addition of the prefix 'Brady-', meaning 'slow'.

Familiar medical terms using suffixes include 'dermatitis' (an inflammation of the skin), where '-itis' is added to the root word term 'dermo', meaning skin. Note that in this case the combining vowel is an 'a' not an 'o.' The suffix '-itis' is common and appears in a wide range of medical terms describing inflammation, including gastritis (inflammation of the stomach) and laryngitis (inflammation of the larynx).

Root words can also have both a prefix and a suffix, creating what may appear to be a complex word but often has a simple meaning. For example, 'pericarditis' means 'inflammation of the area surrounding the heart'. This is made up of a prefix ('peri' meaning surrounding), a root word ('cardi' meaning heart), and a suffix ('itis' meaning inflammation).

Prefixes and suffixes can be combined to form a medical term, without the need for a root word. Anaemia is a term used in medicine to describe reduced red blood cells. This term is created by the combination of the prefix 'an-', meaning no without, and the suffix '-aemia', meaning

TABLE 16.3 Common prefixes.

Prefix	Meaning
an/a-	Without/lack of
ab-	Away from
ad-	Towards, near
ante-	Before
brady-	Slow
dys-	Bad/difficult
ec-, etc-	Out, outside of
end-	In, within
epi-	Upon/over/above
hyper-	Excessive/high
hypo-	Under/below/low
intra-	Within
mon-	One
peri-	Surrounding
poly-	Many, much
post-	After, behind
tachy-	Fast
trans-	Across, through
supra-	Above

condition of the blood. Tachypnoea is a medical term used to describe fast breathing. It is created by combining the prefix 'tachy-', meaning fast, with the suffix '-pnoea', used to describe breathing.

Linking back to the origins of words, many of the root words and affixes come from Latin and Greek origins. However, it is important to understand that in modern medical terminology there is often a combination of more than one origin. Let us go back to our word hypertension. The prefix 'hyper-' has links back to Greek origins meaning 'over/high', whereas 'tension' comes from Latin to mean 'stretch'.

TABLE 16.4 Common suffixes.

Suffix	Meaning
-aemia	Blood
-algia	Pain
-centesis	Puncture, tap
-desis	Binding, fusion
-ectomy	Excision, surgical removal
-graphy	Act of recording data
-itis	Inflammation
-ology	Study of
-pathy	Disease
-pexy	Surgical fixation
-phagia	Eating/swallowing
-phasia	Speech
-plegia	Paralysis
-phobia	Fear
-rrhagia	Flow
-rrhage	Burst
-scopy	Examine
-sclerosis	Hardening

TABLE 16.5 Prefixes relating to colour.

Prefix	Meaning
alb-	White
cirr-	Yellow
cyan-	Blue
erthr-	Red
glauco-	Grey
leuk-	White
melan-	Black

Combining vowel

The final word component is a combining vowel. This is usually the letter 'o', which is added to a word root. An example is the medical term laryngoscopy. The root word 'laryng', meaning the larynx, is combined with the letter 'o' to form laryngo, which is then combined with the suffix '-scopy', meaning to examine. Despite the letter 'o' being the most common combining vowel, 'a and i' are occasionally found in medical terms, with 'e and u' being less common. You can only really ascertain which vowel to use by practicing these words and finding such examples in comprehensive medical dictionaries.

Our understanding and recall of medical terminology can be enhanced by recognising that the building blocks of medical terms are typically a root word and either a prefix and/or a suffix, and that where the process of affixation has taken place, there will often be the use of an adjoining vowel. Once we are aware of these principles, we can break down and comprehend quite difficult and lengthy terms such as those in Table 16.6.

Pronunciation of medical terms

For healthcare professionals it is essential that the correct pronunciation of medical terms is used. Information that is being provided needs to be clearly understood and this helps to avoid any errors or confusion from occurring. Despite appearing daunting at first glance, medical terminology is not difficult to grasp with practice and exposure. The systematic use of component words allows for ease in pronunciation. The complexity occurs with some letters being pronounced differently in some words, where pronunciation rules are not the same for all terms. Many terms can be pronounced phonetically, though there are exceptions that are best discovered with experience. There are many different study tools that will assist with pronunciation such as apps and websites. However, the best way to get an understanding of the pronunciation is through discussions with medical professionals.

Forming plurals

Although forming plurals in medical terminology can be problematic, most plurals will follow normal English language guidelines such as changing words ending in *y* to *ies* (pregnancy/pregnancies). However, it is important to be aware of exceptions to these rules that are accepted in common medical terminology. Table 16.7 provides some examples of nonconventional plurals.

TABLE 16.6 Putting it all together.

Word	Prefix	Root word	Combining vowel	Suffix
Intravenous	Intra	-ven	No combining vowel	-ous
Osteoarthritis	Oste,	-arthr, pertaining to limbs	'o' in this instance	-Itis, inflammation

TABLE 16.7 Forming plurals.

Singular word	Singular word ending	Plural rule	Plural word
Deformity	-y	Drop the *y* and add *ies*	Deformities
Stimulus	-us	Drop the *us* and add *i*	Stimuli
Lumen	-en	Drop the *en* and add *ina*	Lumina
Enterobacterium	-um	Drop the *um* and add *a*	Enterobacteria

TABLE 16.8 Eponym examples.

Eponym	Meaning	Named after
Down syndrome	A genetic disorder affecting the twenty-first chromosome	John Langdon Down (1828–1896)
Fallopian tubes	The tubes that carry the ova to the uterus	Gabriele Falloppio (1523–1562)
Wrigley's forceps	Obstetric forceps used to provide traction when the baby's head is on the perineum	Arthur Wrigley (1904–1984)
Alzheimer's disease	A chronic neurodegenerative disease	Alois Alzheimer (1864–1915)
Pratt's sign	Pain on compression of the calf suggestive of deep vein thrombosis	Gerald H Pratt (1928–2006)
Beck's triad	Three symptoms including hypotension, muffled heart sounds, and increased jugular venous pressure suggesting cardiac tamponade	Claude Beck (1894–1971)

Eponyms

An eponym is a word derived from the name of a real person, mythical character, or fictitious person. These are often words that identify a specific medical procedure, disease, body part, or medical instrument (Duque-Parra et al. 2006). Usually, an eponym is associated with a significant person linked with the identification of the procedure, instrument, body part, or disease. Within medical terminology, we also have eponyms to describe a single symptom/finding, or a range of symptoms.

Although widely employed in English-speaking countries, the use of eponyms can cause problems in identification and meaning, as some eponyms have multiple meanings and others do not describe the location, shape, or structure of a feature, like so many other medical terms.

Despite being discouraged, the use of eponyms is sufficiently widespread in the medical field that clinicians must be familiar with their usage. In Table 16.8 you will find a small number of eponyms to increase your awareness of the notion.

Interestingly, the word *eponym* itself, like so much of the medical terminology we have already covered, originates from ancient Greek. The Greek word eponymous means 'giving name' (Duque-Parra et al. 2006). There are thousands of eponyms in common usage today and a study of their origins often yields a fascinating insight into historical culture and development.

Anatomical positions

In order to map injuries and ailments to the body, a number of anatomical positions exist, which are described in Table 16.9. These allow medical professionals to be able to describe a part of the body accurately and enable other medical personnel to know exactly what they are describing. First, we need one view of a body position to refer to, this is known simply as 'the anatomical position'.

The anatomical position is when a person is presenting facing forwards, feet flat on the floor, arms by their side, and palms facing forward (Figure 16.1). From this position, any movement or location of the body can be precisely described without any confusion using common medical

TABLE 16.9 Anatomical positions.

Position	Description
Supine	Body is lying face up
Prone	Body is lying face down
Lateral	Body is lying on either side (left or right)
Semi-recumbent	Partially reclined, head of bed at 45°
Sitting	You are probably doing it right now

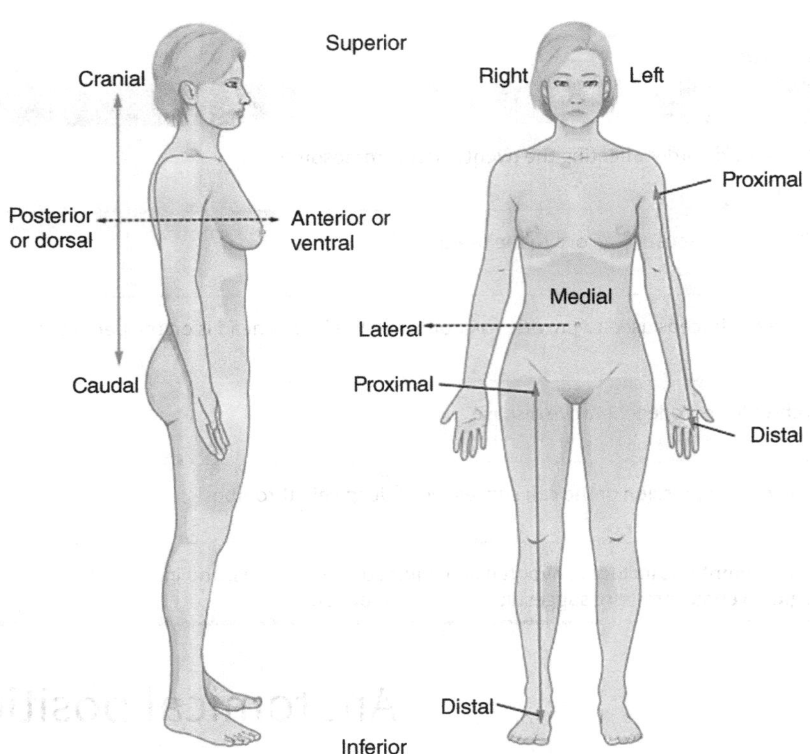

FIGURE 16.1 The anatomical position.

terminology. It is important to note at this stage that any description of the body should be from the patient's perspective. So the right side of the body refers to the patient's right, not the right of the person examining the patient (this will be their left).

Other medical terms are used to describe patient positions that differ from the anatomical position. This can be helpful when describing the position a patient was found in or might be used to assist in treating a patient with a certain diagnosis. For instance, a patient with a head injury will ideally be transported in a supine position with the head slightly elevated; a patient who is having trouble maintaining their own airway may be transported in the lateral position. It is important to include positions in any reports on the patient.

Anatomical directional terms

Anatomical directional terms are used to locate or describe specific body regions. Despite the patient's position, directional terms are derived from a patient in the anatomical position (see previous section and Table 16.10). These terms are often used to describe an injury in relation to another body part.

As a general rule, these terms are paired with their opposite:

TABLE 16.10 Anatomical directional terms.

Superior	Above
Inferior	Below
Medial	Towards the middle/midline
Lateral	Towards the side
Anterior/ventral	Towards the front
Posterior/dorsal	Towards the back
Proximal	Towards the core of the body/origin of limb
Distal	Away from the core of the body/origin of limb
Superficial	Towards/close to the body surface
Deep	Away from the body surface
Internal	Inside
External	Outside

- *Superior and inferior*. Superior means above, whilst inferior means below. The knee is superior (above) the foot, the hand is inferior (below) the elbow.
- *Medial and lateral*. Medial indicates towards the midline of the body, whilst lateral indicates away from the midline. A common term you may hear is the anatomical position of the 'medial malleolus' in relation to intraosseous access. This means that it is the ankle bone (malleolus refers to the ankle bone) on the inside of that leg. A patient may have swelling to the lateral malleolus when sustaining an inversion ankle injury.
- *Anterior and posterior*. Anterior means towards the front, whilst posterior means towards the back. The sternum bone in the chest is anterior, whilst the spine is posterior.
- *Proximal and distal*. Proximal means closest to the point of origin or the trunk of the body, whilst distal means farther away, towards the extremities. When describing an arm, the elbow is proximal compared to the distal wrist.
- *Superficial and deep*. Superficial means towards the body surface, whilst deep is away from the body surface. When describing cuts and lacerations, you may refer to one being superficial (often minor, scratches a few layers of skin) or deep (involving adipose tissue or lacerations cutting into a muscle).
- *Internal and external*. Internal describes inside the body, whilst external is on the outside of the body. A patient may be bleeding internally after a blunt injury, suggestive of bleeding inside the body that you cannot see from the outside.

Anatomical planes

A plane is an imaginary line, vertical or horizontal, that dissects through the body (see Figure 16.2). The division of the body or parts allows us to describe the view from which we study the patient:

- A sagittal or median plane runs from front to back, dividing the body into left and right.
- A frontal or coronal plane runs from side to side, dividing the body into dorsal (back) and ventral (front) parts.

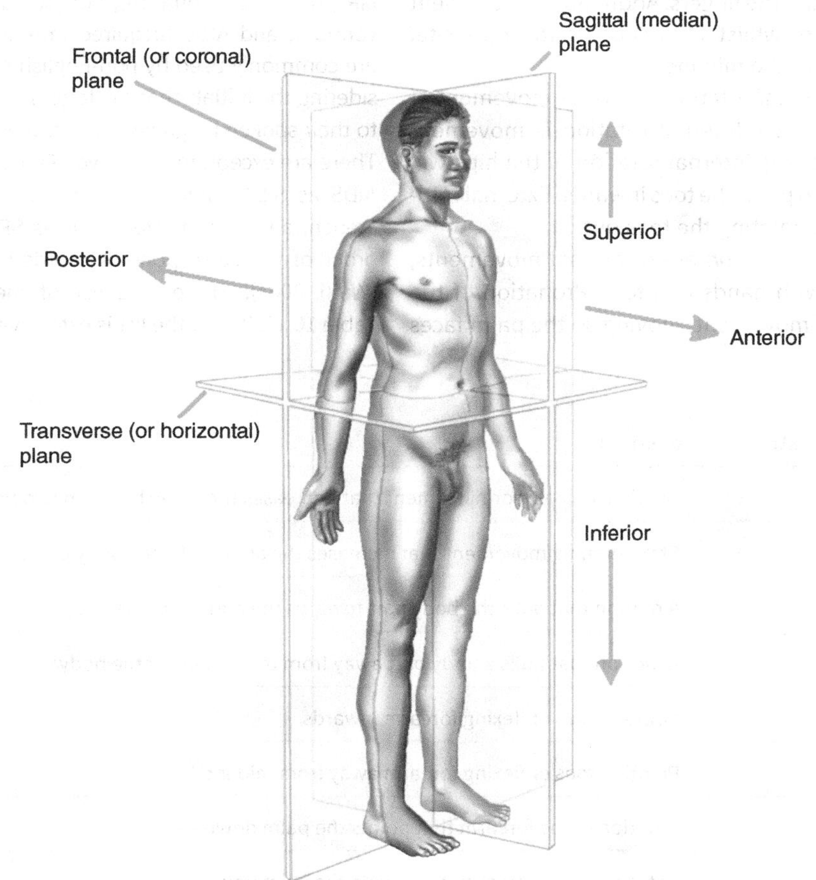

FIGURE 16.2 Anatomical planes.

- A transverse or axial plane is a cross-section through the body or limb, dividing the body into upper and lower.

Movement terminology

Muscles contract and relax to produce movement of joints and subsequently mobility of the skeleton. These actions can be accurately described using anatomical movement terminology (Table 16.11). As a reference point, we use the anatomical position, as stated earlier.

Flexion and *extension* describe the decreasing and increasing of angles between two body parts. Flexion describes the movement that decreases the angle between two parts, e.g. the movement of the forearm towards the shoulder, decreasing the angle between the ulna and radius and the humerus. Extension is the opposite, increasing the angle between two parts. So, in this example, straightening of the arm increases the angle between the forearm and the humerus.

Adduction and *abduction* are terms used to describe the movement *towards* and *away* from the midline of the body. They can also be used in relation to fingers and toes, for example, spreading the fingers. Adduction is movement towards the midline, whilst abduction is the opposite, movement away from the midline.

Internal and *external* rotation describes movement of limbs on their long axis. Internal rotation is movement towards the midline, e.g. internal rotation of the hips will rotate a straight leg to point the toes inwards. External rotation is the opposite, pointing the toes out.

Pronation and *supination* are rotational movements, mostly associated with hands and feet. Pronation of the hand is a rotational movement, moving so the palm faces down. Within the feet, pronation describes the movement of weight on the inside of the foot. This becomes useful in describing ankle injuries caused by inversion. Supination is the opposite, so in the hands rotating the hand so the palm faces up. Or in the ankle that the weight is distributed to the outside of the foot.

Circumduction is a special term that describes a specific movement that is a circular (or conical) motion in a limb. Often this involves a ball and socket joint. Looking at the hips, if you stood on one foot and moved your hip in a circular motion, this may be misidentified as rotation. This is actually circumduction. If you sat with your legs in front of you, and rotated your feet so they pointed inwards, this would describe hip rotation.

Medical abbreviations and acronyms

Some English acronyms have actually become accepted nouns. Acronyms such as CT (computed tomography), MR (magnetic resonance), PCI (percutaneous coronary intervention), and AIDS (acquired immunodeficiency syndrome) are commonly used by non-English-speaking clinicians. Considering the initials that the letters represent do not translate to their spoken language, the acronyms have become nouns. There are exceptions, however. France, for example, refers to AIDS as SIDA, which represents the translated acronym in French, and Russia refers to it as SPID, again reflecting the order of the corresponding words in the Russian language (Wulff 2004). There is a list of medical abbreviations in Table 16.12. Whilst the list is extensive, it is not exhaustive.

TABLE 16.11 Anatomical movement.

Flexion	Bending of a part or movement that decreases the angle between two body parts
Extension	Straightening movement that increases the angle between body parts
Adduction	A motion that pulls the body part towards the midline of the body
Abduction	A motion that pulls a body part away from the midline of the body
Internal rotation	Pointing toes or flexing forearm inwards
External rotation	Pointing toes or flexing forearm away from midline
Pronation	Rotation of the forearm that points the palm downwards
Supination	Rotation of the forearm that points the palm upwards

TABLE 16.12 Medical abbreviations and acronyms.

Abbreviation	Meaning
AAA	Abdominal aortic aneurysm
ABG	Arterial blood gas
ACS	Acute coronary syndrome
AED	Automatic external defibrillator
AF	Atrial fibrillation
AICD	Automated implantable cardioverter defibrillator
ALS	Advanced life support
AV	Atrioventricular
BGL	Blood glucose level
BLS	Basic life support
BP	Blood pressure
bpm	Beats per minute
BSA	Body surface area
BVM	Bag-valve-mask
CAD	Coronary artery disease
CNS	Central nervous system
c/o	Complaining of
CO	Carbon monoxide
CO_2	Carbon dioxide
COPD	Chronic obstructive pulmonary disease
CPAP	Continual positive airway pressure
CPR	Cardiopulmonary resuscitation
CSF	Cerebrospinal fluid
CT	Computerised tomography
CVA	Cerebrovascular accident
DIB	Difficulty in breathing
DKA	Diabetic ketoacidosis
DM	Diabetes mellitus
DVT	Deep vein thrombosis
ECG	Electrocardiogram
ENT	Ear, nose, and throat
$EtCO_2$	End-tidal carbon dioxide
ETT	Endotracheal tube
FAST	Focused assessment with sonography for trauma
FiO_2	Fractional inspired oxygen concentration
FRC	Functional residual capacity
GA	General anaesthetic
GABA	Gamma amino butyric acid
GCS	Glasgow coma scale
GI	Gastrointestinal
GTN	Glyceryl trinitrate
Hb	Haemoglobin
HI	Head injury
HR	Heart rate
Hx	History
IM	Intramuscular
IO	Intraosseous
IV	Intravenous
ICD	Implantable cardioverter defibrillator
ICP	Intracranial pressure
ICU	Intensive care unit
ILCOR	International Liaison Committee on Resuscitation
INR	International normalised ratio

(*Continued*)

TABLE 16.12 *(Continued)*

Abbreviation	Meaning
IPPV	Intermittent positive pressure ventilations
J	Joules
JVP	Jugular venous pressure
kg	Kilogramme
LBBB	Left bundle branch block
LLQ	Left lower quadrant
L/min	Litres per minute
LOC	Loss of consciousness
LUQ	Left upper quadrant
LVF	Left ventricular failure
LRTI	Lower respiratory tract infection
MAP	Mean arterial pressure
mg	Milligramme
MI	Myocardial infarction
min	Minute
ml	Millilitre
mmHg	Millimetre of mercury
mmol	Millimole
MOI	Mechanism of injury
MV	Minute ventilation
Mx	Manage/management
NAD	No abnormality detected
NEB	Nebulised
NG	Nasogastric
NMDA	N-methyl D-aspartate
NOF	Neck of femur
NP	Nasopharyngeal airway

Abbreviation	Meaning
NSAID	Nonsteroidal anti-inflammatory drug
NSR	Normal sinus rhythm
NSTEMI	Non-ST-elevation myocardial infarction
O/A	On arrival
O/E	On examination
OP	Oropharyngeal airway
PAC	Premature atrial contraction
$PaCO_2$	Partial pressure of carbon dioxide (arterial)
PaO_2	Partial pressure of oxygen (arterial)
PCI	Percutaneous coronary intervention
PE	Pulmonary embolus
PEA	Pulseless electrical activity
PEARL	Pupils equal and reactive to light
PEEP	Positive end expiratory pressure
PMHx	Past medical history
PPE	Personal protective equipment
PPH	Postpartum haemorrhage
Pt	Patient
PVC	Premature ventricular contraction
RBBB	Right bundle branch block
RLQ	Right lower quadrant
ROSC	Return of spontaneous circulation
RSI	Rapid sequence induction
RTC	Road traffic collision
RUQ	Right upper quadrant
RV	Right ventricle
Rx/Tx	Treatment

TABLE 16.12 *(Continued)*

Abbreviation	Meaning
SA	Sinoatrial
SAH	Subarachnoid haemorrhage
SCI	Spinal cord injury
SOB	Short of breath
SpO_2	Saturation of haemoglobin with oxygen
SSRI	Selective serotonin reuptake inhibitor
STEMI	ST-elevation myocardial infarction
SUBCUT	Subcutaneous
S/S	Signs/symptoms
SV	Stroke volume
SVT	Supraventricular tachycardia
TBI	Traumatic brain injury
TCA	Tricyclic antidepressants
TIA	Transient ischaemic attack
TPT	Tension pneumothorax
URTI	Upper respiratory tract infection
UTI	Urinary tract infection
VF	Ventricular fibrillation
VT	Ventricular tachycardia
WOB	Work of breathing
#	Fracture
1/24	One hour
1/7	One day
1/52	One week
1/12	One month

Similarities in terminology

There are several word roots in medical terminology that can be easily confused without a degree of attention. This means it is imperative to pay close attention to the root words to ensure the correct message is communicated. Table 16.13 lists some commonly confused medical word roots.

Spelling: British versus American English

There are often two acceptable ways of spelling medical terms in British and American English (Australia adopts the British spelling).

Spell checks will often autocorrect words to the American spelling and will not adopt or acknowledge any silent vowels in British English (meaning that the silent 'o' or 'a' is not spelt out, a common example is paediatric). The other major difference to note is that American spelling will spell words with a 'k' whereas British spelling will utilise a 'c'.

Although these differences are easy to identify and pose no real threat of miscommunication, an awareness of these differences is paramount for accurately communicating in medical language.

You will find some common examples in Table 16.14.

Conclusion

In order to communicate accurately and effectively in a healthcare setting, paramedics and emergency medical technicians need to possess an understanding of medical terminology. By exploring and familiarising ourselves with common grammatical rules and word structure, we can understand medical terms and use them more efficiently and accurately, thus improving patient care in the OOH setting.

This chapter has introduced medical terminology, describing its origins in Greek, Latin, and Arabic; the building blocks by which different medical terms are constructed; an overview of some of the principles for identifying and understanding medical terms; and a guide to some of the acronyms widely employed. In the process, we have seen that medical terminology is a rich and multi-layered language whose roots in other cultures continue to influence and shape the way medicine is studied today.

TABLE 16.13 Common similarities.

Agonist – a type of pharmacological agent that stimulates cellular activity	Antagonist – a substance that inhibits or counters the action of another substance	
Cyst/o – cyst or sac of fluid	Cyt/o – the word root for cell.	
Dysphasia – disorder of speech	Dysphagia – difficulty swallowing	
Ileum – part of the intestinal tract	Ilium – the pelvic bone	
My/o – muscle	Myc/o – fungus	Myel/o – spinal cord or bone marrow

TABLE 16.14 British versus American spellings.

British	American
Oedema	Edema
Haematology	Hematology
Paediatrician	Pediatrician
ECG	EKG

Activities

Now review your learning by completing the learning activities in this chapter. The answers to these appear at the end of the book. Further self-test activities can be found at **www.wileyfundamentalseries.com/paramedic/3e.**

Test your knowledge

1. What is a prefix?
2. What is a suffix?
3. What does the word root '-itis' mean?
4. Which body part is represented by cardi/o?

Activity 16.1

Break down the following medical terms to decipher their meaning:

Tachycardia ______________________
Gastritis ______________________
Dyspnoea ______________________
Cardiovascular ______________________

Activity 16.2

Describe a circumstance where inappropriate pronunciation or misspelled medical terminology could be detrimental to a patient's condition.

Activity 16.3

Can you break down the word?

Dysuria?
Dys meaning ____________
Uria meaning ____________

Now let us try one that is not included in the lists above. These will be found in most medical textbooks:

Rhinoplasty
Rhino meaning ____________
Plasty meaning ____________
Dysuria: Difficulty passing urine; *Rhinoplasty:* The surgical repair of the nose.

Want to try more? Take a look at Cohen and Depetris (2013), with lots of theory and examples of medical terminology.

Glossary

Affixation: This is the process of adding prefixes, suffixes to a base word to create a new word with a modified meaning or grammatical function.

Anatomical landmark: A specific point or structure on the human body that serves as a reference point for anatomical or medical purposes.

Eponym: A word or name derived from the name of a specific person, typically a real historical figure, who is associated with the concept, object, discovery, or invention that the word represents. In paramedicine, the 'Heimlich manoeuvre' is an eponym, named after Dr Henry Heimlich.

Phonetic: Phonetic refers to the study or representation of the sounds of human speech, particularly how speech sounds are produced, transmitted, and perceived. (Phonetically is an adverb referring to something being related to or in a manner that pertains to phonetics.)

Prefix: A word part that is added to the beginning of a base word to create a new word with a modified meaning.

A root word: Also known as a base word, a word in its simplest form, before any prefixes or suffixes are added to it.

Suffix: A linguistic element added to the end of a word or word root to modify its meaning or form.

References

Cohen, B. and DePetris, A. (eds.) (2013). *Medical Terminology: An Illustrated Guide*. Baltimore: Wolters Kluwer Health.

Craik, E. (2015). *The Hippocratic Corpus: Content and Context*. Oxon: Routledge.

Duque-Parra, J.E., Llano-Idarraga, J.O., and Duque-Parra, C.A. (2006). Reflections on eponyms in neuroscience terminology. *Anatomical Record B: New Anatomist* **289** (6): 219–224.

Koch-Weser, S., Dejong, W., and Rudd, R.E. (2009). Medical word use in clinical encounters. *Health Expectations* **12** (4): 371–382.

Stepheson, T. (2022). Hazards of medical terminology from classical languages: it's all Green (and Latin!) to me! *Archives of Diseases in Childhood* **108** (5) 316–362. doi: 10.1136/archdischild-2022-324107. Epub ahead of print. PMID: 35477647.

Walker, S., Wood, M., and Nicol, J. (2013). *Mastering Medical Terminology*. Edinburgh: Churchill Livingstone.

Wulff, H.R. (2004). The language of medicine. *Journal of the Royal Society of Medicine* **97** (4): 187–188.

CHAPTER 17

Essential toxicology for out-of-hospital clinicians

Jack Matulich

Intensive Care Unit, Gold Coast University Hospital, Southport, Queensland, Australia

Simon Menz

Clinical Support Paramedic, St John Ambulance, Western Australia, Australia

Contents

LEARNING OUTCOMES

On completion of this chapter the reader will be able to:

- Discuss the importance of toxicology in the out-of-hospital (OOH) setting.
- Identify key pharmacological processes involved in overdose.
- Understand how advanced life support may be modified in poisoned patients.
- Identify the eight most pertinent toxidromes to paramedic practice.
- Understand the importance of public health and prevention in toxicology.

Fundamentals of Paramedic Practice: A Systems Approach, Third Edition. Edited by Sam Willis and Ian Peate.

Companion website: www.wiley.com/go/willis/paramedic3e

Case Study

You are called to a thirty-five-year-old female, found at home by her partner, unresponsive. The caller statement reads:

'I think my partner has taken an overdose'

On arrival at the house you are greeted by the partner who escorts you to a lady lying on her back on a couch with snoring respirations. Your initial vital sign survey finds:

GCS – 8 (E2 V2 M4)
RR – 8/min
HR – 34/min
BP – 102/58mmHg
SpO2 – 89% RA
BGL – 6.2mmol/L
Temp – 37.3°C
Pupils – Sluggish, equal, 3mm
12 lead ECG – Sinus bradycardia with peaked T waves

You ask the patient's partner what medications are available in the house. They hand you a box of medications that includes:

Tapentadol
Escitalopram
Panedine forte
Metoprolol
Lorazepam

Reader tasks:

1. Consider what your management plan for this patient might be followed by what the expected course of hospital management will be when you arrive at the emergency department.
2. What safety concerns do you need to be aware of for this type of case?
3. What else may you want to be asking the partner to gather relevant history?
4. Does this patient need to be transported priority 1 with pre-notification to the emergency department?

Introduction

It is of paramount importance for out-of-hospital (OOH) practitioners to be able to recognise and treat toxins in their patients. There are very few clinical presentations that will not include toxicity as a differential diagnosis, and being able to confidently assess for toxic symptoms and respond appropriately will undoubtedly save lives. Consider that every presentation from altered level of consciousness to chest pain to polyuria could be attributable to toxins. Even cases that seem clear in aetiology such as road traffic crashes could be caused by toxins. Often it is these clouded circumstances that lead to a missed diagnosis and a later scramble to explain and treat a deteriorating patient. Further, toxins may render some treatments inert unless they are addressed first, which is especially pertinent to critically unwell patients. The paramedic who understands toxicology can pick up on the subtle and obvious cues that might indicate toxins. Many common toxicology presentations have a significant direct impact on the patient in the short term, and all toxicology presentations put the patient at risk of significant lifelong disability or death due to the sequelae associated.

This chapter provides the paramedic with useful information relating to toxicology that can be used in the assessment and management of their patients.

What is a toxin?

It is important for paramedics to understand that any ingested, injected, inhaled, or otherwise absorbed substance that exceeds the human body's ability to adequately neutralise and excrete it is considered a toxic substance. It is not the substance itself that determines toxicity, but its dose in the context of the patient's ability to cope with it. Many substances traditionally regarded as toxic (think cyanide) are regarded as such due to their common availability in easily absorbed, toxic doses. The common culinary herb parsley contains considerable quantities of arsenic (Madeira et al. 2012). However, the doses typically ingested by people are far below the necessary amounts to create a toxic effect and the human body is able to adequately cope with its ingestion. In contrast, there are many substances automatically regarded as inert by most people that can become toxic if absorbed in enough quantity. Indeed, even water can become a toxic substance with a high enough dosage (Tilley and Cotant 2011). This concept is especially pertinent in the paediatric population, where just one pill or sip can be fatal (Table 17.1). The key learning point is that the beginning paramedic practitioner must be vigilant to the signs of toxicity and understand the relationship between dose and toxicity, so as to avoid complacency clouding sound clinical judgement based on substance alone.

TABLE 17.1 Paediatric high-risk substances.

One to two pills can kill	One sip can kill
Amphetamines	Organophosphates
Baclofen	Paraquat
Calcium channel blockers	Hydrocarbons
Carbamazepine	Camphor
Chloroquine and hydroxychloroquine	Corrosives (bleaches/drain cleaners)
Clozapine	Naphthalene (moth balls)
Dextropropoxyphene	Strychnine
Opioids	Pesticides
Propranolol	
Sulphonylureas	
Theophylline	
Tricyclic antidepressants	
Venlafaxine	
Oral hypoglycaemics	
Beta blockers	
Alpha adrenergics such as clonidine and imidazolines	
Chloroquine	
Salicylates	
Clonidine	

Pharmacokinetics in toxicology

Whilst pharmacology has been explored thoroughly elsewhere in this text, it is useful to revisit the concepts of absorption, distribution, metabolism, and excretion in the context of toxicology. Each stage of this process can determine the toxicological risk, outcomes, and management of toxicology patients.

Absorption

Absorption describes the route via which a substance enters the human body. Examples of routes common in the OOH setting include inhalation (into the lungs), ingestion (into the gut), parenteral (into the circulatory system), and topical (onto skin and membrane). However, further routes exist such as intranasal (into the nose), intraocular (into the eye), and intrathecal (into the brain). This is pertinent to know for all patient care interactions, and especially as paramedics are commonly required to transfer patients between hospitals and must therefore understand that each route of absorption carries implications for each substance. Topical administration is typically slow to absorb, and a low percentage of the total substance applied finds the central circulation. Ingested substances depend on factors such as stomach acidity, digestion, and gut perfusion as to the speed and quantity of the substance that will be absorbed. The risk inherent in ingested substances is the ongoing absorption of the substance as it is dissolved. This is particularly important for slow-release medications, which may continue to diffuse over hours to days. As such, anticipating the trajectory of a long duration of supportive care should influence the decision-making on appropriate facilities for transfer.

The paramedic, in their inquiries with the patient should establish if they are taking a delayed release medication. It's important to note how the patient is taking this medication because if the medication was crushed prior to ingestion, this will impact the absorption rate. Some medications are designed for the exterior coating of the tablet to slowly break down, resulting in a 'slow release' of the medication. If these medications are crushed before being taken, the full dose of the medication will be available for absorption immediately rather than over an extended period of time.

Absorption of medications is crucial for a paramedic to understand as particular medications administered by paramedics will have different times of onset based on the route of administration. Some routes of administration will result in faster absorption than others. For example, Aspirin is commonly administered to patients with suspected acute coronary syndrome (ACS). The recommended route of administration is buccal (chewed) as this results in faster absorption than if the tablet was swallowed and absorbed through the GI tract. Each medication will differ in the fastest route of administration. Figure 17.1 is an image that outlines the different routes of medication administration and the abbreviations that are used to describe them.

Distribution

The topic of distribution is concerned with the movement of chemicals through the bloodstream to their target receptors. Remember that chemicals only exert their effect when free in blood plasma and able to attach to their target; and when they are stored or bound to other molecules, they are not activating their receptors. The allotment of chemicals to receptors and

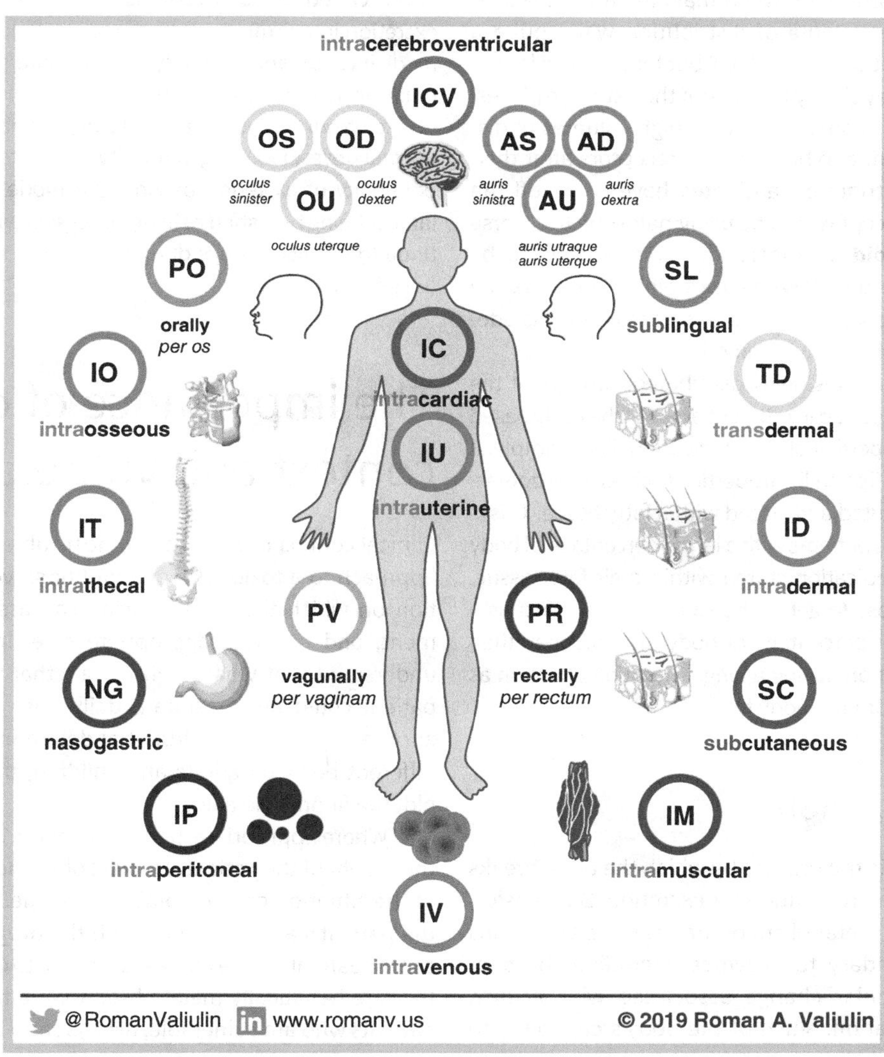

FIGURE 17.1 Routes of medication administration.

storage areas within the body depends on their solubility in different tissues, acidity, and physical size. Some chemicals will easily infiltrate all tissues of the body, whilst some will only enter certain compartments. Some chemicals can pass the blood–brain barrier and affect the central nervous system directly, whilst others cannot. Consider being called to a child who has potentially overdosed on antihistamines. Imagine how your management might change if you found that the agent was a first-generation antihistamine that crosses the blood–brain barrier and sedates, compared to a second generation that does not.

Exactly how far chemicals will disperse in the body is represented by their volume of distribution. This is a complex concept to understand, but in brief the volume of distribution represents the theoretical amount of tissue the chemical will disperse into, represented in litres. A drug with a lower volume of distribution will remain mainly in plasma. Drugs with a larger volume of distribution will require a larger dose to reach therapeutic level but tend to take longer to be excreted as they slowly leach from their storage places. This is important, as some drugs with high volumes of distribution may continue to bind to their receptors after their low volume of distribution antidotes have worn off. An example of this concept would be using naloxone to reverse a slow-release **opioid** overdose. Naloxone is likely to be metabolised before the slow-release opioid. This puts the patient at risk of lapsing back into a toxic state unless adequate antidote levels are maintained.

When a medication is being distributed throughout the body, it's commonly stored in different areas of the body based on the chemical properties of the medication. For example, a medication that has lipophilic properties such as a benzodiazepine, will be distributed and stored within fatty tissue. This is important to know as patients with a larger percentage of body fat will have the medication stored within their fatty tissue, requiring a larger dose to get to the same desired effect as a patient with a lower percentage of body fat. This may then result in the medication having a longer duration of action as it is then released from the body fat.

Biotransformation

Biotransformation is the process by which the body breaks down a chemical in preparation for excretion. Biotransformation is a part of metabolism of medications and toxins and may be secondary to enzymes degrading the substance, and molecular change associated with acidity, hydrolysis, or oxidation. Much of the body's capability to prepare drugs to be excreted is vested in the liver. An impairment in these processes will lead to either the drug or a by-product accumulating and creating a toxic level of the substance. Where a dose of a substance exceeds the capability of the liver to keep up with excretion, this principle will also apply. There are many chronic conditions too that affect the ability of the body to biotransform substances in preparation for excretion.

Excretion

Excretion is the physical removal of the substance or its derivatives from the body. Most excretion is performed by the kidneys, intestinal tract, or sweat glands. Where an impairment in one of these vehicles exists, toxicity may form due to non-excreted poisons building up. Where chronic or acute excretion impairment exists, doctors will down-titrate regular medicines to appropriately compensate for the inevitable build-up. However, where sudden changes in the body's ability to excrete drugs occur, patients may continue to take their normal doses, resulting in toxicity. A final consideration is the possibility of excretion becoming a mode of absorption for infants being breastfed or in utero, as seen when mothers continue to use illicit drugs during pregnancy and breastfeeding (Vajjah et al. 2012).

The importance of clinical context and vulnerability

Clinical context is perhaps the most subjective factor of the approach to a toxicology patient but serves as the foundation on which the OOH clinician can assess, plan, implement, and evaluate appropriate care. It is important to understand that what might be a lethal toxic dose to one patient could be a standard daily dose of a medicine to another. The dose of a drug that determines toxicity will be different between adults and children, the young and the old, the fit and the ailing.

Where appropriate, first consider the dose compared to the weight of the patient. This will often indicate the severity of the situation or deterioration to come. Further, consider the patient's ability to cope with the drug. A terminal liver cancer patient will be more susceptible to overdose on drugs that are hepatically metabolised than a healthy person. In patients who are vulnerable, always carry a low threshold to escalate their care, and either bring the patient to a facility that can provide critical management or arrange for critical care back-up to come to the patient.

Remembering all possible toxic doses and their associated at-risk patient cohorts is not feasible for the general OOH practitioner, and there is no easy metric to apply to all patients to simplify the question of clinical context. Instead, the beginning practitioner should learn common **toxidromes** and agents well, approach all toxic patients with a low threshold for calling for help, and appreciate that any toxic presentation has the potential to become life-threatening very quickly and often in subtle and unpredictable ways. The experience of the OOH practitioner will define how the clinical context is interpreted, and it is important to continually reflect, seek new knowledge, and maintain a humble stance in the face of toxic presentation.

The initial resuscitative approach in toxicology

The OOH environment is the least resourced but often the most critical part of a toxicology patient's medical journey. It is imperative for the OOH practitioner to use their knowledge and understanding of toxicology as the key to good outcomes for the patient. The goal should always be to stabilise the patient for safe transport and to proceed to the most appropriate facility quickly. Toxicity can manifest rapidly, and it is best to have as narrow a window of opportunity for this to happen OOH as possible. The following segment is an adaptation of the contemporary framework for toxicology management abridged to the resource-limited paramedic setting (Daly et al. 2006; Sivilotti et al. 2018).

As with all OOH cases, the primary survey and primary response form the first step to treating a toxicology patient. Where immediate life-threatening complications are present, approach the patient according to your advanced cardiac life support (ACLS) scope and protocols, with supplementary adjustments for toxicology as follows.

Resuscitation

Airway

A thorough assessment of the airway is always pertinent in the toxicology patient. Risks to the airway could include swelling from caustic agents, airway collapse in obtunded patients, airway spasm, inhaled foreign bodies, aspirated vomitus, and exacerbation of pre-existing conditions. Management is as with any other patient and the possibility of complicating or worsening pathology should be considered. Advanced practitioners often consider the clinical context of the patient's toxicity and may opt to gain advanced airway control to pre-empt airway deterioration that might make securing an airway risky later on.

Breathing

A proper assessment of the presence, rate, rhythm, and effort of breathing should be conducted to assess the potential need for respiratory support. **Sedative** toxidromes may depress respiratory drive, which could be detrimental to the obtunded patient, whilst other toxidromes such as the **sympathomimetic** may have a hyperventilation effect that could be just as harmful. When assuming control or support of respiration, it is important to consider the effects of ventilation on the toxin present. Some overdoses such as those from sodium channel blockers may benefit from more aggressive ventilation as an antidote. Further, auscultation of the lungs should be performed to assess for risks such as excessive secretion in **cholinergic** overdose, wheeze indicative of bronchospasm, or aspiration.

Circulation

Ensuring adequate blood flow is important in the toxic patient, as without adequate circulation the sequelae of toxicity will exponentially worsen. The usual primary check and monitoring of the patient's pulse is necessary, noting rate, regularity, and strength followed by blood pressure, heart rate, and electrocardiogram (ECG) monitoring. When presented with an aggressive patient and where an overdose was intentional, safer and less invasive circulation assessments such as visual observation, skin temperature assessed by touch, and capillary refill time (CRT) assessments may be all that can be achieved in the early stages of assessment. Most toxidromes can eventuate in significant or catastrophic reduction in cardiac output, making access for intravascular medicine important but also difficult to obtain. Where safe access is not precluded by agitation, seizure, or other clinical issues, early intravenous access is imperative. When cardiac complications exist, both acute and critical, it is important to consider the likely toxins involved, as some toxidromes may make resuscitation futile without appropriate antidotes in parallel with standard advanced life support.

Hypotension should be addressed with intravenous fluid challenge as a first port of call. Inotropic medications may be required where hypotension persists; however, clinical consultation is recommended to ensure the agent is not contraindicated by interactions with differential poisons.

Symptomatic bradycardia, in isolation, should be treated according to local protocol and is usually addressed with an **anticholinergic** agent such as atropine. Bradycardia may present in a toxidrome that necessitates an anticholinergic response, and therefore close attention should be paid to developing toxic signs. Other causes of symptomatic hypotension in poisoned patients may include digoxin toxicity, beta blocker toxicity, calcium channel toxicity, or sodium channel blocker toxicity.

Wide complex tachycardias are masked enormously by toxins. What may look like ventricular tachycardia may actually be supraventricular tachycardia that has been augmented by sodium channel blockade. In these cases, sodium bicarbonate is often used to stabilise the sodium channels. Cardiotoxic drugs can induce **Torsades de Pointes**; however, treatment remains the same, with magnesium sulphate to stabilise the myocardium.

Narrow complex tachycardia is usually associated with sympathomimetic drugs such as cocaine and amphetamines. Rate control should be approached with titrated benzodiazepines and beta blockers should generally be avoided.

Asystole and ventricular fibrillation are managed according to standard ACLS protocols. If a wide complex tachycardia deteriorates to fibrillation with reasonable suspicion of sodium channel blocker overdose, then sodium bicarbonate may assist in resuscitation.

Seizure control

Many toxins can eventuate in seizures. Even substances that cannot cross the blood–brain barrier may have secondary effects that can induce seizure or make underlying seizure risk more prominent. As a rule of thumb, toxic seizures are generalised and a patient presenting in a toxidrome with focal seizures should be assessed thoroughly for alternative causes for the seizure. Initial management should be responsive to the seizure, ensuring safety of the patient and bystanders, ensuring adequate oxygenation, and reducing seizures through use of benzodiazepines or other anticonvulsants. Whilst indicated in some other seizure groups, phenytoin is contraindicated in seizures secondary to acute poisoning.

Correct hypoglycaemia

Some medications such as insulin can deplete available blood glucose. Other situations may include excessive metabolism of glucose due to a process secondary to toxicity, such as seizures. Hypoglycaemia should be immediately treated in the most appropriate way for the clinical scenario. Use standard protocol but be mindful of the patient's ability to tolerate oral input without aspirating. Closing the treatment loop by reassessing blood glucose after treatment should be conducted to ensure a blood sugar level of >4 mmol/l is achieved and maintained. The paramedic should be aware that patients who have taken an intentional overdose of insulin will often respond to paramedic interventions before becoming hypoglycaemic again. This is a consideration in the patient care plan, for example, reassessing the patient at appropriate intervals and ensuring they are conveyed to hospital.

Achieve normothermia

Poisoned patients may present in both hypothermic and hyperthermic states, depending on the agent. The goal should always be normothermia and the mode of treating an elevated temperature should be determined by its severity. The risks associated with hyperthermia are seizure and organ failure, with risk increasing greatly as hyperthermia increases. Hypothermia may precipitate or mimic cardiac arrest. Whether hypothermia stems from the toxidrome, the environment, or a mix, it should be treated to achieve normothermia, especially in apparent arrest.

Resuscitation antidotes

Whilst emergency antidotes are listed last in this approach to poisoned patients, they should be considered in parallel to all resuscitation. Some critical complications will not be able to be resolved using standard resuscitative practice without antidotes. For example, in severe cardiac compromise from tricyclic antidepressant (TCA) overdose, lethal arrhythmias will generally be extremely difficult to revert without sodium bicarbonate administration and hyperventilation to alkalise the blood and decrease the effect of sodium channel blockade. These antidotes will often be in the critical care practitioner scope of practice and should be considered when assessing the reversible causes of cardiac arrest, referred to as the 'Hs and Ts'. Finally, whilst it may seem like common sense to withhold antiemetics in case of oral overdose, in the case of the paediatric patient, vomiting is not beneficial (The Royal Childrens Hospital Melbourne 2017) and therefore for the benefit of patient comfort the paramedic should administer an antiemetic for the paediatric patient who is presenting with nausea and vomiting.

Risk assessment and disposition

As soon as the patient is stable enough for the clinician to divert their thinking away from resuscitation, a thorough risk assessment should be conducted. Each poisoned patient will have a unique response to their toxin based on their dose, weight, habitus, and organ function. The risk assessment in toxicology is a considered, holistic analysis of the patient and their likely clinical trajectory. A risk assessment in the OOH setting will aid in determining which facility to transport to, which pre-emptive treatments to initiate, and what further resources may be necessary, both OOH and once the patient is handed over. It is always better to overestimate needs and prepare resources greater than the needs of the patient than to underestimate and be unable to treat the patient appropriately.

The five key components to risk assessment are agent(s), dose(s), time since ingestion, clinical progression, and patient factors (Cameron et al. 2015).

Most assessment data in toxicology risk assessment is either subjective or objective, with a large possibility of inaccuracy; as such, critical thinking is paramount at this stage. If the patient is able to communicate what they ingested, the paramedic may be able to get a guide as to what agent and doses are involved. Be cautious of any altered mental status, indication of recreational drug use, or deliberate overdose, as these factors may influence the patient's willingness and ability to give an accurate account of what they have taken. Other information that may assist could lie in empty pill packets, signs of drug use, medical records, and conversations with family or bystanders. Remember that whilst primary information can be inaccurate, secondary information should be taken with even more diligence, as it has an increased likelihood of not being accurate.

Where it is unclear what has been ingested, the OOH clinician must synthesise their patient assessment and their environment to find likely agents. For example, music festivals may give rise to stimulant recreational drugs, older farms may hold organophosphates improperly, and a whisky home brewer may be prone to methanol poisoning. Paracetamol should always be considered in the event of intentional overdose as it is a readily available medication, commonly used in overdose with potentially fatal consequences. In all of these cases a thorough history is required, and the paramedic should be direct when asking what the substance of overdose is.

The time since ingestion is another key influencer of prognosis in the context of clinical progression. Whilst paramedic practice has limited use for this information due to the symptomatic treatment of the patient and high index of transport to hospital regardless, this is extremely useful for the hospital team to know. Many agents have defined time-related courses, which can determine risk at given points in the patient's progression. For example, it is known that in TCA overdose critical instability is most likely to occur within the first six hours of ingestion, and that if the patient remains stable at six hours, they are unlikely to deteriorate. This may influence where the patient will be treated in the emergency department and where they will be transferred to from there.

Paediatric patients pose an escalated susceptibility to poisoning. A smaller habitus, developing organ capability, and inability to understand the risk of ingesting agents make children high-risk toxicology patients. Most paediatric poisoning is also unwitnessed and may not become apparent until symptomology is advanced and critical. A worst-case scenario should always be employed in the paediatric toxicology patient, and drawing on available resources should occur very early, pre-empting a complex paediatric resuscitation.

Differential diagnosis

When assessing a patient with an altered conscious state, toxidromes should be considered as one of the many differential diagnoses (see discussion below on toxidromes). The mnemonic AEIOU-TIPS (Sanello 2018) is useful for helping the paramedic recognise toxicological conditions causing altered conscious states:

A – Alcohol
E – Epilepsy with seizure activity
I – Infection
O – Overdose
U – Uraemia
T – Trauma
I – Insulin
P – Poisoning
S – Stroke

Trauma

Trauma should be considered in any patient who has lost consciousness, including those who have lost consciousness due to a toxidrome. Identifying what the person was doing prior to the loss of consciousness is therefore important. For example, were they standing, which may indicate a possible head strike, if so, did they put their hand out in front of them when they fell, or were they sitting down comfortably? Spinal precautions should be implemented in any patient who meets the criteria for spinal immobilisation using the NEXUS tool. This includes those who are intoxicated with alcohol.

Carbon monoxide poisoning

Carbon monoxide poisoning also needs to be considered in this space. Some forms of carbon monoxide poisoning may be obvious to the paramedic such as intentional self-harm via a vehicle gassing. In this situation the car engine will be running and there will most likely be a pipe leading from the car exhaust and into the cabin, whilst other forms of carbon monoxide poisoning may be more subtle such as a person who has inhaled smoke having been removed from a house fire or a person who has a faulty boiler at home.

Toxicology sequelae

The dangers of toxicity are not isolated to the toxin itself. Most toxic presentations will have the potential for significant sequelae that could cause more damage than the toxin. Sequelae generally pertain to symptoms and are logical complications of how the patient has presented. An example of a sequela would be the possibility of long downtime in an overdose causing **rhabdomyolysis** secondary to tissue breakdown. This may cause electrolyte disturbances and may need preventative and resuscitative care. It is not possible to explore all possible sequelae, because every patient and presentation will host its own set of risks. Consider history, environment, behaviour, drug, and dose when looking for potential sequelae. As with most toxicology understanding, these skills will build as your experience builds. Often verbalising your thought processes with other clinicians to collaborate each individual's knowledge and experience will yield better results.

Toxidromes

Toxidromes are groups of symptoms that are specific to certain classes of overdose. The term toxidrome was established by Mofenson and Greensher (1970) as a way of quickly and accurately identifying paediatric overdose substances. In contemporary practice, toxidromes are used on all age groups and are especially useful for OOH clinicians, who often do not have drug screening capabilities in their work environment yet need to make informed treatment decisions. This section will highlight the key toxidromes to remember, how to identify them, and what treatment goals are appropriate. First, the fundamentals of physiology and pharmacology behind toxidromes must be briefly reviewed (Volle 1963).

Physiology

A toxidrome is a combination of signs and symptoms that can be used to isolate a group of toxins likely to be the culprit of overdose based on the receptors on which they act. The foundation of toxidrome signs and symptoms is the **autonomic nervous system (ANS)**. By sending information between the body and the brain, the ANS regulates most involuntary processes of the body such as breathing, heart rate, blood pressure, and digestion.

The ANS has two divisions, the **sympathetic** and **parasympathetic** nervous systems.

The sympathetic nervous system, otherwise known as the fight-or-flight system, is responsible for preparing the body for maximal exertion by increasing the capacity for high-intensity activity and decreasing nonessential processes. The sympathetic nervous system increases heart rate, dilates pupils, relaxes airways, relaxes the bladder, and prevents digestion.

In contrast, the parasympathetic nervous system, otherwise known as the rest-and-digest system, prepares the body for periods of restoration and digestion. The parasympathetic nervous system decreases heart rate, constricts pupils, tightens airways, contracts the bladder, and promotes digestion. Both the sympathetic and parasympathetic nervous systems work competitively around the body and appropriate physiological response is mediated by balancing both divisions. To do this, the central nervous system uses information from the afferent (information heading to the brain) part of the ANS to regulate the efferent (information heading away from the brain) sending of neurotransmitters to the receptor sites around the body.

The parasympathetic nervous system exerts its effect in a cholinergic manner, meaning that its primary neurotransmitter is acetylcholine. Acetylcholine activates muscarinic and nicotinic receptors around the body to produce the rest-and-digest effect. Acetylcholinesterase is an enzyme that cleans up the acetylcholine and ceases its effect on target receptors.

Whilst acetylcholine is also part of the process of sympathetic innervation, the sympathetic nervous system is adrenergic as opposed to cholinergic, and its primary neurotransmitters are adrenaline and noradrenaline. Both the sympathetic and parasympathetic nervous systems can be influenced positively and negatively by drugs.

Pharmacology

Drugs that encourage the action of a receptor and its associated neurotransmitter are called agonists. A drug that agonises a receptor will elicit a toxic response that is appropriate for the receptors division of the ANS. For example, cocaine is an agonist of adrenergic receptors. Therefore, an increase in sympathetic activity is expected in overdose and signs such as tachycardia and dilated pupils are anticipated. In contrast, drugs that inhibit the action of a receptor and its associated neurotransmitter are called antagonists. An antagonist will elicit the opposite effect of the intrinsic receptor on which it acts. For example, a muscarinic antagonist such as atropine will also increase heart rate and dilate the pupils. It does this by suppressing the parasympathetic nervous system and allowing the sympathetic nervous system to dominate. For this reason, antagonists of the parasympathetic system will have the same effects as agonists of the sympathetic nervous system and vice versa.

In paramedic practice there are five key toxidromes to understand comprehensively: cholinergic, anticholinergic, sedative, opioid, and sympathomimetic. Additionally, there are three further toxidromes that can develop with drugs commonly used in the OOH setting: serotonin syndrome, malignant hyperthermia, and neuroleptic malignant syndrome.

Cholinergic toxidrome

Cholinergic toxins are few and far between in paramedic practice. They are usually isolated to two environments: agricultural settings and terrorist attacks. Cholinergic agents are found in organophosphate pesticides as well as chemical nerve agents. Whilst organophosphate pesticides are slowly being removed from farming practice, there is ongoing use of nerve agents in terror attacks.

Pharmacology

Cholinergic poisons work by either enhancing the ability of acetylcholine to exert its effect or by blocking acetylcholinesterase. In essence, these drugs will increase parasympathetic activity either directly or indirectly.

Signs and symptoms

- *Central*: agitation, respiratory depression, disorientation, coma, seizures.
- *Peripheral*: urinary incontinence, abdominal cramping, bradycardia, bronchoconstriction, diarrhoea, lacrimation, **miosis,** vomiting.
- *Nicotinic* (reserved only for nicotinic agents): muscle cramps, tachycardia, weakness, fasciculations.

Possible agents

Key agents involved in cholinergic syndromes fall into either acetylcholinesterase inhibitor or acetylcholine agonist categories. In the acetylcholinesterase inhibitor category there are organophosphate pesticides, carbamate pesticides, and chemical nerve agents, as well as drugs used for dementia and myasthenia gravis. Acetylcholine agonists include muscarinic agents, nicotinic agents, and mushrooms.

Treatments

Treatment for cholinergic toxidromes focuses on rapid response to symptoms and pre-emptive management of respiratory decline. Any muscarinic signs or symptoms that indicate airway, breathing, or circulation compromise should be challenged with an anticholinergic agent such as atropine. Administration should be responsive to the patient's condition, with increasing dosages and frequency as needed. Continued administration may be required in order to maintain a safe condition. Where adequate gas exchange is not achieved quickly, advanced airway placement and ventilation will be necessary.

Mnemonics and insights

As a rule of thumb, any patient with an altered level of consciousness and excessive output from many orifices should be suspected of a possible cholinergic crisis. The mnemonic SLUDGE or DUMBELS is useful for remembering muscarinic signs and symptoms, whilst MTWTF is useful for nicotinic signs and symptoms (see Table 17.2).

Anticholinergic toxidrome

Anticholinergics are typically associated with 'anti' medicines. The symptomatology is largely the opposite of

TABLE 17.2 Mnemonics for cholinergic toxidrome.

Muscarinic symptoms		Nicotinic symptoms
S – Salivation	D – Diarrhoea	M – Muscle cramps
L – Lacrimation	U – Urinary incontinence	T – Tachycardia
U – Urinary incontinence	M – Miosis	W – Weakness
D – Diarrhoea	B – Bronchospasm	T – Twitching
G – Gastrointestinal upset	E – Emesis	F – Fasciculations
E – Emesis	L – Lacrimation	
	S – Salivation	

cholinergics, meaning if you can remember one the other is simply the opposite. Take extra care when treating patients with chemical restraints, as often these agents can worsen the situation.

Pharmacology

Anticholinergic agents work by competitively blocking central and peripheral cholinergic receptors. The outcome of this is disproportionate sympathetic activity to parasympathetic activity and therefore sympathetic signs.

Signs and symptoms

- *Central:* restlessness, fluctuating mental status, confusion, hallucinations, and fidgeting.
- *Peripheral:* **mydriasis,** dry mucous membranes, tachycardia, flushing of the skin, hyperthermia, urinary retention, and decreased gut motility.

Possible agents

Key agents involved in anticholinergic syndromes are antiparkinsonian drugs, antihistamines, antidepressants, antipsychotics, anticonvulsants, antispasmodics, and some mushrooms.

Treatments

Key treatments for anticholinergic syndromes include treating seizures, correcting hypoglycaemia, and correcting hyperthermia. Maintenance of staff, public, and patient safety is paramount during the period of delirium. It is important to treat delirium and agitation with agents that will not add to the anticholinergic effect, such as haloperidol or droperidol. Instead, benzodiazepines are key to management.

Mnemonics and insights

A simple way to remember anticholinergic symptoms is a simple Alice in Wonderland poem:

Hot as a hair
Hyperthermic
Dry as a bone
Dry membranes/urinary retention
Blind as a bat
Mydriasis
Red as a beet
Flushing of the skin
Mad as a hatter
Agitation/delirium

Another simple phrase to remember is:

'Can't see, can't pee, can't sit, can't poo'.

Opioid toxidrome

Opioids are analgesics that are widely used and abused. Whilst identifying opioid toxicity in a patient on arrival may seem easy, it is often harder to detect approaching opioid toxicity when the clinician is administering analgesics such as fentanyl or morphine. Always be vigilant for the signs and symptoms.

Pharmacology

Opiates bind to four subtypes of opioid receptors with the intention of providing analgesia to moderate to severe pain. In opioid-naive patients or when taken in excess, they can cause depression of the central nervous system.

Signs and symptoms

Signs and symptoms include decreased mentation, euphoria, sedation, apnoea/respiratory depression, miosis, decreased heart rate, decreased blood pressure, and decreased gut motility.

Possible agents

Agents include short- and long-release oral opioids, over-the-counter combined opioids, intravenous opioids, inhaled opioids, and heroin.

Treatments

Key treatments for opiate overdose are supportive. Maintaining a patent airway and adequate ventilation are paramount in treating opiate overdoses. The competitive opioid receptor antagonist naloxone can be administered to reverse the effects of opioid overdose. Naloxone works by having a higher affinity to opioid receptors than the overdose substance without the negative side effects. Care must be taken where the biological lifespan of the overdose lasts longer than the relatively short duration of action of naloxone (thirty to sixty minutes) because patients may become re-narcotised as the substance rebinds to opiate receptors. For this reason it is not appropriate for administration without transport to an appropriate facility for close observation. Further, the effect of clearing the opioid receptors of someone dependent on opiates is immediate progression to withdrawal. This may include vomiting, diarrhoea, aggression, and seizures.

Mnemonics and insights

The signs and symptoms of opioid overdose are quite vague and vary depending on the dose and agent. Any patient with pinpoint pupils, altered level of consciousness, and signs of respiratory depression should have opioid overdose considered as a differential diagnosis.

Sedative toxidrome

The sedative toxidrome is very similar in presentation to the opioid toxidrome. The distinction is made due to the differences in treatment in each toxidrome, necessitating the ability to distinguish between the two. Sedative toxidrome can sometimes also be referred to as sedative-hypnotic toxidrome.

Pharmacology

The pharmacology of sedative agents varies based on what class of drug is causing the sedation. Typically, sedatives depress the reticular activating system (RAS) by affecting gamma-aminobutyric acid (GABA) neurotransmitter activity in a variety of ways.

Signs and symptoms

The signs and symptoms include decreased mentation, sedation, ataxia, stupor, apnoea/respiratory depression, coma, nystagmus, diplopia, lack of coordination, and flaccidity.

Possible agents

Possible agents for sedative overdoses are benzodiazepines, barbiturates, GHB/Fantasy, baclofen, and clonidine.

Treatments

Supportive care is paramount in sedative overdose. Maintaining a patent airway and adequate ventilation are primary measures for treating sedative overdose. Enhanced elimination is possible for some sedatives in the hospital setting; however, there is a limited range of available treatments in the OOH setting at present. Flumazenil has previously been advocated as a naloxone equivalent for benzodiazepines, although its significant risk of inducing seizures usually means that its costs are greater than its benefits (Sivilotti 2015). Where the benzodiazepine overdose is induced by the clinician and benzodiazepine withdrawal risk is minimal, there is some scope for its use.

Mnemonics and insights

Whilst most sedatives are anticonvulsant, GHB lowers the seizure threshold and may induce paradoxical seizures in patients in overdose. Care should be taken to monitor for seizure activity in such patients.

Sympathomimetic toxidrome

Most sympathomimetic overdoses will be recreationally abused stimulants. Take care to observe for signs of worsening toxicity or development of further toxic signs such as serotonin syndrome.

Pharmacology

Sympathomimetic drugs are mimics of sympathetic adrenergic neurotransmitters. They work by agonising alpha and beta receptors, creating excessive sympathetic drive.

Signs and symptoms

The general toxidrome of sympathomimetics is very similar to an anticholinergic toxidrome. The characteristic hyperactive bowel sounds and sweating of sympathomimetics, in contrast to the hypoactive bowel sounds and dry skin of anticholinergics, are used to differentiate them.

Other signs and symptoms are agitation, paranoia, delusions, hyperreflexia, seizures, mydriasis, tachycardia, hypertension, diaphoresis, piloerection, sweating, hyperthermia, and increased gut motility.

Possible agents

Agents include amphetamines, cocaine, stimulants, and monoamine oxidase inhibitors (MAO-Is).

Treatments

Treatment of sympathomimetic toxicity is centred around responding to the symptoms of the toxin and preventing seizure. Cooling hyperthermia with non-invasive methods or cool intravenous fluid and providing a low-stimulus environment are primary responses. Like anticholinergic toxicity, staff, public, and patient safety becomes an issue in sympathomimetic toxicity. Benzodiazepines and/or antipsychotics may be required to manage delirium in a safe manner. Where tachycardia or hypertension becomes an issue, it is best to titrate intravenous benzodiazepines to effect. In general, it is best to avoid beta blockers due to a risk of unopposed alpha stimulation, causing dangerous paradoxical hypertension.

Mnemonics and insights

One way to remember the sympathomimetic toxidrome is using the mnemonic GET SMASHD. The first letter of each element is imperative for differentiating sympathomimetic toxicity from anticholinergic toxicity:

G - Gut sounds increased
E - Erection
T - Tachycardia
S - Sweats
M - Mydriasis
A - Agitation
S - Seizures
H - Hyperthermic, hypertensive
D - Delusional

Hallucinogenic toxidrome

There are many drugs or medications with hallucinogenic effects, some of the most commonly used are illicit in many parts of the world. The hallucinogenic effect of drugs and medications is often desired by the individual taking the medication. However, it can also be an unwanted side-effect or manifest in a way that is undesirable for the individual.

Signs and symptoms

Hallucinogenic agents can produce a wide variety of effects that may differ between each individual. These include numbness, disorientation, loss of coordination, nausea and vomiting, paranoia, visual and auditory hallucinations, anxiety, agitation, and aggression. Some people may experience an increase in their heart rate and respiratory rate, whilst others may experience a decrease. The skin may also present as hot or flushed.

The effects of the hallucinogenic toxidrome can be exacerbated by other medications, especially alcohol. These patients are also at risk of physical injury, which needs to be considered when assessing the safety risk that these individuals pose to themselves.

Possible agents

Many hallucinogenic drugs are illicit in parts of the world and include marijuana, LSD, psilocybin and mescaline (found in some mushrooms). Some other prescribed drugs with a dissociative effect can also present with hallucinogenic effects including PCP, ketamine, and occasionally morphine.

Treatments

The most effective treatment for hallucinogenic toxidrome is time and reassurance. Waiting for the body to metabolise the substance and have the effects diminish over time is common, however, the safety of the individual needs to be ensured during this time. De-escalation techniques are the first line of management with the removal of additional external stimuli being effective as well. Occasionally physical or chemical restraint may be required if attempts at de-escalation have been unsuccessful.

Insights

Not all individuals with hallucinations will be the result of hallucinogenic toxidrome. Some illnesses such as schizophrenia or post-traumatic stress disorder may manifest with hallucinogenic symptoms with the presence of any substance use or abuse.

Serotonin syndrome

Serotonin syndrome occurs when serotonin builds up in the blood and varies from mild to critical. It overlaps significantly with other toxidromes and, as always with toxicology, a worst-case scenario mindset will prevent patients being undertreated or under prioritised.

Aetiology

Serotonin syndrome is an excess of central nervous system serotonin secondary to overagonism of serotonergic receptors. It is usually associated with ingestion of multiple serotonergic agents, although it can be caused by single-agent ingestion.

Signs and symptoms

Signs and symptoms include agitation, aggression, seizures, mydriasis, increased reflexes, hyperthermia, clonus, tremor, sweating, and diarrhoea.

Possible agents

Agents that precipitate serotonin syndrome are vast and diverse; however, all are serotonergic in some way. These agents include selective serotonin reuptake inhibitors (SSRI), ecstasy (methylenedioxymethamphetamine, MDMA), monoamine oxidase inhibitors (MAOI), cocaine, tramadol, antiemetics, serotonin noradrenaline reuptake inhibitors (SNRI), St John's wort, TCAs, amphetamines, and pethidine.

Treatments

The first response to serotonin syndrome should be to discontinue the agent(s) causing excess serotonin. Agitation may need to be managed with benzodiazepines. Butyrophenones (haloperidol/droperidol) should be avoided, as their anticholinergic properties may reduce the body's ability to regulate hyperthermia. Responding to hyperthermia using active cooling may be necessary. If the patient's condition warrants, further measures such as serotonin antagonists, intubation, and paralysis may be required. Opiates such as fentanyl or morphine can exacerbate the effects of serotonin syndrome; therefore administration of fentanyl and morphine should be avoided when suspecting serotonin syndrome (Scotton 2019).

Mnemonics and insights

One tool that has been validated as a simple, accurate identifier of serotonin syndrome is the Hunter criteria. To be positive for serotonin syndrome according to the Hunter criteria, the patient must have ingested a serotonergic agent and have at least *one* of the following:

- Spontaneous clonus.
- Inducible clonus *plus* agitation or diaphoresis.
- Ocular clonus *plus* agitation or diaphoresis.
- Tremor *plus* hyperreflexia.
- Hypertonia *plus* temperature above 38 °C *plus* ocular clonus or inducible clonus.

Malignant hyperthermia

Malignant hyperthermia is rare but life threatening. It is only relevant to paramedic practice due to the use of **inhaled anaesthetics** for acute pain. The best treatment for malignant hyperthermia is prevention. Taking a proper history before administration can determine whether someone may be safer receiving alternative modes of analgesia. Avoid complacency and ask for a familial history first.

Aetiology

Whilst little is known about the exact pathophysiology of malignant hyperthermia, it is understood that it is caused by continuous skeletal muscle activation due to a genetic condition. People susceptible to malignant hyperthermia have been found to have abnormal skeletal muscle receptors. When under the influence of certain anaesthetic agents, susceptible patients may accumulate calcium around skeletal muscle receptors, leading to cellular hypermetabolism, rhabdomyolysis, acidosis, and anaerobic metabolism.

Signs and symptoms

- *Early:* tachypnoea, tachycardia, muscle rigidity, spasms aches/cramps with no explanation.
- *Late:* extreme hyperthermia (sometimes >40 °C), dark urine.

Possible agents

Possible agents are inhaled anaesthetics, and the key perpetrators OOH are methoxyflurane (green whistle/penthrox) and depolarising muscle relaxants (succinylcholine).

Treatments

Key treatments for malignant hyperthermia are active cooling and commencing high-flow oxygen therapy, removing the offending agents, and removing the patient from hot environments. Ice packs should be applied in the axilla and groin along with cool saline intravenously.

Methoxyflurane and malignant hyperthermia

Before administering methoxyflurane, ensure that the patient is asked about familial cases of malignant hyperthermia. Parents, siblings, and children with a history of malignant hyperthermia impose a 50% risk of malignant hyperthermia, whilst other close relatives impose a 25% risk. Other analgesics will generally be more appropriate for patients with a family history due to the significant risk of malignant hyperthermia.

Whilst the condition is called malignant *hyperthermia*, hyperthermia is a late sign. By having a baseline set of observations along with an assessment of muscle tone, the paramedic can identify early signs that may be suspicious of malignant hyperthermia and escalate care appropriately.

Neuroleptic malignant syndrome

Neuroleptic malignant syndrome is a serious reaction to antipsychotic medication. Wherever there has been a change in dose or new agent started, there lies a risk. 'Lead pipe rigidity' is a hallmark sign.

Aetiology

Neuroleptic malignant syndrome is poorly understood, and most current theories do not fully explain the entire symptomatology. The most comprehensive explanation to date is that the syndrome involves central dopamine receptor blockade in the hypothalamus, leading to dysautonomia.

Signs and symptoms

Signs and symptoms include tachycardia, confusion, agitation, labile blood pressure, muscle rigidity ('lead pipe rigidity'), hyperthermia, sweating, and bradykinesia.

Possible agents

Agents include neuroleptics, including typical and atypical antipsychotics as well as some antiemetics. First-generation (typical) antipsychotics are most likely. The syndrome also occurs on withdrawal of antiparkinsonian drugs.

Treatments

Treatment of neuroleptic malignant syndrome should start with ceasing the offended agent. Supportive care should be followed. Active cooling may be necessary and in this case ice packs should be applied in the axilla and groin, along with cool saline intravenously. Care should be taken to maintain normotension whilst being mindful of the lability of blood pressure in neuroleptic malignant syndrome. If treatment of agitation is necessary, benzodiazepines are first-line treatments, whilst antipsychotics should be avoided.

Mnemonics and insights

The key to distinguishing neuroleptic malignant syndrome from other toxicities is 'lead pipe' muscle rigidity. Table 17.3 and Figure 17.2 provide quick reference guides to toxidromes.

TABLE 17.3 Toxidrome quick guide.

	Essential			Useful			
	Mental Status	Eyes	Lungs and Skin	Vitals	Bowels	Reflexes	Tone
Cholinergic	Normal	Miosis	Wet	Stable	Increased	Normal/ Reduced	Fasciculations
Anticholinergic	Agitated	Mydriasis	Dry	Increased	Reduced	Normal	Reduced (late)
Sedative	Lethargic	Normal	Dry	Reduced	Reduced	Reduced	Reduced
Opioid	Lethargic	Miosis	Dry	Reduced	Reduced	Normal	Normal
Sympathomimetic	Agitated	Mydriasis	Wet	Increased	Increased	Increased	Normal
Serotonin syndrome	Agitated	Mydriasis	Wet	Increased	Increased	Lower > upper	Increased
Neuroleptic malignant syndrome	Agitation	Normal	Wet	Increased	Normal	Reduced	Lead pipe rigidity
Malignant hyperthermia	Agitation	Normal	Wet	Increased	Normal	Reduced	Normal/rigidity

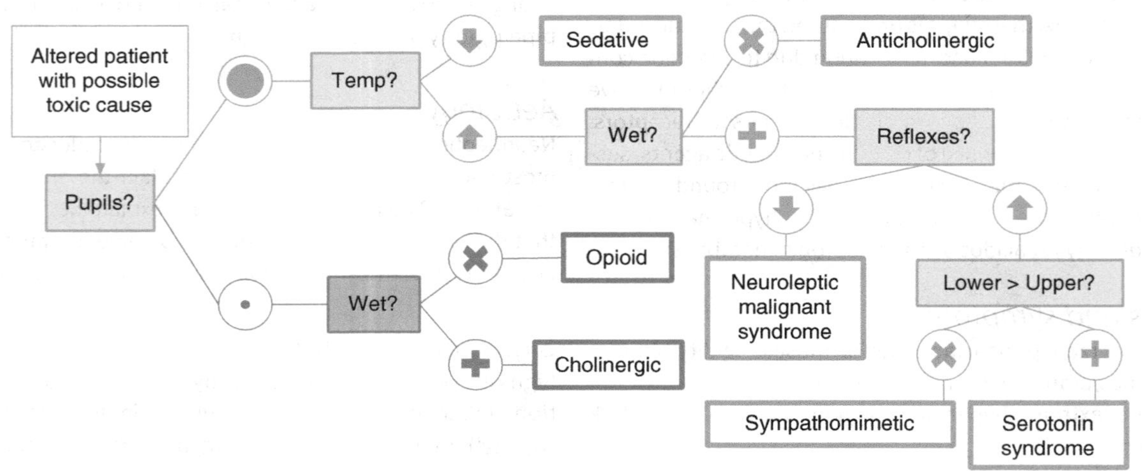

FIGURE 17.2 Toxidrome flowchart.

Activities

Now review your learning by completing the learning activities in this chapter. The answers to these appear at the end of the book. Further self-test activities can be found at **www.wileyfundamentalseries.com/paramedic/3e.**

Test your knowledge

1. You are called to a music festival where the medical team have initiated treatment on a twenty-six-year-old male who was brought in by security for agitated behaviour that has persisted despite verbal de-escalation. The festival medics state on handover that he has become increasingly hypertensive, tachycardic, and hyperthermic, as well as delusional. Given the context of the presentation, what is the likely toxidrome he is facing? What agents could be to blame? Considering how illicit drugs could be brought into a music festival, how could you explain the escalating clinical symptoms?
2. As a military medic on tour, you are tasked to medivac as many patients as possible following an enemy attack on a village. On arrival at the village, you notice the local people are vomiting, sweating profusely, and have constricted pupils. As you triage victims, you see most patients are having difficulty breathing due to excessive secretions. What is the likely toxidrome affecting the victims? What kind of agent could be causing these symptoms? What would be the primary class and an example of an antidote to treat this toxidrome?
3. At 7:15 a.m. you are called to a residential aged care facility, where the nurse on shift gives handover on a seventy-six-year-old female who was found with an altered level of consciousness by a carer. She has a history of depression, Parkinson's disease, and hypertension. The nurse reports she has been reusing her medicines for the past three days, including her antiparkinsonian agent. She was increasingly agitated yesterday, and a dose of sublingual antipsychotic medication was administered to settle her for bed last night. On assessment the patient is tachycardic, hypertensive, febrile, and completely rigid. What syndrome could be implicated in this scenario? How would you manage this OOH?
4. You are called to a forty-seven-year-old female by her husband late at night. He awoke to find his wife in the living room, slumped on the couch with an empty bottle of wine next to her. He states this is a normal behaviour for his wife since her mother's funeral but became worried when he could not rouse her. On assessment she withdraws to pain but does not open her eyes or respond verbally. Her respiratory rate is 6, heart rate is 45, and you notice she is holding an empty packet of Valium. What toxidrome is she displaying? What assessments would help you gauge what level of supportive care she needs?
5. Whilst off duty at the beach, you notice the lifeguards are treating a twelve-year-old male by their buggy. The patient has a triangle bandage on his left arm and is holding a methoxyflurane whistle. He is flushed and inconsolable. His mother is trying to settle him whilst the lifeguards arrange a meeting place for an ambulance. You introduce yourself and clinical background to the lifeguards, and they reveal the boy was previously settled and has started getting worked up in the last ten minutes. The mother calls the lifeguards over because she feels the boy is becoming rigid, just like when his younger sister had a reaction to anaesthetic when having her tonsils out. Given this presentation, what toxic process could be occurring? What would your first action be? Thinking about the environment and resources likely to be available to you, what could you do to begin treating the toxidrome?

Activity 17.1

As a primer for situations you may face, consider the following scenarios, and note possible sequelae for these patients:

1. Seventy-five-year-old John has a history of myocardial infarction and ventricular fibrillation. He accidentally ingests his grandson's attention deficit hyperactivity disorder (ADHD) medication, dexamphetamine.
2. Four-year-old Isobel has found her nan's 'blister pack' of medications. She has consumed two-days-worth of medications, which include metoprolol, paracetamol, metformin, and frusemide.
3. Seventeen-year-old Tim tried gammahydroxybutyrate (GHB) at a friend's house for the first time. He felt unwell and decided to ride his bike home. He has a new bruise to his left temporal region.
4. Eighty-four-year-old Betty had a fall last week and suffered a skin tear on her right shin. She has cognitive disabilities and has accidentally taken 3g of aspirin.

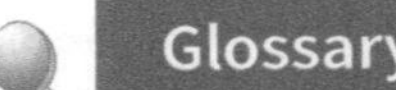

Glossary

Anticholinergic: Drugs that enhance the effects of the sympathetic nervous system by blocking acetylcholine.

Autonomic nervous system (ANS): The part of the body's nervous system that controls bodily functions not consciously directed, such as heart rate, breathing, and digestion.

Cholinergic: Drugs that either enhance the neurotransmitter acetylcholine or block its breakdown, causing increase in parasympathetic activity.

Inhaled anaesthetic: Anaesthetic agents used to induce anaesthesia, reduce pain, and calm patients. Most notably methoxyflurane (green whistle/penthrox) in the OOH setting. Key instigator of malignant hyperthermia.

Miosis: Constriction of the pupil.

Mydriasis: Dilation of the pupil.

Opioid: Analgesic and anaesthetic drugs that act on opioid receptors throughout the body to reduce pain, produce euphoria, and depress the central nervous system.

Parasympathetic nervous system (PNS): The branch of the ANS that handles 'rest-and-digest' functions. When activated it increases peristalsis, causes bronchoconstriction, moistens mucous membranes, and constricts pupils, amongst other effects.

Rhabdomyolysis: Systemic syndrome characterised by vomiting, confusion, darkened urine, and renal failure as a result of muscle breakdown due to sustained compression, excess muscle activation, and some medications.

Sedative: Broad category of drugs that can include barbiturates and benzodiazepines, with the intention of inducing sleep, central nervous system depression, or induced coma.

Sympathetic: The branch of the ANS that handles 'fight-or-flight' functions. When activated it increases heart rate, stops digestion, and causes bronchodilation, amongst other effects.

Sympathomimetic: A drug that mimics or instigates a sympathetic response, e.g. cocaine.

Torsades de Pointes: A form of ventricular tachycardia where the cardiac electrical pattern revolves around the centre of the heart. The pattern of the outer edges of the ECG trace looks like sine waves.

Toxidrome: A syndrome comprising a collection of signs and symptoms that can identify toxicity from specific groups of drugs.

References

Bar-Oz, B., Levichek, Z., and Koren, G. (2004). Medications that can be fatal for a toddler with one tablet or teaspoonful. *Pediatric Drugs* **6** (2): 123–126. doi: 10.2165/00148581-200406020-00005.

Cameron, P., Jelinek, G., and Kelly, A. (2015). *Textbook of Adult Emergency Medicine*. 4e. London: Elsevier Saunders.

Daly, F., Little, M., and Murray, L. (2006). A risk assessment based approach to the management of acute poisoning. *Emergency Medicine Journal* **23** (5): 396–399. doi: 10.1136/emj.2005.030312.

Jenkins, G. and Tortora, G.J. (2013). *Anatomy and Physiology: From Science to Life*. 3e. Chichester: Wiley.

Madeira, A., de Varennes, A., Abreu, M. et al. (2012). Tomato and parsley growth, arsenic uptake and translocation in a contaminated amended soil. *Journal of Geochemical Exploration* **123**: 114–121. doi: 10.1016/j.gexplo.2012.04.004.

Michael, J.B. and Sztajnkrycer, M.D. (2004). Deadly pediatric poisons: nine common agents that kill at low doses. *Emerg Med Clin North Am* **22** (4): 1019–1050. doi: 10.1016/j.emc.2004.05.004.

Mofenson, H. and Greensher, J. (1970). The nontoxic ingestion. *Pediatric Clinics of North America* **17** (3): 583–590. doi: 10.1016/s0031-3955(16)32453-1.

Sanello, A., Gausche-Hill, M., Mulkerin, W. et al. (2018). Altered mental status: Current evidence-based recommendations for prehospital care. *West J Emerg Med* **19** (3): 527–541. doi: 10.5811/westjem.2018.1.36559.

Scotton, W.J., Hill, L.J., Williams, A.C. et al. (2019). Serotonin syndrome: pathophysiology, clinical features, management, and potential future directions. *Inter J Tyyptophan Research* **12.** doi: 10.1177/1178646919873925.

Sivilotti, M. (2015). Flumazenil, naloxone and the 'coma cocktail'. *British Journal of Clinical Pharmacology* **81** (3): 428–436.

Sivilotti, M., Traub, S., and Grayzel, J. (2018). *UpToDate: Initial Management of the Critically Ill Adult with an Unknown Overdose.* 18e. Waltham, MA: Walters Kluwer.

The Royal Childrens Hospital Melbourne. (2017). Poisoning – acute guidelines for initial management. Available at: https://www.rch.org.au/ (accessed 10 August 2022).

Tilley, M. and Cotant, C. (2011). Acute water intoxication during military urine drug screening. *Military Medicine* **176** (4): 541–453. doi: 10.7205/milmed-d-10-00228.

Vajjah, P., Isbister, G., and Duffull, S. (2012). Introduction to pharmacokinetics in clinical toxicology. *Methods in Molecular Biology* **18** (4): 289–312. doi: 10.1007/978-1-62703-050-2_12.

Volle, R. (1963). Pharmacology of the autonomic nervous system. *Annual Review of Pharmacology* **3** (1): 129–152. doi: 10.1146/annurev.pa.03.040163.001021.

CHAPTER 18

Trauma

Charlie Gadd

Ambulance Paramedic, Ambulance Victoria, Victoria, Australia

Contents

LEARNING OUTCOMES

On completion of this chapter the reader will be able to:

- Identify the prevalence of minor and major trauma.
- Summarise the most common forms of trauma a paramedic is likely to encounter.
- Recognise key symptoms of minor and major trauma relating to the head, face, neck and back, abdomen, pelvis, and limbs.
- Reflect on the connection between external signs of trauma and the possibility of associated imperceptible injury.
- Identify key out-of-hospital treatments and interventions for each of these forms of trauma.

Case Study

You have been dispatched to a motorcycle versus car road traffic collision (RTC). On arrival you note the speed limit is 80 kmph, and the motorcyclist is lying still, with his motorbike approximately 50 metres further down the road. On closer assessment, the motorcyclist is conscious, pale, and has a Glasgow Coma Score (GCS) of 15. He has severe pain to his pelvic region and is finding it difficult to breathe. You suspect that he has a tension pneumothorax and a pelvic injury. You apply oxygen, decompress his chest, place a pelvic binder on and administer strong analgesia. He is extricated with full spinal immobilisation and is transported lights and sirens to the nearest major trauma centre (MTC).

Fundamentals of Paramedic Practice: A Systems Approach, Third Edition. Edited by Sam Willis and Ian Peate.

Companion website: www.wiley.com/go/willis/paramedic3e

Introduction

Paramedics attend many traumatic incidents across the span of their career, involving both minor and major trauma. This chapter will provide an overview of the trauma cases that a paramedic is most likely to encounter, including traumatic injury to the face, neck, back, abdomen, pelvis, and limbs.

Prehospital trauma bypass

Major trauma centres (MTCs) are hospitals that are staffed with specialist medical and nursing teams and equipped with high-level diagnostic and treatment equipment. These hospitals provide the highest level of trauma care possible and ensure that patients have the best chance of survival, rehabilitation, and quality of life. When attending trauma patients, paramedics must ensure they transport to the correct level of trauma care. Many ambulance services now include trauma time-critical guidelines and prehospital trauma bypass guidelines, to ensure there are minimal delays to lifesaving intervention and definitive care. Within the Victorian State Trauma System (VSTS) in Australia, patients meeting trauma time-critical criteria should be transported to the highest level of trauma service possible within sixty minutes (Ambulance Victoria 2023). This may include bypassing smaller regional trauma centres and increasing transport time to ensure that the patient receives specialist care. This enables the patient to receive the highest level of care as soon as possible and may remove the need for secondary transport. Within the VSTS, there are three types of time criticality. These are outlined in Table 18.1.

If the patient meets any of these criteria, the guidelines direct paramedics to bypass lower-level hospitals to get to the highest level of trauma service possible within 60 minutes.

A tool that can be used in addition to the trauma time-critical guidelines in patients with head injuries is the 5HEDS tool (Ambulance Victoria 2023). Patients with blunt force trauma to the head that are still GCS 13–15, with or without loss of consciousness or amnesia, can be categorised as having a serious blunt force head injury if they meet the following criteria:

- Any loss of consciousness exceeding 5 minutes
- Head or skull fracture
- Emesis more than once
- Neurological deficits
- Seizure

TABLE 18.1 Three types of time criticality in the VSTS.

	Definition	Examples
Actual	Actual physiological distress as seen by deranged vital signs	HR >120 or <60 RR >30 or <10 Systolic BP <90 SPO2 <90 GCS <13 if 16 years old or over GCS <15 if <16 years old
Emergent	No physiological distress, but the patient has a pattern of injury that has a high likelihood of deteriorating into actual physiological distress	Penetrating injuries Serious blunt force injuries Major burns Crush injury Pelvic fractures Major fractures or dislocations
Potential	No physiological distress or pattern of injury, but the patient has a mechanism of injury that has the potential to deteriorate into actual physiological distress	Motor vehicle impact >60 kmph Motorcycle impact >30 kmph Explosion Fall over 3 m

Head injuries

Each year in the UK 1.4 million people attend accident and emergency (A&E) departments with a head injury, with males making up more than 70% of reported head injuries (NICE 2014). Around 90% of head injuries are classified as minor and are often caused by cuts and bruises (NICE 2014). Less than 0.2% prove to be fatal. Major injuries can include a fractured skull or intracranial haemorrhage, which requires intensive treatment and can be potentially life threatening.

Minor head injuries

Minor head injuries do not cause any long-term damage to the brain, a common example being scalp wounds, which may or may not lead to concussion, depending on the mechanism of injury (MOI). Minor head injuries are common in people of all ages and can be caused by the following mechanisms:

- **Falls** – estimated as causing 22–43% of minor head injuries.
- **RTCs** – estimated as causing 25% of minor head injuries.
- **Assaults** – estimated as causing 30–50% of all minor head injuries (NHS Choices 2015).

Injuries to the scalp often look worse than they actually are. For example, a small laceration to the skin of the highly vascular tissues of the scalp may bleed profusely, even when the wound is less than 1 cm long.

Scalp injuries generally stop bleeding with a dressing and firm pressure to the site. Even though the head injury may appear minor, a full neurological assessment must be performed in order to confirm this.

Major head injuries

In the UK, the largest cause of major head injuries is RTCs. Other causes include falls, accidents, and assaults (NHS Choices 2015). Serious injuries to the head often cause internal damage with no signs of external injury, making them more difficult to assess. It is important for the paramedic to utilise all the information available when assessing head-injured patients. Look specifically at the patient's level of consciousness, patients with GCS of 9–12 or <8 are the majority of fatalities from a major head injury (NICE 2014). Establish if high-impact forces were involved in the injury. Where the patient has been involved in an RTC, check for a bullseye in the vehicle windscreen – a clear sign that the patient's head has collided with the glass.

Major head injuries can also elicit a systemic (whole-body) response due to the control centres of the brain being either directly or indirectly involved. Systematic responses can be present in many head-injured patients, including those with skull fractures, base-of-skull fractures, subdural haematomas, and subarachnoid haemorrhage.

In major head trauma patients with systemic responses, we have management targets to aim for to reduce the chance of secondary injury. Secondary injuries evolve over hours to days after the primary incident, and can involve hypoxia, ischaemia, cerebral oedema, hypotension, or hypertension. As a result, we should aim for a systolic blood pressure of 100–120 mmHg, oxygen saturations >95%, and end tidal carbon dioxide of 30–35 mmHg, whilst managing any other complications such as seizures or hypoglycaemia.

Skull fracture

Skull fractures occur with direct, blunt, and penetrating trauma to the skull, for example, in RTCs, sporting injuries, or assaults. A skull fracture can occur anywhere around the cranium and can be a simple fracture with only one break or a multiple fracture with depressed sections of skull that could damage the brain. A simple fracture that does not involve the brain may be difficult to spot. You may find localised bruising and a small amount of bleeding, but body systems will not be affected. Skull fractures are generally caused by high-impact blunt forces and are often not apparent without in-hospital investigations (e.g. X-ray and computerised tomography [CT] scan).

Base-of-skull fracture

The base of the skull comprises a network of bones located slightly above and behind the nasal cavity that surround, protect, and support the brain. Base-of-skull injuries generally occur with blunt force trauma to the face or to the sides of the skull. As these injuries are associated with high-impact forces, patients will usually present with additional injuries and may be unconscious. There are many indicators that can help form a provisional diagnosis, such as:

- History of trauma to the head or face.
- Major bruising behind the ears (late sign).

- Bruising around both eyes ('Battle's sign'; late sign).
- Bleeding from the ears or nose with cerebrospinal fluid (CSF) present. CSF gives the blood a glossy look and does not mix with the blood but instead separates from it.

These patients are often seriously ill and require rapid packaging and transport. Diagnosis of a base-of-skull fracture is usually by signs and symptoms; they are difficult to identify using medical imaging (Morgan 1999), making the importance of history taking and assessment paramount.

Subdural haemorrhage

Also known as a subdural haematoma, a subdural haemorrhage is a collection of slow-moving blood below the inner layer of the **dura mater,** which forms around the surface of the brain. Often the result of trauma and sometimes forming spontaneously, these injuries can be slow in progression and patients may appear without symptoms initially (Meagher and Young 2013). The increasing pressure on the brain can lead to:

- Confusion
- Agitation
- Slurred speech

Any patient presenting with these symptoms or other neurological deficiencies (such as poor balance, nausea, or lack of coordination) that are of new onset since a trauma requires transport to hospital to ensure that appropriate scans are completed, and if necessary, surgery performed to repair the bleed.

Subarachnoid haemorrhage

Subarachnoid haemorrhage is bleeding between the brain surface and the fine membranes that surround it. This is generally fast-flowing blood and patients will often present with decreased levels of consciousness, nausea, seizures, and confusion. In this type of injury blood can form rapidly within the **subarachnoid space** and force the brain downwards. This pushes the cerebrum into the brain stem and the body's control centres. It can therefore produce a rapid systemic reaction known as **Cushing's triad** (Figure 18.1), which is a clear sign of raised intracranial pressure (ICP). The three aspects of Cushing's triad are:

- Hypertension
- Bradycardia
- Altered breathing

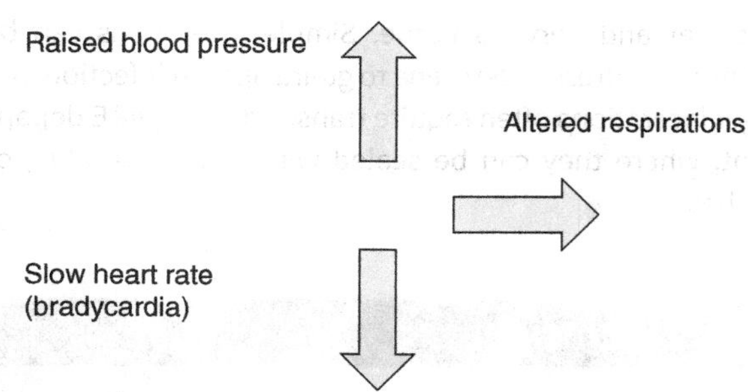

FIGURE 18.1 Diagrammatic representation of Cushing's triad.

Cushing's triad is a late sign of increased ICP within the skull, and the patient should be transported rapidly to the nearest trauma unit for assessment.

Practice insight

When managing a patient with a significant head injury, *listen carefully* to the bystanders. In all the noise and chaos it is easy to miss vital clues from those who were there when it happened. History taking is critical when managing a patient with a head injury, as it will not only help the paramedic decide what actions to take and how quickly to apply these – for example, to immobilise or not immobilise the patient – but will also allow the receiving hospital to take the necessary course of action, e.g. perform a CT scan.

Facial injuries

Paramedics will treat many facial injuries, ranging from simple lacerations to serious fractures with airway compromise. Injuries to the face include:

- Soft tissue lacerations.
- Temporary or permanent blindness due to trauma affecting the eyes.
- Nasal injuries including epistaxis (nosebleed) and septal deviation following a fight or other high-energy trauma.
- Le Fort fractures of the mid-face involving the mandible.
- Tooth damage and/or tooth loss.

Nasal and mandible fractures can impede the use and efficacy of airway adjuncts, making airway management a challenge in patients with facial injuries.

Laceration

Lacerations can present as small, simple cuts to the skin or deep, long wounds that involve damage to underlying muscular and nervous tissue. Simple lacerations can be cleaned and dressed on scene to guard against infection, but larger lacerations often require transport to the A&E department, where they can be sealed with steristrips, glue, or stitches.

> **Practice insight**
>
> Avoid applying a steristrip or glue to a wound if you have not had the appropriate training. Applying a steristrip is simple, but if the wound is not assessed accurately or cleaned well enough, it could become infected. In the case of an isolated minor laceration that requires assessing for minor intervention, refer such minor injuries to the most appropriate unit – such as general practice or urgent care centre – and avoid referring the patient to the A&E department.

Nasal injury

The nose is highly prone to sustaining trauma due to both its protuberance and the cartilaginous make-up of its main structure. When the nose sustains trauma, it often causes rupturing of internal blood vessels and lacerations. Fractures often cause the nose to be swollen and misshapen. Prehospital treatment of nasal injuries mainly concerns airway management, control of blood loss, neurological assessment, and pain management.

Facial fracture

Jaw fractures can be extremely painful and debilitating, reducing the patient's ability to move and clench the jaw. Fractures of the jaw often involve damage to the teeth and airway compromises due to blood loss or foreign-body airway obstructions. Most jaw fractures are relatively simple in nature and require minimal intervention, but more serious injuries such as a Le Fort fracture may require manual airway management or postural drainage to ensure that the airway is maintained. Fractures to the cheekbone or brow can cause compromises to the eye sockets and severely affect eyesight if mismanaged. Fractures may present with palpable pain, and localised swelling and bruising, which can mask damage to underlying structures through loss of palpable landmarks. As such, any facial injury displaying significant swelling or bruising should be treated as a potentially major injury and the patient transported to hospital for further assessment and treatment, until proven otherwise within A&E. Patients with significant pain, regardless of their condition, should have their pain managed using strong pain relief as soon as possible to make them comfortable.

> **Practice insight**
>
> When assessing for any fracture, use the mnemonic SLIPDUCT B: Swelling, Loss of movement, Irregularities, Pain, Deformity, Unnatural movement, Crepitus, Tenderness, Bruising.

Neck and back injuries

Patients with neck or back injuries must be assessed with the utmost care. Injuries in this region can range from strains of the musculature that supports the neck and back, creating nothing more than discomfort, to serious fractures with the potential for life-changing or life-threatening consequences. It is vital that the paramedic assesses and manages these patients correctly to prevent permanent disability or death.

Ambulance services have begun to apply commonsense approaches to spinal immobilisation in order to minimise harm to patients by putting them through lengthy and unnecessary spinal immobilisation procedures. A commonly used cervical spine (C-spine) clearance tool based on evidence-based criteria was formed by the National Emergency X-Radiography Utilisation Study (NEXUS; Ackland and Cameron 2012). As part of this guideline, patients who present with any of the following should receive spinal immobilisation:

- Midline cervical tenderness.
- Altered mental status.
- Focal neurological deficit.
- Evidence of drug or alcohol intoxication.
- Presence of other injury considered painful enough to distract from neck pain.

Spinal immobilisation

There remains an absence of strong evidence for the use of spinal immobilisation. The decision to provide spinal immobilisation should be based on clinical findings, patient history, by reading the scene (mechanisms of injury), knowledge of local guidelines, and best available evidence as to which is the best method for spinal immobilisation. Generally speaking, spinal immobilisation requires the following equipment:

- Cervical collar.
- Immobilisation device such as a rescue board, scoop stretcher, or ambulance trolley.

- Straps (stretcher or rescue board).
- Head blocks and tape.

Practice insight

The difference between spinal shock, neurogenic shock, and autonomic dysreflexia is important to understand, but can be a sticking point for many students.

Neurogenic shock occurs immediately after injury due to disruption of the sympathetic outflow tracts above T6 vertebrae. Often caused by fractures or dislocations within the spinal column, this leads to unopposed parasympathetic drive. As a result, the patient presents as warm and pink, hypotensive, with paradoxical bradycardia. This occurs quickly after initial injury and can last weeks.

Spinal shock also occurs immediately after injury, shock in this case refers to a transient period of depressed reflexes and loss of sensorimotor function below the level of injury. It is characterised by paralysis, loss of bowel and bladder control, and reduced reflex activity, and can last from days to months.

Autonomic dysreflexia is permanent but does not develop until late after the period of initial injury and spinal shock, when reflexes have recovered. Often occurring in injuries to T6 and above, unopposed reflex sympathetic innervation caused by noxious stimuli such as pain, causes an exaggerated vasoconstrictive response below the level of injury. A maximal vasodilatory parasympathetic response will then occur, but this cannot travel below the level of injury, and therefore cannot counteract the sympathetic drive. This leads to cool pale skin below the injury, flushed warm and pink skin above, with hypertension and bradycardia.

C-spine fractures

Fractures of the c-spine are potentially life threatening due to this area being the exit point for many important nerves. The nerves that exit the spinal cord along the neck are responsible for the control of the diaphragm and intercostal muscles, and therefore of respiration. If the cord is severed high in the neck, there is a high likelihood that the patient will not survive; if the fracture is lower in the spine, the patient can be left without mobility of the lower limbs. Fractures to the neck or back often present as central spinal pain that worsens on palpation of the cervical spinal processes (the protruding part of each vertebra). If any centralised neck or back pain is present, then the patient should undergo full spinal immobilisation to prevent further damage to the spinal cord, and pain management should always be administered. Fractures where the spinal cord has been damaged may also present with neurological changes such as:

- Loss/altered sensation when applying a light touch to the patient (spinal shock).
- Weakness or loss of movement (spinal shock).
- Peripheral vascular dilation below the injury site without rebound tachycardia (neurogenic shock).
- Tingling, burning, or numbness anywhere in the body (spinal shock).

Practice insight

Remember, nerves C3–C5 keep the diaphragm alive. Be extra cautious when suspecting a patient may have an injury to C3–C5. Even in the absence of neck pain, C-spine immobilisation may be necessary in cases in which there is a high MOI. Manual in-line stabilisation of the head can be achieved with your hands or knees and is important before a cervical collar can be placed on the patient.

Cervical collars and immobilisation

A number of ambulance services have moved towards immobilising the spine with soft collars, away from traditional hard or semi-rigid collars, due to reported cases of patient discomfort, tissue ulceration, time delays when measuring the collar, and the potential for increased ICP (Figure 18.2).

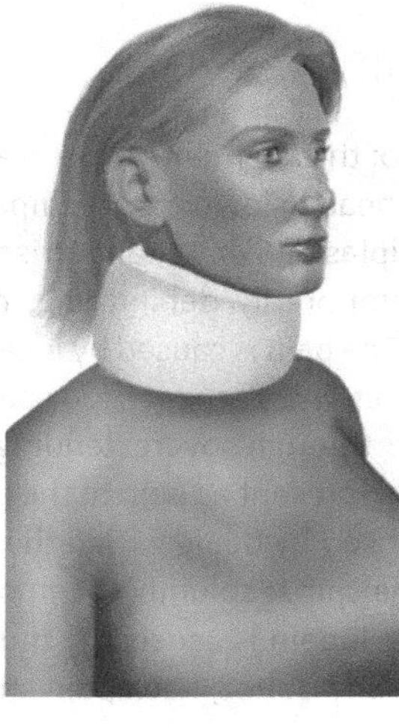

FIGURE 18.2 Application of a soft collar.

When making the decision to immobilise the patient, be sure to consider how long they will need to spend on a hard board. If the time spent on a rescue board is to exceed twenty minutes, consider using a vacuum mattress or immobilising straight onto the ambulance bed to minimise the possibility of pressure sores.

During extrication, patients may be able to self-extricate if they are conscious and cooperative, not intoxicated, and not prevented from doing so by injury (Ambulance Victoria 2023). In patients requiring specialist extrication such as entrapment in a motor vehicle, critical interventions should be given whilst fire and rescue work on extrication. Any patients with evidence of injury, or meeting trauma time-critical guidelines, should be considered time sensitive, requiring rapid extrication (Nutbeam et al. 2022). In this instance, extrication and transport to definitive care is a priority and clinical care should be limited to necessary critical interventions to expedite extrication time.

Historically, emergency services have focused on absolute movement minimisation, however, due to the rarity of spinal injuries and high frequency of other time-critical injuries, the goal of extrication should be to reduce time on scene and use gentle patient handling (Nutbeam et al. 2022).

Practice insight

If your patient receives full spinal immobilisation, consider giving an antiemetic (anti-sickness medication) for the transport to hospital if this is indicated by your ambulance service. If the patient vomits whilst they are lying flat and strapped to a board, there is an increased risk of airway obstruction and aspiration.

Muscular injuries

Muscular injuries of the neck can be incurred through rapid movement of the head in low-velocity impacts, sometimes referred to as 'whiplash' (Skinner and Driscoll 2013). These injuries, whilst temporarily debilitating, rarely have life-changing effects. The pain is caused by localised inflammation of muscle fibres within the neck or back muscles due to tearing/strain through overextending the muscles. These injuries often present as pain to the sides of the neck or back, characterised by being within the muscle with no involvement of the spinal column. It can often be difficult to determine if neck pain is caused by muscular or spinal involvement. If in any doubt, neck pain should be treated as a C-spine injury.

Practice insight

When palpating a patient's spine for tenderness, remember that there are large muscles around the neck area, so be sure to palpate the central vertebral column and not the musculature. Someone with a pulled muscle in the neck should not receive spinal immobilisation.

Chest injuries

Chest injuries caused by high-impact **velocity** can be very serious due to the life-sustaining nature of the contents of the chest. Chest injuries can range from rib fractures to sucking chest wounds or ruptured blood vessels. Due to the difficulties in assessing chest injuries in a prehospital environment, life-threatening injuries can often be misdiagnosed or mismanaged. Amongst the more serious chest injuries are:

- Rib fractures (due to associated complications)
- Flail segment
- Pneumothorax
- Tension pneumothorax
- Haemothorax
- Ruptured blood vessels

Rib fractures

A rib fracture on its own is not considered an emergency. As a stable rib fracture will not be likely to cause any damage to underlying tissues, these are mainly treated with pain management, support, and rest. Rib fractures often present with localised bruising and pain that worsens on inspiration, movement, and palpation. If a patient presents with a rib fracture as well as other signs, such as shortness of breath, hypoxia, or diminished breath sounds on the affected side, suspect damage to the underlying lung.

Flail segment

Flail segment is defined as a fracture of two or more ribs in two or more places. This injury can present with abnormal chest movement (a seemingly floating segment of chest wall that moves separately to surrounding areas), shortness of breath, and acute pain. In the prehospital setting it should be considered a serious injury, with airway support and pain relief being applied promptly.

Pneumothorax

A pneumothorax is an abnormal build-up of air in the pleural space (between the lung and the chest wall). There are many different types, including:

- Simple pneumothorax
- Open pneumothorax
- Tension pneumothorax
- Haemo-pneumothorax

A pneumothorax can be caused by underlying pathologies (such as a severe asthma attack) or by surgical or traumatic injuries such as a flail segment or penetrative injury. A *simple pneumothorax* may present with shortness of breath, mild pain, and minimally reduced air entry and hyper-resonance on the affected side. A simple pneumothorax does not require needle thoracocentesis (needle chest decompression).

A *tension pneumothorax* is a severe life-threatening emergency, and this patient can rapidly deteriorate. A tension pneumothorax occurs when air collects within the **potential space** between the visceral and parietal pleura, usually due to penetrating trauma to the chest or through the progression of a simple pneumothorax. During a tension pneumothorax, inhaled air does not escape through the normal mechanisms of respiration (through the trachea via exhalation) but remains within the potential space due to a skin flap that prevents exhalation. The collection of air within the potential space starts to increase the pressure exerted onto the lung. As a result, the lung collapses and can shift the mediastinum to the opposite side. This will compromise respiration and blood flow. The most common symptoms include chest pain and respiratory distress, with decreased air entry and hyper-resonance on the side of the pneumothorax. The prehospital treatment of this injury is primarily respiratory support, needle thoracocentesis (Figure 18.3), chest

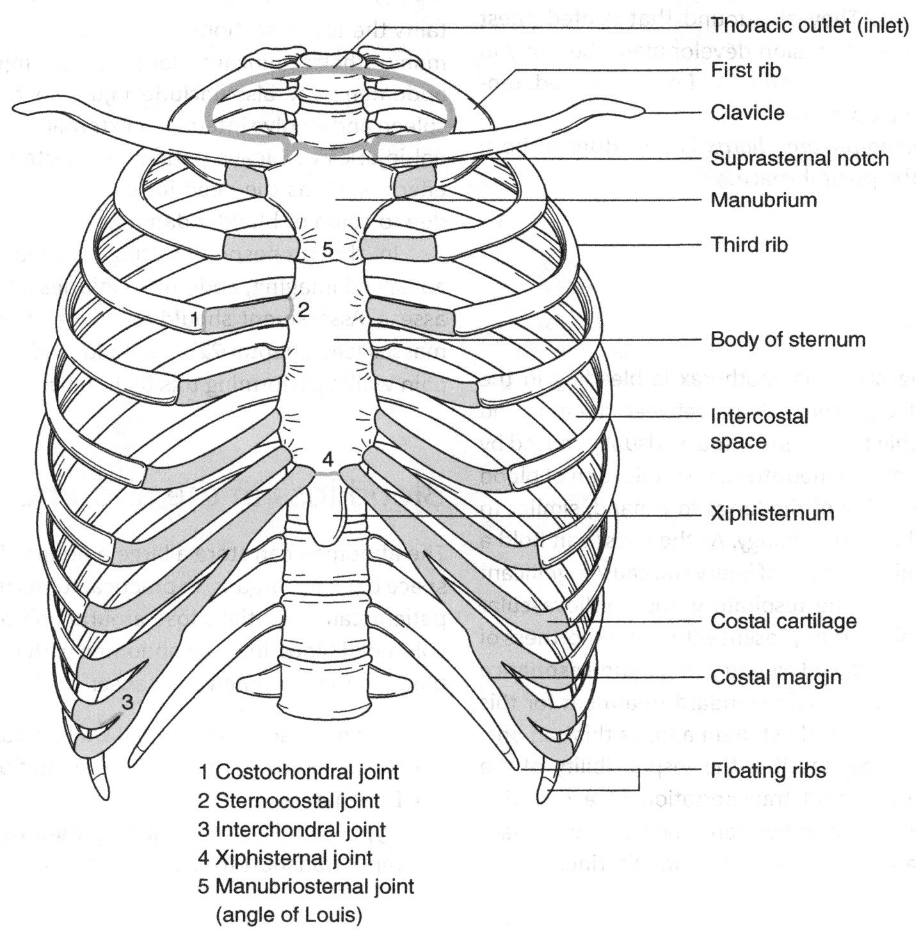

FIGURE 18.3 Needle thoracocentesis. Source: Gregory and Mursell 2010 (p. 277, Figure 14.1 Sternal landmarks for needle thoracentesis).

decompression, and rapid transportation to an A&E department. In-hospital treatment includes a surgical chest drain or further surgical interventions.

An *open pneumothorax* occurs in any situation where there is a hole in the chest wall and air enters the pleural space through the open hole in the chest instead of through the usual route. Specific treatment for this condition is not conclusive, with some ambulance services treating with a non-occlusive dressing, whilst others apply occlusive three-sided or vented dressings. Theoretically, three-sided occlusive or vented dressings allow air to escape during exhalation, but will occlude the open wound during inhalation, reducing the chance of a tension developing. However, the lungs still have a high chance of tensioning, especially if the dressing becomes clotted with blood, or poorly adheres to the skin (Butler et al. 2013). In this case, there should still be continual monitoring for tensioning, and either decompression via needle/finger, or burping of the dressing.

In addition, the 2013 Tactical Combat Casualty Care guidelines state there is no evidence for or against the use of improvised three-sided dressings, but they may be time consuming to apply. They also found that vented chest seals reduce the risk of tension development, but only in animal models, and that regardless of dressing used, tensions may still develop (Butler et al. 2013).

Finally, a *haemo-pneumothorax* is a mixture of both blood and air in the pleural space.

Haemothorax

As the name suggests, a haemothorax is bleeding in the thorax or chest. It is a haemorrhage between the lung and the chest wall, within the potential space. Usually caused by trauma (either blunt or penetrative), this collection of blood can decrease the ability of the lungs to expand, similar to tension pneumothorax physiology. As the chest can hold a large amount of fluid, this type of injury can cause significant compromises to both the respiratory and cardiovascular systems. This condition may present with acute shortness of breath, severe pain, reduced air entry, and **hypo-resonance** on the affected side. The gold standard treatment for this type of injury is a surgical chest drain and, as this can only be enacted within hospital, it is the responsibility of the paramedic to ensure rapid transportation to a receiving centre and to provide supportive care, such as airway management, pain management, and close monitoring.

Ruptured blood vessel

The chest contains many important blood vessels, including the aorta and pulmonary veins. In high-velocity trauma these vessels can be highly vulnerable to tearing or rupturing; vast internal bleeding can occur in a short time and death can follow almost instantly. The only way the paramedic will know this is happening is through physical signs and symptoms of shock. Therefore, treatment focuses around managing ABCs (airway, breathing, circulation), including arresting any external haemorrhage and providing fluid and oxygen therapy, in accordance with current guidelines.

Abdominal injuries

Abdominal injuries due to high-velocity trauma have the potential to be fatal due to the density and make-up of the organs within the abdominal cavity. The abdomen contains the lower sections of the aorta and vena cava, and many other significant blood vessels. Injuries within the abdomen may also include injury to the liver and the spleen and involve internal or external blood loss. Abdominal injuries can leave patients subjected to life-changing effects such as the need for colostomy bags or catheters due to colon or bladder damage.

In the prehospital setting, without the benefit of advanced imaging, abdominal injuries are very difficult to assess. Assessment should focus mainly on palpation for masses (see Chapter 22), free fluid, and the assessment of pain whilst performing this technique.

Blood loss in the abdomen

The abdomen can store a large amount of fluid in the free space between organs. In practical terms this means that a patient can potentially lose around half of the circulating volume of blood into the abdomen with relative ease. Free blood in the abdomen can cause:

- An almost solid abdominal wall on palpation.
- Reduced bowel sounds on auscultation.
- Extreme pain.
- Hypovolemic shock requiring **fluid replacement** with rapid transport to the nearest MTC.

Practice insight

The aggressive approach to fluid resuscitation in haemorrhagic hypovolaemia patients is outdated and harmful for patients. Resuscitation with blood products is the gold standard, however, this is not often achievable prehospitally. As a result, crystalloids such as normal saline are often used.

Poor outcomes of fluid resuscitation using crystalloids include:

- Coagulopathy (dilutional), metabolic acidosis, hypothermia (lethal triad of death in trauma) (Ramesh et al. 2019).
- Disruption of blood clots due to increased blood pressure (Ramesh et al. 2019).
- Dilutional anaemia.

As a result, the minimal amount of crystalloid fluid administration should be given to maintain perfusion to the brain and heart. This is referred to as permissive hypotension.

Most guidelines advocate for a degree of hypotension in patients with haemorrhagic hypovolaemia resulting from trauma, gastrointestinal haemorrhage, or aortic rupture. Blood pressure, conscious state, and peripheral pulses are often used to guide the amount of fluid given (Ambulance Victoria 2023).

Open abdominal injury

Some abdominal injuries involve an open cavity in the abdomen, usually caused by penetrating trauma such as stab or slicing wounds. These injuries leave the abdomen exposed to major risk of infection. The rupture of the **peritoneal membrane** and the muscle tissues that ensure that the organs remain in place can allow the intestines to protrude through the wound. Any organs that protrude outside the abdominal cavity should be kept moist and covered by either clingfilm or a blast dressing to ensure that minimal damage is caused. Close monitoring, pain management, and immediate transport to a MTC are required.

Pelvic injuries

The pelvis is a ring-like structure of bone that supports standing, walking, and most simple movements. Pelvic injuries are amongst the most life-threatening injuries and must be assessed and handled carefully. Many major blood vessels run through or around the pelvis, and genito-urinary organs are also contained within and around this structure. Surgical interventions are often required in the case of pelvic fractures such as 'open-book' fractures and hip dislocations. Historically, paramedics were taught to 'spring the pelvis' during an assessment to check for pain and movement, but this practice is now outdated. Signs of a fractured pelvis are sought instead, which include:

- Establishing the MOI.
- Urinary incontinence.
- Bleeding (including from the urethra, vagina, or rectum).
- Deformity.
- Neurological and vascular deficits in the lower limbs.
- The patient will be heavily guarding the area.
- Other lower limb injuries such as a fractured femur.
- Pelvic asymmetry or limb shortening.

Splinting the pelvis with a pelvic binder has been shown to reduce pelvic fractures and provide stabilisation (Clarke and Stewart 2013), making it more comfortable for the patient and minimising any further damage. However, it is important to do so with the minimal amount of movement possible, and the strongest pain relief will be required prior to applying the device. Splinting is also an extremely important haemorrhage control device. Multiple litres of blood can be lost into the pelvic and retroperitoneal space without significant tamponading ability (Lee and Porter 2007). As a result, reducing the fracture will stabilise the bones, and prevent further disruption of clots during movement (Lee and Porter 2007).

Open-book pelvic fracture

An open-book fracture is usually caused by high-velocity trauma to the front of the pelvis in the pubic region, as seen in a motorcycle accident. The pelvis is separated at both the front and the back, and this may cause one or both sides of the pelvis to open 'like a book' at the front. Patients with this injury may present with external rotation of the legs, extreme pain, and also life-threatening internal bleeding. Other significant injuries should also be expected, and the patient will require rapid packaging and transport. The pelvis will require stabilising using a pelvic splint. Intravenous (IV) fluid in the presence of shock should be administered to maintain radial pulses, and strong pain relief will also be required. This patient should receive full spinal immobilisation.

Hip dislocation

Hip dislocation occurs when the ball-shaped head of the femur comes out of the cup-shaped acetabulum. This injury can often present in a similar way to a neck-of-femur fracture (see next section), with shortening and rotation of the leg on the affected side and pain in the region of the hip joint. It may be possible to feel deformity in the area of the joint, although this is not always present. Paramedic intervention should focus on immobilising the affected leg in the same way as with a neck-of-femur (NOF) fracture and pain management, preferably with the strongest drug available.

Neck-of-femur fracture

The NOF is located at the proximal point of the femur (Figure 18.4). NOF fractures largely affect the ageing population and are more common in elderly women (Filipov 2014). In Australia, there were approximately 16,518 patients over the age of 40 who had experienced an NOF fracture (ANZHFR 2014). Rates of NOF fractures are expected to increase by 15% every five years until 2026 (ANZHFR 2014). NOF fractures are often the result of falls, although they can occur after minor trauma in patients with osteoarthritis and other systemic diseases affecting bone density (NHS Choices 2016). Elderly patients, especially those with osteoporosis, who suffer falls and potentially minor trauma require a higher level of suspicion for NOF fractures.

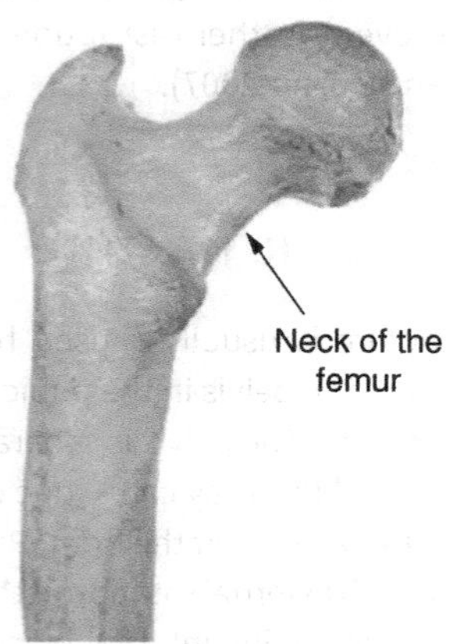

FIGURE 18.4 Neck of femur.

Mid-shaft femur fractures

Mid-shaft femur fractures are often the result of major trauma such as an RTC, due to the amount of force required to fracture dense bone through substantial muscle mass (Griffin et al. 2015). These fractures occur below the NOF and above the knee and can be spiral, **comminuted,** or open/compound (Keany and McKeever 2015). The femur itself is extremely vascular and is surrounded by major blood vessels, nerves, large muscles, and tissues (Keany and McKeever 2015). Fractures to this bone can therefore lead to life-threatening hypovolaemia, fat embolism, nerve damage, and in a compound fracture, **exsanguination.** Mid-shaft femur fractures can present with bruising, swelling, deformity, crepitus, and extreme pain to the mid-thigh area (Keany and McKeever 2015). In the absence of considerable blood loss and other life-threatening injuries, management involves the strongest available pain relief, traction splint, and timely transport to an appropriate health facility.

When assessing all fractures or dislocations, it is important to check for neurovascular compromise distal to the injury. If neurovascular compromise is evident, applying traction to realign the fracture and then splinting may be indicated. Neurovascular assessment includes sensation, colour, temperature, strength, peripheral pulse, and capillary refill.

Reducing a fracture using a traction splint, for example, stops further damage to surrounding tissues and reduces pain by pulling the fractured bones closer to the correct anatomical position (Griffin et al. 2015). Reduction can also resolve neurovascular compromise.

Practice insight

When presented with a compound fracture (open fracture), where possible, prior to applying a traction splint, cleaning the wound thoroughly with normal saline can potentially decrease the patient's infection risk.

Limb injuries

The limbs of a human provide the apparatus for undertaking almost all tasks and physical processes. As such, the arms and legs can be subject to many injuries when involved in trauma.

Limb lacerations

Minor limb lacerations can be a common injury and are also simple to treat. After making sure the wound is clean and ensuring major vessels are not damaged, the wound can be dressed, and wound closure effected on site by the paramedic practitioner (where appropriate) or in hospital. By contrast, major lacerations of the limb can damage blood vessels, muscular tissues, and also the underlying bones and tendons. With wounds such as this, bleeding is to be expected but can often be halted by firm, direct pressure at the injury site and the wound can be dressed for transport to hospital. Wound assessment should primarily focus on the length, width, and depth of the injury, with an assessment of distal motor and sensory function and pulses. History taking is also vital, as this will help establish whether the injury was caused by mechanical (accidental injury) or medical means.

De-gloving

De-gloving is an injury where the skin and some of the soft tissues are fully removed from the underlying structures like a 'glove'. This can be isolated to one finger or might involve a whole hand, foot, or arm or leg, in some cases leading to surgical amputation of the affected digit/limb. Primary prehospital treatment is to keep the affected area moist and appropriately dressed, and to address any pain the patient may be suffering.

Crush injuries

Crush injuries can result in massive damage to both the soft tissues and the skeletal structures of the limb. Caused by huge pressures on a relatively small area, crush injuries often result in serious blood loss, and need surgical intervention and sometimes amputation. Treatment should focus on controlling any bleeding and managing the patient's pain. Prolonged crush injuries can lead to *crush syndrome* or rhabdomyolysis.

This is the release of myoglobin into the bloodstream from damaged muscle fibres. Myoglobin can cause kidney failure. Recurrent examples of crush injury include the trapped car-crash victim. But consider the elderly person who has fallen and cannot move. They may also be affected by rhabdomyolysis. These patients may require treatment of dialysis and bicarbonate. Some ambulance services encourage paramedics to deliver crystalloids to flush the kidneys.

Amputations

An amputation is a traumatic removal of the distal end of a limb. This injury can be severely life threatening and can result in massive blood loss. Such injuries, resulting from high-impact trauma, leave an open-ended wound with a high risk of contamination and infection. The control of blood loss may require indirect pressure or the use of a tourniquet. Once bleeding is under control, the wound should be dressed with a tight-fitting blast bandage and appropriate fluid (refer to local or national fluid guidelines) and pain relief given. These patients require advanced surgical techniques and should be transported to the nearest MTC.

Upper limb injuries

Fractured/dislocated clavicle

Injuries such as this may present with localised bruising and swelling, along with palpable pain and/or deformity of the bone. A fractured, dislocated clavicle is extremely painful, and the patient may not allow you to touch them. Strong pain relief is needed early on. The arm on the affected side should be immobilised with a large arm sling in whatever position the patient finds most comfortable, and distal pulses should be carefully monitored.

Fractured/dislocated shoulder

As the shoulder is a complex collection of joints, it can be difficult to assess whether it is dislocated or broken. The focus of the assessment should be based on pain response, range of movement, and deformity. If the patient is experiencing any pain in the joint, particularly on movement, after experiencing some form of trauma to the upper body or arms, it should be assumed that there is either a fracture of the joint or a dislocation of some or all the components of the joint. Prior to moving the patient, it may be necessary to administer pain relief and immobilise the affected arm in a comfortable position using a sling.

Shock

Shock is a physiological response to inadequate tissue oxygenation. The results of such inadequate tissue perfusion end in the same way, but there are a number of causes, as outlined in Table 18.2.

TABLE 18.2 Shock classifications and their origins.

Classification	Origin
Hypovolaemic	Decreased intravascular volume. For example, in haemorrhage or dehydration
Cardiogenic	A reduction in the heart's pumping ability, often caused by a reduced ejection fraction or impaired ventricular filling. Can be due to myocardial infarction, myocarditis, arrhythmias etc
Distributive	A relative hypovolaemia due to pathological redistribution of body fluids from the intravascular space to another space within the body. This can be caused by anaphylaxis, sepsis, or spinal cord injury (neurogenic shock)
Obstructive	Caused by physical obstruction of the great vessels or the heart itself. Can be caused by tension pneumothorax, cardiac tamponade, aortocaval compression during positive pressure ventilation, and high PEEP

Conclusion

Paramedics routinely face patients who present with some form of trauma. Whilst it will be clear from this chapter that treatment of trauma is central to paramedic practice, it is worth noting that the majority of trauma cases will be *minor* cases. However, each paramedic must be prepared to encounter and respond to major trauma. Regardless of severity, the paramedic must provide interventions that are based on careful assessment and diagnosis and the latest evidence.

Activities

Now review your learning by completing the learning activities in this chapter. The answers to these appear at the end of the book. Further self-test activities can be found at **www.wileyfundamentalseries.com/paramedic/3e.**

Test your knowledge

1. Identify the three major signs of Cushing's triad.
2. What is the mnemonic used to assess fractures and what does each letter stand for?
3. What type of injury describes two or more rib fractures which can cause abnormal chest movement?
4. Describe the major differences between a pneumothorax and a tension pneumothorax.
5. Which type of fracture is most common in elderly women after a fall?
6. Name the type of injury that causes rhabdomyolysis.

Activity 14.1

Ambulance services across the world use different criteria for suspected cervical spine (C-spine) injuries. The NEXUS criteria and the Canadian C-Spine Rule are commonly used both prehospitally and in hospital to determine whether imaging is necessary. Compare and contrast the NEXUS criteria and the Canadian C-Spine Rule. Do they differ to those used by your local (national) ambulance service?

Activity 14.2

According to the National Institute of Health and Clinical Excellence (NICE), prehospitally in the presence of an uncontrolled haemorrhage, fluid replacement should only be used to maintain a palpable central pulse (https://www.nice.org.uk/guidance/ng39/chapter/recommendations#management-of-haemorrhage-in-prehospital-and-hospital-settings). What are the fluid replacement guidelines for an uncontrolled haemorrhage in your local (or national) ambulance service?

Activity 14.3

Increasingly, ambulance services are decompressing chests prehospitally in the presence of tension pneumothorax. What is the practice of your local (or national) ambulance service? What are the major differences between services and their procedures?

Glossary

Comminuted fracture: A fracture segmenting the bone into two or more fragments.

Cushing's triad: A triad of symptoms widely recognised as associated with raised intracranial pressure (raised blood pressure, lowered pulse, and altered respirations).

Dura mater: A thick membrane; the outermost layer of the meninges.

Exsanguination: Severe blood loss causing death.

Fluid replacement: The process of replacing lost bodily fluids through methods such as oral intake or intravenous methods.

Hypo-resonance: A loud, low-pitched, resonant sound.

Hypovolaemia: Decreased blood volume.

Major trauma centre (MTC): A hospital that has specialist facilities to deal with major trauma patients.

Percuss: The process of tapping a certain part of the body to compare percussion notes.

Peritoneal membrane: A serous membrane that covers the peritoneum of the abdomen.

Potential space: A space that can exist between two features, for example, between the visceral and parietal pleura of the lung.

Subarachnoid space: A space located between the arachnoid membrane and the pia mater.

Surgical emphysema: The presence of gas or air within the subcutaneous tissue.

Velocity: A force of motion.

References

Ackland, H. and Cameron, P. (2012). Cervical spine: assessment following trauma. *Australian Family Physician* **41** (4): 196–201.

Ambulance Victoria. (2023). Ambulance Victoria clinical practice guidelines for ambulance and MICA paramedics. Melbourne: Ambulance Victoria. Available at: https://www.ambulance.vic.gov.au/paramedics/clinical-practice-guidelines/ (accessed 4 May 2023).

Australian and New Zealand Hip Fracture Registry (ANZHFR) Steering Group (2014). Australian and New Zealand guideline for hip fracture care: improving outcomes in hip fracture management of adults. Available at: http://anzhfr.org/wp-content/uploads/2016/07/ANZ-Guideline-for-Hip-Fracture-Care.pdf (accessed February 2018).

Butler, F.K., Dubose, J.J., Otten, E.J. et al. (2013). *Management of Open Pneumothorax in Tactical Combat Casualty Care: TCCC Guidelines Change 13-02*. Fort Sam, Houston, TX: Army Inst of Surgical Research.

Clarke, D. and Stewart, M. (2013). Stabilisation of pelvic fractures. *Emergency Medical Journal* **30** (5): 424–426.

Filipov, O. (2014). Epidemiology and social burden of the femoral neck fractures. *Journal of IMAB* **20** (4): 516–518. doi: 10.5272/jimab.2014204.516.

Gregory, P. and Mursell, I. (2010). *Manual of Clinical Paramedic Procedures*. Chichester: Wiley.

Griffin, X.L., Parsons, N., Zbaeda, M.M. et al. (2015). Interventions for treating fractures of the distal femur in adults. *Cochrane Database of Systematic Reviews* **(8)**: CD010606. doi: 10.1002/14651858.CD010606.pub2.

Keany, J.E. and McKeever, D. (2015). Femur fracture. *Medscape.* Available at: https://emedicine.medscape.com/article/824856-overview (accessed February 2018).

Lee, C., and Porter, K. (2007). The prehospital management of pelvic fractures. *Emergency Medicine Journal* **24** (2): 130–133.

Meagher, R.J. and Young, W.F. (2013). Subarachnoid haematoma. *Medscape.* Available at: http://emedicine.medscape.com/article/1137207-overview (accessed February 2018).

Morgan, B. (1999). Basal skull fractures. London Health Sciences. Available at: http://www.lhsc.on.ca/Health_Professionals/CCTC/edubriefs/baseskull.htm (accessed January 2013).

NHS Choices (2015) Head injuries: minor head injury/lump on head. Available at: http://www.nhs.uk/Conditions/Head-injury-minor/Pages/Causes.aspx (accessed February 2018).

NHS Choices (2016). Severe head injury. Available at: https://www.nhs.uk/conditions/severe-head-injury http://www.nhs.uk/Conditions/Head-injury-minor/Pages/Causes.aspx (accessed January 2018).

NICE (2014). Head injury: assessment and early management. Clinical Guideline CG176. Available at: https://www.nice.org.uk/guidance/cg176/chapter/Introduction (accessed January 2018).

Nutbeam, T., Fenwick, R., Smith, J.E. et al. (2022). A Delphi study of rescue and clinical subject matter experts on the extrication of patients following a motor vehicle collision. *Scandinavian Journal of Trauma, Resuscitation and Emergency Medicine* **30** (1): 41.

Ramesh, G.H., Uma, J.C., and Farhath, S. (2019). Fluid resuscitation in trauma: what are the best strategies and fluids? *International Journal of Emergency Medicine* **12** (38): 1–6.

Skinner, D.V. and Driscoll, P.A. (eds.) (2013). *ABC of Major Trauma.* 4e. Oxford: BMJ Books/Wiley-Blackwell.

CHAPTER 19

Prehospital electrocardiography

Alexander Olaussen

Department of Paramedicine, Monash University, Victoria, Australia; School of Public Health and Preventive Medicine Research, Monash University, Victoria, Australia; National Trauma Research Institute, Melbourne, Australia; Alfred Health, Victoria, Australia; Centre for Research and Evaluation, Ambulance Victoria, Victoria, Australia; ILCOR EIT Task Force

Contents

LEARNING OUTCOMES

On completion of this chapter the reader will be able to:

- Evaluate the components of a basic electrocardiogram (ECG).
- Identify the relationship between the ECG and the cardiac conduction pathway.
- Identify abnormal ECG rhythms.
- Discuss acute coronary syndromes.
- Identify treatments for some of the abnormal cardiac rhythms.

Fundamentals of Paramedic Practice: A Systems Approach, Third Edition. Edited by Sam Willis and Ian Peate.

Companion website: www.wiley.com/go/willis/paramedic3e

Case study

An ambulance has been called to a male complaining of chest pain. On arrival you find the male is pale, sweaty, clammy, and feeling nauseous. Once an ECG has been obtained, it is noted there is ST-segment elevation above 3 mm in the anterior leads. The patient is treated for an ST-elevation myocardial infarction (STEMI) and taken to the local cardiac catheter lab.

Introduction

The electrocardiogram (ECG) is a valuable tool in the assessment of a patient with a variety of clinical conditions. It is cheap, poses negligible risks to the patient and is readily available. The ability to use and accurately acquire and interpret an ECG to suggest a range of cardiac conditions is a vital skill. This chapter will give you the skills to examine and identify what a normal ECG should look like, and what abnormal ECGs are worthy of further investigations and management. The chapter will also discuss how the ECG is formed, thereby allowing you to understand the ECG, rather than merely recognise its waveform patterns.

Background: what is an ECG?

An ECG is a pictorial view of the electrical activity of the heart. Cardiac cells are depolarised and repolarised by moving electrically charged ions in and out of their cell membrane. This electrical activity can be captured on the skin surface with electrodes, and then displayed graphically on paper or a screen. This gives an insight into both the electrical pathway through the heart and whether certain areas are getting enough or reduced blood supply.

The first ECG machine was developed in 1911, when Willem Einthoven immersed each of his own limbs in a container of salt solution, enabling him to chart electrical activity and thus create a rudimentary ECG (Snellen 2008). Einthoven assigned letters to the various positive and negative deflections of the ECG so that they could be charted and measured. He arbitrarily selected the letters P, Q, R, S, and T, which are now used universally to describe ECG waves (Figure 19.1). Each letter refers to an electrical 'wave' (whether it be a **depolarisation** or **repolarisation** wave) located within the heart. Measuring and charting each wave helps to evaluate how the heart is working and to confirm whether it is working normally or there is a pathology that needs attention.

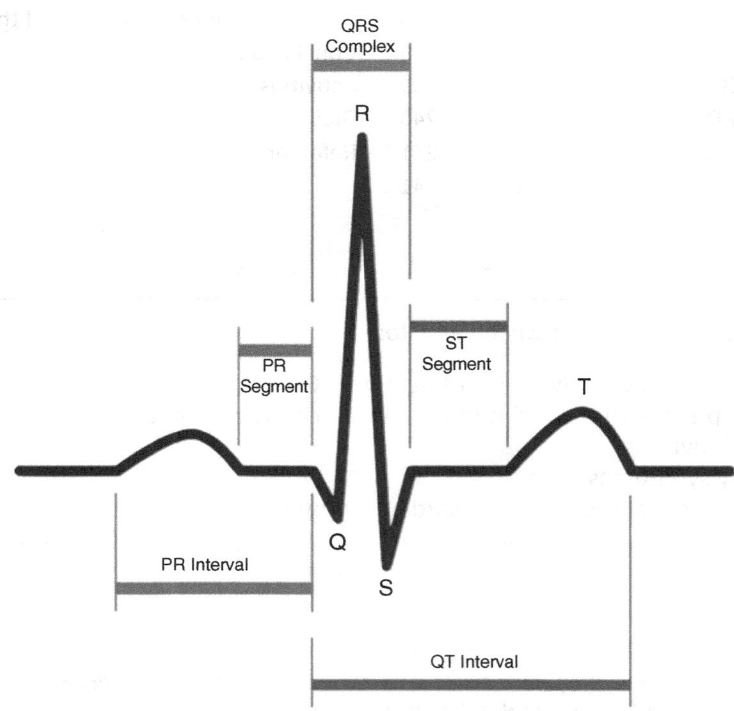

FIGURE 19.1 Letters code the different waveform deflections of the ECG.

Electrical conduction system of the heart

The heart's natural pacemaker is known as the sinoatrial (SA) node. The SA node is a cluster of highly specialised cells capable of generating an electrical impulse. Once the SA node has discharged the electrical signal, this leads to atrial contraction. The contraction is caused by a depolarisation of the cardiac cells. The signal then travels to the next phase of the conduction system known as the atrioventricular (AV) node bundle of His, which then travels down the left and right bundle branches and into the **Purkinje fibres** leading to contraction of the ventricles. When the cardiac cells are resting (or recovering) this is known as repolarisation. During repolarisation the heart is not contracting (Figure 19.2).

Capturing the ECG

Accurate and consistent capturing is a critical first step in interpreting the ECG. The ECG is collected by placing electrodes on the patient's skin. It is important to place the electrodes in the right position and to ensure the patient is lying still when ready to capture the ECG. The standard three-lead ECG is obtained by placing four electrodes on the patient as shown in Figure 19.3. Avoid placing the electrodes over bone as this will diminish the ability to pick up the heart's electrical activity. By placing another 6 leads across the chest (i.e. the precordial leads, or chest leads) a total of 12 views of the heart become available. This can be confusing at first, but the student should take relief from the fact that the ECG machine can generate 12 'views' (also called leads) from 10 electrodes (i.e. the sticky dots on the patient), through complex vector maths. A 12e-lead ECG is a way of viewing the heart from 12 different viewpoints.

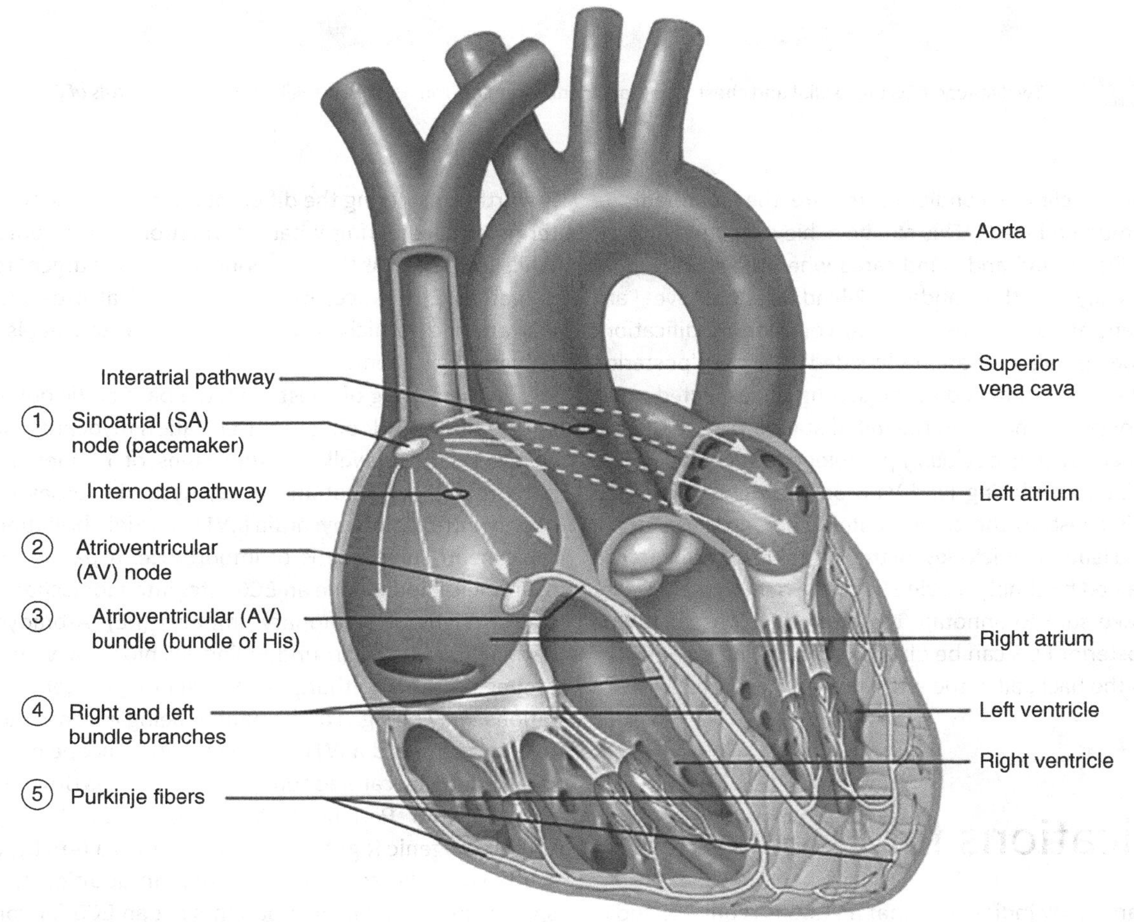

FIGURE 19.2 Electrical conduction of the heart.

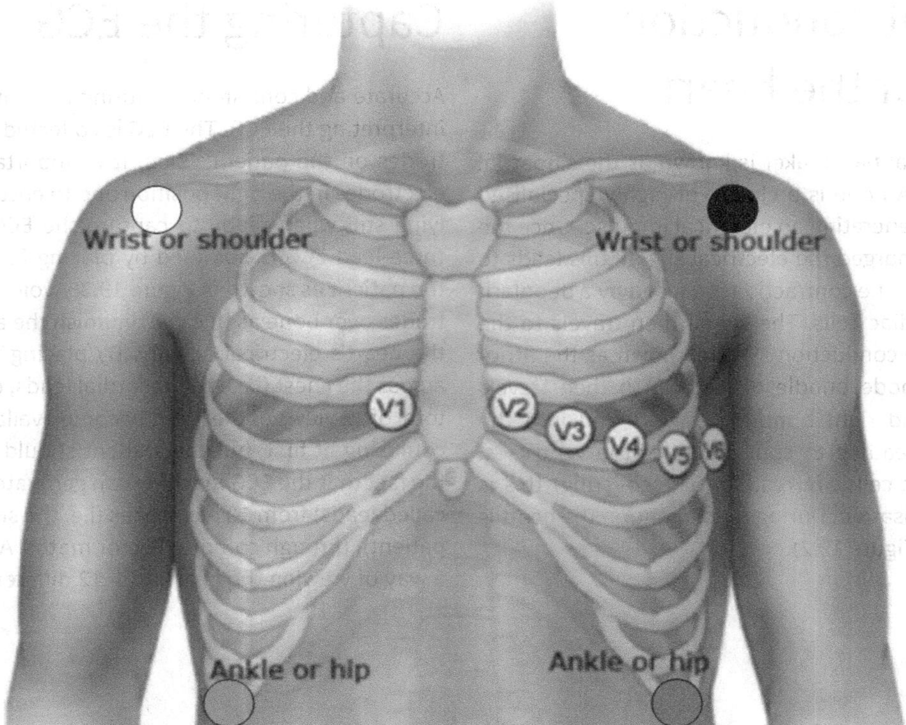

FIGURE 19.3 Twelve-lead ECG precordial and chest lead placement. Source: From Peate and Hill 2023, *Fundamentals of Critical Care*.

Certain clinical conditions require the paramedic to obtain modified leads. This can be achieved by moving the electrodes around and is indicated when the suspicion for STEMI is high but the standard 12-lead does not reveal any significant abnormalities. The two common modifications worth being aware of are 'right-sided' ECG and 'posterior' ECG. These are obtained in the setting of suspected acute coronary syndrome when the initial standard 12-lead does not reveal anything obviously pathological. Right-sided ECG is obtained by placing lead V4-6 on the right side of the patient's chest, in the same anatomical landmarks as for standard leads. A quick view of the right side of the heart can be obtained by simply moving V4 to the right mid-clavicular line. Make sure to annotate the printed ECG as such with V4R. Posterior ECG can be obtained by moving V4-6 further around the back, all in the sixth intercostal space.

Indications for ECG

There are many indications that an ECG is required, and in practice, most patients end up getting an ECG. However, it is worth considering the different indications for an ECG in terms of considering what information can be obtained. Whilst chest pain is the commonest and most urgent reason to get an ECG trace, many other clinical presentations warrant one – which may provide clues as to what is going on with the patient.

In the setting of chest pain, the paramedic obtains an ECG to primarily look for a ST-elevation myocardial infarction (STEMI), as well as other signs of ischaemia. In a patient with palpitations or tachycardia, assessing for supraventricular tachycardia (SVT) or atrial fibrillation with rapid ventricular rate is of importance. A patient who is dyspnoeic should have an ECG integrated for ischaemia as well as signs of pulmonary embolus (PE). A bradycardic patient may have an underlying AV block or ventricular escape rhythms. Lethargy and weakness, as well as palpitations, may be signs of the patient being in conscious ventricular tachycardia (VT). A patient with syncope may have rare underlying cardiac abnormalities such as Brugada syndrome, Wolff Parkinson White (WPW) syndrome, and Arrhythmogenic Right Ventricular Dysplasia (ARVD), which are beyond the scope of this book. In addition to these specific indications, most patients get an ECG for continuous monitoring en route to hospital.

The ECG paper

Knowledge of the ECG paper is crucial for accurate interpretation. The ECG recording is printed on special paper with set gridlines. The standard paper speed rate is 25mm/second and with a voltage of 10mm/mV. This leads to the following intervals and amplitudes which the student must commit to memory (Table 19.1).

The standard strip is longitudinally broken up into three-second portions, denoted with small thick lines at the top of the strip. Each three-second bracket consists of fifteen sets of 0.2-second brackets, which are again broken up into five sets of 0.04-second blocks. Regarding amplitude (i.e. the height), each small square is 1 mm in height. Ten small squares – which is the same as two large squares – is equal to 1 mV of electricity detected from the heart's electrical conduction system. When discussing ECGs with colleagues or other health care providers on the phone (e.g. cardiologists), longitude is commonly described in milliseconds and amplitude in millimetres (Figure 19.4).

TABLE 19.1 ECG paper speed.

Paper	Interpretation
1 small square = 1 mm	0.04 seconds (i.e. 40 ms)
5 small squares = 5 mm = 1 large square	0.20 seconds (i.e. 200 ms)
5 large squares	1 second
1 small square in amplitude	1 mm = 0.1 mv

The components of the ECG

It is important to recognise how P, QRS, and T waves 'normally' present in an ECG and what they represent to identify 'abnormal' presentations.

P wave

The normal P wave should be upright, rounded, and each of them in Lead II all looking the same. The P wave represents the discharge of energy (or depolarisation) from the SA node and throughout the atrium. The SA node lies in the wall of the right atrium and when depolarised sends electricity down the inter atrial pathways throughout the right and left atrium.

This electrical discharge causes atrial contraction. Any alterations from normal potentially mean the pacemaker origin is somewhere else within the atrial pathways or atrial tissue. This could be as subtle as P waves changing shape (instead of upright, rounded, and mostly symmetrical) or displaying irregular rhythms due to multiple sites firing in order to compensate for the poorly discharging SA node (Houghton and Gray 2008).

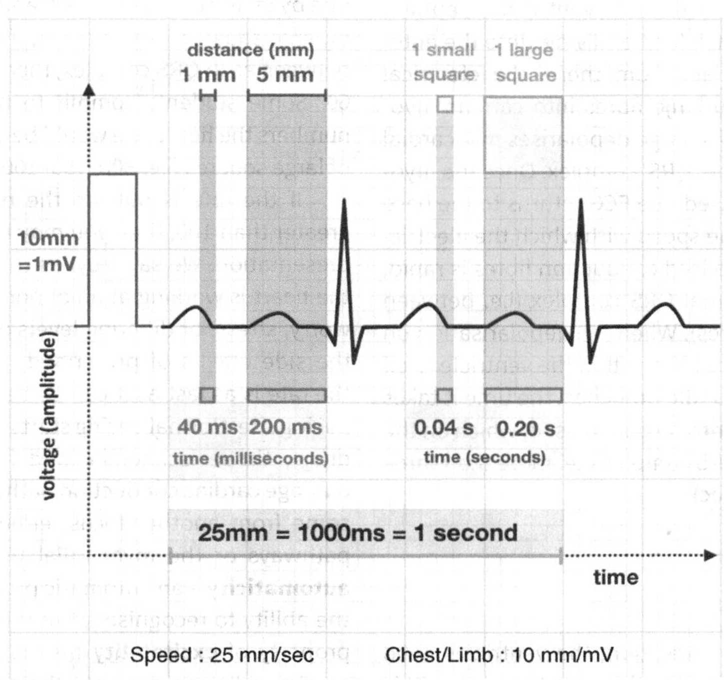

FIGURE 19.4 Paper speed. Source: Life in the Fast Lane / https://litfl.com/ecg-rate-interpretation (accessed 28 July 2023).

PR interval

Once the electrical discharge from the atria reaches the AV node there is a deliberate slowing down of the electricity, in order to allow the blood to travel from the atria down to the ventricles. This slowing can be seen on the ECG as the flat isoelectric PR segment. The PR interval is measured from the start of the P wave to the start of the QRS complex and should be between 0.12 and 0.2 seconds (i.e. between three and five small squares).

If there is any delay in the time from when the SA node fires (P wave) to when the ventricles depolarise (QRS complex), the PR interval will be greater than 200 ms and you should seek out the pathology. The causes of pathology to the AV node can be numerous, and range from **ischaemia,** injury, or **infarction** to medicinal and drug interaction (such as digoxin, most **beta blockers,** and some **calcium-channel blockers**). Whatever the reason, if there is a delay in AV conduction, consider AV block.

QRS complex

Once the stimulus leaves the AV node, it passes down to the next part of the conduction pathway, known as the bundle of His (Houghton and Gray 2008). The bundle of His passes into the **interventricular septum** and divides into the left and right bundle branches. These bundle branches then pass downwards, into the interventricular septum, where the left bundle branch further divides into the anterior and posterior **fascicles.** From there, the electrical signal passes from the Purkinje fibres into cardiac myocytes, and the electrical discharge depolarises myocardial tissue as represented by the 'QRS' complex. Once the myocardium has fully depolarised, the ECG returns to the base line or **isoelectric line.** The speed with which the electricity travels down the specialised conduction fibres is rapid, resulting in a narrow normal QRS complex (i.e. between one and three small squares). When the depolarisation on the other hand commences from within the ventricle itself or there is a block in the bundle branches, the time it takes to depolarise the entire ventricle is increased, which on the ECG manifests as a wide QRS complex (i.e. more than three small squares or ≥ 120msec)

T wave

Following ventricular depolarisation, the ventricles need to repolarise; in preparation for the next heartbeat. This movement of the ions back across the semipermeable membrane to their normal resting is seen on the ECG as the T wave. Changes to the T wave (such as hyperacute T waves) are often times the first sign of concerning ischaemia to the myocardial tissue. The normal T wave should be upright, slightly rounded, and asymmetrical – meaning it should be slightly slanted on the upstroke and shortened or sharper on the downstroke.

The rate and rhythm of an ECG

Heart rate

Knowledge of the ECG paper speed (see Table 19.1) helps us calculate a cardiac rate. To calculate the rate of an ECG there are a number of different methods for counting. If the rhythm is irregular, then printing out a long strip (e.g. 6 or 10 seconds) and counting the number of QRS complexes gives the best estimate of the rate. If the rhythm, however, is regular, there are shortcuts that can be taken.

Because each large square is the same as 0.2 seconds, it follows that if there was a QRS on every large square, there would be 5 beats in a second and 300 per minute. Noone has this heart rate, but it demonstrates the principle behind the '300-method'. In the '300-method', you will get the cardiac rate by taking the number 300 and dividing it by the number of large squares. For instance, if there are 5 large squares between each QRS complex, then the rate is 300/5, which is 60. Some students commit to memory the sequence of numbers the heart rate would be depending on the number of large squares (i.e. 300–150–100–75–60–50–43–37).

If the rate is outside the norms of less than 60 or greater than 100, then you *may* have an abnormal cardiac presentation. We say *may,* as there could be reasons why the heart is working at an abnormal rate (such as anxiety, worry, stress, or differing levels of fitness, or as a result of the side effects of prescribed medications). Sometimes, the rate is as fast as it can go because of the origin of the pacing site. Normal pacing starts in the SA node, but certain drugs, tissue ischaemia, and infarction or disease can damage cardiac conduction pathways. The pacing site may come from another focus, either within the conduction pathways or the myocardial tissue itself. This is called **automaticity** – an automatic property of cardiac cells with the ability to recognise when things are going wrong. The property of **excitability** means that, when irritated, the cardiac cells can generate their own electrical signal and take over the pacing of the heart.

Practice insight

Remember, a piece of paper doesn't have a heart rate – the patient does, so always feel the radial pulse when recording an ECG. Correlate what you feel with what you see!

Heart rhythm

The biggest question to ask is: is there a pattern to the rhythm? Is it regular, is there a regular (or repeating) irregularity, or is it 'all over the place' with no identifiable pattern? Whilst we sometimes make assumptions regarding heart rhythm based on patient age, to do so can be dangerous. It is important to be as sure as you can that the reason for the call/admission you are attending is not the initiating event of any dysrhythmia. Take time to establish whether there is any history of dysrhythmia, or whether a dysrhythmia or irregularity has been clinically detected before. From the ECG, you can observe for any inconsistencies in the 'QRS complex' whether **cardiac conduction** is regular and thus effective. The blood pressure and oxygen saturation will assist in your assessment of whether cardiac output is sufficient. Always correlate what you see with what you feel by palpating the patient's pulse; asking the patient 'how do you feel?' may also assist in making your decision regarding the sufficiency of the cardiac work.

Practice insight

The key to successful ECG interpretation is practice, practice, practice. Be sure to discuss the ECG findings with your crewmate and other staff members and follow this up with plenty of research and reading. Know the time limits for each section of the QRS – if anything is out of the ordinary, consider it to be abnormal and worthy of further investigation.

Now that you understand what each wave represents, you can move onto to systematically interpret the ECG in a structured way.

A structured interpretation approach

Reading the ECG successfully relies on a structured approach. Whilst many resources will suggest different templates, what they all have in common is that they stress the importance of a structure. This is important for a few reasons. For instance, a good structure is something to fall back on in times of fatigue or stress, as well as an invaluable tool when confronted with an ECG that looks bizarre. A good structure can also help avoid the missing of important findings when at first glance the ECG appears normal.

Many texts will advocate for an 8-, 10-, or 12-step process. However, in reality, for the out-of-hospital (OOH) practitioner, four key questions sufficiently address all ECGs. The questions to ask (and answer) with every ECG are given in Table 19.2.

A more extended template for analysing an ECG is presented in Table 19.3.

It should be noted that whilst there are many different ECG diagnoses, the paramedic must be particularly aware of those that can and should be treated urgently in the OOH environment such as bradycardia, tachycardia (including SVT and VT), drug overdoses, acute coronary syndromes, and cardiac arrests. ECG diagnoses beyond these are 'nice to know' and can help paint a more holistic picture of the patient's presentation. However, given the volume of subtle and rare ECG findings, it is important that these do not deter students from engaging with the core ECG topics.

AV heart blocks

There are four main types: a) first-degree, b) second-degree type 1, c) second-degree type 2, and d) third-degree (also called complete heart block). Their naming corresponds to progressing severity.

First-degree AV block

This is technically not a block, as no beats are missed, rather there is a conduction delay. There is always a QRS after the P wave – it is just delayed (i.e. ≥ 200 ms). This is often an incidental finding and of minimal clinical significance.

Second-degree AV block

This *is* a block because some of the P wave activity does not innervate the bundle of His and therefore there is no QRS. There are two types of second-degree AV blocks.

TABLE 19.2 Questions to ask with an ECG.

	Question	How to tell	Interpretation	Potential pathologies
1	Is it regular or irregular?	Map out the QRS on a piece of paper. Ignore the occasional ectopic beats when making this assessment	Irregular rhythms require further careful assessment to see whether there is a relationship between the P wave and the subsequent QRS complexes	Pathologies of irregularities include atrial fibrillation, AV blocks beyond first degree, and some rare atrial arrhythmias such as multifocal atrial tachycardia and wandering atrial pacemaker
2	Is it fast or slow?	The normal rate is between 60 and 100. If the rhythm is regular, then use the 300-method, otherwise, calculate the number of QRS over a 3- or 6-second strip and multiply by 20 or 10 respectively	A slow rate (<60bpm) is called bradycardia and can lead to a lack of vital organ perfusion. A fast rate (>100) is called tachycardia and may lead to cardiac ischaemia as there is not enough time for the coronary arteries to fill	Bradycardias can be asymptomatic in the setting of sinus bradycardia in fit and healthy people, otherwise bradycardias are often associated with complete heart blocks or idioventricular rhythms. Tachycardias can range from sinus tachycardia in the anxious person to SVT, rapid atrial fibrillation, and VT
3	Is it wide of narrow?	This refers to the width of the QRS	Between 1 and 3 small squares is considered normal	≥ 120 ms (i.e. ≥ 3 small squares) indicate pathology. The patient may be in cardiac arrest (with rhythms like VF and VT), the patient may be in conscious VT (which is a true emergency), or there may simply be pre-existing bundle branch blocks or paced rhythms, which is of minimal clinical concern
4	Is it a STEMI, or other signs of ischaemia?	Identify the J point (where the QRS finishes), and then determine if there is ST elevation. See separate section further down on STEMIs	Depending on the lead and the age and sex of the patient, what constitutes significant ST Elevation varies	A STEMI is a serious subtype of Acute Coronary Syndrome that may indicate coronary occlusion, which requires thrombolysis and coronary artery imaging +/– stenting

Type 1 (known as Wenckebach phenomenon or Mobitz type 1)

Here the PR interval increases in time and the distance between the P wave and the QR wave progressively becomes longer and longer until eventually a QRS beat is dropped and the P wave fails to pass through the AV node to the bundle of His. Once this happens, the process is reset, and the same cycle continues.

Type 2 (known as Mobitz type 2)

The PR interval, unlike in type 1, is constant; however, occasionally the P wave is not followed by a QRS complex, failing in its conduction to the bundle of His. This rhythm can be difficult to detect, therefore a long rhythm strip may be needed in order to evaluate it.

Third-degree AV block

This is where there is no associative conduction between the atria and the ventricles. In this condition, both atria and ventricles depolarise independently and bear no resemblance to each other. This condition should be easier to identify than a second-degree AV block, as although the P waves and QRS complexes are autonomous, they are usually regular. Therefore, if you were to identify the P waves on the rhythm strip, they would be regular, as would the QRS complexes; however, as they work independently of each other, they appear to be irregular. See Figure 19.5 for an example.

TABLE 19.3 Template for analysing an ECG.

Component	Answer
Atrial rate	
Atrial rhythm	
Ventricular rate	
Ventricular rhythm	
Axis	
P wave	
PR interval	
QRS complex duration	
Q wave	
J point	
T wave	
ST segment	
QTc interval	
Additionals	
Ectopics?	
Other signs?	
Interpretation	
DCCS?	
STEMI?	
ICP backup?	
In summary	

DCCS = Direct Current Counter Shock; STEMI = ST-Elevation Myocardial Infarction; ICP = Intensive Care Paramedic.

Third-degree/complete AV block

Analogy to remember the types of AV blocks

It might be helpful to understand the concept of these AV blocks in terms of analogy. Imagine the P wave is someone's alarm clock and the QRS is them arriving at work. In a first-degree AV block, the worker is predictably always late, but never misses a day of work. In a Wenckebach AV block, as the week progresses, the worker arrives later and later each day, until they – predictably – don't turn up at all on a Friday. In a Mobitz type 2, they may or may not be on and miss days at random. In a third-degree AV block, there is no correlation at all between when the alarm goes off and when they arrive at work. It should therefore be clear that the seriousness of the blocks increases as a QRS beat (or work) is increasingly unreliable.

Heart blocks and the QRS width

The time it takes the electrical impulse to travel from the AV node and down to the end of the Purkinje fibres (i.e. systole) should not be any longer than 120 ms (0.12 seconds). This represents normal ventricular discharge. If the ventricular discharge time is longer, it will widen the QRS complex (as the X-axis is time), indicating the presence of potential pathology. Thus, it is important to measure the width of the QRS complex. Remember, the QRS complex represents cardiac conduction: if cardiac conduction is disrupted, so is muscle contraction and cardiac output, which may mean cerebral hypoxia and almost certain disruption of other key systems.

The QRS becomes wider as the normal conduction pathway is disrupted. Accordingly, the only way in which the electrical signal can discharge the ventricles is abnormally, i.e. through cellular depolarisation, as opposed to conduction pathway depolarisation.

Idioventricular rhythm

Widely recognised as any rhythm originating from within the ventricle, an idioventricular rhythm is identified as a 'wide and bizarre' QRS complex that exceeds the normal QRS limits (<120 ms). The conduction is delayed and distorted due to the fact that the affected ventricle relies on the functioning ventricle to depolarise it *indirectly,* **myocyte** to myocyte, rather than through the

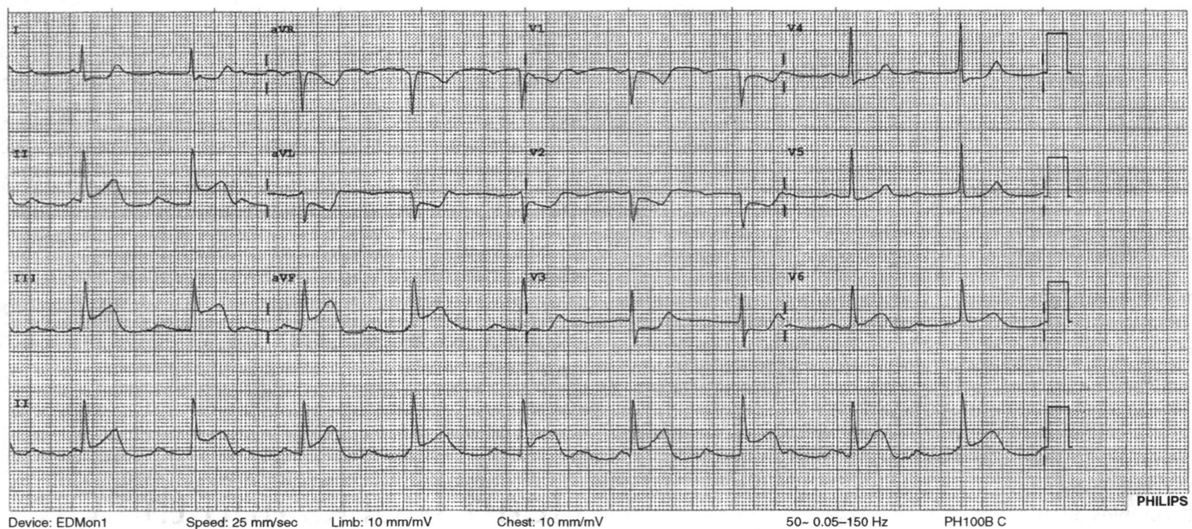

FIGURE 19.5 Example of complete heart block (i.e. no relationship between the P wave and the QRS). In this case, a complication of the underlying STEMI.

conduction pathways, which results in a wide QRS complex.

The rate is often bradycardic. If the rate is <50 bpm, the naming is idioventricular. If the rate is a little quicker, i.e. >50bpm, but less than 100bpm, the rhythm is known as accelerated idioventricular rhythm (AIVR). If the rate is >100bpm, it is most likely (or at least safest to assume) that the patient has VT. These rhythms may or may not produce a pulse, and management should be guided by clinical assessment.

Bundle branch blocks

One abnormality clearly visible on the 12-lead ECG is bundle branch block (either left or right), manifested by a high degree of aberrant conduction. Bundle branch block is essentially the loss of the conduction pathway somewhere in the bundle branch (or, at times, the fascicle of the left bundle branch). In terms of severity, left bundle branch block (LBBB) is far more severe than right bundle branch block (RBBB), and is associated with much higher mortality and **morbidity.** Recognising RBBB and LBBB on the ECG takes practice. A useful mnemonic is 'WiLLiaM MaRRoW'. This mnemonic spells out the shape of the RBBB and LBBB in leads V1 and V6. In an LBBB, a W pattern is often seen in V1 and an M pattern in V6. This is reversed in RBBB, in which an M is seen in V1 and a W in V6.

Left bundle branch block

Interruption of the left bundle branch deprives the ventricle of its intrinsic conducting pathway. As the left bundle branch (including the fascicle) is unable to conduct, it relies on the right bundle branch to cellularly conduct the signal from myocyte to myocyte (Houghton and Gray 2008), stimulating contraction and *usually* showing as a wide QRS. Remembering that the septum normally depolarises from left to right can help decipher some of the features of LBBB. A LBBB means that the septum now has to depolarise right to left. This produces a negative wave in V1 and positive wave in V6. The right ventricle is then depolarised, seen as a small notch, followed by the electricity being spread cell to cell across to the left ventricle (Figure 19.6).

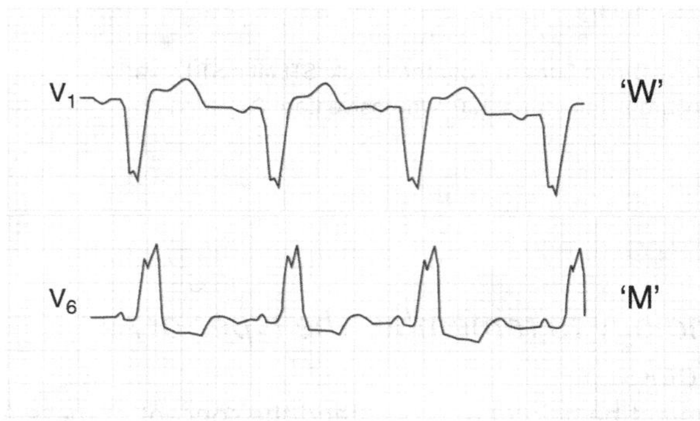

FIGURE 19.6 Schematic representation of LBBB. Source: https://litfl.com/left-bundle-branch-block-lbbb-ecg-library

Right bundle branch block

For RBBB, the right ventricle is not stimulated by activation impulses travelling down the right bundle branch. Instead, the signal travels down the left bundle branch – as per normal – then depolarises the left ventricle before cell-to-cell conduction travels across to the right ventricle. Imagine you are standing in lead V1 and looking at this. The electricity first travels towards you (i.e. the septum depolarising from left to right, indicated by a positive wave), the electricity then heads away from you (depolarising the left ventricle), before it eventually comes back towards you, indicated by a second positive wave. This gives rise to the characteristic M shape – or rabbit ears – in V1. RBBB does sometimes have a pathological cause, although it can be seen in healthy individuals. Compared with LBBB, RBBB does not represent such a high mortality rate.

Incomplete bundle branch block

Usually caused by the same pathology, a partial blockage in one of the bundle branches can cause an incomplete bundle branch block. More difficult to recognise than a complete bundle branch block, the delay causes abnormal shapes and complexes without exceeding the 120-ms boundary in an idioventricular presentation.

Ectopic beats

Single ventricular ectopic beats are common and appear as isolated wide and bizarre QRS complexes. In isolation they are not of concern but frequent PVCs of many different shapes (i.e. multifocal) may be a sign of ischaemia and should be weighed carefully in the setting of clinical presentation suspicious for cardiac event.

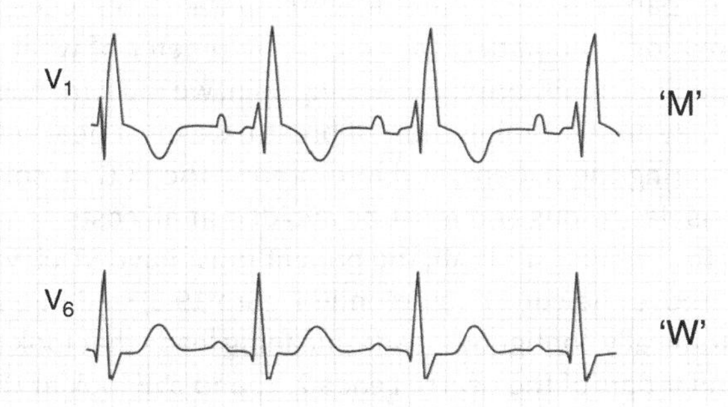

FIGURE 19.7 Schematic representation of RBBB. Source: https://litfl.com/right-bundle-branch-block-rbbb-ecg-library.

Acute coronary syndromes and the ECG

Paradigms in acute coronary syndrome detection

Before delving into STEMIs, the current era, it is worth understanding where this terminology has come from in order to understand where we have been and where we are heading. In the 1990s, a large meta-analysis of randomised trials on fibrinolytic therapy for AMI (acute myocardial infarction) showed a clear benefit of thrombolysis (Trialists 1994). That is to say, although there was a slight increase in strokes, the benefits of breaking up the clot in the coronary artery (i.e. thrombolysis) far outweighed the risks and saved a large number of lives.

It was then noticed that a subgroup of these patients – those who had elevation of their ST segment – did even better with this treatment. Following these findings, we moved from the 'Q wave era' into the new 'STEMI' era.

However, keep in mind what we are really trying to detect with our clinical history and ECG interpretation whether there is any coronary artery occlusion. Because a large proportion of patients with said occlusion do not display ST elevation – just as many patients who display ST elevation have open clean coronary arteries – dichotomising acute coronary syndromes into STEMIs or not is misleading and patients can be missed both by false negatives and false positives.

A new movement is occurring and has been coined occlusion myocardial infarction (OMI; McLaren et al. 2022). This encompasses even more ECG signs, beyond ST elevation, that are predictive of coronary occlusion and will benefit from thrombolysis. Despite emerging evidence of OMI's superiority in detecting occlusion compared to STEMI, and a strong push towards including more ECG patterns under the umbrella of OMI, most current clinical practice guidelines and jurisdictions operate under the STEMI paradigm.

ST segment

The ST segment should be isoelectric. The isoelectric line is from the end of the T wave to the start of the next P wave. Draw this line through the QRS complex and notice whether the ST segment is above, below, or on the isoelectric line. ST Depression (i.e. below the line) may indicate ischaemia or injury to the myocardium, whereas ST elevation may indicate infarction (although this is not definitive, as we have just discussed).

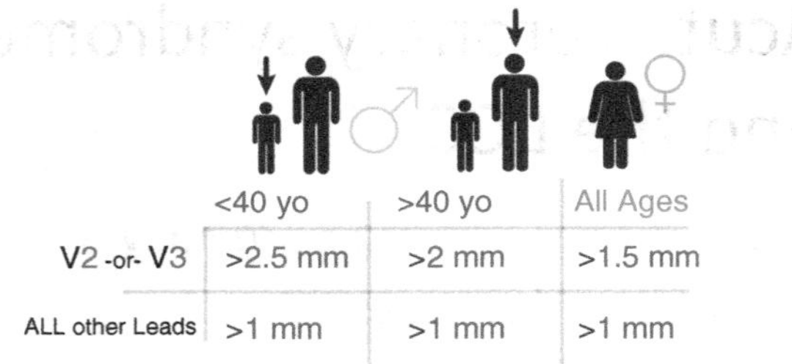

<40 yo
>40 yo
All Ages
V2 -or- V3
>2.5 mm
>2 mm
>1.5 mm
ALL other Leads
>1 mm
>1 mm
>1 mm

FIGURE 19.8 Graphical representation of the different cut-offs for abnormal ST elevation depending on age and sex. Source: https://www.tamingthesru.com/blog/grand-rounds/stemi.

How many millimetres constitute 'serious' myocardial damage (i.e. a STEMI)? The answer to this question has evolved extensively over the last three decades. The current definition takes age and sex into account. For females, elevation above 1.5 mm in V2 and V2, and above 1 mm in all other leads constitute elevation. For males less than 40 years of age, up to 2.5 mm in V2 and V3 is acceptable, beyond which elevation is significant. That cut-off is 2 mm for males above the age of 40. A visual representation of this is worthwhile and can be seen in Figure 19.8.

Given the rapid change of these cut-offs, be guided by local recommendations. It is important to note that if the ST depression or elevation does not equal 2 mm and the patient's condition suggests a cardiac event, it should still be considered an important finding and referred to an appropriate medical practitioner.

Practice insight

When conducting a 12-lead ECG, it can sometimes be difficult to place the leads on the patient due to clothing or positioning. Ideally the patient should be in a private environment such as an ambulance or their own home and should be lying comfortably. This is not always possible. Ask your crewmate to assist, when necessary, by holding clothes or preparing the patient.

Acute coronary syndromes and the ECG

Correctly identifying an acute coronary syndrome (ACS) through ECG interpretation is a fundamental skill. ECG changes are sometimes clear with this condition and sometimes not.

ACS are currently divided into three categories:

- Unstable angina pectoris (UA)
- Non-ST-elevation myocardial infarction (NSTEMI)
- ST-elevation myocardial infarction (STEMI)

All three types are classified as an ACS. UA and NSTEMI present the same and are only differentiated based on the presence or absence of troponin biomarker (which is done in hospital). For practical purposes, the prehospital paramedic clinician could therefore separate patients presenting with cardiac chest pain into one of two categories: STEMI or UA/NSTEMI

The signs and symptoms of an ACS are those of myocardial ischaemia/injury: retrosternal pain (sometimes disguised/reduced by progressive diabetic neuropathy, which is important to consider), sometimes referring into the jaw/arm, as well as diaphoresis, nausea and vomiting, and shortness of breath. There are of course atypical presentations, which should always be considered when evaluating the patient. Remembering that females are more likely to present atypical and may present with different symptoms such as dyspnoea and tiredness is important.

The ECG findings of UA and NSTEMI can be normal or can present with signs that are recognised as ischaemia (such as hyperacute T waves, ST Depression, T wave inversion, etc). Regardless, the treatment in these patients is the same. That is, analgesia, nitrates, supportive therapies, and keeping a close eye on whether it progresses to STEMI. STEMI should receive thrombolysis or urgent percutaneous coronary angiography therefore being able to identify a STEMI is critical.

When diagnosing a STEMI, it should be made clear yet again that the clinical presentation must be taken into consideration. The STE part of **STE**MI comes from the ECG. The MI part of STE**MI** comes from the paramedics' clinical impression. The patient is the best barometer of what is happening: if they are experiencing pain, we must manage it; if they are becoming short of breath, we must deal with it. Ignoring the patient, and interpreting the ECG in isolation, is dangerous and must be avoided at all costs.

To diagnose a STEMI, the patient must have ST elevation above the cut-off (as seen in Figure 19.8) and in two anatomically contiguous leads (meaning leads that look at a similar part of the heart). Leads 2, 3, and aVF look at the inferior part of the heart. V1–V4 look at the anteroseptal part. Leads 1, aVL, V5, and V6 look at the lateral part of the heart.

Conclusion

Throughout this chapter we have discussed and examined different ECG presentations, and the associated pathology. We have introduced a structure for 'reading' ECGs, so as to know when an abnormality is present. Being able to recognise a 'normal' ECG and decipher it through logical progression is a fundamental skill. It is, however, appropriate to remember that attached to the 10 electrodes is a patient: often frightened, in pain, vulnerable, and utterly reliant on the care being provided to them. Focusing on translating and interpreting an ECG is important but does not exceed the importance of attentive patient care.

Identifying a STEMI is important for the purpose of acute thrombolytic therapy. Other ECG presentations with some exemptions can largely be managed based on the symptoms and the effect on the perfusion.

Activities

Now review your learning by completing the learning activities in this chapter. The answers to these appear at the end of the book. Further self-test activities can be found at **www.wileyfundamentalseries.com/paramedic/3e.**

Test your knowledge

1. What does the P wave represent?
2. What does the QRS complex represent?
3. What does the T wave represent?
4. What is a dysrhythmia?
5. List three dysrhythmias.
6. What is a LBBB?

Activity 19.1

Answer the following questions:

1. What is the correct paper speed of an ECG?
2. How many squares does this paper speed represent?
3. Name one method for calculating the rate of an ECG.

Activity 19.2

What three conditions comprise an ACS?

Activity 19.3

When the left bundle branch becomes blocked, why is this significant?

Glossary

Automaticity: The ability of the cardiac cells to send an electrical signal independently of any stimulation.

Beta blockers: A class of drugs that target beta cells, thus reducing the sympathetic response, which in turn can help reduce hypertension and cardiac arrhythmias.

Bradycardic: A slow cardiac output, determined as 60 beats per minute or below.

Calcium-channel blockers: A class of drugs that reduces the movement of calcium through calcium channels, thereby reducing hypertension and heart rate.

Cardiac conduction: The pathway of electrical movement through the heart.

Cardiac output (CO): The volume of blood ejected from the heart over one minute: stroke volume (SV) × beats per minute (BPM) = cardiac output (CO).

Cardiogenic shock: Inadequate tissue perfusion to the cardiac muscle due to the heart's inability to function properly, thereby causing an inadequate pumping mechanism, resulting in multisystem shock and multi-organ failure.

Cerebral perfusion: A net pressure gradient that allows adequate oxygenated blood to flow to the brain.

Depolarisation: A move in a cell's membrane, allowing more positive or negative agents through it, thus allowing it to discharge, creating a cellular reaction.

Epicardial: The outer layer of the heart.

Excitability: The ability to excite a cardiac myocyte to cause a contraction.

Fascicle: A cluster, collection, or bundle.

Infarction: Death of tissue (otherwise known as necrosis), which can be due to ischaemia or injury.

Interventricular septum: The wall separating the ventricles.

Ischaemia: An interruption of oxygen and glucose to the tissues, usually characterised by reduced blood flow to an area of the body.

Isoelectric line: The baseline of the ECG.

Morbidity: The degree to which the condition the patient suffers from affects them.

Myocyte: Tubular muscle cells that are found in cardiac, skeletal, and smooth muscle masses.

Pacemaker: A cluster of highly specialised cells located in the right atria, responsible for starting the cardiac contractions.

Purkinje fibres: A group of myocytes that are responsible for conducting cardiac impulses across a large area of myocardium; thereby creating and propagating synchronous contractions of the myocardium.

Repolarisation: A move, following depolarisation, where the membrane potential returns to a resting phase; thereby allowing the cell to depolarise again.

Subendocardial: Positioned below the endocardial layer of the heart.

Tachycardic: A fast cardiac output, determined as 100 beats per minute or above.

Transmural: Pertaining to full thickness.

References

Houghton, A.R. and Gray, D. (2008). *Making Sense of the ECG: A Hands-on Guide.* 3e. London: Hodder Arnold.

Kaier, T.E., Twerenbold, R., Puelacher, C. et al. (2017). Direct comparison of cardiac myosin-binding protein C with cardiac troponins for the early diagnosis of acute myocardial infarction. *Circulation* **136** (16): 1495–1508.

McLaren, J.T., Meyers, H.P., Smith, S.W. et al. (2022). From STEMI to occlusion MI: paradigm shift and ED quality improvement. *Canadian Journal of Emergency Medicine* **24** (3): 250–255.

Snellen, H.A. (2008). *Willem Einthoven (1860–1927) Father of Electrocardiography: Life and Work, Ancestors and Contemporaries*. London: Springer.

Trialists, F.T. (1994). Indications for fibrinolytic therapy in suspected acute myocardial infarction: collaborative overview of early mortality and major morbidity results from all randomised trials of more than 1000 patients. *The Lancet* **5** (343(8893): 311–322.

CHAPTER 20

Assessing the cardiovascular system

Matt Campbell

Registered Paramedic, St John WA, Western Australia, Australia

Contents

LEARNING OUTCOMES

Upon completion of this chapter, you will be able to:

- Name and locate key anatomical features of the heart.
- Understand normal cardiac physiology.
- Describe the components of the cardiac electrical conduction system.
- Identify common cardiac pathologies and the associated clinical presentations.
- Describe the components of the cardiovascular examination in the out-of-hospital setting.
- Explain the out-of-hospital management priorities of the cardiac patient .

Case study

You have been called to a 56-year-old male who is complaining of chest tightness. He reports to you that he has an ongoing cardiac history whereby he had a myocardial infarction (MI) in June last year leaving him with permanent damage to parts of his heart muscle (myocardium). He is now experiencing chest tightness again, which feels like his previous MI.

Fundamentals of Paramedic Practice: A Systems Approach, Third Edition. Edited by Sam Willis and Ian Peate.

Companion website: www.wiley.com/go/willis/paramedic3e

Introduction

Patients presenting with some form of cardiac pathology represents a large volume of out-of-hospital (OOH) work. Recognising common pathologies and providing timely treatment is key to patient outcomes. The paramedic needs to have a solid understanding of the cardiovascular system including what constitutes normal cardiac anatomy, physiology, and electrophysiology. Developing an understanding of cardiac pathologies will assist the clinician in conducting a thorough and focused cardiac assessment, leading to timely interventions. This chapter will provide an overview of cardiac anatomy, physiology, common cardiac conditions, cardiac assessment considerations, and cardiac management principles.

Cardiac anatomy and physiology

Function and location of the heart

The heart is a hollow muscular organ comprising of four chambers (Figure 20.1). It serves to circulate blood via the circulatory system to perfuse the entire body. Through this process it contributes to the other roles of the cardiovascular system, which include tissue oxygenation, removal of carbon dioxide and waste products, circulation of nutrients, and thermoregulation through warmth and cooling distribution. The heart lies centrally in the thoracic cavity behind the sternum and in front of the spinal column. It sits above the diaphragm, below the clavicles, and between the two lungs. The top of the heart is referred to as the base and is at the level of the second intercostal space. The bottom part of the heart, referred to as the apex, lies to the left of the sternum at approximately the fifth intercostal space midclavicular line. The average human heart is slightly larger than a fist and weighs approximately 200 to 425 g (Huff 2012).

Cardiac regions

The heart can be classified into five regions or territories, which are useful during patient assessment because they allow paramedics to describe the location of injuries or illness such as myocardial infarctions.

The five main cardiac regions/territories are:

1. Septal (between the atria and the ventricles)
2. Anterior (the front of the heart)

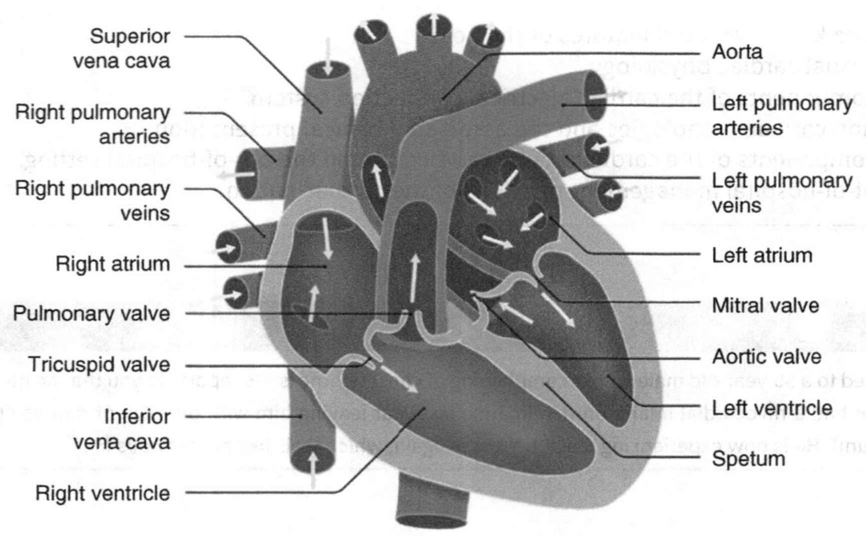

FIGURE 20.1 Anatomy of the heart. Source: Healthline Media UK Ltd / https://www.medicalnewstoday.com/articles/180986#definition (accessed 28 July 2023).

TABLE 20.1 Cardiac regions/territories

I Lateral	aVR	V1 Septal	V4 Anterior
II Inferior	aVL Lateral	V2 Septal	V5 Lateral
III Inferior	aVF Inferior	V3 Anterior	V6 Lateral

3. Posterior (the back of the heart)
4. Lateral (the side of the heart)
5. Inferior (the bottom of the heart)

(Huff 2012)

Figure 20.1 shows how paramedics can use a 12-lead ECG when combined with knowledge of the regions of the heart to identify exactly which part of the heart is impacted.

Structure of the heart

The heart is enclosed in a layer called the **pericardium.** This layer consists of a fibrous outer sac known as the fibrous pericardium and an inner dual layered fluid membrane known as the serous pericardium. The fibrous pericardium provides attachment to other structures and anchors the heart in the thoracic cavity. The serous pericardium consists of two layers (parietal and visceral) between which is the pericardial space. The space is filled with a lubricating clear fluid allowing for resistant free contractility (Arackal and Alsayouri 2019). An understanding of this fluid-filled space is important as fluid or blood accumulation in the settings of infection or trauma can impair this contractility.

The middle layer of the heart is the **myocardium.** This layer is predominately made up of myocytes that contribute to the contractility of the heart. There is variable thickness to this layer corresponding with the heart chambers involved. The greatest thickness is seen in the ventricles.

The innermost layer is the **endocardium.** This thin layer contributes to the valves found within the heart.

Chambers and valves

The heart's upper chambers, the right and left atrium, are separated by the interatrial septum. The lower chambers, the right and left ventricle, are separated by the interventricular septum. The septa provide a delineation between the right and left sides of the heart, allowing us to discuss two separate pumping systems. The right heart forms part of the pulmonary circuit and is responsible for pumping deoxygenated blood via the pulmonary arteries to the lungs for oxygenation. Gas exchange occurs in the lungs and the oxygenated blood returns via the pulmonary veins to the left heart. The thicker walled left heart forms part of the systemic circuit and pumps the oxygenated blood to the rest of the body (Yoganathan et al. 2004).

Four valves are responsible for separating the chambers of the heart. The tricuspid valve consists of three leaflets and directs blood flow from the right atrium to the right ventricle. The mitral valve (sometimes referred to as the bicuspid valve) consists of two leaflets and directs blood flow from the left atrium to the left ventricle. In a healthy system the valves also prevent the backflow of blood. The tricuspid valve and the mitral valve are known as the atrioventricular valves. Connected to the valves are pieces of fibrous tissue called chordae tendineae. The chordae tendineae then attach to the papillary muscles on the walls of the ventricles. The opening and closure of these valves is facilitated by pressure changes in the heart. During the diastolic filling phase, the atrioventricular valves are open and blood flow into the ventricles is facilitated. With increased pressure the valves close and backflow of blood is prevented by the contraction of the papillary muscle pulling on the chordae tendineae. Damage to the ventricular wall or valvular abnormalities can present with various myocardial pathologies. The other two valves in the system are the semi-lunar valves. These half-crescent shaped valves consist of three cusps and are known as the aortic valve and the pulmonary valve. The pulmonary valve provides forward direction of blood flow from the right ventricle to the pulmonary artery. The aortic valve provides forward flow from the left ventricle to the aorta. These valves work in opposition to the atrioventricular valves, opening during ventricular contraction (systole) and closing during ventricular relaxation (diastole) (Yoganathan et al. 2004).

Circulatory flow and coronary perfusion

Two large vessels, the superior vena cava and the inferior vena cava, return systemic circulation to the right atrium. Circulation from the upper portion of the body is returned via the superior vena cava and circulation from the lower portion of the body is returned via the inferior vena cava. The filling of blood into the right atrium increases the pressure within this circuit and blood is forced into the right ventricle. A further increase in pressure then forces blood through the pulmonic valve to the pulmonary arteries and to the lungs. Gas exchange occurs in the lungs at a capillary level and oxygenated blood is then returned to the left atrium via the pulmonary veins. The filling of the left atrium causes an increase in pressure resulting in the opening of the mitral valve and forward flow into the left ventricle. As the pressure increases in the left ventricle the aortic valve is forced open and blood is ejected through the aorta and into the systemic circulation (Wesley 2011; Huff 2012). The filling of the ventricles is largely a passive process; however, the atria provide an additional 30% of filling through atrial contraction. This process known as atrial kick can be lost in certain cardiac pathologies such as atrial fibrillation (Namana et al. 2018). It is also important to recognise that the right side of the heart and the left side of the heart are co-coordinating simultaneously during the filling and ejection phases. A pathology or abnormality on one side of the heart may therefore influence the other side.

Perfusion to the heart itself is supplied via the coronary arteries (Figure 20.2). The right coronary artery and the left coronary artery have various branches that perfuse specific regions of the heart. Knowing what branches supply what areas of the heart is important as it can help clinicians predict culprit vessels based on patient presentation. Both the left and right coronary artery arise from the aorta. In approximately 60% of patients the right coronary artery supplies blood to the sinoatrial node and 90% of patients have blood supply to the atrioventricular node from the right coronary artery (Kumar and Clark 2017). The key branches of the left coronary artery include the left circumflex, the left diagonal, and the left anterior descending (LAD). The LAD perfuses a large portion of the left heart and pathology in this vessel can have significant consequences for the patient. Approximately 80–90% of the population are deemed right coronary artery dominant, meaning their right coronary artery gives rise to the posterior descending artery. The remaining 10–20% of the population are left coronary artery dominant (Huff 2012).

Cardiac electrophysiology

An understanding of cardiac electrophysiology is important as it underpins our knowledge of how the heart works and how deviations from normal conduction can manifest clinically in our patients. A sound understanding on electrophysiology is also required to interpret 12-lead ECGs. This section provides a general overview of the cardiac conduction system, but readers are encouraged to read Chapter 19 to examine this topic in more depth.

Cardiac electrophysiology involves the movement of the ions sodium, potassium, and calcium. It is the movement of these ions across cell membranes that generates the electricity that is then converted into the mechanical heart contraction. The movement of sodium ions into the cell creates a polarised state, which is then propagated across to adjacent cells. The depolarisation of cells triggers an electrical impulse (or stimulus) in a wave-like fashion across neighbouring cells. As potassium ions leave the cell it enters a repolarised state lowering its threshold and preparing itself for another stimulus (Wesley 2011). The action potential of the cardiac cell is fundamental to understanding how electrophysiology influences cardiac behaviour. Different cardiac cells behave differently because of differences in their action potential and thresholds for stimulus.

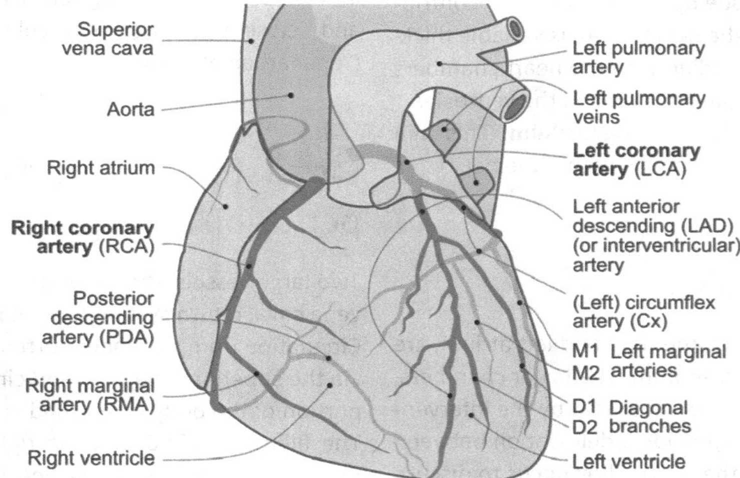

FIGURE 20.2 Coronary arteries. Source: https://en.wikipedia.org/wiki/Coronary_arteries (accessed 28 July 2023).

In a healthy heart the sinoatrial node (SA) is deemed the primary pacemaker of the heart and controls the rate of electrical firing (Kumar and Clark 2017). In certain conditions and pathologies, surrounding cells may take over this role. This can manifest in clinically significant consequences the further away from the SA node this occurs.

In a normal healthy heart, the electrical signal will travel from the SA node down the internodal conduction tracts and interatrial conduction tract. It will reach the atrioventricular (AV) junction with a brief pause at the AV node and bundle of His. The impulse will then continue along the right bundle branch and the left bundle branch into the terminating Purkinje network. A co-ordinated cardiac contraction should follow each impulse down this pathway (Walraven 2011). See Figure 20.3. The heart is innervated by both sympathetic and parasympathetic control. These systems work in opposition and influence control over heart rate, stroke volume and blood pressure (Wesley 2011).

Abnormalities can be seen along the entire conduction pathway described above. In certain conditions such as atrial fibrillation there are multiple foci in the atria firing rather than a single impulse from the SA node. In some conditions there is an additional pathway to the AV node, which can cause significant tachydysrhythmias such as Wolf Parkinson White (WPW) syndrome. Some patients may have a delay or block in one of the left or right branches, as is the case in right bundle branch blocks (RBBB) and left bundle branch blocks (LBBB). The latter are more significant in the context of chest pain (Tan et al. 2020). In some patients there may be complete dissociation between the conduction system of the atria and ventricles, as is seen in patients with a complete (or third-degree) heart block.

Treatment for pathologies associated with the conduction system vary greatly and are often case specific. Some patients are best managed with a wait and see approach, others will require pharmaceutical therapy (e.g. adenosine, amiodarone, atropine), and others may require electrical pacing or cardioversion (Chat and Farooq 2021). Some of these treatments may be available to the OOH clinician depending on your level of training and service provider.

Cardiac pathologies

There are a range of cardiac pathologies that the paramedic will see during their work. With an aging population it is likely some of these presentations may increase.

Acute coronary syndromes

The term acute coronary syndromes (ACS) relates to three very distinct conditions. These are unstable angina, ST-segment elevation myocardial infarction (STEMI) and non-ST-segment elevation myocardial infarction (NSTEMI). The term ACS is reserved for these three conditions only. Each

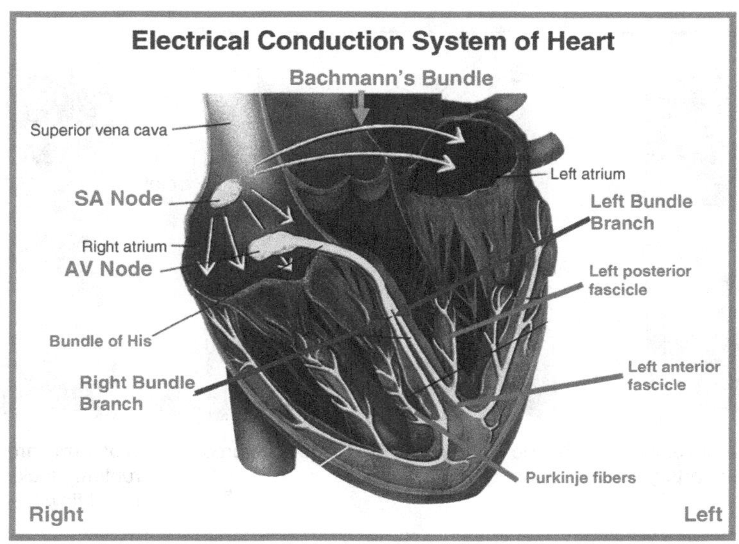

FIGURE 20.3 Electrical conduction system of the heart. Source: The University of New Mexico Albuquerque / https://www.unm.edu/~lkravitz/EKG/electricalconduction.html (accessed 28 July 2023).

of these terms relates to a condition whereby there is a lack of blood flow to the heart muscle, the myocardium caused by a build-up of fatty plaque also known as atheroma (Figure 20.4).

Unstable angina is a partial occlusion of one of the coronary arteries by the atheromatous fatty plaque, leading to intermittent chest tightness and other symptoms without warning, hence the term unstable. Unstable angina requires urgent treatment, as it can lead to a STEMI or NSTEMI.

A STEMI relates to a serious occlusion in one or more of the coronary arteries and requires urgent treatment whereas a NSTEMI is a partial occlusion of one or more of the coronary arteries but still requiring urgent treatment to reperfuse the coronary arteries.

Remember: Time is myocardium

The Myocardium does not tolerate hypoxia and will die without an adequate supply of oxygen/ Therefore the paramedic should act fast and do everything possible to reduced myocardial oxygen demand such as carrying the patient to the ambulance in a carry chair or stretcher instead of walking them.

Ischaemic heart disease

Ischaemic heart disease or IHD (sometimes referred to as myocardial ischaemia) is characterised by a reduction in oxygenated blood supply to the myocardium (the heart muscle). This reduction in blood supply may be due to several causes but vessel disease and atherosclerosis are commonly the main culprits. IHD is more often seen in the elderly, diabetic patients, cigarette smokers, and those with high levels of cholesterol (hypercholesterinaemia). IHD contributes to significant morbidity and mortality in the general population and may present itself on the ACS continuum from angina through to unstable angina and MI. It typically presents with chest pain +/– associated symptoms, although there are increasing presentations of ACS in the absence of any chest pain. Be aware of subtle signs such as breathlessness particularly in females and diabetics (Fulde and Fulde 2014).

Heart failure

Heart failure is the inability of the ventricles to pump blood effectively to the rest of the body. The ventricles initially become enlarged (hypertrophic) as they attempt to pump against increased resistance. Over time this hypertrophy eventually weakens the ventricular wall and a dilation occurs further inhibiting the ventricle to provide the forceful contraction required to pump blood forward. As a result of this failure to pump blood there is a backflow of blood in the circuit and fluid accumulation in the pulmonary and/ or systemic circuit. A left-sided failure leads to engorgement of the pulmonary vessels and to sodium and water being forced into the interstitial space (Kumar and Clark 2017). Pulmonary oedema develops due to this fluid shift.

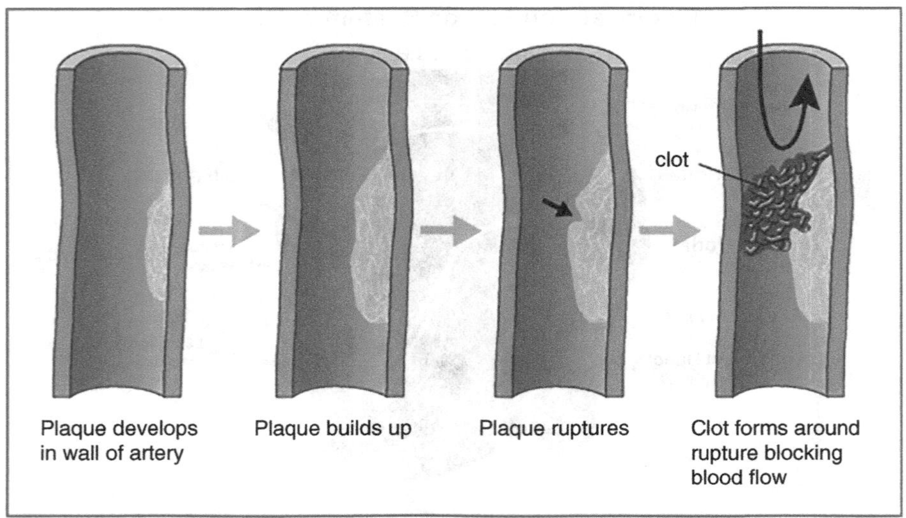
clot
Plaque develops in wall of artery
Plaque builds up
Plaque ruptures
Clot forms around rupture blocking blood flow

FIGURE 20.4 Progression of atheroma build up in the coronary arteries. Source: NurseRN.com / https://www.registerednursern.com/pulse-points-nursing-assessment (accessed 28 July 2023).

The subsequent fluid leakage may be seen clinically as shortness of breath, orthopnoea, cyanosis, and crackles on auscultation. A right-sided failure may present with fatigue, jugular venous distension (JVD), and peripheral oedema. There are numerous reasons for heart failure. A previous MI causing damage to the ventricle and chronic hypertension causing a progressive weakening of the ventricle muscle are two possible causes. Right-sided failure is often caused by left-sided failure. The right ventricle is forced to constantly contract against increased resistance and over time develops the dilation and subsequent inability to contract efficiently. Patients with heart failure may be prescribed a range of pharmaceutical therapies to assist with their symptoms and minimise further deterioration of the heart muscle. Therapies may include beta blockers, angiotensin-converting enzyme (ACE) inhibitors, and diuretic agents (Kumar and Clark 2017). The goal of these therapies is to minimise the strain on the heart and remove excess fluid from the circulation.

Atrial fibrillation

Atrial fibrillation (AF) is the most common and clinically significant cardiac dysrhythmia that is seen in emergency departments (Fulde and Fulde 2014). It is therefore a common presentation paramedics will encounter in their clinical practice. AF is characterised by its irregularly irregular rhythm as seen on the ECG. Rather than the co-ordinated singular electrical pathway from the SA node to the AV node, there are multiple foci firing in the atria. This chaotic electrical firing causes the irregularity seen on the ECG. Patients may be presenting with AF for the first time or as a recurrent episode of known AF. These presentations may be further classified as paroxysmal (self-terminates in <24 hours), persistent (sustained AF >7 days), or permanent. AF can also present with symptoms, including palpitations, chest discomfort, or shortness of breath. Patients may also be asymptomatic. There are various causes for AF including heart failure, IHD, sepsis, and heavy alcohol consumption (Morin et al. 2016). The treatment goals for AF include identifying and treating the causative agent, rate or rhythm control, and preventing the risk of thromboembolism (Fulde and Fulde 2014). Due to the poor atrial contraction, blood can pool in the atria and mural thrombi can develop due to the blood stasis. These are small pieces of thrombi that adhere to the atrial wall and may dislodge causing vessel occlusion. AF is a significant risk factor for stroke development and needs to be managed accordingly.

Valvular heart disease

There are a range of valvular heart conditions. We will briefly discuss two of the more significant conditions: aortic stenosis and mitral stenosis. Both conditions are caused by a narrowing of the valve, which leads to impeded blood flow through the valve.

Aortic stenosis affects the aortic valve and impairs blow flow from the left ventricle to the aorta. This structural abnormality forces the left ventricle to pump harder to overcome the resistance leading to ventricular hypertrophy. Common causes and risk factors include rheumatic fever and increasing age. Like the disease progression itself, symptom onset is usually gradual and occurs over time. Patients may present with chest pain, dyspnoea, and syncope. Some patients may be completely asymptomatic (Marquis-Gravel et al. 2016).

Mitral stenosis involves abnormality to the mitral valve and is commonly caused by rheumatic disease. The inflammatory process caused by rheumatic fever can affect the mitral leaflets and with time the inflammation can result in scarring and adhesions to the valve cusps. Inability of the valve to close properly leads to increased left atrial pressures and ultimately right ventricular failure. Treatment for mitral stenosis involves management of symptoms and valve replacement for some patients (Shah and Sharma 2021).

Tip

Some rural and remote communities are more susceptible to rheumatic fever, particularly where access to healthcare is limited. Consider the societal and demographic factors of your patient when conducting your clinical assessment and whether rheumatic fever could be a possible contributing factor.

OOH cardiovascular examination

Paramedics must be able to identify the early signs of serious cardiac illness and/or abnormality. Early identification and symptom recognition may prevent patient deterioration and lead to the initiation of timely interventions. Adopting a systematic approach to your assessment can provide the structure needed to identify these early signs of illness. The structured cardiovascular examination includes many of the elements used when assessing other body systems. There are, however, some cardiovascular-specific considerations the clinician should include. A thorough cardiovascular examination should involve the following:

- Identifying the chief complaint using a thorough history.
- Body systems review.
- Assessing past medical history and medication/drugs.
- Looking at social and family history.
- Physical examination.

Identifying the chief complaint using a thorough history

The chief complaint is usually what prompted the patient to call for paramedic assistance. Common presenting complaints include chest pain, palpitations, dyspnoea, and peripheral oedema (Maria et al. 2022). It is worth remembering that the chief complaint may not be the most serious condition that you identify in your clinical assessment. It is important to ask the patient to explain their presenting complaint and make considerations for difficulties in communicating this information (e.g. age, language barriers, etc). It is vital that the clinician delves into the history of the chief complaint (Blaber and Harris 2021). Thorough questioning alone is often enough to reveal the likely diagnosis. Two commonly adopted mnemonics to assist in this questioning process are **OPQRST ASPN** and **SOCRATES** (Maria et al. 2022):

TABLE 20.2 **Pain assessment mnemonics.**

OPQRST ASPN	SOCRATES
Onset	**S**ite
Provocation/palliative factors	**O**nset
Quality	**C**haracteristics
Region and radiation	**R**adiation
Severity	**A**ssociated Symptoms
Time	**T**iming
Associated **S**ymptoms	**E**xacerbates/alleviates
Pertinent **N**egatives	**S**everity

The following are examples of questions to ask the patient:

- What were you doing when the pain started?
- How long did the pain last for?
- Describe the quality of the pain. Is it sharp, crushing, tearing?
- Does the pain radiate anywhere? E.g. down your arm, into your neck, into your back
- Is there anything you do that makes the pain better or worse? E.g. lying flat, taking deep breaths. Do your symptoms resolve at rest?
- What time did the pain/breathlessness start?
- Did you or do you currently have any other symptoms? E.g. dizziness, vomiting, diaphoresis, breathing difficulties?
- Have you had any recent illness, injury, or trauma?

Body systems review

Cardiovascular disease and pathology can manifest in seemingly unrelated complaints from the patient. For example, the patient may deny chest pain or palpitations and instead complain of syncope or fatigue. These subtle signs and symptoms may be clues as to an underlying cardiac pathology such as heart block or cardiac failure. A systematic review of the body systems can assist the OOH clinician in 'ruling-in' certain cardiac conditions (Maria et al. 2022):

- Do you ever have trouble lying flat at night due to breathlessness?
- Do you ever get short of breath on mild exertion?
- Do you ever get pain in your calves?
- Have you noticed any swelling around your lower legs and ankles?
- Have you noted any change in skin colour? E.g. foot or leg looking grey or blue.
- Do you ever get dizzy or feel like you will pass out when exercising?
- Have you noticed any change in your urine output?

Past medical history and medications/drugs

Patients with previous cardiac emergencies (e.g. MI) are at a greater risk of cardiac conditions and complications (Yousuf et al. 2020). The patient may also describe similarities of their current symptoms to previous episodes. By asking questions about their medical history these red flags can be identified early. Linking the patient's current presentation to previous episodes can also help to streamline your interventions and form a provisional diagnosis of what is most likely occurring to the patient. It is also important to enquire about previous clinical investigations. Ask the patient if they have previously had an ECG, angiography, angioplasty, etc and the reasons why these investigations were undertaken.

Reviewing the patient's medications can provide great insight into their medical history. Common classes of cardiac medications include anti-hypertensives, beta blockers, glycosides, nitrates, diuretics, and anticoagulants (Yousuf et al. 2020). The OOH clinician must be able to identify these medications, the reason they are prescribed, and how they work in the body. Improving your pharmacy recognition will help to identify the patient more likely to be suffering from a cardiac condition in your differential diagnoses. Your questioning surrounding medications should also include enquiries about the use of illicit substances and non-prescription medication. Cocaine, methamphetamine, pre-workout preparations, and others can lead to acute and chronic cardiac pathology.

As with any patient examination, ask questions about medication allergies, for example:

- Do you have a cardiovascular past medical history? Are you or have you ever been treated for a MI ('heart attack'), cardiac dysrhythmia, hypertension, angina, cardiac failure?
- Do you have a pacemaker or implantable cardioverter defibrillator (ICD)?
- Have you had any previous cardiac surgery?
- Do you have any history of stroke, peripheral vascular disease (PVD), diabetes, chronic obstructive pulmonary disease (COPD), renal disease, asthma, high cholesterol?
- What medications are you currently taking?
- How long have you been taking these medications and what conditions are you taking them for?
- Have there been any recent changes to your medications? E.g. a new medication, cessation of a medication, change in dose.
- Are you compliant with taking your medications?
- Do you take any recreational drugs?
- Do you take any herbal remedies or supplements?
- Do you have any allergies to food or medications?

Remember

One of the quickest and easiest ways to identify potential cardiac pathologies is simply to ask the patient about their past and current medical history.

History taking accounts for approximately 80% of paramedic care.

Social and family history

There are a range of modifiable and fixed risk factors that can pre-dispose a patient to cardiovascular disease. Many of these risk factors can be identified through focused questioning. Modifiable risk factors that are worth asking about include use of cigarettes, alcohol consumption, and level of physical activity. Some cardiovascular conditions have a familial and genetic link (fixed risk factors) so enquiring about the health of immediate family members should form part of your questioning (Yousuf et al. 2020). For example:

- Do you smoke? If yes, how many cigarettes a day and for how many years?
- Do you drink alcohol? If yes, how much do you consume in a week?
- Do you engage in regular physical activity?
- Have you had any recent dramatic weight loss or gain?
- Has anyone in your family been treated for a cardiac condition before?
- Has anyone in your family died suddenly under the age of 45?
- Have you done any recent travel?
- What is your occupation? Are you or have you previously been exposed to any hazardous dust, chemicals, or fibres?

Physical examination

The physical examination of the patient should involve both hands-on and hands-off approaches and utilise a range of clinical assessment diagnostic tools discussed here. The information you have obtained from your patient questioning will assist in the physical examination and guide your assessment approach. Prior to the physical examination it is worth noting the patient's surrounds as this can provide useful information.

Environmental assessment

What can you note in the surrounding environment that may give clues to the patient's general wellbeing? For example, is there evidence of cigarette butts on the table, are there mobility aids in the room, is the patient receiving supplemental oxygen, etc (Blaber and Harris 2021)? Taking in the patient's surrounds will help prime your brain for the rest of the patient examination. Whilst the temptation may be to focus only on the chest during your cardiovascular assessment, it is worth reiterating the importance of a whole-body systematic assessment. Cardiac pathologies can present in changes involving the neck, mouth, eyes, feet, and hands. We will discuss some key assessment items to look for in these areas during your assessment.

Talk to the patient

The first component of the physical examination involves simply talking to the patient. At the same time you should be observing the 'global signs'. These are generalised impressions about the patient's appearance such as the size of the patient, any notable peripheral swelling, work of breathing, colour of skin (e.g. pale, jaundiced), etc (Blaber and Harris 2021). By introducing yourself to the patient you can elicit a range of information. A verbal response from the patient can help to determine their level of responsiveness. You may also note changes in voice or difficulties speaking.

Assess the pulse

An early assessment of the patient's pulse is important in the context of the cardiovascular examination. A surprising amount of information can be obtained from simply taking the time to check the pulse. Generally the radial pulse will be used but other sites including the brachial, carotid, and apical pulse may be assessed. The femoral pulse and the pedal pulse may also be examined as part of your lower limb assessment. When taking a pulse we are assessing for rate, regularity, and volume/character (Kumar and Clark 2017). With the rate we are determining if it is fast, slow, or normal. It is worth remembering that some patients may have pulse rates that are normally slow or slightly fast. It is worthwhile asking the patient if they know what their heart rate normally is when you detect a deviation from the norm. Use your index finger and middle finger to apply pressure to the specific pulse site. Avoid using your thumb. Refer to Figure 20.5 for the various locations of pulse assessment. To assess the rate count the number of beats over a 15 second period and multiply that number by four. If you detect

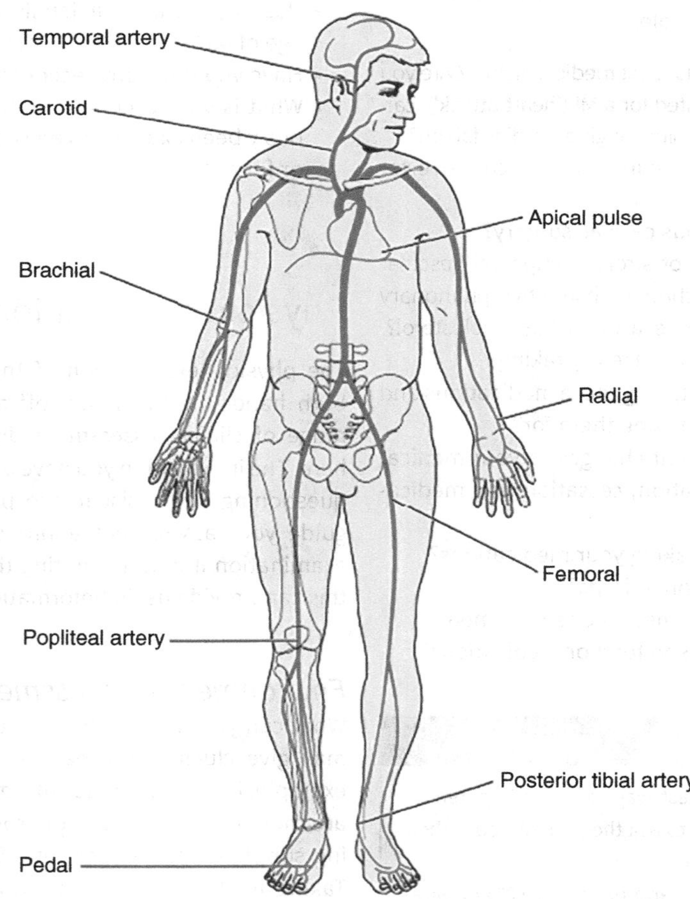

FIGURE 20.5 Pulse points. Source: NurseRN.com / https://www.registerednursern.com/pulse-points-nursing-assessment (accessed 28 July 2023).

irregularities when taking the pulse, then a full 60 second assessment should be conducted. When assessing the regularity of the pulse you are noting if the pulse is regular, regularly irregular, or completely irregular. Some specific conditions present with these patterns (e.g. AF is the classic irregularly irregular rhythm) and should prompt further assessment. When assessing the character of the pulse you are determining if the pulse feels bounding, strong, weak, or thready. This can give information regarding the volume status of the patient.

Tip

For a more advanced OOH assessment you may consider comparing the pulse at different sites on the body. Narrowing of the aorta can represent with pulse delays. A delay between the left and right radial pulse can indicate an abnormality between the brachiocephalic trunk and the left subclavian artery. A radial/femoral pulse delay may indicate an abnormality between the thoracic aorta and the iliac arteries.

Assess the hands

Whilst assessing the radial pulse the clinician should also examine the patient's hands and fingers. Note the colour and temperature of the hands. Cold peripheries may be a sign of poor perfusion. When assessing the nails you are examining for evidence of cyanosis, clubbing or splinter haemorrhages. Clubbing is when the nail bed adopts a rounded appearance and is likely due to increased small vessel growth beneath the nail (Figure 20.6). Cardiac causes of clubbing may include

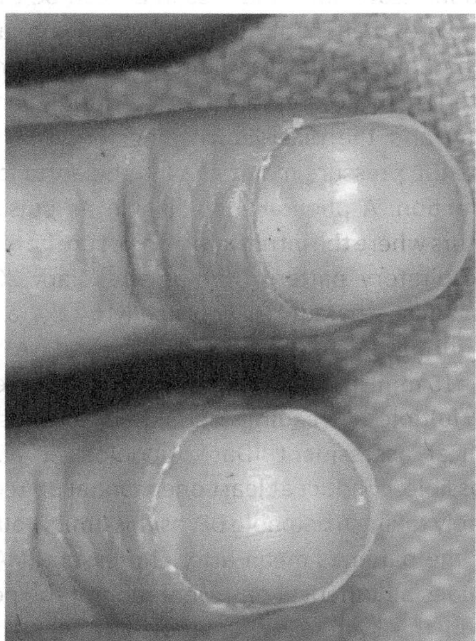

FIGURE 20.6 Clubbing. Source: Used with permission of Mayo Foundation for Medical Education and Research.

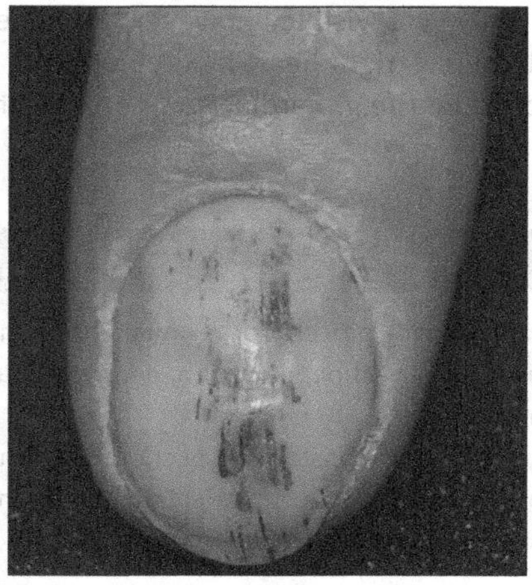

FIGURE 20.7 Splinter haemorrhages. Source: Parveen Kumar et al. 2017. Reproduced with permission from Elsevier.

congenital heart disease or bacterial endocarditis. Splinter haemorrhages are small areas of bleeding that run underneath the nail in parallel lines (Kumar and Clark 2017) (Figure 20.7). This can be a sign of bacterial endocarditis. When assessing the hands you may also note nicotine staining, which is suggestive of extensive cigarette use and a key risk factor for cardiovascular pathology.

Assess the face

When assessing the patient's face you should observe for abnormalities around the eyes. Patients may present with a condition called Xanthelasma, which are cholesterol filled skin lesions (Akyüz et al. 2016). See Figure 20.8. Assessment of the oral cavity may reveal poor dental hygiene, which is a risk factor for the development of bacterial endocarditis (Carinci et al. 2018). Around the patient's neck you need to assess for the presence of JVD. Place the patient in a semi-recumbent position with a head angle of approximately 45^0. Normally the jugular

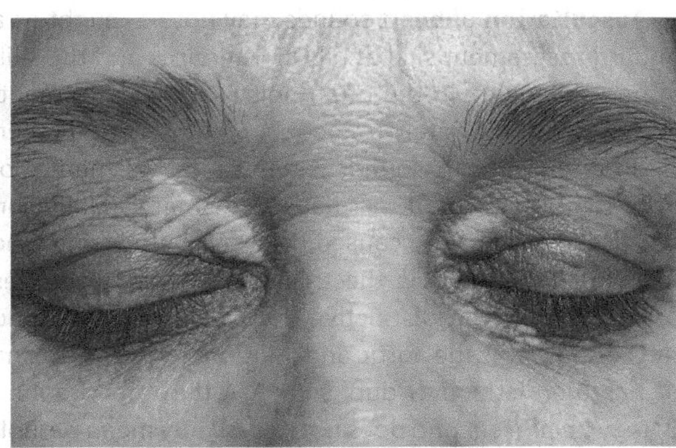

FIGURE 20.8 Xanthelasma. Source: Nau Nau / Shutterstock.

veins are only just visible, however, in patients with fluid overload (e.g. right heart failure) or in the presence of cardiac trauma (e.g. cardiac tamponade) there may be JVD.

Tips

A commonly taught process for examining the chest and thorax involves inspection, palpation, percussion, and auscultation (listening).

Always inspect the posterior aspect of the chest as well as the anterior chest. This is particularly important in the setting of penetrating trauma to the chest.

Assess the thorax (the chest)

The thorax can be assessed using the mnemonic IPPA. Place the patient in the most appropriate position, for example, upright during times of dyspnoea, or in a comfortable position determined by the patient all other times.

Inspection is the visual examination of the chest. Ensuring patient dignity and privacy is maintained, you should expose the chest to ensure nothing is missed. Inspect for bruising or deformity (may indicate underling chest trauma), scars (may indicate previous cardiac surgeries), rashes (may indicate shingles or another painful rash), and discolouration of the skin (may indicate inadequate oxygenation).

Palpation of the chest is used to detect any pain or crepitus. Assessing for equal chest rise and fall can also be done by placing your hands on the anterior chest during the respiratory cycle. Palpation of the apex of the heart may also reveal enlargement or anatomical displacement.

Percussion of the chest is a skill that is likely to be performed during a cardio-respiratory workup, for example, when undertaking a respiratory exam or to determine consolidation or air in the lungs.

Auscultation of heart sounds may not be taught as a standard assessment skill at all OOH services and the skill can be challenging in the often noisy OOH environment. However, if appropriately trained and if time permits then auscultation for heart sounds is a useful assessment tool when completing your cardiac assessment (Mallinson 2017). Heart sounds are caused by the valves closing. The first heart sound (S1) is the tricuspid and mitral valves closing and has the distinctive 'lub' sound. The second heart sound (S2) is the aortic and pulmonary valves closing and has the distinctive 'dub' sound. A third heart sound (S3) may be present and does not necessarily mean pathology particularly in healthy young people. In patients over the age of 35 years it should warrant further investigation (Fulde and Fulde 2014). On auscultation it would sound like 'lub-da-dub'. A fourth heart sound (S4) represents a pathological condition. It is caused by the atria contracting against a noncompliant ventricle. As such S4 is heard before S1 and would sound like "da-lub-dub". Systolic and diastolic murmurs may also be heard on auscultation. The presence of turbulent blood flow may be suggestive of a regurgitation or narrowing in the valves. It can also be a completely normal finding in a healthy heart. This is a skill and observation most likely to be assessed for and detected at hospital.

Tip

'Listen with intent'. Based on your clinical questioning, assessment, and observations you are likely to have already formed some differential diagnoses. When auscultating the chest and heart listen with intent and expect to hear what you think may be occurring. Adopting this mindset will make it easier to detect when you hear an abnormal sound. Be systematic with the areas and order you auscultate. Kept it standardised for all your patient assessments.

Assess blood pressure

Blood pressure (BP) is defined as the amount of pressure exerted on the walls of the arteries by the circulating blood volume. BP must be assessed during your cardiovascular examination. Acute abnormalities in BP can be treated in the OOH environment and can reveal underlying cardiac or vascular pathology. The systolic reading (top number) is representative of the pressure exerted during ventricular contraction and the diastolic reading (bottom number) represents the pressure maintained in the aorta following the contraction. A phenomenon known as pulsus paradoxus occurs where the intrathoracic pressure is influenced by the respiratory pattern (Kumar and Clark 2017). To assess for pulsus paradoxus you need to take a systolic reading during inspiration and expiration. A systolic decrease >15 mmHg during inspiration is considered pathological. Multiple BP readings should be taken as part of your clinical assessment (Daskalopoulou et al. 2015). Where possible, conduct at least one manual BP recording. Avoid simply taking a palpable BP, as this limits your ability to assess the patient's mean arterial pressure (MAP). The MAP provides a numerical representation of the perfusion pressure in the systemic circulation. A MAP of at least 65 mmHg is required to perfuse the brain and other vital organs. An optimal MAP may need to be higher and should be individualised for patients (e.g. elderly patient with co-morbidities such as atherosclerosis or hypertension) (Leone et al. 2015). Many of the cardiac monitors available provide the MAP following an automated BP recording. To work out the MAP you can use the following equation:

$$\text{MAP} = \text{Diastolic Pressure} + 1/3(\text{Systolic Pressure} - \text{Diastolic Pressure})$$

E.g.

$$\text{BP of } 120/90 \text{ mmHg. MAP} = 90 + 1/3(120 - 90)$$

$$\text{MAP} = 90 + 10$$

$$\text{MAP} = 100^{\circ}\text{mmHg}$$

Tip

It is good practice to take BP recordings on bilateral arms to compare and note any differences. A subclavian steal syndrome may cause a significant difference in BP recordings between arms.

OOH management of the cardiac patient

It is best to keep the goals of managing the cardiac patient in the OOH environment simple. The clinician should focus on maintaining oxygenation, maintaining perfusion, managing pain, and transporting the patient to the most appropriate facility to manage their condition. Cardiac presentations will require further investigation +/– further treatment at hospital. As OOH clinicians, the responsibility is to provide a high standard of initial care to maximise the long-term outcome for our patients.

This section does not intend to address the management principles for all the cardiac presentations you may encounter. Depending on the country you work in and the service you work for, your treatment protocols and guidelines may differ. This is a general discussion on some key interventions that OOH providers can offer.

Pharmacological treatment

The number of medications available to paramedics to treat cardiac conditions has drastically increased over the last couple of decades. Many of the interventions and medications given OOH are similar to those the patient would likely receive if they walked straight into an emergency department. Let's examine some of these medications:

Antiplatelets: *Aspirin* has been shown to reduce mortality associated with acute MI by inhibiting platelet aggregation and thrombus formation. This is achieved through the inhibition of prostaglandin production and the disturbance in the production of thromboxane A2.

Heparin Sodium is an anticoagulant agent that inhibits clot formation. It inactivates factors IIa and Xa through its binding to antithrombin III. Action is immediate following IV administration. This is likely to be administered to patients with a STEMI requiring percutaneous intervention at a Cardiac Catheterisation Laboratory (Fulde and Fulde 2014).

Venodilation: *Glyceryl Trinitrate* exhibits a number of actions on vascular smooth muscle including vasodilation, reduced venous return, reduced left ventricular pressure, reduced systemic resistance, and reduced myocardial oxygen demands (Maria et al. 2022). It may be administered for various cardiac conditions such as acute MI and Acute Cardiogenic Pulmonary Oedema (ACPO). This comes in a range of presentations including sublingual tablets, sublingual sprays, transdermal patches and IV infusions.

Pain relief: *Fentanyl* and *Morphine* are narcotic analgesics for pain control. They may be used as a multi-modal pharmaceutical regime to manage cardiac related pain. These should be observed for respiratory depression and caution in elderly patients.

Nausea management: *Anti-emetics* may be administered for symptomatic relief of nausea and vomiting associated with a cardiac complaint.

Blood pressure and dehydration management: *Intravenous crystalloid solutions* provides fluid replacement for those exhibiting cardiogenic shock or profoundly hypotensive. Caution should be taken in those patients who may already be displaying signs of fluid overload. Judicial fluid administration in patients with oedema or on fluid restriction.

Managing hypoxia: *Oxygen* provides a means of reversing hypoxia and maintaining adequate oxygenation via various flow rates and oxygen delivery systems. Depending on your scope of practice you may also have access to inotropes and the ability to provide haemodynamic support through inotropic infusions, which increase BP through vasoconstriction. Examples include metaraminol, dopamine, noradrenaline, and adrenaline.

Non-pharmacological treatment

Standard care for cardiac patients should involve plenty of reassurance; minimising patient exertion; 12-lead ECG acquisition; ongoing cardiac monitoring; IV access if administering a medication; and pre-notification to the receiving facility for patients who are unstable, deteriorating, or have a confirmed STEMI. Early notification to the receiving hospital has been shown to improve door to balloon times and patient outcomes for those needing primary percutaneous coronary intervention (PPCI) treatment.

Tip

It is important not to forget the psychological care these patients may require and that you can provide. Patients who have called an ambulance for a cardiac condition are often quite scared and your words and actions have an impact. Do not neglect the humane side of your practice when attending to this patient cohort.

Conclusion

Patients presenting with acute or chronic cardiac conditions is a common occurrence in OOH medicine. An understanding of the signs and symptoms of these conditions and the skills necessary to conduct a thorough clinical assessment are vital for OOH care providers. Knowledge of these conditions and timely interventions will result in improvement in overall patient outcomes. This chapter has provided an overview on some of these key elements and how to translate this into your clinical practice.

Activities

Now review your learning by completing the learning activities in this chapter. The answers to these appear at the end of the book. Further self-test activities can be found at **www.wileyfundamentalseries.com/paramedic3e.**

Test your knowledge

1. Heart failure is a type of ACS – true or false?
2. Aspirin is a blood thinner – true or false?
3. What is the name of the middle muscular layer of the heart where the myocyte cells are located?

Activity 20.1

Describe the flow of blood through the heart.

Activity 20.2

Complete the missing words:

_____________ is the visual examination of the chest. Ensuring patient dignity and privacy is maintained you should expose the chest to ensure nothing is missed. Inspect for _____________ or deformity (may indicate underling chest trauma), scars (may indicate previous cardiac surgeries), rashes (may indicate shingles or another painful rash) and discolouration of the skin (may indicate inadequate oxygenation).

Palpation of the chest is used to detect any pain or _____________. Assessing for equal chest rise and fall can also be done by placing your hands on the anterior chest during the respiratory cycle. Palpation of the apex of the heart may also reveal enlargement or anatomical displacement.

_____________ of the chest is a skill that is likely to be performed during a cardio-respiratory workup for example when undertaking a respiratory exam or to determine consolidation or air in the lungs.

_____________ of heart sounds may not be taught as a standard assessment skill at all OOH services and the skill can be challenging in the often noisy OOH environment. However, if appropriately trained and if time permits then auscultation for heart sounds is a useful assessment tool when completing your cardiac assessment (Mallinson 2017). Heart sounds are caused _____________.

Glossary

Atrial Fibrillation (AF): A common cardiac dysrhythmia characterised by an irregular and often rapid rate. Originates in the upper chambers of the heart.

Contractility: The innate ability of the cardiac muscle to contract and eject blood.

Inferior vena cava: A large vein that carries deoxygenated blood from the lower portion of the body and returns it to the right atrium.

Interatrial septum: A thin wall of tissue that separates the right atrium from the left atrium.

Interventricular septum: Wall of tissue that separates the right ventricle from the left ventricle.

Leaflets: Flaps of tissue that make up the valves of the heart.

Myocardium: Middle muscular layer of the heart where the myocyte cells are located.

Polarised: The state of the cell at rest when no electrical activity is occurring.

Pulmonary veins: Veins that carry deoxygenated blood from the lungs and return it to the heart.

Rheumatic fever: Inflammatory disease that can cause inflammation at multiple sites in the body including the heart. Caused by the bacteria group A Streptococcus.

Serous: Fluid that resembles serum. Typically pale yellow to transparent in nature.

Superior vena cava: A large vein that carries deoxygenated blood from the upper portion of the body and returns it to the right atrium.

References

Akyüz, A.R., Ağaç, M.T., Turan, T. et al. (2016). Xanthelasma is associated with an increased amount of epicardial adipose tissue. *Medical Principles and Practice* **25** (2): 187–190.

American Academy of Ophthalmology. (2023). What is xanthelasma? [Image]. Available at: https://www.aao.org/eye-health/diseases/what-is-xanthelasma (accessed 11 January 2023).

American Family Physician. (2010). Aymptomatic Linear Haemorrhages. [Image]. Available at: https://www.aafp.org/pubs/afp/issues/2010/0601/p1375.html (accessed 11 January 2023).

Arackal, A. and Alsayouri, K. (2019). *Histology, Heart*. StatsPearl Publishing.

Blaber, A. and Harris, G. (2021). *Assessment Skills for Paramedics*. 3e. McGraw-Hill Education.

Carinci, F., Martinelli, M., Contaldo, M. et al. (2018). Focus on periodontal disease and development of endocarditis. *J Biol Regul Homeost Agents* **32** (2) (Suppl 1): 143–147.

Chat, M.H. and Farooq, B. (2021). Cardiac dysrhythmias. In: *Perioperative Anaesthetic Emergencies* (ed. U.U.G. Salmani, K. Benazir, and J.S. Khan), pp. 109–123. AkiNik Productions

Daskalopoulou, S.S., Rabi, D.M., Zarnke, K.B. et al. (2015). The 2015 Canadian Hypertension Education Program recommendations for blood pressure measurement, diagnosis, assessment of risk, prevention, and treatment of hypertension. *Canadian Journal of Cardiology* **31** (5): 549–568.

Fulde, G. and Fulde, S. (2014). *Emergency Medicine. The Principles of Practice*. 6e. Sydney: Elsevier.

Huff, J. (2012). *ECG Workout. Exercises in Arrhythmia Interpretation*. 6e. Philadelphia, PA: Wolters Kluwer.

Kumar, P. and Clark, M. (2017). *Kumar & Clark's Clinical Medicine*. 9e. Sydney: Elsevier.

Leone, M., Asfar, P., Radermacher, P. et al. (2015). Optimizing mean arterial pressure in septic shock: a critical reappraisal of the literature. *Critical Care* **19** (1): 1–7.

Maria, S.J., Micalos, P.S., and Ahern, L. (2022). Recognising, assessing and managing chest pain. *Journal of Paramedic Practice* **14** (1): 16–24.

Marquis-Gravel, G., Redfors, B., Leon, M.B. et al. (2016). Medical treatment of aortic stenosis. *Circulation* **134** (22): 1766–1784.

Mallinson, T.E. (2017). A survey into paramedic accuracy in identifying the correct anatomic locations for cardiac auscultation. *British Paramedic Journal* **2** (2): 13–17.

Morin, D.P., Bernard, M.L., Madias, C. et al. (2016). The state of the art: atrial fibrillation epidemiology, prevention, and treatment. *Mayo Clinic Proceedings* **91** (12): 1778–1810.

Namana, V., Gupta, S.S., Sabharwal, N. et al. (2018). Clinical significance of atrial kick. *QJM: An International Journal of Medicine* **111** (8): 569–570

Shah, S.N. and Sharma, S. (2021). Mitral Stenosis. In *StatPearls [Internet]*. StatPearls Publishing.

Tan, N.Y., Witt, C.M., Oh, J.K. et al. (2020). Left bundle branch block: current and future perspectives. *Circulation: Arrhythmia and Electrophysiology* **13** (4): e008239.

Walraven, G. (2011). *Basic Arrhythmias. 7e*. NJ: Pearson Education

Wesley, K. (2011). *Huszar's Basic Dysrhythmias and Acute Coronary Syndromes. Interpretation and Management.* 4e. Missouri: Elsevier.

Yoganathan, A.P., He, Z., and Casey Jones, S. (2004). Fluid mechanics of heart valves. *Annual Review of Biomedical Engineering* **6** (1): 331–362.

Yousuf, O., Chrispin, J., Tomaselli, G.F. et al. (2015). Clinical management and prevention of sudden cardiac death. *Circulation Research* **116** (12): 2020–2040.

CHAPTER 21

Assessing the nervous system

Charlie Gadd
Ambulance Paramedic, Ambulance Victoria, Victoria, Australia

Jemmima Bowd
Ambulance Paramedic, Ambulance Victoria, Victoria, Australia

Contents

LEARNING OUTCOMES

- Describe the anatomy and physiology of the nervous system.
- Understand the importance of a systematic approach to assessing neurological conditions.
- Identify key points of history taking to gain a comprehensive overview of the patient.
- Perform a thorough physical examination and utilise focussed assessments to generate differential diagnoses.
- Link neurological assessment findings to common neurological presentations in the out-of-hospital setting.

Case Study

You are dispatched to a 56-year-old male with slurred speech and facial drooping. The patient lives independently with his wife and scores a '0' on the Modified Rankin Scale (MRS). The symptoms started (onset) approximately 60 minutes prior to your arrival. On arrival the patient is sitting upright and slumped to the left side. His eyes open spontaneously, and he responds with words that don't make sense (inappropriate words). He can obey commands to squeeze your fingers with obvious weakness to the left side. The patient's airway is patent and self-maintained, breathing is normal, and he is well perfused. The patient has no allergies and is currently medicated with atorvastatin and candesartan for hypercholesterolemia and hypertension. On examination, the patient has a heart rate of 75, is hypertensive at 180/70 mmHg, respiration rate of 24, Glasgow Coma Scale (GCS) of 13. He is afebrile, and normoglycaemic. The 12-lead **electrocardiogram** (ECG) shows atrial fibrillation, lung sounds are clear with equal air entry, pupils are equal and reactive to light (PEARL). The patient is recognition of stroke in the emergency room (ROSIER) and Ambulance Clinical Triage For Acute Stroke Treatment (ACT-FAST) positive. You load the patient onto the ambulance and proceed to hospital using lights and sirens to a nearby endovascular clot retrieval (ECR) capable hospital, pre-notifying them en route.

Fundamentals of Paramedic Practice: A Systems Approach, Third Edition. Edited by Sam Willis and Ian Peate.

Companion website: www.wiley.com/go/willis/paramedic3e

Introduction

Neurological conditions are a group of diseases that impact the brain and spinal cord tissues. These conditions can be acute and traumatic (stroke, traumatic brain injury, or spinal cord injury), or chronic and degenerative (dementia, Parkinson's disease, or multiple sclerosis). The development of neurological conditions can be influenced by many factors including genetics, congenital defects, immune system dysfunction, or social and environmental factors (Farooqui 2016).

Globally, neurological conditions are the second leading cause of death, accounting for nine million (16.5%) deaths per year (Carroll 2019). Between 2001 and 2014, there was a 39% increase in neurological related deaths (The Neurological Alliance 2019). Furthermore, neurological conditions are the leading cause of disability, contributing to 276 million (11.6%) disability adjusted life years (Carroll 2019). Between 2016 and 2017, more than one million people were admitted to emergency departments in the UK with a neurological concern, which is a 21% increase over five years (The Neurological Alliance 2019). These statistics represent a significant burden to healthcare that is seen worldwide in the out-of-hospital (OOH) setting. Common neurological conditions seen OOH include stroke, seizure, dementia, and Parkinson's disease. In this chapter, we will explore the general anatomy and physiology of the neurological system before diving deeper into the central and peripheral nervous systems. We will then discuss a systematic approach to history taking and physical examination of a patient presenting with a neurological concern, with direct reference to certain neurological conditions and their abnormal findings.

Structure and function of the nervous system

The nervous system is a complex network of nerves and cells that carry impulses between the brain, the spinal cord, and other parts of the body. The primary function of the nervous system is to detect changes in the external and internal environments and trigger appropriate responses (Marieb and Hoehn 2019). The nervous system is responsible for the regulation of vital body functions, voluntary and involuntary movement, learning and memory, and the senses. The nervous system is vulnerable to various disorders caused by structural defects or developmental abnormalities, disease, and trauma. Assessment, examination, and preliminary diagnosis of neurological conditions requires knowledge of the anatomy and physiology of the nervous system.

The nervous system consists of two main divisions: the central nervous system (CNS) and the peripheral nervous system (PNS) (Marieb and Hoehn 2019). The PNS is further divided into the somatic nervous system (SNS) and the autonomic nervous system (ANS). Within the nervous system, there are two types of cells: neurons and glial cells.

Neurons are the main structural and functional units of the nervous system. Neurons are responsible for receiving sensory input and transmitting motor commands. Each neuron consists of a cell body (soma), dendrites, and an axon (Figure 21.1).

The cell body contains cellular organelles and is where the cellular DNA is stored. From the cell body, there are many branch-like extensions known as dendrites. Dendrites contain receptors that are responsible for receiving input from other neurons in the form of neurotransmitters (NTs). These signals cause electrical changes in the neuron that are interpreted in the cell body. If the signal is strong enough, it is transmitted to and received by an axon as an action potential (AP). The AP travels to the axon terminal, causing the release of NTs and continuing the process. The site where the axon connects to another neuron is the synapse. Each neuron is surrounded by a layer of lipid, known as the myelin sheath. The myelin sheath provides insulation for the nerve cell and allows electrical impulses to travel quickly and efficiently without loss of signal (Stadelman et al. 2019).

Glial cells are smaller, non-excitatory cells. Glial cells are divided into two classes: microglia and macroglia (Jäkel and Dimou 2017). Microglia are responsible for the immune defence of the CNS by removing damaged neurons and pathogens. Macroglia are also responsible for myelinating neurons, as well as providing structural support, protection, and nutrition.

Central nervous system

The CNS is the processing centre of the body and is composed of two parts: the brain (located in the skull) and the spinal cord (located in the vertebral column) (Marieb and Hoehn 2019). The brain is made up of the cerebrum, cerebellum, diencephalon, and brainstem. The brain is surrounded by three protective layers known as the meninges: the pia mater (inner layer), arachnoid mater (middle layer),

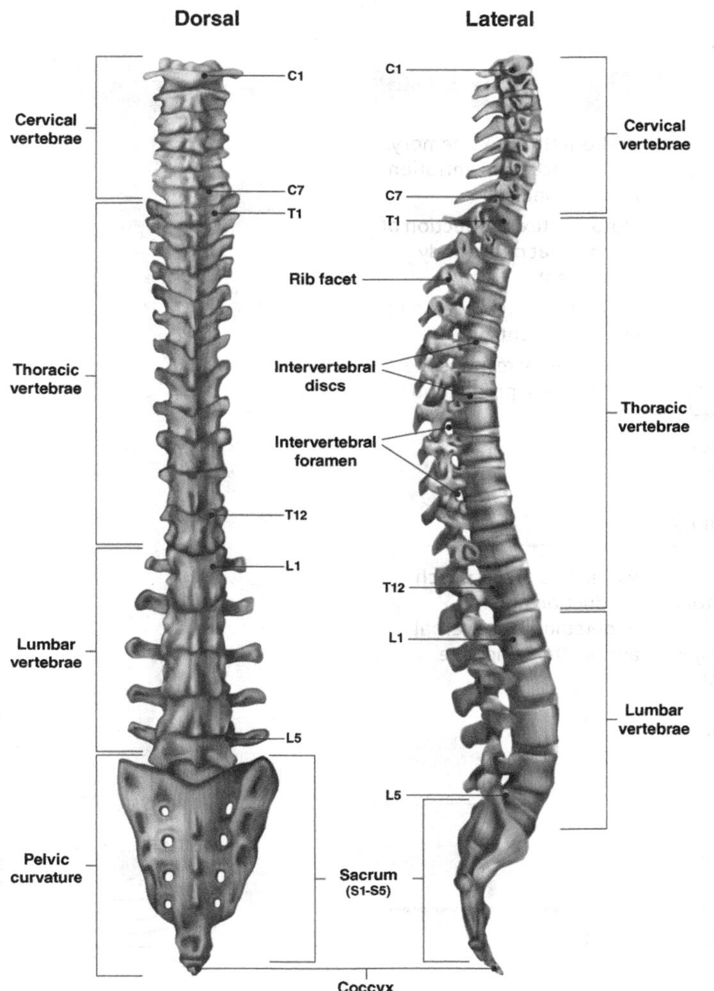

FIGURE 21.1 A neurone.

and dura mater (outer layer). The brain and spinal cord are also covered in a colourless fluid called cerebrospinal fluid, which functions to protect from physical and chemical damage.

Cerebrum

The cerebrum is the largest part of the brain and is divided into the left and right cerebral hemispheres (Gupta 2017). The hemispheres are separated by a groove known as the great longitudinal fissure. The two hemispheres are joined by the corpus callosum, which delivers messages from one hemisphere to the other. The cerebral cortex is the outer layer that lies on top of the cerebrum and is involved in reasoning and emotions, thought and memory, and language (Molnár et al. 2019). The cerebrum can be further divided into four lobes that each have their own primary functions (Table 21.1).

Cerebellum

The cerebellum is located below the occipital lobes, separated from the cerebrum by the tentorium (D'Angelo 2018). The cerebellum is responsible for various fine motor skills such as the movement of fingers. The cerebellum is also responsible for muscle coordination, balance, posture, muscle tone, and performing rapid, repetitive actions.

Diencephalon

The diencephalon is located between the cerebrum and the midbrain (Moini and Piran 2020). Within the diencephalon are the thalamus and hypothalamus. The thalamus is responsible for directing sensory impulses into the cerebrum, as well as motor function and sleep cycle regulation. The hypothalamus is involved in the regulation of temperature, appetite, water balance, sleep, blood vessel constriction and dilation, and emotions.

TABLE 21.1 Function of the cerebral lobes.

Lobe	Function	Special features
Frontal	Voluntary movement, speech, reasoning and thought	Prefrontal cortex: memory, intelligence, concentration, and personality Motor cortex: production of signals that direct body movement Premotor cortex: head and eye movements Broca's area: responsible for language production
Parietal	Integrating sensory information such as vision, hearing, motor, and memory	
Temporal	Receiving and processing auditory information, recognition of objects and faces, verbal memory, and interpretation of emotions and reactions	Wernicke's area: speech production and understanding of verbal and written language
Occipital	Receiving and processing visual information	

Source: Adapted from Marieb and Hoehn 2019.

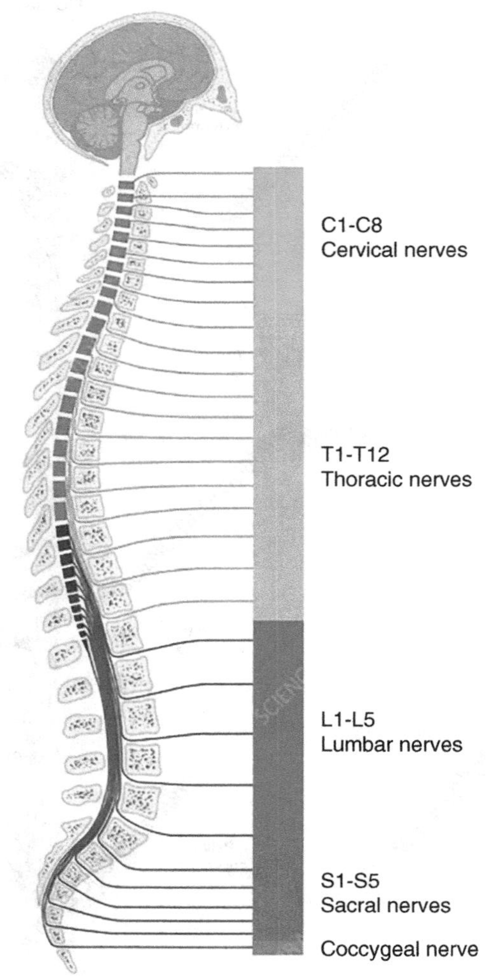

FIGURE 21.2 Spinal cord.

Brainstem

The brainstem consists of the midbrain, pons, and medulla oblongata. The midbrain is located below the cerebrum and at the top of the brainstem (Sciacca et al. 2019). It is responsible for visual and auditory reflexes, movement, and regulating autonomic functions. The pons is located below the midbrain. It is responsible for multiple reflex actions, including chewing, tasting, saliva production, bladder control, and facial expressions (Moini et al. 2021). The medulla oblongata is the lowest part of the brainstem and connects with the spinal cord. It is responsible for regulating vital body functions including heart and blood vessel function, digestion, respiration, swallowing, coughing, and sneezing (Diek et al. 2022).

Spinal cord

The spinal cord continues from the medulla oblongata. It acts as the link between the brain and peripheral nerves. The spinal cord is separated into five regions: cervical, thoracic, lumbar, sacral, and coccyx, as well as afferent and efferent spinal nerves (Marieb and Hoehn 2019). Afferent and efferent spinal nerves merge to form peripheral nerves. Afferent nerves carry information from the peripheries to the brain, and efferent nerves carry information from the brain to the peripheries.

Peripheral nervous system

The PNS refers to the parts of the nervous system outside of the brain and spinal cord. The PNS is made up of 12 pairs of cranial nerves, 31 pairs of spinal nerves, peripheral nerves, and neuromuscular junctions. Within the PNS, bundles of nerve fibres (axons) are responsible for conducting information to and from the CNS. The PNS is subdivided into two systems: the SNS and the ANS.

Somatic nervous system

The SNS is informally referred to as the voluntary system. It is composed of nerves that connect to the skin, sensory organs, and skeletal muscle. The SNS is responsible for most voluntary muscle movements and for processing sensory information from the external environment such as hearing, touch, and sight via afferent and efferent neurons.

Autonomic nervous system

The ANS is informally referred to as the involuntary system. It can be further subdivided into the sympathetic nervous system and the parasympathetic nervous system. The sympathetic nervous system is responsible for the 'fight-or-flight' response (Bankenahally and Krovvidi 2016). The parasympathetic nervous system acts as a counterbalance to sympathetic responses to danger, returning the body back to equilibrium.

Cranial nerves

The 12 pairs of cranial nerves connect the brain to different parts of the body, including the head, neck, and torso (Marieb and Hoehn 2019). Each pair of cranial nerves is numbered and named based on their function. Functions of the cranial nerves include smell, vision, movement, taste, facial expression, balance, and sensation. The function and assessment of cranial nerves will be further discussed below in physical examination.

Spinal Nerves

The 31 pairs of spinal nerves are grouped based on spinal region. There are 8 cervical nerve pairs, 12 thoracic nerve pairs, 5 lumbar nerve pairs, 5 sacral nerve pairs, and 1 coccygeal nerve pair (Marieb and Hoehn 2019). Each of the spinal nerves are composed of both sensory and motor fibres. The spinal nerves interact directly with the spinal cord to communicate information to and from the peripheries. For the purpose of assessing sensory function, the area of skin and subcutaneous tissue supplied by a single spinal nerve is referred to as a dermatome.

History taking and physical examination

Neurological presentations can be broad and complex and require thorough history taking and physical examination. This section will outline a systematic approach to enable paramedics to perform a thorough history and physical examination on the neurological patient.

History

History taking is the first step in the assessment of a neurological patient. A thorough history will allow the paramedic to understand why an ambulance has been called and what the primary concerns are.

Begin by asking open-ended questions that allow the patient to explore their concerns. This will provide a broad overview of the patient's current condition from which we can begin to ask more targeted questions. It is important to note that many patients presenting with neurological complaints may not be able to answer questions or provide a detailed history. Patients with neurological concerns may be unable to speak, have a poor memory, or be confused. It is important to consider history gathering from bystanders or the patient's family and carers.

Table 21.2 gives some examples of history taking questions that can be applied to the neurological patient.

Patient presentations are becoming increasingly complex. Many patients we encounter have multiple chronic health conditions (referred to as co-morbidity), as well as compounding social and environmental risk factors. It is important that paramedics perform a complete secondary survey including past history and risk factors.

Table 21.3 outlines examples of secondary history taking questions for the neurological patient.

Physical examination

Most neurological conditions are not visible and require a physical examination to determine a differential diagnosis. A thorough and systematic approach to the physical examination is essential to rule-in and rule-out differential diagnoses and to limit diagnostic error.

General inspection

An initial visual inspection of the patient enables you to assess the patient's current presenting problem and history. Look for scars indicating previous injuries or surgeries, or muscle wastage and tremors indicating a potential neurodegenerative condition. Observe posture, paralysis, and symmetry for signs of an acute stroke.

Conscious state assessment

GCS is a widely used assessment tool used to evaluate changes in conscious state in response to defined stimuli. Its

TABLE 21.2 Example questions for history taking.

Topic	Example questions
Chief concern	What are you concerned about today?
Onset	When did this start? Is this condition acute, subacute, chronic, or insidious?
Character	What does it feel like? Has it come on suddenly or gradually? What region on your body is most affected?
Prodromal signs and symptoms	Have you been feeling well recently? Did you experience any palpitations, light-headedness/dizziness, or any visual/auditory/verbal changes beforehand? Have you had any recent trauma, falls, or illnesses? Have you seen a doctor for anything recently?
Associated symptoms	What other symptoms do you have? Have you experienced any pain, weakness, or loss of consciousness? After the episode did you feel weak, fatigued, or confused?
Aggravating and relieving factors	Has anything made your condition better or worse?
History of similar episodes	Has anything like this ever happened before? Were any attempts at a diagnosis successful? Have you had any treatment and was it effective?

original intended use was for repeated bedside assessment; however, it has since been applied to the OOH setting (Mehta and Chinthapalli 2019). The GCS is used as an objective assessment tool in the primary survey to assess initial conscious state, in the secondary survey to compare against their usual baseline, and during reassessment to identify trends. The scale examines three components of responsiveness: eye-opening, verbal, and motor responses (Teasdale and Jennett 1974).

Scoring is done on a scale of 3–15, with individual scores given to each of the 3 components. Eye-opening assesses arousal mechanisms in the brainstem. This is performed by assessing the patient's eye movement. If the patient's eyes are not opening spontaneously, the paramedic will speak to the patient and then apply pressure to the patient to initiate an eye-opening response (Mehta and Chinthapalli 2019). The three validated sites of pressure stimulus include nail-bed pressure, trapezius squeeze, or supraorbital pressure (Mehta and Chinthapalli 2019). It is important that a verbal and pressure stimulus is not applied at the same time.

Verbal response tests the patient's ability to comprehend, process, and reply appropriately. The paramedic will speak to the patient and assess their responses. It is common for paramedics to ask 'time, person, and place' questions to assess this (Mehta and Chinthapalli 2019).

Motor response assesses the patient's ability to interpret and perform simple instructions. It is common for paramedics to ask a patient to squeeze their fingers (Mehta and Chinthapalli 2019). When assessing motor response, especially in the neurological patient, it is important to remember that unilateral weakness does not necessarily equate to a lower score. If a patient can squeeze fingers on the right side but has left-sided weakness, they can obey commands.

Patients that have language barriers, an intellectual or neurological disability, or are drug/alcohol affected may be difficult to accurately assess. Thus, it is important to consider the entire clinical picture. Table 21.4 outlines the components and scores of the GCS.

If patients are assessed to have an altered conscious state, the AEIOUTIPS mnemonic can be used as a memory aid to generate differential diagnoses (Table 21.5).

Pupillary assessment

The pupils are a gateway to the central and PNS. Characteristics of the pupils will change based on sympathetic and parasympathetic innervation in the body (Mathôt 2018). These changes can be indicative of trauma and brain injury, or damage to the optic nerves and pathways surrounding it.

Normal pupils will be round, equal in size, appropriate in size to the available light, and reactive to changes in ambient light (Talley and O'Connor 2019). Normal pupils are commonly handed over as PEARL (pupils equal and reactive to light). To perform a pupil assessment, initially inspect the pupil and note any abnormalities or injuries. Assess the size, equality, and shape of each compared to the available light – in darker light the pupils will dilate (Mathôt 2018). Then, perform a lighted inspection by shining a light into the lateral side of one eye for one to three seconds and inspect for size, response (normal, sluggish, unresponsive), and consensuality (light shone in one eye will cause a reaction in both). Once the light stimulus is removed, both pupils should return back to their original state. Repeat this in the alternate eye and note any abnormalities.

TABLE 21.3 Example questions for secondary survey.

Topic	Example questions	Examples in neurological patients
Allergies	Do you have any allergies? What type of reaction does it cause?	Does this allergen cause neurological symptoms such as headaches, dizziness, altered consciousness, or visual disturbances?
Medications	What medications do you take? What do you take these medications for? Have you been taking your medications as directed? Have you had any recent changes to your medications, doses, or timing?	Does the patient take any medications that are consistent with a neurological history (e.g. anticonvulsants, Parkinson's medication)? Is the patient on any anticoagulants or antiplatelets?
Medical history	Do you have any medical history? Do you have any issues with your brain/heart/lungs/kidneys/liver? Do you have issues with your blood pressure, cholesterol, diabetes?	Consider how conditions that are not neurological in nature can impact a patient's neurology. Does this patient have a persistent arrhythmia or a clotting disorder? Does this patient's medical condition cause a sedentary lifestyle? Does this patient have diabetes?
Family history	Did either of your parents, grandparents or siblings have any medical or genetic conditions?	Some neurological conditions can be hereditary. These include Alzheimer's disease, Parkinson's disease, and epilepsy.
Alcohol and other drugs	Do you drink? (If so, how many per week?) Do you take any recreational drugs (including type, frequency, routes)? Does your alcohol consumption or recreational drug use impact other aspects of your personal life?	Consider how excess alcohol consumption can lead to hypertension, heart disease, and stroke. Consider intravenous drug use and the risk of blood clots or infection.
Social history	Do you live alone? Are you able to perform your activities of daily living by yourself or with the support you have? How do you mobilise at home and in the community? Do you think you need any help with your daily life? What is/was your occupation?	Does your family know the signs and symptoms of stroke and other neurological conditions to look out for? Are you able to seek appropriate healthcare when required? Did your occupation expose you to any toxins?
Environmental history	Does the patient's residence appear clean and well kept? Have there been any recent natural or manmade disasters in the area? Has the patient noticed any strange odours within their residence or water, any changes in water colour?	If the patient's residence appears unclean and unkept, why? Consider any exposure to toxins and pollution.

Abnormal pupil responses can be a sign of impaired neurological function. Conditions that can cause aberrant pupil changes include drug toxicity, trauma, stroke, brain or brainstem injury, and poor perfusion or oxygenation.

Motor and sensory assessment

Motor and sensory assessment for paramedics OOH is simple and used to find gross irregularities in the patient's condition. Initially, paramedics must assess bilateral limb

TABLE 21.4 Glasgow Coma Scale.

Component tested	Response	Score
Eye-opening	Spontaneous	4
	To sound	3
	To pressure	2
	None	1
Verbal response	Orientated	5
	Confused	4
	Words	3
	Sounds	2
	None	1
Motor response	Obeys commands	6
	Localising	5
	Normal flexion	4
	Abnormal flexion	3
	Extension	2
	None	1

Source: Adapted from Mehta and Chinthapalli 2019.

TABLE 21.5 AEIOUTIPS mnemonic.

A	Alcohol/drug intoxication
E	Epilepsy (postictal)
I	Insulin (diabetic) or other metabolic problem
O	Overdose or oxygen (hypoxia)
U	Underdose (of medication or drug/alcohol withdrawal)
T	Trauma to the head
I	Infection
P	Pain or psychiatric symptoms
S	Stroke/TIA

strength. The three components of the strength test are the push, pull, and grasp for the upper extremities, and push (plantarflex), pull (dorsiflex), and leg raise for the lower extremities. Make sure to test these at the same time to feel for equality.

In the motor component, you must include a gait assessment if the patient is able to walk. Walking is essential for many activities of daily living (ADLs). As a result, immobility and poor gait will have substantial effects on our patients (Middleton and Fritz 2013). Before assessing gait, ask the patient for any subjective issues they have with walking, ascertain how many falls they have had in the past 12 months, and enquire about the use of walking aids such as a walking stick or wheelie walker. Assess the patient's ability to independently stand up from a seated position, walk a short distance, and seat themselves again. Inspect for speed and balance issues. Patients are at an increased risk of falls if they have balance or mobility problems, cognitive impairment, continence problems, home hazards, or when taking certain medications (Lusardi et al. 2017; Pellicer-García et al. 2020).

For sensory, we want to assess neurovascular observations such as temperature, colour, soft and hard sensation, or the presence of numbness, tingling, or burning. An adapted cranial nerve assessment for the OOH setting should also be performed at this stage (Table 21.6).

Focussed assessment

Focussed assessments are clinical decision tools or memory aids that allow us to further modify our patient care. The most important focussed assessments for the

TABLE 21.6 Adapted cranial nerve assessment.

Nerve no.	Function	Assessment
II, III, IV, VI	Pupils, vision, eye movement	Test pupils as per pupil assessment. With the patient's head still, have them follow your finger in an 'H' pattern
V	Facial sensation, jaw movement	Lightly tap forehead, cheeks, and chin to assess sensation. Place fingers on the mandible and have the patient bite down
VII, XII	Facial muscle and tongue movement	Have the patient smile, raise eyebrows, shut eyelids, puff out cheeks, and poke tongue out
VIII	Hearing	Rub your fingers together next to the patient's ears to assess hearing
IX, X	Uvula and swallowing	Have the patient open their mouth and observe that the uvula is midline, have the patient swallow
XI	Shoulder and head movement	Have the patient shrug and turn their head against resistance from your hand

Source: Talley and O'Connor 2019, with permission of Elsevier.

neurological patient in the OOH environment surround stroke identification.

OOH stroke triage

Delay to definitive care in the context of ischaemic stroke is associated with poor clinical outcomes, increased financial burden for the healthcare system, and reduced functional independence at 90 days (Kim et al. 2022). Secondary transfer from hospitals that cannot perform thrombolysis or ECR also contributes negatively to these outcomes (Froehler et al. 2017). As a result, it is important that paramedics can recognise strokes, and triage to the appropriate facility.

Strokes are characterised by a sudden and rapid onset of weakness or loss of movement to parts of the body, especially on one side. Patients may also have difficulty speaking or swallowing, visual disturbances, headaches, or an altered level of consciousness. Strokes can be classified as ischaemic or haemorrhagic. Whilst it is impossible to differentiate between ischaemic and haemorrhagic strokes without imaging, certain findings increase the likelihood of a haemorrhagic stroke (Lumley et al. 2020).

TABLE 21.7 **ROSIER tool breakdown.**

With blood glucose >3.5mmol/L:		
Symptom	**Score**	
Loss of consciousness or syncope	Y = −1	N = 0
Seizure activity	Y = −1	N = 0
New acute onset of:		
Asymmetric facial weakness	Y = +1	N = 0
Asymmetric arm weakness	Y = +1	N = 0
Asymmetric leg weakness	Y = +1	N = 0
Speech disturbance	Y = +1	N = 0
Visual field defect	Y = + 1	N = 0
Total score: −2 to +5		

Source: Adapted from Nor et al. 2005.

Face–arm–speech test and recognition of stroke in the emergency room tool

An OOH stroke identification screen is recommended as standard practice (Glober et al. 2016). Commonly, the face–arm–speech test (FAST) is used, assessing facial and arm weakness and/or paralysis, and speech problems such as slurred speech or the inability to speak.

An alternative tool that can be used in the OOH setting is the recognition of stroke in the emergency room (ROSIER) tool (Table 21.7). ROSIER, much like FAST, assesses facial, arm and speech deficits, but also includes visual field defects. It is scored between −2 and +5, with a score of +1 or above indicating a higher likelihood of stroke (Nor et al. 2005).

OOH stroke-identification tools are good at selecting patients with strokes, however, false positives from mimics such as migraine, seizure, infection, or hypoglycaemia will often inadvertently be picked up (Lumley et al. 2020). As a result, it is important to have a large differential of possible mimics (Gibson and Whiteley 2013).

Stroke severity scales

There are multiple stroke severity scales employed around the world. Some give a numerical score to indicate stroke severity, whilst others use binary yes/no algorithms. Each assessment tests various components of the neurological examination that are predictive of large vessel occlusions (LVOs) and allows patients to be triaged to ECR hospitals.

The National Institute of Health Stroke Scale (NIHSS) is the most commonly used stroke severity scale and is used in-hospital and in the OOH space. The ACT-FAST triage tool is a relatively new scale used within the Victorian healthcare system in Australia.

The NIHSS

The NIHSS is the gold standard for in-hospital acute stroke assessment (Larsen et al. 2022). It is a quantitative measure of stroke deficit that measures level of consciousness, language, visual field deficits, neglect, and motor and sensory function. A higher score on the NIHSS indicates a higher likelihood of LVO that may be responsive to ECR, as opposed to thrombolysis alone (Larsen et al. 2022).

Several adaptations of the NIHSS have been developed, with some applied to the OOH setting. For example, the shortened-NIHSS-8 is a simplified version of the full NIHSS exam that is easier to use for OOH clinicians. This scale has similar rates of sensitivity and specificity to the full NIHSS but is easier to complete in the time sensitive and often resource lacking OOH environment (Purrucker et al. 2015). It also has the advantage over other non-NIHSS derived scores as it uses the same assessments and grading. Therefore, trends in the patient condition can be formed from symptom onset during the OOH phase, right through to the patient's rehabilitation phase. The shortened-NIHSS-8 is outlined in Table 21.8.

TABLE 21.8 Shortened-NIHSS-8 breakdown.

Measurement	Scoring Definition	Score	Result
Level of consciousness	Alert	0	
	Rousable to minor stimulation	1	
	Rousable to painful stimulation	2	
	Unrousable	3	
Level of consciousness questions Age and current month	Both correct	0	
	One correct or dysarthria	1	
	Neither correct	2	
Commands open/close eyes, grip and release hands	Both correct (ok if impaired by weakness)	0	
	One correct	1	
	Neither correct	2	
Best gaze Test horizontal eye movements tracking object-face	Normal	0	
	Partial gaze, abnormal gaze in 1 or both eyes	1	
	Forced eye deviation or total paresis which cannot be overcome	2	
Facial palsy Show teeth, close eyes tightly, raise eyebrows	Normal	0	
	Minor paralysis, asymmetrical smile	1	
	Partial paralysis	2	
	Complete paralysis	3	
Motor arm Arm outstretched 90 degrees if sitting and 45 degrees if supine Score left and then right arm	No drift for 10 seconds	0	Left score = Right score = Total score =
	Drift but does not hit bed	1	
	Some effort against gravity but cannot sustain	2	
	No effort against gravity	3	
	No movement at all	4	
	Unable to assess due to amputation etc	x	
Dysarthria Ask patient to slowly count to 5	Normal	0	
	Slurred speech but intelligible	1	
	Unintelligible or mute	2	
	Intubation or mechanical barrier	x	
Extinction/neglect Simultaneously touch patient on both hands or legs with eyes closed Show fingers in both visual fields	Normal, no neglect	0	
	Neglect or extinction of double simultaneous stimulation in any modality	1	
	Profound neglect in both visual and sensory modalities	2	
Total score:			

Source: Adapted from Demeestere et al. 2017.

ACT-FAST

The ACT-FAST tool is another stroke triage tool used by OOH clinicians. It consists of a three-step algorithm that tests unilateral arm drift, severe language deficits, and gaze deviation or hemineglect (Zhao et al. 2021). It then sieves patients through an eligibility and stroke mimic screen (Zhao et al. 2018). This has the same end goal as the shortened-NIHSS-8, and has performed favourably compared to other tools, with the added benefit of ease of use (Patrick et al. 2021) (Table 21.9).

Modified Rankin Scale

The Modified Ranking Scale (MRS) is a measure of pre-morbid function and assesses a patient's dependency on others for care and their ability to carry out their usual ADLs such as walking, bathing, and continence (Banks and Marotta 2007).

TABLE 21.9 ACT-FAST tool breakdown.

Step	Assessment	
Step 1: Arms	Have the patient hold arms out at 45–90°s. If one arm falls to the stretcher <10 seconds, or one arm not moving, move to step 2.	
Step 2: Chat/tap	CHAT If right arm weak, assess for severe language deficit Mute Gibberish Unable to follow commands	TAP If left arm weak, assess obvious gaze deviation away from left side or inappropriate response to shoulder tap and name call (for example, failing to notice examiner)
Step 3: Eligibility	Deficits are new or significantly worse Onset <24 hours Independent at home with minimal assistance Exclude mimics (hypoglycaemia, seizure, coma, brain malignancy) No rapid improvement of symptoms at scene	

Source: Adapted from Zhao et al. 2021.

Most ECR guidelines such as the UK's National Institute for Health and Care Excellence guidelines require patients to have an MRS <3 to be eligible for ECR (Table 21.10). This is because highly dependent patients are unlikely to have meaningful functional recovery after treatment (Smith and Schwamm 2015).

TABLE 21.10 MRS breakdown.

Score	Description
0	No symptoms
1	Has some symptoms but still able to carry out usual duties and activities
2	Unable to carry out all activities but able to walk independently
3	Requiring some help but still able to walk independently
4	Unable to walk or tend to bodily needs without assistance
5	Bedridden, incontinent, requiring constant care and attention

Source: Adapted from Banks and Marotta 2007.

Conclusion

This chapter has described the basic structure and function of the nervous system, providing the foundation knowledge needed to perform a neurological assessment. A range of history taking and physical examination techniques have also been explained, enabling paramedics to thoroughly and systematically assess patients presenting with neurological conditions.

Activities

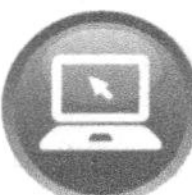

Now review your learning by completing the learning activities in this chapter. The answers to these appear at the end of the book. Further self-test activities can be found at **www.wileyfundamentalseries.com/paramedic/3e.**

Test your knowledge

1. Neurological conditions are the leading cause of death globally – true or false?
2. The myelin sheath slows down nerve conduction so that no information is lost
3. The spinal cord is the link between the CNS and the PNS.
4. Paramedics should apply a verbal and pressure stimulus at the same time when assessing the GCS so that the patient is more likely to respond.
5. Ischaemic and haemorrhagic strokes can be differentiated by clinical signs and symptoms alone.
6. Patients with an MRS <3 are more likely to have meaningful functional recovery from ECR treatment compared to highly dependent patients.

Activity 21.1

Short answer:

1. Compare the signs and symptoms of ischaemic and haemorrhagic strokes and explain why they may present differently.
2. Explain why it is important to ask open ended questions at the beginning of history taking.
3. Reflect on some neurological patients you have attended. How did your communication change, what parts of the assessment were particularly difficult, how can you improve in the future?

Activity 21.2

Practice:

1. Using peers or colleagues, perform ROSIER, s-NIHSS-8, and ACT-FAST as part of a practical simulation.
2. Using peers or colleagues, practise the adapted cranial nerve exam.

Glossary

Action potential: A spike of electrical activity that allows cells to send signals around the body.

Activities of daily living (ADLs): Essential tasks that humans need to perform to live safely and have adequate quality of life. These tasks include basic ADLs such as ambulating, feeding or toileting. Higher order ADLs include cooking, navigating transportation, or managing medications.

Disability adjusted life year: An epidemiological value that represents overall disease burden. It is shown as the number of years lost to disease, ill health, or death.

Endovascular clot retrieval: Removal of a blood clot using imaging and a catheter that can suction the clot out of the blood vessel or break the clot into small pieces.

Gaze deviation: In stroke patients: bilateral eye deviation away from weak/paralysed side.

Hemineglect: In stroke patients: unilateral deficit of awareness or attention to the weak/paralysed side.

Large vessel occlusion (LVO): A type of ischaemic stroke consisting of a blockage to a major blood vessel in the brain.

Secondary transfer: The transfer of a patient from one medical facility to another. This is often performed to improve the management of the patient by transferring them to a facility with better equipment, facilities, or specialists.

Thrombolysis: Breakdown of a blood clot using medication.

References

Bankenahally, R. and Krovvidi, H. (2016). Autonomic nervous system: anatomy, physiology, and relevance in anaesthesia and critical care medicine. *BJA Education* **16** (11): 381–387. doi: 10.1093/bjaed/mkw011.

Banks, J.L. and Marotta, C.A. (2007). Outcomes validity and reliability of the modified rankin scale: implications for stroke clinical trials. *Stroke* **38** (3): 1091–1096. doi: 10.1161/01.STR.0000258355.23810.c6.

Carroll, W. (2019). The global burden of neurological disorders. *The Lancet Neurology* **18** (5):418–419. doi: 10.1016/S1474-4422(19)30029-8.

D'Angelo, E. (2018). Physiology of the cerebellum. In: *Handbook of Clinical Neurology* (ed. M. Manto and T.A.G.M. Huisman), pp. 85–108. Elsevier.

Demeestere, J., Garcia-Esperon, C., Lin, L. et al. (2017). Validation of the National Institute of Health stroke scale-8 to detect large vessel occlusion in ischaemic stroke. *Journal of Stroke & Cerebrovascular Diseases* **26** (7): 1419–1426. doi: 10.1016/j.jstrokecerebrovasdis.2017.03.020.

Diek, D., Smidt, M.P., and Mesman, S. (2022). Molecular organization and patterning of the medulla oblongata in health and disease. *International Journal of Molecular Sciences* **23** (16): 9260. doi: 10.3390/ijms23169260.

Farooqui, A.A. (2016). Neurological aspects of neurological disorders. In: *Trace Amines and Neurological Disorders* (ed. T. Farooqui and A.A. Farooqui), pp.237–256. Academic Press.

Froehler, M.T., Saver, J.L., Zaidat, O.O. et al. (2017). Interhospital transfer before thrombectomy is associated with delayed treatment and worse outcome in the STRATIS registry (Systematic evaluation of patients treated with neurothrombectomy devices for acute ischaemic stroke). *Circulation* **136** (24): 2311–2321. doi: 10.1161/CIRCULATIONAHA.117.028920.

Gibson, L.M. and Whiteley, W. (2013). The differential diagnosis of suspected stroke: A systematic review. *The Journal of the Royal College of Physicians in Edinburgh* **43** (2): 114–118. doi: 10.4997/JRCPE.2013.205.

Glober, N.K., Sporer, K.A., Guluma, K.Z. et al. (2016). Acute stroke: current evidence-based recommendations for out-of-hospital care. *The Western Journal of Emergency Medicine* **17** (2): 104–128. doi: 10.5811/westjem.2015.12.28995.

Gupta, D. (2017). Neuroanatomy. In: *Essentials of Neuroanesthesia* (ed. H. Prabhakar), pp. 3–40. Academic Press.

Jäkel, S. and Dimou, L. (2017). Glial cells and their function in the adult brain: a journey through the history of their ablation. *Frontiers in Cellular Neuroscience* **11:** 24. doi: 10.3389/fncel.2017.00024.

Kim, B.D., Morey, J.R., Marayati, N.F. et al. (2022). Out-of-hospital stroke triage to route patients directly to a thrombectomy center: New York City first-year experience. *Stroke: Vascular and Interventional Neurology.* **3** (2). doi: 10.1161/svin.122.000409.

Larsen, K., Jæger, H.S., Hov, M.R. et al. (2022). Streamlining acute stroke care by introducing national institutes of health stroke scale in the emergency medical services: A prospective cohort study. *Stroke* **53** (6): 2050–2057. doi: 10.1161/STROKEAHA.121.036084.

Lumley, H.A., Flynn, D., Shaw, L. et al. (2020). A scoping review of pre-hospital technology to assist ambulance personnel with patient diagnosis or stratification during the emergency assessment of suspected stroke. *BMC Emergency Medicine* **20** (1). doi: 10.1186/s12873-020-00323-0.

Lusardi, M.M., Fritz, S., Middleton, A. et al. (2017). Determining risk of falls in community dwelling older adults: a systematic review and meta-analysis using post-test probability. *Journal of Geriatric Physical Therapy* **40** (1): 1–36. doi: 10.1519/JPT.0000000000000099.

Marieb, E.N. and Hoehn, K.N. (2019). *Human Anatomy & Physiology, Global Edition*. 11e. Pearson International.

Mathôt, S. (2018). Pupillometry: psychology, physiology, and function. *Journal of Cognition* **1** (1): 16. doi: 10.5334/joc.18.

Mehta, R. and Chinthapalli, K. (2019). Glasgow coma scale explained. *BMJ* **365** (1): 1296. doi: 10.1136/bmj.l1296.

Middleton, A. and Fritz, S. L. (2013). Assessment of gait, balance, and mobility in older adults: Considerations for clinicians. *Current Translational Geriatrics and Experimental Gerontology Reports* **2** (1): 205–214. doi: 10.1007/s13670-013-0057-2.

Moini, J. and Piran, P. (2020). Diencephalon: thalamus and hypothalamus. In: *Functional and Clinical Neuroanatomy* (ed. S.G. Waxman), pp. 267–292. McGraw Hill.

Moini, J., Koenitzer, J., and LoGalbo, A. (2021). Brain structures and functions. In *Global Emergency of Mental Disorders* (ed. J. Moini, J. Koenitzer, and A. LoGalbo), pp. 3–30. Academic Press.

Molnár, Z., Clowry, G.J., Šestan, N. et al. (2019). New insights into the development of the human cerebral cortex. *Journal of Anatomy* **235** (3): 432–451.doi: 10.1111/joa.13055.

Nor, A. M., Davis, J., Sen, B. et al. (2005). The recognition of stroke in the emergency room (ROSIER) scale: development and validation of a stroke recognition instrument. *The Lancet Neurology* **4** (11): 727–734. doi: 10.1016/S1474-4422(05)70201-5.

Patrick, L., Smith, W., and Keenan, K.J. (2021). Large vessel occlusion stroke detection in the out-of-hospital environment. *Current Emergency and Hospital Medicine Reports* **9** (3): 64–72. doi: 10.1007/s40138-021-00234-9.

Pellicer-García, B., Antón-Solanas, I., Ramón-Arbués, E. et al. (2020). Risk of falling and associated factors in older adults with a previous history of falls. *International Journal of Environmental Research and Public Health* **17** (11): 4085. doi: 10.3390/ijerph17114085.

Purrucker, J.C., Hametner, C., Engelbrecht, A. et al. (2015). Comparison of stroke recognition and stroke severity scores for stroke detection in a single cohort. *Journal of Neurology, Neurosurgery, and Psychiatry* **86** (9): 1021–1028. doi: 10.1136/jnnp-2014-309260.

Sciacca, S., Lynch, J., Davagnanam, I. et al. (2019). Midbrain, pons, and medulla: Anatomy and syndromes. *RadioGraphics* **39** (4): 1110–1125. doi: 10.1148/rg.2019180126.

Smith, E.E. and Schwamm, L H. (2015). Endovascular clot retrieval therapy. *Stroke* **46** (6): 1462–1467. doi: 10.1161/STROKEAHA.115.008385.

Stadelmann, C., Timmler, S., Barrantes-Freer, A. et al. (2019). Myelin in the central nervous system: structure, function, and pathology. *Physiological Reviews* **99** (3): 1381–1431. doi: 10.1152/physrev.00031.2018.

Talley, N.J. and O'Connor, S. (2019). *Talley & O'Connor's Clinical Examination Essentials: An Introduction to Clinical Skills (and How to Pass Your Clinical Exams*. 5e. [ebook]. Elsevier Health Sciences.

Teasdale, G. and Jennett, B. (1974). Assessment of coma and impaired consciousness. A practical scale. *The Lancet* **304** (7872): 81–84. doi: 10.1016/S0140-6736(74)91639-0.

The Neurological Alliance. (2019). *Neuro Numbers 2019: A report by the neurological alliance*. Available at: https://www.neural.org.uk/assets/pdfs/neuro-numbers-2019.pdf (accessed 20 October 2022).

Zhao, H., Pesavento, L., Coote, S. et al. (2018). Ambulance clinical triage for acute stroke treatment. *Stroke* **49** (4): 945–951. doi: 10.1161/STROKEAHA.117.019307.

Zhao, H., Smith, K., Bernard, S. et al. (2021). Utility of severity-based out-of-hospital triage for endovascular thrombectomy. *Stroke* **52** (1): 70–79. doi: 10.1161/STROKEAHA.120.031467.

CHAPTER 22

Assessing the abdomen

Matthew Faulkner*
Anaesthetics North/Western Training Scheme, Melbourne, Victoria, Australia

Clare Sutton
School of Biomedical Sciences – Paramedicine, Charles Sturt University, Bathurst, New South Wales, Australia

Georgina Pickering
School of Biomedical Sciences – Paramedicine, Charles Sturt University, Bathurst, New South Wales, Australia

Contents

LEARNING OUTCOMES

On completion of this chapter the reader you will be able to:

- Describe the anatomical borders of the abdomen.
- Recognise the difference between visceral and parietal pain.
- Define the acute abdomen.
- Consider the many causes of abdominal pain.
- Describe the components of a clinical assessment required to perform an appropriate evaluation of the abdomen.

Case Study

An emergency call has been received for a 25-year-old male complaining of severe abdominal pain. He is vomiting and curled up in a ball on the floor. His mum explains that the pain came on suddenly and has got progressively worse over the last few hours. He has a mild fever but no other associated symptoms.

*With contributions from Rachel Jones-Lumby.

Fundamentals of Paramedic Practice: A Systems Approach, Third Edition. Edited by Sam Willis and Ian Peate.

Companion website: www.wiley.com/go/willis/paramedic3e

Introduction

Acute abdominal pain represents one of the top three symptoms prompting patient presentation to emergency departments (EDs), accounting for up to 7% of ED cases. It is the main presenting complaint in patients over 65 years, where it accounts for 13% of ED visits (AACE and Joint Royal Colleges Ambulance Liaison Committee 2016). Causes of abdominal symptoms include appendicitis, cholecystitis/biliary colic, gastritis, urinary/renal colic, intestinal obstruction (including constipation), gastroenteritis, pancreatitis, diverticulitis, peptic ulcer perforation, mesenteric adenitis (especially in children), and gynaecological conditions in women (Manterola et al. 2011; Abdullah and Firmansyah 2012).

A systematic and thorough clinical examination of the abdominal system should thus be part of every paramedic's repertoire. This chapter will review the anatomy of the abdomen and outline a thorough and detailed approach to abdominal examination and assessment.

Abdominal anatomy and physiology

The abdominal cavity represents the largest bodily cavity and is filled by the abdominal viscera and the following major organ systems:

- *Gastrointestinal (or alimentary) system,* comprising distal oesophagus, stomach, duodenum, ileum, caecum, appendix, ascending/transverse/descending colon, and sigmoid colon (Figure 22.1).
- *Hepatobiliary and pancreatic system,* comprising liver, gall bladder, pancreas, and related ducts (Figure 22.2)
- *Spleen and lymphatics.*
- *Urinary system,* comprising kidneys, ureters, and urinary bladder (Figure 22.3).

An abdominal **viscus** may be hollow or solid. Hollow organs include those of the gastrointestinal tract (oesophagus, stomach, small and large intestines, appendix), gallbladder and bile ducts, pancreatic duct, fallopian tubes, ureters, and urinary bladder. Solid organs include the liver, pancreas, spleen, kidneys, adrenals, uterus, and ovaries.

It is helpful to have some understanding of the early development of the abdomen and its contents, as it assists in explaining how certain pain syndromes come to present in the way they do. In embryonic development, the primitive *gut tube,* through sequences of folding and division, gives rise to the **peritoneum,** a tough layer of tissue similar to that of lung pleura and pericardium, which is similarly made up of a parietal and visceral layer. These layers are separated by a thin film of fluid in the peritoneal cavity, which lubricates, stores fat, allows for selective diffusion of water and solutes, and assists in infection control (Kumar and Clark 2017; Martini et al. 2017). As the name suggests, the visceral layer envelopes the visceral organs, and is formed by a complex series of outpouchings off the

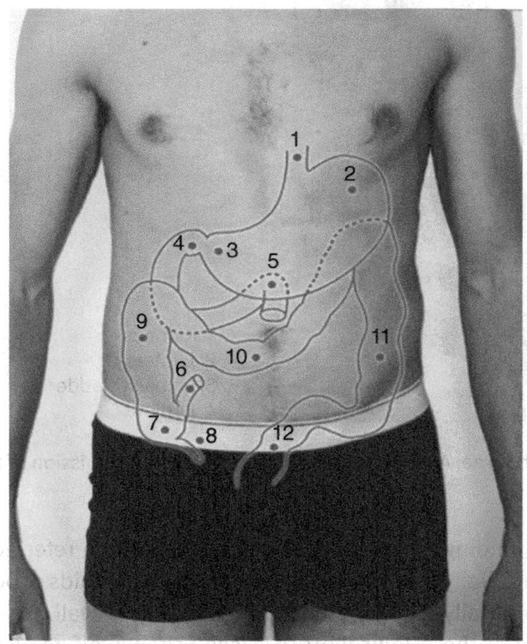

FIGURE 22.1 Gastrointestinal system. Source: M. Magain, Melbourne, Australia, 2014. Reproduced with permission of M. Magain.

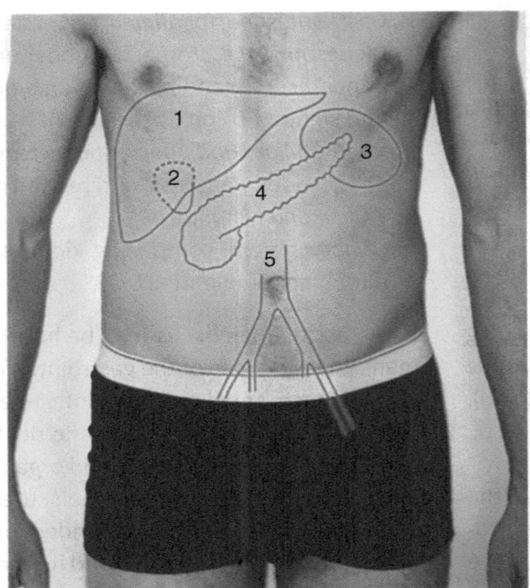

FIGURE 22.2 Hepatobiliary and pancreatic system. Source: M. Magain, Melbourne, Australia, 2014. Reproduced with permission of M. Magain.

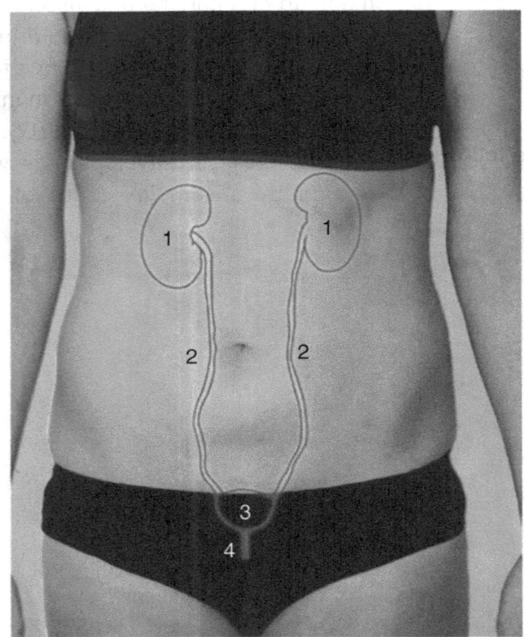

FIGURE 22.3 Urinary system. Source: M. Magain, Melbourne, Australia, 2014. Reproduced with permission of M. Magain.

posterior abdominal wall. Imagine, if you will, suspending a taut piece of clingfilm, then placing on it a tube. Gradually allow the clingfilm to become slack, until it eventually adheres to itself, with the tube enveloped within it at the bottom. The suspended, self-adhered section from which this tube now hangs would be referred to in the gut as a **mesentery** – two suspensory folds of peritoneum reflected off the posterior abdominal wall. This complex embryological process (see Schoenwolf and Larsen 2009) leads to a division of organs that are suspended intraperitoneal

TABLE 22.1 Distribution of the abdominal organs.

Intraperitoneal	Retroperitoneal	Secondarily retroperitoneal
Abdominal oesophagus	Thoracic oesophagus	Pancreas
Stomach	Rectum and anus	Duodenum
Spleen		Ascending colon
Liver (with gallbladder)		Descending colon
Jejunum		
Ileum		
Caecum and appendix		
Sigmoid colon		

organs, and to those that are retroperitoneal or secondarily retroperitoneal (Table 22.1), and thus are essentially adherent to the posterior abdominal wall.

The peritoneum allows for free movement of most of the abdominal viscera. With the enveloping of each organ in visceral pleura and their suspension from their mesentery (or adherence to the posterior abdominal wall) comes their associated blood supply and, importantly to this chapter, their nerve supply. When we refer to types of pain, keep in mind the underlying anatomy, and hopefully *why* a patient experiences a particular sensation will become more evident.

Genitourinary causes of abdominal pain

It is important to always consider that (especially younger) patients presenting with abdominal pain may have symptoms originating from reproductive organs and referring to other parts of the abdomen.

Females

Always consider gynaecological causes of pain in females (especially of childbearing age), which may include pain relating to menstrual periods, endometriosis, ruptured ovarian cysts, pelvic inflammatory disease, ovarian torsion, or ruptured ectopic pregnancy (see Brown and Cadogan 2011, section XII). As discussed later in the chapter, targeted history gathering may be required depending on the level of suspicion and given presentation.

Most gynaecological conditions will present with lower abdominal pain. Some may also include vaginal discharge or blood loss. Some gynaecological presentations such as ruptured ectopic pregnancy with haemodynamic instability can be life threatening. It may be difficult to differentiate between, say, a right-sided ectopic pregnancy and appendicitis, thus careful consideration of all differential diagnoses should be the practice of an astute paramedic.

Males

It is important to remember that abdominal pain in (especially young) males may well be referred from the reproductive organs. It may be necessary to specifically enquire about (and where appropriate, examine for) testicular pain, as some patients may not volunteer such information on general questioning. Dividing conditions by age is often useful:

- In males under 25 years (and especially aged 12–14 years), acute testicular torsion should always be considered (Meckler et al. 2016). There is usually acute onset of testicular and lower abdominal pain, and often associated nausea and vomiting, and one testis may sit high (and very painfully) in the scrotum. The testis becomes nonviable after approximately six hours of torsion.
- Acute epididymo-orchitis, with pain beginning gradually in the testis and sometimes referring to the abdomen, may be a cause in the sexually active male.
- In those further advanced in age, one should always consider acute urinary retention as a result of prostate pathology, urethral stricture, pelvic tumours, or even constipation. Although the distended urinary bladder is often palpable, elderly patients may present only with delirium or restlessness, so this condition can be easily missed.

The abdomen can be divided into quadrants (Figure 22.4) by passing a dividing median line vertically though the umbilicus, and a second line at right angles to this line transversely, with each segment named accordingly. This will assist with describing findings and locating landmarks.

One can also divide the abdomen into nine regions (Figure 22.5). When we overlay a diagram of organ locations (Figures 22.1–22.3 and 22.6), we begin to build up a picture of how surface anatomy relates to underlying structures.

The nature of abdominal pain

There are three pathways by which a patient may experience abdominal pain: visceral, somatic, and referred.

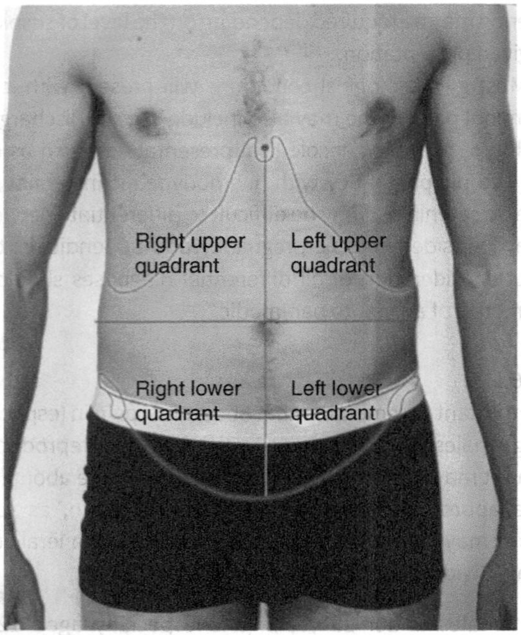

FIGURE 22.4 The four abdominal quadrants. Source: M. Magain, Melbourne, Australia, 2014. Reproduced with permission of M. Magain.

Visceral pain tends to be elicited by stretching and distension and is mediated by afferent C fibres (a type of autonomic nerve fibre) located in the walls of hollow viscera and in the capsules of solid organs. Each organ is supplied by a pair of nerve bundles (see Netter 2006, pp. 318–328), and they can be divided into the cardiopulmonary, thoracic, lumbar, sacral, and pelvic branches (corresponding to where they join the spinal canal).

The visceral structures, encased by the peritoneum and suspended from their mesenteries, tend to be associated with different sensory levels in the spine (Figure 22.7). Given that they possess bilateral paired nervous innovations, increased luminal distension (say, in the bowel due to obstruction), forceful smooth-muscle contractions ('colic'), or capsular stretching (such as acute hepatitis) is most often poorly localised, centralised to the midline, and referred to other regions, also supplied by that same division of the **splanchnic system.** When the paramedic takes a history, they may find that discomfort began as a vague, centralised ache (visceral pain). As the pathology progresses, this pain may become parietal in nature, leading to signs of peritonism that ought to ring alarm bells for the paramedic.

Practice insight

Here is a handy way to remember the direction of nerve fibres: Afferent fibres Arrive at the central nervous system. Efferent fibres Exit the central nervous system.

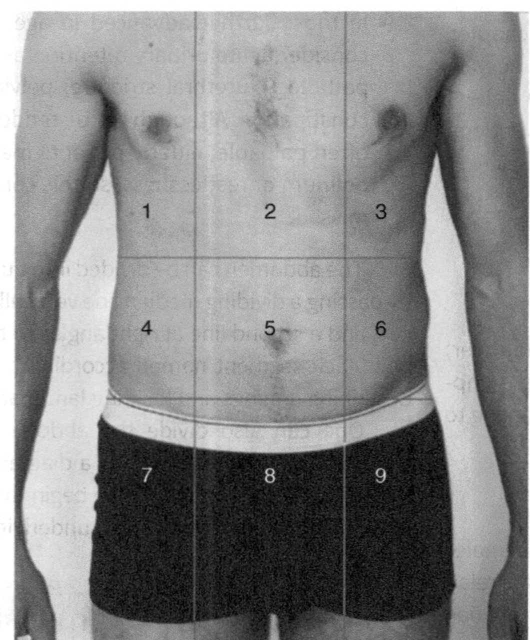

FIGURE 22.5 The nine abdominal regions. Source: M. Magain, Melbourne, Australia, 2014. Reproduced with permission of M. Magain.

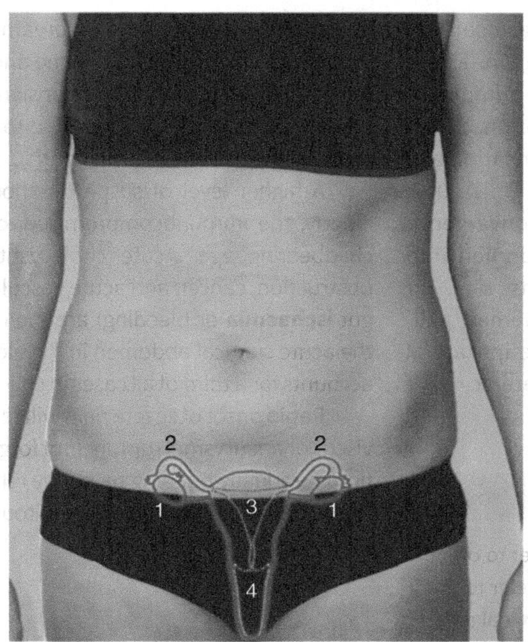

FIGURE 22.6 Location of the ovaries. Source: M. Magain, Melbourne, Australia, 2014. Reproduced with permission of M. Magain.

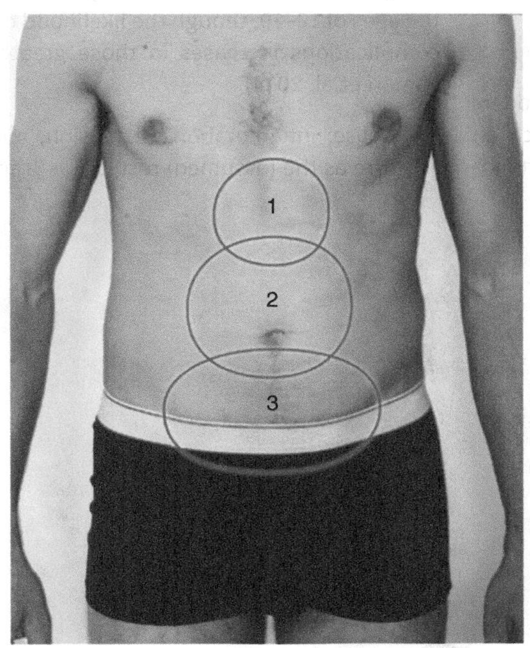

FIGURE 22.7 Visceral structures. Source: M. Magain, Melbourne, Australia, 2014. Reproduced with permission of M. Magain.

Parietal pain is mediated by a different set of nerve fibres, called C and A delta nerve fibres, which form part of the somatic nervous system, responsible for detecting sensory modalities such as touch, temperature, and pain. These fibres are responsible for the transmission of rapid, localised, sharp, and more acute signals, and the somatic afferent fibres are directed to only one side of the nervous system (in contrast to visceral pain sensations). Thus, any irritation of the parietal peritoneum by the likes of blood, pus, bile, urine, gastrointestinal contents, or inflammatory mediators released in response to a pathological insult will be transmitted as a localised, sharp, stabbing pain. This is what doctors often refer to as 'peritonitic', and it implies a condition that may well need surgical intervention.

Referred pain denotes the perception of sensation at a site distant from the pain stimulus (Kumar and Clark 2017; Martini et al. 2017). This is due to the complex convergence of afferent fibres from wide areas in the abdomen into small areas of the spinal cord. This explains why, for example, diaphragmatic irritation (by an inflamed gallbladder, for instance) is often perceived in the ipsilateral (that is, the right side) shoulder, because the phrenic nerve serves both of these areas (Figure 22.8).

Practice insight

Remember that although abdominal pain can refer to other areas of the body, so too can pain in other areas refer to the abdomen. Cardiac pain may be reported as abdominal pain, so always consider 'abdominal pain' that may be referring from the chest.

The acute abdomen

The 'acute abdomen' refers to any nontraumatic sudden, severe abdominal pain of unclear aetiology for which an urgent operation may be necessary. It is of utmost importance to start with the ABCs (airway, breathing, circulation): signs of reduced circulating blood volume and hypoperfusion may be reflected by tachycardia, hypotension, tachypnoea, diaphoresis, and pallor. Shock may be due to bleeding, to substantial fluid losses (as seen in pancreatitis), or to sepsis.

A higher level of suspicion should be reserved for the elderly, the immunocompromised, children, and women of childbearing age. Acute cholecystitis, appendicitis, bowel obstruction, cancer, and acute vascular conditions (leading to gut **ischaemia** or bleeding) are the most common causes of the acute surgical abdomen in the elderly, whilst appendicitis accounts for a third of all cases in children (Meckler et al. 2016).

Rapid onset of severe pain will tend to suggest perforated viscus or aneurysmal rupture (not forgetting myocardial infarction). Gradually building pain may reflect worsening appendicitis, bowel obstruction, or a genitourinary or gynaecological issue.

Important abdominal pathologies

Appendicitis

The greatest incidence of acute appendicitis occurs around the ages of 10–19, though the likelihood of perforation and complications increases in those greater than 65 years (Omari et al. 2014).

- *Cause:* inflammation, distension, and potential rupture as the (assumed) result of entrapped bacteria.

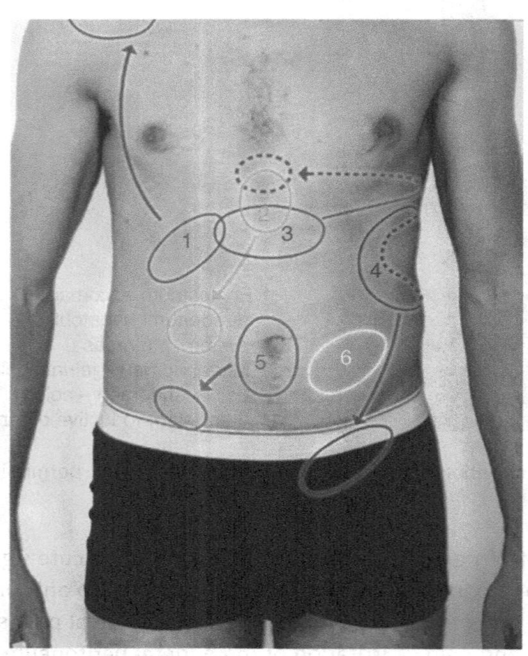

FIGURE 22.8 Referred pain. Source: M. Magain, Melbourne, Australia, 2014. Reproduced with permission of M. Magain.

- *Presentation:* starts as poorly localised central or epigastric abdominal pain, usually periumbilical, which shifts to the right iliac fossa.
- *Associated symptoms:* low-grade fever, anorexia, nausea, vomiting, and either diarrhoea or constipation.
- *Examination:* localised right iliac fossa tenderness on palpation.
- *Specific signs and symptoms:*
  - McBurney's sign – point tenderness over a place two-thirds of the distance along a line taken from the anterior superior iliac spine to the umbilicus.
  - Rovsing's sign – assessing for any tenderness in the right illiac fossa arising from palpation of the opposite, left illiac fossa.
  - Psoas sign – the ileopsoas is a retroperitoneal hip flexor muscle, lying under the appendix at the edge of the peritoneum. Flexion of the right hip may cause right iliac fossa irritation when the appendix is inflamed.
  - Obturator sign – likewise, flexion and internal rotation of the right hip may cause spasm, and resultant right iliac fossa pain, as the obturator muscle (in part responsible for this movement) sits close to the appendix.

Intestinal obstruction

- *Causes:* adhesions (especially due to prior surgeries), incarcerated hernia, volvulus (twisting), intussusception (telescoping), carcinomas, diverticulitis, mesenteric infarction (as may be seen in the setting of emboli secondary to atrial fibrillation), Crohn's disease, or neurological disorders affecting peristalsis.
- *Presentation:* in high obstruction, there tends to be early vomiting, colicky ('wave-like') pain, and distension. In low obstruction, there is constipation and inability to pass flatus, resulting in distension.
- *Associated symptoms:* nausea, vomiting (sometimes feculent in the case of small bowel obstruction), and possible shock.
- *Specific signs and symptoms:* always consider hernia entrapment, especially in the inguinal regions or beneath scars from previous surgeries. Always ask about stools (specifically looking for evidence of altered bowel habits and/or bleeding).

Diverticulitis

- *Cause:* diverticula are dead-end pouches most commonly within the descending colon wall. The process is termed diverticulosis. The reason sudden inflammation occurs remains uncertain (Peery et al. 2012).
- *Presentation:* lower abdominal pain radiating to the left iliac fossa, often with guarding on palpation.
- *Associated symptoms:* bloody diarrhoea, fever.
- *Specific signs and symptoms:* sometimes presents with profuse frank rectal blood loss.

Biliary colic, acute cholecystitis, and pancreatitis

We can group these under the one banner because, although they represent different processes, they may nonetheless be related to inflammation of, or blockages within, the biliary tree.

Gallstones form within the gallbladder (which stores bile made by the liver) in 5–25% of the population and this number is higher in Western populations (Gurusamy and Davidson 2014). Whilst often asymptomatic, gallstones are well known to potentially lead to presentations of biliary colic, acute or chronic cholecystitis, as well as potentially life-threatening pancreatitis, obstructive jaundice, or gallbladder cancer (Stringer et al. 2013). Let us break them down into each entity.

Biliary colic

- *Cause:* interruption of normal bile flow by stones or sludge, causing the muscular distended gallbladder to repeatedly try to squeeze bile past the blockade.
- *Presentation*: episodic right upper quadrant colicky (wave-like and intermittent) pain.
- *Associated symptoms:* may be jaundiced if there is blockade of the common bile duct (most visible as scleral icterus – the yellowing of the white parts of the eyes), combined with dark urine (due to high levels of bilirubin). There may be nausea and vomiting.
- *Specific signs and symptoms:* may describe right scapula and shoulder tip discomfort. Pain tends to be poorly localised. Episodes may occur after fatty meals and pain tends to subside over a number of hours. Episodes may become more intense and frequent over time.

Acute cholecystitis

- *Cause:* ongoing prevention of bile outflow, leading to distension, irritation, inflammation, infection, and potentially perforation of the gallbladder.
- *Presentation:* constant, severe right upper quadrant pain that refers to the right scapula and shoulder.
- *Associated symptoms:* anorexia, nausea, vomiting, fever, and occasional jaundice.

- *Specific signs and symptoms:* Murphy's sign – painful splinting of respiration (patient suddenly stops breathing) at deep inspiration, whilst the examiner is placing gentle pressure over the gallbladder region, due to severe sharp right upper quadrant pain. There will be localised tenderness and involuntary guarding.

Acute pancreatitis

- *Cause:* most easily remembered by the mnemonic (alluding to alcoholism as a leading cause) IGETS-MASHED – idiopathic, gallstones, ethanol, trauma, steroids, mumps (and a variety of other infections), autoimmune, scorpion sting (of all things), hyperthermia/hyperlipidaemia/hyperparathyroidism, ERCP (endoscopic retrograde cholangio-pancreatography – a procedure used to clear biliary obstructions), drugs.
- *Presentation:* sudden, severe mid-epigastric abdominal pain that tends to radiate to the back and sometimes chest. It is normally associated with guarding.
- *Associated symptoms:* repeated vomiting, dehydration, fever, shock if severe.
- *Specific signs and symptoms:* may derive some relief from sitting forward. May have absent bowel sounds on auscultation and describe offensive or fatty stools (due to poor digestion).

Ruptured abdominal aortic aneurysm

- *Cause:* weakening of the vessel wall through a variety of postulated causes (Chaikof et al. 2009).
- *Presentation:* sudden onset of left abdominal pain, often tearing or knifelike, and radiating through to the back.
- *Associated symptoms:* syncope, collapse, or unexplained shock.
- *Specific signs and symptoms:* classic triad of abdominal pain, hypotension, and pulsatile, tender abdominal mass. Note that, given this condition is life threatening, it must always be considered, especially in vulnerable groups such as previously known abdominal aortic aneurysm or men over 45 years of age (Brown and Cadogan 2011).

Patient assessment

Once you have completed the primary survey and established the patient is not time critical, you may begin the secondary survey, which includes the patient interview (history taking), a clinical examination, and a full set of vital signs.

The process outlined in this chapter is based on a medical model approach, which is a systematic process consisting of a comprehensive history and a structured clinical examination. Before commencing the assessment, ensure you have identified and managed any immediate threats to life. Patients found to be time critical during the primary survey will require a limited, focused exam. The medical model approach should only be utilised for patients determined not to be time critical.

The abdominal system is interlinked with other body systems and abdominal conditions may sometimes only be detected through abnormal presentations in other systems. For this reason, it is often necessary to undertake an integrated clinical examination. The two most common integrated examinations are the cardio-respiratory and cardio-abdominal examinations.

History taking

Accurate diagnosis of an abdominal complaint will be almost impossible without a history. History taking may occur prior to examination and treatment of the patient or concurrently with other activities. A suggested structure for obtaining the history is listed here and questions are listed in Table 22.2.

Presenting complaint and history of presenting complaint

The presenting complaint refers to the main reason the patient sought help in the first place. The chief complaint for abdominal conditions may often not present typically, and it may take further investigations to exclude the involvement of other systems. Some of the most common signs and symptoms associated with abdominal complaints are listed in Table 22.3.

Other factors that can help to generate a more definitive list of *differential diagnoses* are related to a more detailed exploration of the type and duration of the pain. Helpful mnemonics are explained in Table 22.4.

Practice insight

Particular care should be taken in higher-risk populations such as pregnant or childbearing-age females, elderly, or immunocompromised patients.

TABLE 22.2 Questions for abdominal patients.

Type of history	Lines of enquiry (questions to ask)
History of presenting complaint	When did it begin?
	How severe is it? Does it affect functionality (walking upstairs/to the bathroom, washing/dressing)?
	What were you doing when it started?
	Are there any relieving or aggravating factors?
	Were you eating during onset?
	Are there any associated symptoms?
	Is the onset acute, subacute, or chronic?
	Any recent illness/infection?
	Have you taken any medication to attempt to resolve these symptoms and how effective was it?
Previous medical history	Any history of previous abdominal problems?
	Any abdominal surgery?
	Any cardiac history?
	Any history of renal calculi or urinary tract infection?
	Any history of diabetes, hypertension, gout, hepatitis, peptic ulcers, colitis, bowel cancer?
	Any previous hospital admissions? Similar episodes or recent investigations?
Medication history	Do you take any medications on a regular basis? Note dosage and compliance
	Length of time on current medication regime? Date of last medication review?
	Do you take any 'over-the-counter' medication?
	Any history of recreational drugs?
	Any use of herbal remedies?
Social history	Any history of smoking? Number and years?
	Alcohol consumption?
	Any history of recreational drug use?
	Patient's occupation? Retired or still employed?
	Any anxiety-related symptoms or history of depression?
	Travel history?
	Nutrition and diet?
	Attitude to health and physical activity?
	Any social support needed/in place for activities of daily living?
Family history	Health of siblings?
	Cause and age at death – parents and siblings?
	Family history of hypertension or diabetes?
	Family history of renal disease?
	Family history of polycystic kidney disease?

TABLE 22.2 *(Continued)*

Type of history	Lines of enquiry (questions to ask)
Review of systems: gastrointestinal	Any history of indigestion or heartburn? Any difficulty swallowing (dysphagia)? Any abdominal pain or discomfort? Any bloating or swelling of the abdomen? Any signs of jaundice? Have you noticed any sudden/unexplained weight gain or weight loss? Sore tongue or mouth ulcers? Any change in bowel motions or abnormal colour? Have you vomited blood (haematemesis) or had black bowel motions (melaena)? Any change in frequency or effort of urination? Any blood in urine?

Past/previous medical history

It is important to gain a comprehensive *surgical* history in addition to the usual *medical* history. Prior abdominal surgeries can predispose to **adhesions** leading to strictures and obstructions, or to fistula formation. It may be necessary to ask specifically about previous conditions such as ulcers, gallstones or renal stones, diverticulitis, hernias, or appendicitis. In particular:

- It is often necessary to ask females discreetly about past pregnancies, terminations, and potential for current pregnancy.
- Also ask about menstrual periods, endometriosis, ovarian cysts, and pelvic inflammatory disease.
- In males, it may be important to ask about testicular pain or prostate issues.

Drug history

Drug history should be explored during the history taking and this should include questions around compliance and concordance, and whether or not the patient is taking any additional 'over-the-counter' medication, herbal remedies, or recreational drugs. Establish whether the patient has had any recent review of their medication and whether they have recently started or stopped taking any medication. It is good to develop a working knowledge of the commonly prescribed medications for abdominal conditions, especially as the patient may not always be able to communicate this information to you during an acute presentation (Talley and O'Connor 2017).

Practice insight

Note medications that may mask symptoms (analgesia) or exacerbate (nonsteroidal anti-inflammatory drugs or **NSAIDs** and bleeding; opiates and constipation) abdominal presentations.

TABLE 22.3 **Signs and symptoms of abdominal pathology.**

Pain
Fever
Nausea and/or vomiting
Reflux/heartburn
Loss of appetite; early postprandial satiation
Unintentional weight loss
Bloating and/or distension
Altered bowel habitus (diarrhoea, constipation, or both; dark or pale stools, mucous)
Dysuria/haematuria
Bleeding (haematemesis, malaena, frank rectal blood loss, vaginal bleeding)
Jaundice

TABLE 22.4 **Mnemonics for taking a symptom/pain history.**

OPQRST-ASPN	SOCRATES
Onset	**S**ite
Provocation or **P**alliation	**O**nset
Quality	**C**haracteristics
Region and **R**adiation	**R**adiation
Severity	**A**ssociated symptoms
Time	**T**iming
Associated **S**ymptoms	**E**xacerbating factors
Pertinent **N**egatives	**S**everity

Allergies

Questions around allergies relate to medication, food, and other factors (insect bites, animals). Further questions should be asked around any identified allergies to determine what the exact nature of the response was and whether the patient suffered a minor allergic reaction or an anaphylactic reaction.

Social history

Social history incorporates a wide range of information, from day-to-day activities to occupation, travel history, physical activity, nutrition, and alcohol and tobacco consumption. The responses to these questions may provide important clues to the presence of risk factors for specific conditions, as well as providing you with a good overview of the patient's general health status (Douglas et al. 2013). Additional social history questions in need of further investigation in the abdominal patient are those around pregnancy (or potential pregnancy), sexual history (if appropriate), and the ongoing use of analgesics. Potential occupational, sexual, or travel exposure to potential pathogens such as hepatitis-causing viruses should be specifically addressed.

Family history

Always consider abdominal disorders that may have a genetic component, such as cancers in family members (e.g. bowel, ovarian), autoimmune diseases (see Cojocaru et al. 2011), or inflammatory bowel disease (Crohn's disease, ulcerative colitis).

Practice insight

Remember, a *symptom* is something the patient feels, and is able to describe. A *sign* is something you uncover on examination. The two are commonly confused.

Clinical examination

Clinical examination of the abdominal system starts with an end-of-bed assessment to provide a general impression of the patient. This considers factors such as the patient's gender, weight, and body shape (any evidence of obesity, wasting, or other features of note), as well as a consideration of environmental clues. Whilst the chief anatomical area for abdominal examination focuses on the abdomen, it is important to undertake a systematic examination starting from the patient's hands and nails, moving up to their arms, neck, and face, including examination of the eyes and mouth (Talley and O'Connor 2017). A more detailed examination of the abdomen would follow utilising the IAPP (inspection, auscultation, palpation, and percussion) structure (Douglas et al. 2013).

Patients should be observed for the following behaviours:

- *Restlessness* is often noted with presentations of acute cholecystitis or renal colic.
- *Reluctance to move,* where a foetal position may be maintained, can be seen in the setting of peritonitis.
- *Shallow breathing* may be notable when abdominal pain is exacerbated by deep inspiration or, for example, when the diaphragm itself is irritated by peritonitis or a markedly inflamed gallbladder impinging on it.

Hand assessment

Much information about the patient's level of perfusion can be obtained through a brief examination of the hands. Examine for palmar erythema (reddened palms) and a hepatic flap (asterixis) caused by liver failure. Check also for finger clubbing, cyanosis, and any other abnormalities present in the nails such as leukonychia (white nails due to kidney disease). You should also take note of the temperature and texture of skin (warm and dry or cool and clammy).

The radial pulse is located at the wrist. Described as a peripheral pulse, it is the most commonly palpated pulse by the paramedic and helps determine cardiovascular efficiency due to its presence and strength. When assessing a pulse, take note of:

- Presence/absence
- Rate
- Regularity
- Strength

Head and neck assessment

Inspect the eyes to exclude any pallor of the conjunctiva, which may suggest anaemia, or any signs of jaundice. Check also for any signs of pallor or cyanosis in the face and mouth, and for any evidence of poor dentition, halitosis, or mouth ulcers (Douglas et al. 2013; Talley and O'Connor 2017). Check the neck for any signs of increased jugular venous pressure.

Abdominal examination

Following the IAPP format, examination of the abdomen starts with inspection of the thorax and abdomen.

Inspection

The abdomen should ideally be examined with the patient supine, hands by their sides, though clearly this may not always be achievable. This helps facilitate abdominal muscle relaxation (lifting the patient's knees may also help). The abdomen should be fully exposed (preserving privacy and dignity), and the patient kept as warm and comfortable as possible.

Inspect the abdomen, observing for previous surgical scars. Recent scars tend to appear pink, old scars white. Small scars around the umbilicus may indicate previous laparoscopic surgeries; lower **Pfannenstiel incision** scars ('bikini-line' scars) may indicate caesarean section or gynaecological surgeries in female patients (Figure 22.9)

Irregularities in shape possibly suggest hernia or enlargement of an underlying organ. Also inspect for skin irregularities such as rashes, prominent veins (possibly suggesting hepatic portal congestion or impedance to inferior vena cava flow from thrombosis or tumour), spider naevi (suggestive of liver cirrhosis), or stretch marks, which may reflect **ascites.** Pulsatile masses could be indicative of an abdominal aortic aneurysm.

Auscultation

During auscultation you will primarily listen for bowel sounds, which should be audible in all abdominal regions in healthy individuals. One tends to report bowel sounds as either

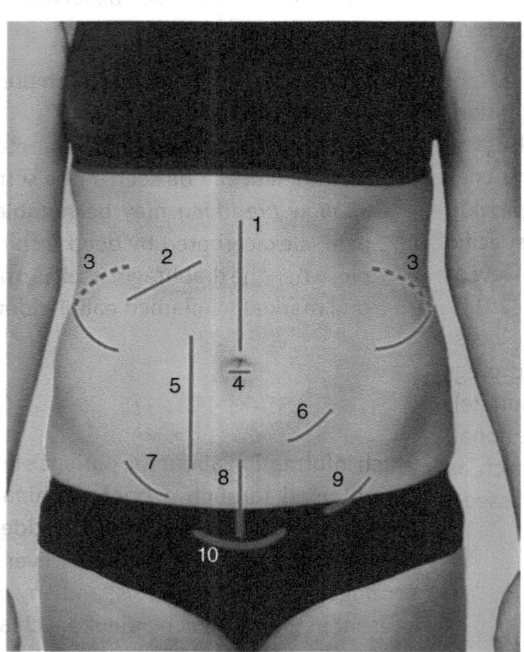

FIGURE 22.9 Surgical scar locations. Source: M. Magain, Melbourne, Australia, 2014. Reproduced with permission of M. Magain.

'present' or 'absent', where an absence of sound suggests bowel paralysis (paralytic ileus). One might also note high-pitched 'tinkling' sounds when an obstruction is present.

Palpation

Palpating the abdomen should be carried out methodically, with the fingers together and pressure distributed across the anterior surfaces of all the examiner's fingers; in the case of examining for a palpable liver or spleen, pressure should be distributed along the thumb side (lateral aspect) of the examiner's hand and fingers. Always ask where the patient is most tender, as this is the area that ought to be examined last. If the paramedic is haphazard in this respect, patient trust may be lost, and the patient may resist further palpation.

Begin with light pressure in the quadrant farthest from the main source of pain. Feel for lumps, masses, or signs of peritonism, moving systematically. Always consider what structures lie beneath your hand during palpation, and regularly watch the patient's facial expressions for suggestions of discomfort. Proceed to deep palpation, following the same pattern and leaving the most tender regions until last.

> **Practice insight**
>
> Signs of peritonism may include:
>
> - *Guarding* – the voluntary or involuntary tensing of the abdominal wall muscles over an inflamed abdominal region to guard the underlying structures against the pain of palpation. Involuntary guarding suggests peritonitis.
> - *Rigidity* – constant involuntary contraction of abdominal muscles.
> - *Rebound tenderness* – sudden release of a slowly compressed abdominal wall causing a rapid stab of sharp pain.

The liver may, on occasion, require specific attention. To palpate for a liver, align your hand with the patient's right costal margin, beginning at the umbilicus (or even the right iliac **fossa** if liver enlargement is suspected), asking the patient to breathe in and out slowly. Use the lateral edge of the hand to press down on expiration; you may sometimes feel the edge of the liver under your hand. Repeat this process, moving about 1–2 cm at a time towards the costal margin on the right (that is, the base of the ribs). Many disorders may cause liver enlargement and/or tenderness, including hepatitis (acute viral, toxic, or alcoholic), right-heart failure (where the liver becomes congested with blood), cancers (which are causing the liver capsule to stretch, or may have started to bleed or infiltrate other vital areas), or perhaps biliary obstruction with cholangitis (infection of the common bile duct).

Percussion

Percussion may be applied to gauge the size of organs, or the location of fluid. It will also tend to elicit pain if peritonitis is present. In general, hollow and mostly air-filled organs such as the intestines will produce a more resonant percussion note, whereas fluid (such as blood or ascites) will sound dull. Percussion involves placing your hand flat on the region to be examined, and then briskly tapping the middle finger of this hand with the tip of the middle finger of your other hand.

> **Practice insight**
>
> There are five 'Fs' of abdominal distension to consider: fat (obesity), fluid (ascites or severe bleeding), foetus (pregnancy), flatus (gaseous distension from causes such as bowel obstruction), and 'filthy' big tumour (Talley and O'Connor 2017).

Conclusion

Paramedics will commonly assess patients with abdominal pain. Rapid identification and treatment of abdominal disorders, along with timely transport to the most appropriate medical facility, are vital to ensure optimal patient outcomes. This chapter provides a thorough overview of abdominal assessment and common abdominal pathologies.

Activities

Now review your learning by completing the learning activities in this chapter. The answers to these appear at the end of the book. Further self-test activities can be found at **www. wileyfundamentalseries.com/ paramedic/3e.**

Test your knowledge

1. Show two ways in which the abdomen can be divided by an overlying grid to help describe signs and symptoms of abdominal pain. Identify the underlying structures in each of these divisions.
2. What is the difference between visceral and parietal pain?
3. What is an acute abdomen? What symptoms, signs, and details in the history of the presenting complaint might assist the paramedic to decide that a patient with abdominal pain is time critical?
4. What additional diagnoses need to be considered in the young female presenting with abdominal pain?
5. Provide a working diagnosis and two possible differential diagnoses for the case study given at the start of the chapter.

Activity 22.1

Draw the abdomen with an overlying grid showing four quadrants or nine regions and include as many anatomical structures as you can (it may help to use different colours for each major organ system). Try repeating this activity over time to improve your anatomical knowledge.

Activity 22.2

Have a fellow student imagine an abdominal condition without your knowledge of its nature. Take a history, focusing down on what you feel the problem may be. Can accurate diagnoses in medicine be made through careful history taking alone?

Activity 22.3

Undertake an abdominal examination of a patient (real or simulated). Practise being systematic, and do not forget to monitor your patient's facial expressions for clues regarding discomfort or pain.

Activity 22.4

Review the anatomy of the biliary tree, including the liver and its hepatic ducts, the gallbladder, the cystic duct, the pancreatic duct, the common bile duct, and the manner in which this system drains into the duodenum (see Netter 2006, pp. 294–296).

Glossary

Adhesions: Past abdominal surgery can cause tissue to adhere to adjoining structures and result in the formation of bands of scar tissue. This can lead to strictures (narrowings in a hollow tube), fistulae (abnormal connection between structures), or obstruction.

Ascites: An accumulation of fluid in the peritoneal cavity, most commonly as the result of severe liver disease.

Fossa: A hollow or depression. Thus, the iliac fossa is an area overlying the ileum (the large wing-shaped sections of the pelvis), either on the left or the right.

Ischaemia: Restriction of blood supply, leading to a lack of nutrients and oxygen needed to sustain normal cellular metabolism.

Mesentery: Two sheets of peritoneum, containing vessels and nerves, which reflect off the posterior abdominal wall to suspend the jejunum and ileum. This term can also be extended to include any double fold of peritoneum that surrounds an abdominal structure.

Nonsteroidal anti-inflammatory drug (NSAID): A class of commonly used anti-inflammatory medications (such as aspirin or ibuprofen), which often produce gastrointestinal side effects (such as gastric erosion and bleeding), especially with continued or high-dose use.

Peritoneum: A lining of the abdominal cavity, comprising serous membrane, forming the parietal (outer) layer, which lines the abdominal and pelvic cavities, and the visceral (inner) layer, which envelops abdominal organs.

Pfannenstiel incision: A low, slightly curved, abdominal incision made to gain access to the pelvic organs. Commonly used for caesarean section deliveries or hernia repair.

Splanchnic system: Paired nerve fibres that supply both autonomic efferent and sensory afferent signals to and from (respectively) the abdominal viscera.

Viscus (pleural = viscera): Any internal organ, whether solid or hollow (usually in reference to abdominal and pelvic organs).

References

Abdullah, M. and Firmansyah, M.A. (2012). Diagnostic approach and management of acute abdominal pain. *Acta Medica Indonesiana* **44** (4): 344–350.

AACE (Association of Ambulance Chief Executives) and Joint Royal Colleges Ambulance Liaison Committee (2016). *JRCALC Clinical Practice Guidelines*. Bridgwater: Class Publishing.

Brown, A.F.T. and Cadogan, M.D. (2011). *Emergency Medicine.* 6e. London: Hodder Arnold.

Chaikof, E.L., Brewster, D.C., Dalman, R.L. et al. (2009). The care of patients with an abdominal aortic aneurysm: The Society for Vascular Surgery practice guidelines. *Journal of Vascular Surgery* **50** (4 suppl): s2–s49.

Cojocaru, M., Cojocaru, I.M., Silosi, I. et al. (2011). Gastrointestinal manifestations in systemic autoimmune diseases. *Maedica (Buchar)* **6** (1): 45–51.

Douglas, G., Nichol, F., and Robertson, C. (2013). *Macleod's Clinical Examination.* 13e. London: Churchill Livingstone.

Gurusamy, K. and Davidson, B. (2014). Clinical review: gallstones. *BMJ* **348**: g2669.

Kumar, P. and Clark, M. (2017). *Kumar & Clarke's Clinical Medicine*. Sydney: Elsevier.

Manterola, C., Vial, M., Muraga, J. et al. (2011). Analgesia in patients with acute abdominal pain. *Cochrane Database of Systematic Reviews* **34** (1): CD005660.

Martini, F., Tallitsch, R., and Nath, J. (2017). *Human Anatomy*. 9e. Sydney: Pearson.

Meckler, G., Quereshi, N., Al-Mogbil, M. et al. (2016). *Tintinalli's Emergency Medicine: A Comprehensive Study Guide*. New York: McGraw-Hill.

Netter, F.H. (2006). *Atlas of Human Anatomy.* 4e. Oxford: Saunders Elsevier.

Omari, A.H., Khammash, M.R., Qasaimeh, G.R. et al. (2014). Acute appendicitis on the elderly: risk factors for perforation. *World Journal of Emergency Surgery* **15;9 (1)**: 1–6.

Peery, A.F., Barrett, P.R., Park, D. et al. (2012). A high fiber diet does not protect against asymptomatic diverticulosis. *Gastroenterology* **142** (2): 266–272.

Schoenwolf, G.C. and Larsen, W.J. (2009). *Larsen's Human Embryology*. Oxford: Elsevier/Churchill Livingstone.

Stringer, M.D., Fraser, S., Gordon, K.C. et al. (2013). Gallstones in New Zealand: composition, risk factors and ethnic differences. *Australia and New Zealand Journal of Surgery* **83**: 575–580.

Talley, N.J. and O'Connor, S. (2017). *Clinical Examination.* 4e. New York: Elsevier.

CHAPTER 23

Assessing the respiratory system

Janie Brown

Curtin School of Nursing, Faculty of Health Sciences, Curtin University, Perth, Western Australia, Australia

Dan Staines

Department of Nursing, Midwifery and Healthcare Practice, Coventry University, Coventry, UK

Samantha Sheridan

School of Biomedical Sciences – Paramedicine, Charles Sturt University, Bathurst, New South Wales, Australia

Georgina Pickering

School of Biomedical Sciences – Paramedicine, Charles Sturt University, Bathurst, New South Wales, Australia

Contents

LEARNING OUTCOMES

On completion of this chapter the reader will be able to:

- Discuss the function and general anatomy of the respiratory system.
- Describe pulmonary ventilation and the mechanism of breathing.
- Recognise the presentation of commonly occurring causes of respiratory conditions in the out-of-hospital setting.
- Describe and discuss the focused history-taking information that is required as part of a comprehensive respiratory assessment.
- Discuss the relevant physical assessment skills required and process for undertaking a comprehensive respiratory assessment.

Fundamentals of Paramedic Practice: A Systems Approach, Third Edition. Edited by Sam Willis and Ian Peate.

Companion website: www.wiley.com/go/willis/paramedic3e

Case Study

You have an emergency call to attend a 20-year-old patient, at a residential address, who is having difficulty breathing. On arrival you meet a patient, sitting on a chair, leaning forward with an inhaler in their hand. They are alert and maintaining their own airway. The breathing pattern is shallow and regular, with an approximate rate of 28 breaths per minute. The patient cannot speak in full sentences but can communicate using two- to three-word replies. There appears to be increased effort of breathing and a subtle wheeze is audible without a stethoscope throughout expiration. Their friends who called for the ambulance are all looking concerned.

Introduction

Respiratory conditions accounted for 6.2% of all presentations to the emergency departments across Australia in 2021–2022, the third most popular reason for presenting to the emergency department (AIHW 2023). Therefore, a comprehensive and systematic respiratory assessment is frequently performed by contemporary paramedics as a component of out-of-hospital (OOH) patient care. This chapter outlines the significant respiratory anatomy and physiological processes a paramedic should be familiar with prior to undertaking a focused respiratory assessment as part of a patient physical assessment. The chapter describes how this assessment involves taking a relevant history and performing an in-depth physical assessment.

Respiratory anatomy and physiology

The respiratory system comprises the nose and mouth, the pharynx (the throat) and larynx (the voice box), the trachea (the throat), bronchi, and the lungs. During normal breathing, air enters the body through the nose (Figure 23.1). Inhaled air is passed from the external to the internal naris, whilst being warmed and humidified. As the air is inhaled, it is also spun and rolled around the nasal cavity, mainly through the presence of the superior, medial, and inferior nasal conchae or turbinate bones. The main role of these bones is to facilitate 'exertional filtration' and prevent foreign bodies from being inhaled into the respiratory tract.

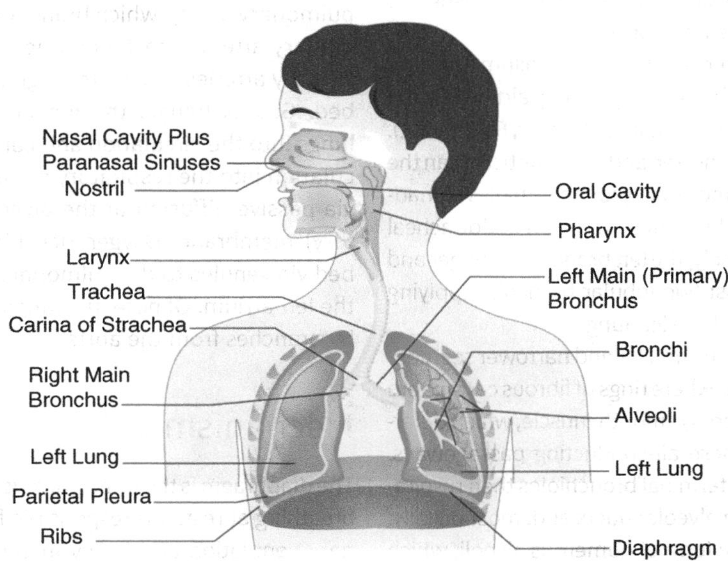

FIGURE 23.1 Anatomy of the respiratory system.

The pharynx is a short muscular tube that starts at the internal nares and extends to the cricoid cartilage at the lower end of the larynx. It can be split into three anatomical areas: nasopharynx, oropharynx, and laryngopharynx. The nasopharynx provides the sole passageway for inhaled air and is anatomically located posterior to the nasal cavity. The oropharynx (soft palate to hyoid bone) and laryngopharynx (hyoid bone to oesophagus posteriorly and larynx anteriorly) have the dual roles of allowing air to pass into the respiratory tract and facilitating swallowing of food.

The larynx is a short vessel connecting the laryngopharynx to the trachea and houses significant anatomical structures associated with the respiratory system. The larynx contains the vocal cords and the epiglottis, a leaf-shaped tissue that has the highly specific function of preventing food from entering the trachea. As swallowing occurs, the larynx rises, causing the epiglottis to move down. The glottis is the space between the vocal folds and is considered the anatomical dividing line between the proximal upper airway and distal lower airway.

The trachea is approximately 12 cm long in adults and anatomically located anterior to the oesophagus. Structurally it comprises 16–20 C-shaped arrangements of cartilage that are incomplete posteriorly. A key function of this cartilage is protection against the total collapse of the trachea but also to allow a transient partial collapse whilst partially digested food dilates the oesophagus. The trachea bifurcates at the carina, which is heavily innervated by the autonomic nervous system, as irritation caused by the presence of foreign bodies instigates coughing reflexes to help clear the obstruction.

The right bronchus enters the lung at the hilum and subdivides into three lobular bronchi, providing airflow to the right lung's three lobes (upper, middle, and lower; Figure 23.1). The right bronchus is wider, shorter, and more vertical than the left bronchus, making it far more likely for paramedics to inadvertently intubate the right bronchus during an endotracheal intubation attempt. Conversely, the left bronchus is longer and narrower, and splits into just two lobular bronchi, supplying the upper and lower lobes of the left lung.

Lobar bronchi branch into smaller and narrower segmental bronchi then bronchioles, where rings of fibrous cartage are replaced by airways enclosed by smooth muscle, which determines the lumen size of these air-conducting passageways. The bronchioles divide into terminal bronchioles then respiratory bronchioles, before the alveolar ducts and, most distally, the airways terminate in the form of numerous alveoli, which are the functional unit of the respiratory system. These pouch-like sacs are elastic and, along with alveolar ducts, serve as the respiratory zone where the diffusion of gases occurs. Surfactant is secreted by specialised cells in the alveolar walls that prevent the alveoli from collapsing during expiration, by reducing the surface tension on the internal surface and allowing the alveoli to expand.

Lungs and pleural membranes

Lungs are cone-shaped organs of respiration. In between the lungs lies the space housing the heart, great vessels, trachea, oesophagus, and bronchi, which is called the mediastinum. The apices of the lungs on the anterior aspect of the chest extend 1–2 cm superior to the clavicles, whereas the bases of the lungs reside approximately on the sixth rib in the mid-clavicular line and the eighth rib on the mid-axillary line. On the posterior aspect, apices can be detected at the T1 vertebrae anteriorly, whereas lung bases can be found at the level of T10 (expiration) and T12 (inspiration) due to inspiratory descent.

The lungs are enclosed within smooth, moist membranes called the pleura, a closed bag of membranes containing the visceral membrane attached directly to the lung, then the parietal membrane attached to the thoracic cavity. Between these membranes is a serous membrane that secretes pleural fluid, allowing friction-free membrane movement during breathing.

Blood supply to lungs and gas exchange

Deoxygenated blood leaves the right ventricular via the pulmonary artery, which branches in the left and right pulmonary arteries, each entering their respective lung. Pulmonary arteries branch through arterioles to the capillary bed. Gas exchange, the movement of oxygen from the lungs into the circulation and carbon dioxide from the circulation into the respiratory system for exhalation, occurs via passive diffusion at the alveolar capillary (or respiratory) membrane. Oxygen-rich blood leaves the capillary bed via venules to the pulmonary veins, which empty into the left atrium. Of note, the lungs themselves are perfused by branches from the aorta.

Mechanism of breathing

The diaphragm is the principal muscle contributing to normal breathing at rest. It is responsible for around 75% of pulmonary ventilation and is key in generating the difference in pressure gradient that is essential for ventilation to occur. During inspiration, the diaphragm contracts and flattens, which increases the size of the thoracic cavity. According to **Boyle's Law,** the increased volume will reduce the pressure of air within the thoracic cavity, thus creating a pressure difference between atmospheric air (outside the lungs) and intrathoracic air (inside the lungs). Due to this pressure gradient, air will move from higher to lower pressure, and consequently the lungs will fill with atmospheric air. Its dependence on muscular activity is the reason inspiration is known as an active process. When an increased depth of ventilation is required, accessory muscles can assist.

Throughout expiration, the diaphragm and external intercostal muscles relax, which subsequently reduces the volume within the thoracic cavity. This increases the intrathoracic pressure above atmospheric pressure. Therefore, air simply moves out of the lungs down its concentration gradient. Expiration is aided by the elastic recoil of lung tissue and no energy is consumed. Thus, exhalation is known as a passive process.

Pathophysiology of respiratory conditions

Prior to respiratory assessment, it is essential for paramedics to have a basic understanding of some of the more common disease pathologies that cause breathing problems in the OOH setting (Table 23.1). This deeper level of understanding allows paramedics to detect potential clinically significant cues during subjective history taking.

Patient assessment

The first priority in any OOH patient environment is risk assessment of the threat of further danger to the patient or danger to paramedics. Once the risk of danger has been assessed and, where necessary, eliminated, a quick scan of the environment may provide additional information regarding the patient's previous respiratory history. Observations may include presence of mobility aids, use of respiratory inhalers, home oxygen tubing, presence of sputum pots, modification to the living environment, and the presence of previously completed patient report forms or clinical care pathways.

Practice insight

The scene survey starts the moment you arrive. Observations may include presence of medication, sputum pots, home oxygen tubing, and completed patient report forms or clinical care pathways, as well as modifications to the living environment and use of mobility aids.

Once a brief scan of the environment has been completed, the paramedic should turn attention to the patient, as significant information regarding the severity of respiratory distress can be immediately identified through simple observation (Table 23.2).

Before any interaction with the patient, it is important the paramedic introduces themself, explains what they are about to do, and gains the patient's consent to proceed. Obtaining informed consent ensures that practice remains professional and legal. Once consent has been obtained, paramedics should conduct a structured primary survey following the steps provided by the Airway, Breathing, Circulation, Disability (ABCD) protocol. The primary survey should be a dynamic process in which the assessment of ABCD should be regularly repeated.

During the primary survey, determine whether a patient is 'primary-survey positive' or 'primary-survey negative'. A 'primary-survey positive' patient suggests that the paramedic has identified a significant abnormal finding or threat to life, which requires further and immediate intervention as indicated. A 'primary-survey negative' patient exhibits no significant threats to ABCD, and therefore a more detailed history and detailed clinical assessment can be conducted.

History taking

Taking the history is an essential part of patient assessment. In this chapter the focus is on respiratory presentations, with a comprehensive question list presented in Table 23.3. To assist in the attainment of a relevant subjective history, the following systematic approach ensures that nothing is missed. Start by asking the patient what is currently wrong with them (presenting complaint), gain as much history of the presenting complaint as possible, gather other relevant previous medical history, their current medications regime, any illicit drug use and allergies, and relevant family and social history.

Presenting complaint and previous medical history

The presenting complaint refers to the key focus of why the patient, or a bystander, called for the ambulance service. Subjective information regarding the history of the breathing problem is clinically significant and replies from the patient can aid in the development of a working diagnosis.

The patient's previous medical history may also be relevant, and it is very important for the paramedic to place the current presenting complaint into the context of the patient's normal health, well-being, and quality of life. For

TABLE 23.1 Common disease pathologies causing breathing difficulty.

Condition	Definition	Signs and symptoms	Pathophysiology
Asthma	Common, reversible chronic inflammatory condition of the lower airways, associated with hypersensitivity	Dyspnoea, cough, unable to speak in full sentences. Wheeze, tachypnoea, tachycardia, hyper-resonant, accessory muscle use	Chronic inflammation of the bronchi which results in narrowing of the airways. Irritation causes smooth muscle to contract and produces respiratory compromise. Inflammatory processes also cause excessive mucus production and swelling
Chronic obstructive pulmonary disorder (COPD)	An umbrella term for chronic lung diseases, most common of which are chronic bronchitis and emphysema. COPD is a progressive pulmonary disease characterised by airflow obstruction that is not fully reversible	Progressive dyspnoea, wheezing, chest tightness, cough, purulent sputum, cyanosis	Airway obstruction results from damage to the alveoli, alveolar ducts, and bronchioles due to chronic inflammation
Pulmonary oedema	Fluid accumulation in the lungs, often as a result of heart failure (cardiogenic pulmonary oedema)	Dyspnoea, decreased exercise tolerance, chest pain. Cough often producing white or pink frothy sputum. Wheezing and crackles. Anxiety and restlessness, associated with feeling of suffocation	Reduced left ventricular function / increased left ventricular pressure allows blood to pool causing engorgement of the pulmonary circulation, with sodium and water forced across the respiratory membrane
Pneumonia	A respiratory infection affecting the alveoli. It can affect either lungs, one lung, or individual lobes	Dyspnoea, fever, cough, tachycardia	Depends on cause. Infection spread by respiratory droplets, causing inflammation via immune response in the lungs. Fluid leaks into the alveoli, affecting gas exchange
Pulmonary embolism	Obstruction of circulation through the pulmonary artery	Dyspnoea, pleuritic chest pain, cough, possible deep vein thrombosis, unilateral leg oedema, tachycardia, tachypnoea, fever	Occlusion of the pulmonary artery by an embolus (blood clot, air, fat, amniotic fluid) usually at multiple sites, preventing forward circulation, resulting in pulmonary infarction
Pneumothorax and Haemo-pneumothorax	Presence of air (and blood) in the plural space, caused spontaneously or by trauma or respiratory conditions	Dyspnoea, sudden-onset pleuritic chest pain	Loss of the normal negative pressure in the pleural space that 'adheres' the visceral pleura (lungs) to the parietal pleura (ribs), causing the affected lung to collapse

example, from a respiratory viewpoint, a patient with chronic obstructive pulmonary disorder (COPD) will always have an element of dyspnoea, which may be exacerbated through exertion, bacterial/viral infections, or stress.

Medication history

Identification of medication specifically prescribed for patients with respiratory disease can be useful to understanding progression and history of respiratory disease and pathology. It is helpful to develop your knowledge of the pharmacology and indications of some of the more commonly prescribed drugs for respiratory problems, especially where the patient cannot talk or communicate due to dyspnoea. Although awkward, the paramedic should ask about illicit drug use if they perceive this may be relevant.

TABLE 23.2 Immediate observations.

Appearance	Age Sex AVPU (Alert, Verbal, Pain, Unresponsive) How interactive is the patient? Generalised overview of general health (body mass index, signs of cachexia, tone, any sign of muscle wasting) Emotional state
Work of Breathing	Is the patient breathing? What is the approximate rate? Depth and pattern of breathing (shallow, regular, deep sighing)? Does the patient look breathless (i.e. forward tripod position)? Is there any supplemental oxygen? Pursed lip breathing Any respiratory sounds (stridor, wheeze, strenuous breathing) Generalised signs of increased effort (accessory muscle use)
Circulation to skin	Pallor? Is the patient cyanosed? Is the patient flushed, ashen, pale?

Allergies

An essential piece of subjective history relates to whether the patient has any known allergies to drugs, animals, or food. It is important to establish the severity of the allergy.

Family and social history

A family and social history considers the patient's day-to-day activities and personal capability. Lifestyle, environmental, and social factors are all pertinent information to gather.

Clinical examination

Respiratory assessment encompasses a focused approach to history taking, asking well-informed questions, to assist the paramedic to 'rule in' or 'rule out' provisional diagnoses. This will allow the paramedic to conduct a more attentive clinical examination, noting clinical signs from other body systems and other anatomical locations other than the chest in isolation.

Patients with respiratory disease can range in severity from those requiring immediate resuscitation to those where respiratory assessment reveals no adverse findings.

TABLE 23.3 Potential questions for history taking from patients with respiratory presentations.

History of presenting complaint	Ask about and explore: • what the patient was doing when symptoms started • onset as acute, subacute, or chronic • relieving or aggravating factors • severity of symptoms • effect of symptoms on functionality • any medication taken to attempt to resolve symptoms and effectiveness
Previous medical history	Ask about and explore: • history of respiratory diseases • family history of atopic and similar diseases • relevant surgical history • previous respiratory hospital presentations
Medication history	Ask about and explore: • respiratory and other medications taken regularly and dosages • 'over-the-counter' medication use • length of time taking the medications • concordance/compliance with the medication regime • illicit substances/recreation drug use
Social history	Ask about and explore: • smoking history • care plans • dependants • carers • community services • alcohol use • occupation • recent travel
Review of systems: respiratory	• Ask about and explore: • cough • sputum • haemoptysis • wheezing • chest pain • other symptoms

A systematic approach to any assessment starts with an assessment of the scene, followed by a primary survey, focused history, and, where appropriate, a more thorough physical examination.

A 'primary survey-negative' patient should have a comprehensive physical examination conducted. Whilst the chief anatomical area for respiratory examination focuses around the chest, it is important to consider other locations such as hands, face, and neck, as these may reveal additional findings specific to the respiratory system. Ensure consent for physical examination is still valid, given that your respiratory assessment involves exposure of the chest and peripheral examination of hands, face, and neck.

Focused respiratory physical assessment

A frequently used format for respiratory examination of the chest is Inspection, Palpation, Percussion, and Auscultation (IPPA). A common mistake made by paramedics in respiratory assessment is that they will examine the anterior chest but overlook the lateral or posterior aspects of the chest. Good practice is thus to undertake IPPA of the anterior chest first and then repeat this format laterally and posteriorly, working from head (superiorly) to toe (inferiorly), comparing left to right.

Inspection

Clinical examination must start with complete and active visualisation of the patient's chest (Figure 23.2). Inspection of the chest is often first performed at a distance before closer inspection. In general, inspection of the chest can be split into two clear subcategories: (i) rate, pattern, and effort of breathing; and (ii) further inspection of chest.

> **Practice insight**
>
> In order to maintain patient dignity whilst exposing their chest, communicate your intentions to your crewmate and those on scene. Protect modesty by keeping the patient covered with a blanket or their own clothes when on scene; and keep the ambulance doors locked if in the back of the vehicle.

Rate, pattern, and effort of breathing

Normal adult respirations typically range between 16 and 25 per minute. Respiratory rate can be an important indicator of disease severity and normal breathing should be unlaboured and regular. In normal breathing it should also take twice as long to breathe out than in, demonstrating a ratio of 1:2 for inspiration and expiration.

Accurate assessment of a patient's respiratory rate can be challenging within the OOH setting. It is recommended that to calculate the most accurate respiratory rate the paramedic needs to count the number of respirations across a whole minute. This may not always be appropriate or practicable, so respiratory rates are often counted over 30 or 15 seconds and then this figure is multiplied ×2 or ×4, respectively.

Eupnoea breathing should be even, coordinated, and regular. Inspect for symmetry and mobility of the anterior and posterior chest. Make note of any impairment of movement or asymmetry. Signs of increased effort of breathing include inability to talk in full sentences and patients adopting the forward tripod position (leaning forward on a chair, often resting their hands on their knees), which facilitates pulmonary ventilation (Figure 23.3).

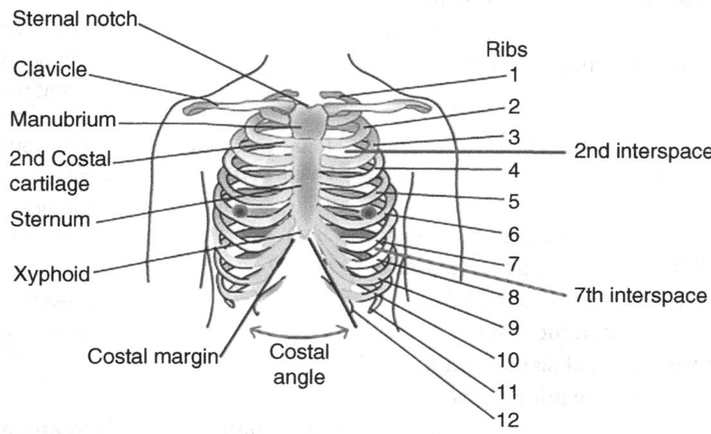

FIGURE 23.2 Anatomical landmarks of the anterior aspect of the chest.

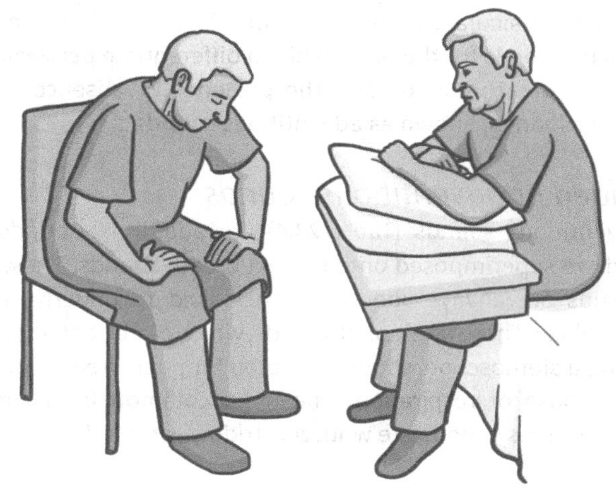

FIGURE 23.3 Patient in tripod position.

Signs of increased effort of breathing can often be displayed through intercostal recession and use of accessory muscles. Intercostal recession is a clinical sign of respiratory distress that occurs because of increasingly negative intrathoracic pressure causing recession or retraction of the chest. This is commonly seen within the intercostal spaces. The degree of contractility and work of accessory muscles (trapezius, scalenus, sternoclomastoid, intercostal) should be noted, as they assist the chest with expansion, thus increasing minute volume.

Further detailed inspection of the thorax

Further inspection should include:

- Checking for presence of scars (thoracotomy, pacemaker, lobectomy, coronary artery bypass graft, heart valve replacement).
- Checking for presence of central cyanosis.
- Checking the chest for trauma to the thorax, namely contusions, abrasions, puncture wounds, lacerations, swellings, burns.
- Inspecting the posterior aspects for sacral oedema, commonly associated with heart failure.
- Checking the pallor.
- Assessing the nutritional state of the patient.
- Determining whether the patient looks frail or there are signs of cachexia.

Palpation

Palpation refers to touching the patient to assess for tenderness (palpate gently), masses, inflammation/warmth, texture, and moisture. Chest palpation can be broadly split into two: palpation of the thorax and assessment of lung compliance/chest expansion.

Palpation of thorax

Begin examination by light palpation across the thorax, which in normal circumstances should not elicit any pain to the patient. The chest should feel warm and dry. The paramedic should lightly palpate over ribs for signs of tenderness or crepitus, especially following traumatic incidents such as falls or road traffic collisions. Palpation can also help exclude the presence of surgical emphysema, fracture, or instability of the larynx, and suspected clavicular injury. Do not neglect to palpate the posterior chest, as well as the spine and vertebral position.

Healthy lungs should be stretchy and distensible. Lung compliance refers to the ease with which the lungs are stretched, as well as the equality and the depth (sometimes known as excursion) of respiration. When compliance is low, more effort is needed to inflate the lungs. Whilst paramedics cannot directly measure lung compliance, we can examine for bilateral thoracic wall compliance to detect excursion of breathing and thoracic compliance.

To assess chest compliance on the posterior aspect of the chest, the paramedic must place their hands directly at the level of the tenth vertebrae with thumbs extended along the lateral rib cage. The paramedic should ask the patient to breathe a maximum inspiration and as the thorax fills with air, the paramedic's thumbs should separate symmetrically in normal lung tissue.

Densities within the lungs can be detected by palpating for tactile fremitus. With the hands placed on the patient's back, fingers pointing towards the patient's head, ask the patient to repeat the words 'ninety-nine' noting the transmission of vibrations, symmetry of vibrations, and any areas of marked increased or decreased fremitus.

Percussion

Percussion of the thorax is a practiced, clinical skill that is both felt and heard as the paramedic attempts to determine the resonance or hollowness of the chest. The paramedic should place the middle finger of their nondominant hand firmly against the patient's chest in a hyper-flexed position within an intercostal space. It is very important to ensure that the paramedic's other fingers do not rest upon the chest, as this has a dampening effect on the resonance generated. The striking action from the middle finger of the paramedic's dominant hand should aim to strike the distal interphalangeal joint using a flick of the wrist in a constant, smooth motion. Finger-to-finger contact time should be kept to a minimum, and often paramedics will strike the nondominant hand a second time, which merely provides confirmation of resonance produced. Percussion of the chest requires considerable practice to achieve competence but when performed accurately can assist OOH paramedics in detecting different grades of resonance that can be sensitive to distinctive pathologies of the underlying lung tissue.

Percussion is performed anteriorly, posteriorly, and laterally. Normal percussion will penetrate approximately 5–7 cm into the chest and a normal chest can be described as 'drum-like' or resonant to percussion. A more 'hollow-sounding' chest can be associated with an increased volume of air within the thoracic cavity, whereas a build-up of fluid within lung tissue can result in a duller resonance. Within the clinical examination context, these are termed hyper-resonant and hyporesonant, respectively.

Auscultation

Auscultation via stethoscope is arguably the most important part of respiratory assessment, as it evaluates the turbulent airflow through the respiratory tract during inspiration and expiration. Airflow is assessed by quality of breath sounds created and the presence or absence of added sounds. The chief objective of prehospital auscultation is to identify differences in sounds produced from larger and smaller airways, as well as whether the air is passing through fluid-filled or narrowed airways, causing increased air turbulence.

Introduction to the stethoscope

The stethoscope is used to listen to the chest by amplifying sounds generated within the respiratory tract. Tubing on stethoscopes can vary in length and, depending on stethoscope manufacturer, stethoscopes may have a different tool that is placed onto the patient's chest, namely a bell or diaphragm. The bell of a stethoscope should be used for low-pitched sounds (like heart sounds), whereas the diaphragm should be considered when sounds are higher in pitch (like breath sounds).

Normal breath sounds

Normal lungs will produce four types of breath sound, depending on where on the thorax the paramedic listens: tracheal, bronchial, broncho-vesicular, and vesicular. Tracheal and bronchial sounds are described as harsh or sharp, whereas vesicular sounds are soft and low, with broncho-vesicular sounds being a mix. The key objective of auscultation is for the paramedic to differentiate between normal breath sounds and the presence or absence of added sounds, known as adventitious sounds.

Added or adventitious sounds

Adventitious sounds (Table 23.4) are additional sounds and are superimposed onto normal breath sounds. These sounds are always abnormal and linked to underlying pathology. These additional sounds, which can be detected using a stethoscope, should be noted for pitch, frequency, and phase of respiration. The most common forms of adventitious sounds are wheeze, stridor, and crackles.

Method of auscultation

Prior to auscultation, the paramedic should ask the patient to cough to help clear the airways and to breathe more deeply and slowly than normal, through an open mouth to minimise additional air turbulence from the nasopharynx. Whilst the paramedic is listening to the anterior chest, it is recommended that the patient rests their hands on their knees; whilst the paramedic is auscultating the posterior region, it is considered good practice to ask the patient to fold their arms and rest their hands on their opposite shoulders. This helps to separate the scapulae to facilitate auscultation.

Begin at the lung apices, superior to the clavicles, and work down inferiorly, comparing right and left sides. Across the thorax, press the diaphragm of the stethoscope firmly

TABLE 23.4 Pathophysiology of advantageous sounds.

Wheeze	A wheeze is typically described as a sharp whistling, mostly on expiration. Wheezing occurs when smooth-muscles contract around the bronchioles, leading to a reduction in lumen size and ability to conduct air distally into the respiratory tract. Wheezing is common in patients with asthma and exacerbation of COPD.
Stridor	Stridor is a high-pitched sound, mostly on inspiration. Stridor occurs when there is partial obstruction of the larynx or trachea. Stridor is common in foreign body inhalation, anaphylaxis, and life-threatening asthma.
Crackles	Crackles, sometimes termed 'crepitations', sound like bubbling or popping (or like rubbing hair between your fingers), occurring mostly on inspiration. Crackles occur when small airways snap open. Crackles are common in pneumonia, pulmonary oedema, and bronchitis.

against the skin and listen for a full inspiration and full expiration in each anatomical location. It is important to move across the chest to enable immediate and direct comparison with the contralateral side.

Practice insight

It can sometimes be difficult to hear normal or abnormal breath sounds due to environmental noise. Therefore, whenever you are going to auscultate a patient's chest, let everyone on scene know and ask bystanders to remain quiet.

Hand assessment

Significant peripheral signs associated with respiratory disease are finger clubbing and nicotine staining. Finger clubbing, a painless enlargement of connective tissue at the nail bed, can be associated with many respiratory diseases. The patient's fingers begin to develop a spoon-like appearance with the loss of nail-bed angle. The cause of finger clubbing is unclear but can be associated with lung abscess, pulmonary fibrous, lung malignancy, asbestosis, and congenital heart defects. The best method of assessing for finger clubbing is by looking across the nail bed and placing the fingers together to determine whether the space in between the fingers is narrowed.

Another clinically significant sign could be the presence of bilateral hand tremor. This can often be a sign of other significant co-morbidities (such as diabetes or Parkinson's disease), so a holistic assessment needs to be considered. However, fine tremors can be associated with excessive selective β2-adrenoreceptor agonist use in the acute dyspnoeic patient. Correspondingly, a coarse tremor may be evident in patients who have a build-up of carbon dioxide in the blood, known as asterixis, common in COPD patients.

Head and neck assessment

A brief inspection of the nose may reveal nasal flaring if increased respiratory effort is present. Check for the presence or absence of central cyanosis by examining the sublingual region of the mouth. The paramedic can smell for previous use of cigarettes on the patient's breath. The presence or absence of pursed lips should be noted, as it can also be indicative of increased respiratory distress. Finally, note the working of accessory muscles around the neck and also inspect for the presence of distended neck veins, which can be more apparent in patients with heart failure.

Conclusion

As outlined in this chapter, respiratory assessment can be split into history taking and physical examination. Through the practice and application of clinical skills, paramedics can form credible provisional respiratory diagnoses and detect more subtle clues to clinical findings on physical examination.

Activities

Now review your learning by completing the learning activities in this chapter. The answers to these appear at the end of the book. Further self-test activities can be found at **www.wileyfundamentalseries.com/paramedic/3e.**

Test your knowledge

1. What are the functions of the respiratory system?
2. What is a primary survey?
3. Describe three acute respiratory illnesses that may require paramedic attendance?
4. List in order, the clinical skills required when undertaking a focused respiratory physical assessment.

Activity 23.1

Consider the case study at the start of the chapter. Describe your approach to the patient and your assessment of their situation.

Activity 23.2

Ask an experienced paramedic colleague to demonstrate percussion on a patient who presents with a respiratory illness.

Activity 23.3

Practise assessing respiratory rate on friends and family. Count their rate without them knowing. Take a note of the features of their breathing including depth, regularity, effort, and chest movement.

Activity 23.4

Use a stethoscope to listen to a 'normal' chest on friends and family in order to establish what is normal, before listening to a patient's chest, who may have added sounds and other abnormal findings. Document your findings in both the normal and acutely unwell presentations.

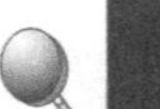

Glossary

Boyle's Law: The pressure of a gas decreases as the volume of the gas increases.

Cachexia: Weight loss and deterioration in physical condition.

Conjunctiva: The membranes which line the inside of the eyelids.

Crepitus: Grating, crackling, or popping sounds and sensations experienced under the skin and joints.

Deglutition: The act of swallowing.

Diffusion: A net movement of molecules or ions from high concentration to lower concentration until equilibrium is reached.

Eupnoea: Normal-parameter breathing rate.

Fissures: Any cleft or groove, normal or otherwise.

Hilum: An area where blood vessels and nerves enter or leave an organ.

Surgical emphysema: The presence of gas in subcutaneous soft tissues.

Turbinate bones: Thin scroll-shaped bones within the nasal cavity that increase turbulent airflow, thus maximising the surface area in contact with cilia and mucous-covered layers of epithelium membrane.

References

Australian Institute of Health and Welfare [AIHW]. (2023). Emergency department care activity. Australian Government: Canberra. Available at: https://www.aihw.gov.au/reports-data/myhospitals/intersection/activity/ed (accessed 25 January 2023).

Baker, C. (2017). Accident and emergency statistics: demand, performance and pressure. House of Commons Library 6964. London: UK Parliament. Available at: https://commonslibrary.parliament.uk/research-briefings/sn06964 (accessed 25 January 2023).

CHAPTER 24

Paramedic assessment skills

Steven Poulton

UK HCPC Paramedic and Senior Lecturer in Paramedic Science, York St John University, UK

Contents

LEARNING OUTCOMES

By the end of this chapter you will be able to:

- Recognise the ABCDE approach to patient assessment.
- Have an understanding of the different variations based on initial assessment.
- Apply the primary and secondary survey to patient care.
- Understand the importance of maintaining assessment skills.

Case study overview

You are being sent to a 58-year-old who has developed acute chest pain following exercise.

You ask yourself a mirage of questions: is the patient breathing, what was the exercise, does the patient have a pulse or are they awake? We can easily get consumed and lost with the vast array of questions we need answers to but we must start somewhere.

Fundamentals of Paramedic Practice: A Systems Approach, Third Edition. Edited by Sam Willis and Ian Peate.

Companion website: www.wiley.com/go/willis/paramedic3e

Introduction

Every paramedic needs to have an advanced understanding of the primary and secondary survey. When starting out as a student paramedic, applying the theory to the practice can be challenging. This chapter provides a theoretical discussion on the primary and secondary survey and uses case-based learning to aid the student paramedic in applying the theory to the practice.

It is important for paramedics to understand the theory of why we do what we do; for example, why do we perform patient assessments, and why do we intervene when we need to, etc. The underpinning theory can help paramedics to systematically process information that our patients provide to us, allowing us to respond appropriately. This chapter focuses on paramedic patient assessment and the core questions we must ask to gain a thorough history, which will allow us to provide appropriate care.

The ABCDE approach applied to patient assessment

The (**ABCDE**) primary survey is well known by paramedics; first-aiders and others who work in emergency care. This systematic approach was first documented in the mid-twentieth century, and stands for:

Airway
Breathing
Circulation
Disability
Exposure

A historical narrative of the ABCDE approach

Safar and McMahon (1958) were the first to document the importance of managing a patient's airway and breathing giving rise to the first two letters of the mnemonic 'A' and 'B', later Kouwenhoven et al. (1960) evidenced cardiac massage introducing 'C'. It wasn't until a tragic plane crash in 1976 when the additional 'D' and 'E' were added to the algorithm. It was 1976 when the creator of the Adult Trauma Life Support (ATLS) courses Dr Styner brought together all the letters into what we know today as the primary survey. Due to Dr Styner's tragic case, the extra letters 'D' and 'E' were added, which we'll explore later.

The ABCDE approach is synonymous with paramedic care but is also widely used in hospital settings, for example, among clinicians in the emergency department. Clinical staff start at the first letter of the alphabet and proceed along to the next, only once the previous letter has been satisfied. During their primary assessment and at each stage a number of questions are asked, for example, is the patient's airway open? (See Table 24.1 for a full range of questions the

Case study 1

You conduct a primary survey on a 57-year-old female, they are talking to you and engaging in full conversation. They are breathing comfortably, have good colour, a steady heart rate, and are fully alert.

If we apply the ABCDE method here we can see, because they are talking to us, the physiology of speech process means their airway is open and they are able to maintain it for themselves. Their breathing is normal, circulation appears normal, they are fully alert. There appears to be no issue relating to 'disability'.

Case study 2

You are called to attend a 89-year-old male who is unconscious and does not appear to be breathing.

Applying ABCDE, we open and check the airway, as the patient is not talking or breathing, and can see that it is clear. We then move onto breathing and note a cessation of breathing; therefore, our patient needs support with their breathing, and we intervene by delivering ventilatory breaths. Moving on to 'C' we also note that they have no palpable pulse, meaning they have no circulating blood (circulation). Our patient is in cardiac arrest, and we perform cardiopulmonary resuscitation (CPR).

TABLE 24.1 Primary survey.

Stage of the mnemonic (most important first)	Questions we can ask
Danger	Are we, our crewmate, the patient, or bystanders in any immediate danger? If yes, how can we remove the danger or mitigate it from causing us harm? If no, we can proceed onto 'R' (response)
Response	How responsive is our patient? Alert – does your patient respond to your presence, are they looking around their environment responding appropriately? Verbal – do they respond only when spoken too? if no, we apply a pressure stimulus Pressure – do they respond when a stimulus is delivered? Unresponsive – if you have arrived at this stage your patient is unresponsive
Airway	Is your patient's airway clear? Do they look like they can manage it for themselves, for example, are they able to swallow? Are they chewing any gum, or do they have dentures? If yes, consider removal of the object to avoid the choking hazard If the patient is not able to manage their own airway, which is the best airway adjunct to use? Do you need to provide suction to remove any fluid obstruction or use magill forceps to remove solids?
Breathing	Is the patient breathing? What is your patient's breathing rate? Is it within normal parameters for your patient's age? Are they using any accessory breathing muscles? If yes, this would indicate your patient is in respiratory distress and needs assistance Can you hear any audible abnormal sounds, for example, a wheeze? (An audible sound can be one that you hear within a short distance from your patient. Other sounds include stridor and bubbling and may only be heard on auscultation)
Circulation	Can you feel a palpable pulse on your patient? (Carotid for central or radial for peripheral, as examples) If you can feel a pulse, what is the rate, is it slow, within normal parameters, fast, regular, or irregular? How does your patient look, do they look pale, in which case they could be losing blood, do they look flushed, indicating a possible rash or feeling too hot? What is the patient's capillary refill time (CRT), <2 seconds is considered normal
Disability	Revisiting the initial responsive level perform a Glasgow Coma Score (GCS) on your patient, which is part of a mini neurological assessment Is your patient exhibiting facial symmetry? Are your patient's pupils symmetrical? What is your patient's blood sugar reading? Do they have any other notable deficits?
Exposure/ environment	If it is appropriate to expose your patient, do you note any abnormal markings, rashes, or non-accidental injuries on visual inspection? Does the environment need any special consideration? Could your patient have been laid in a cold environment for a long period of time and be hypothermic?

**The term pressure replaces the term 'painful'. An example of suitable pressure includes applying pressure to the clavicle or supraorbital of either eye.*

paramedic should ask themselves.) All being well, the clinician is able to move along the mnemonic to the next letter, however, should they not gain the appropriate response then they stop, intervene, and continue. The following set of case studies exemplify the process.

A key difference between the two cases is that in Case study 1, our patient presents to us in a way that allows us to efficiently move through the mnemonic. In Case study 2, however, we must intervene because we have not elicited the desired outcome. It is important to remember that the reason we start with airway is because a blocked airway will cause our patient to go into cardiac arrest and we know irreversible brain damage can occur within minutes (Gräsner et al. 2021).

Staying safe on scene

When paramedics are tasked to any incident the first thing they should consider is 'safety'. Safety for ourselves; safety for our crew members; safety for our students; safety for the patient; and safety for bystanders. Safety requires us to be dynamic therefore we alter this with the term 'danger'.

We can mitigate dangers and remove any potential hazards, which may mean removing the patient or withdrawing ourselves from the scene. Providing there are no dangers, or we have mitigated against them, we can then introduce ourselves to the patient.

In 2013, Dr Kate Granger through her own personal experience of poor bedside communication started the campaign #hellomynameis. In Kate's own experience, staff treating her for cancer failed to introduce themselves before proceeding to deliver care. This basic courtesy of human introduction provides a vital lifeline, it starts trust formation and offers those in vulnerable situations a human connection. Doing so may also help to keep the paramedic safe.

Through introducing ourselves to the patient we can then add the letter 'R' to the mnemonic, which stands for response. Assessing a response requires a stepwise approach using the mnemonic AVPU (alert, vocal, pain, unresponsive; see Table 24.1). Assessing a response helps us decide the severity of our patient's condition.

Clinical consideration

Whilst safety is always the first consideration when working as a paramedic, sometimes we can over assess the situation as dangerous when there really is no threat to the paramedics. Experience will help us to get this balance right. **Discuss this with your mentor.**

Applying the primary survey – a case-based approach

It is important when we are called to incidents that we apply our primary survey to every patient we attend. Rehearsing it en route to the call or discussing it with your crewmate will allow you to mentally prepare prior to arriving on scene, which will aid in allowing you to appropriately manage the patient.

If we apply the primary survey theory discussed in this chapter to these case studies, we can see that the patient in Case study 3 is able to manage his own airway, as he is talking. However, in Case study 4, our construction lady is unconscious and therefore unable to manage her own airway. This patient is critically unwell for a number of reasons.

We are taught as students to treat every patient in isolation. The information we are provided with once we are dispatched can be completely different to what we are presented with when we arrive on scene. Therefore, as paramedics we must be dynamic, always adapting our practice to meet the needs of the patient and the primary survey is no different.

Case study 3

You are dispatched to a residential address for a 68-year-old-male who has developed some chest pain. He communicates to you in full sentences with no abnormal airway or respiratory sounds. The patient explains he was doing some housework when he developed some central crushing chest pain radiating into his left arm. Since the pain started, he has begun sweating profusely, become pale looking, and is very anxious. As a consequence of the pain and anxiety, the patient's breathing rate has risen and is now 24 breaths per minute. His heart rate via a radial pulse is 40 beats per minute.

Case study 4

Dispatch have sent you to a construction site. A 28-year-old-female has fallen off the top of some scaffolding, which is 20 ft high. When you arrive, she is lying on her back and her hard hat has broken into many pieces. She is unresponsive, her breathing rate is slow at 8 beats per minute, her pulse is fast at 120 beats per minute, and whilst taking her pulse you felt she was waxy, clammy, and very pale. You also notice she has a large laceration to her right femur and is haemorrhaging externally.

Adapting the primary survey to trauma

The trauma patient

Any information received either en route to the incident or once you arrive can mean you need to add or subtract elements of the primary survey. Take Case study 4, our patient has a severe bleed and as you will know from your understanding of pathophysiology, they will haemorrhage and die before they become hypoxic, so we must introduce a big 'C' or catastrophic haemorrhage, which is placed prior to airway assessment.

In addition, during suspected trauma, you should consider the patient's c-spine (Table 24.2), which would be managed at the same time as managing the airway.

Managing a trauma patient can increase your cognitive load and it is important to systematically work through the algorithm to help alleviate any built-up nerves and to ensure you methodically address each step of the trauma survey.

The unconscious patient

Any paramedic will tell you that whenever the dispatch information is updated on route to the address to read 'patient is unresponsive and unconscious' they take a big 'gulp' as it shows that the patient has deteriorated. The paramedic will now prepare to deliver advanced life support. It is important, however, to remember our stepwise approach using the primary survey. In this section, we visit the unconscious patient and consider the adaptions we must take.

Like all incidents, safety is of paramount importance therefore the initial danger stage never deviates. We process

TABLE 24.2 The trauma primary survey.

Danger	Are there any immediate dangers to me, my crew, or the patient?
Response	Using AVPU, what is the responsive level of my patient?
Catastrophic haemorrhage	Is there any catastrophic haemorrhaging? If so, how can I stop the bleeding, do I need to apply any military dressings, for example, celox or torniquets?
Airway and c-spine	Is the patient's airway open?
Breathing	Is the patient breathing? What is the rate, rhythm, and depth? Should I auscultate the chest?
Circulation	Does the patient have a pulse? What is the patient's CRT? It is important at this stage to also revisit any dressings you applied during the initial catastrophic phase to ensure no re-bleeding has occurred Is there any other bleeding internally I need to consider? Cavities to be aware off include the thorax, abdomen, pelvis, and long bones.
Disability	What is the patient's GCS? Is my patient fully alert, orientated, and conscious?
Exposure / Environment	Do I need to consider any exposure of my patient to find other injuries? Do I need to consider any environmental conditions?

and mitigate any dangers, and we move onto response. It is at the response stage that we gain our first significant piece of information, how alert is our patient.

A fully unconscious patient will be 'U' on the AVPU scale. Now we know our patient is not alert we must ensure they have everything they need to physiologically stay alive.

Understanding, however, what the possible mechanism of injury is can be relevant. Was it a traumatic or medical cause that has led our patient to be unresponsive? We don't know yet, so you would not be judged for including catastrophic haemorrhage into the mnemonic.

We already know that irreversible brain damage starts around three to four minutes without oxygen, so it is important we assess the patient's airway. A visual inspection is needed of the nasal and oral cavities, so potentially you will need to consider a head tilt–chin lift (Figure 24.1) or a jaw thrust in cases of trauma (figure 24.2).

Airway inspection complete, we assess their breathing, and it is now that we have to consider the possible mechanism of injury (MOI).

Opening the airway

Two techniques for opening the airway are discussed; the head tilt–chin lift (Figure 24.1) and the jaw thrust (Figure 24.2).

The head tilt–chin lift can be used to displace the tongue anteriorly and off the back of the throat in any patient who is unconscious and not suspected of suffering from trauma.

The jaw thrust technique is recommended for any suspected trauma induced injury in an unresponsive patients. When assessing their breathing we perform a jaw thrust at the same time as looking for chest movement to ensure where possible that we prevent further damage of the patient's c-spine. Should there be no suspicion of any trauma inducing injury then the head tilt–chin lift may be applied.

Whichever method of assessing the patient's airway and breathing is chosen, it is during this stage that breathing and circulation are assessed simultaneously.

A patient who is not breathing normally and not responding is considered to be in cardiac arrest. The paramedic should draw on the latest evidence when managing a cardiac arrest and this includes following local procedures combined with the latest guidelines from organisations such as the Resuscitation Councils.

if, however, we felt breath and a palpable central pulse, then we must consider what intervention is appropriate. For example, if your breathing patient has a low respiratory rate, they will require ventilatory support. If the airway was initially occluded, your patient will require suctioning and an airway adjunct. It is important to remain dynamic, always adapting yourself to your patient's needs.

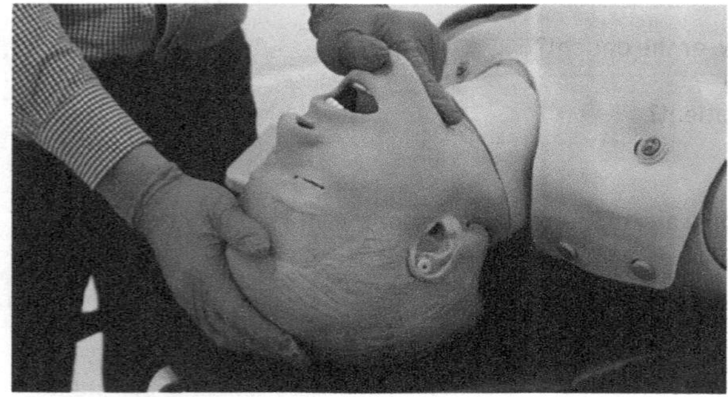

FIGURE 24.1 Head tilt–chin lift.

Reversible causes of cardiac arrest

Should your patient require advanced life support it is important to have a good understanding of the reversible causes, these are known as the '4 Hs and 4 Ts', simply put because there are four within each category that start with either an H or a T. See Table 24.3 for more information.

Secondary survey

The secondary survey is the assessing and treating of non-life-threatening injuries or illnesses. In some circumstances, if your patient presents as time critical you may

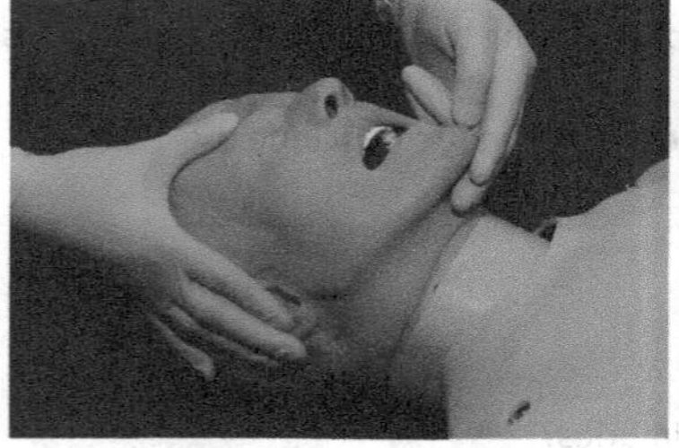

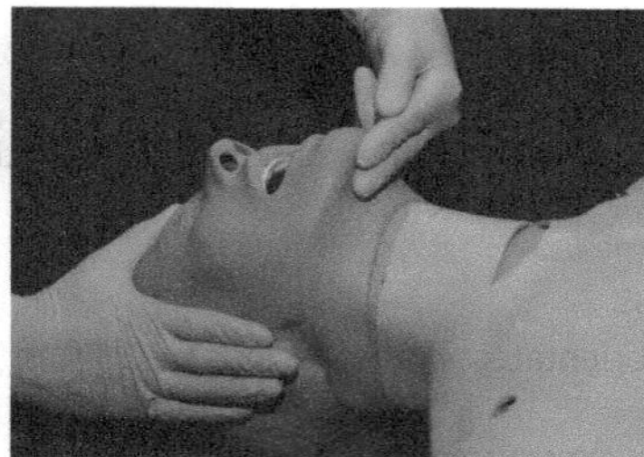

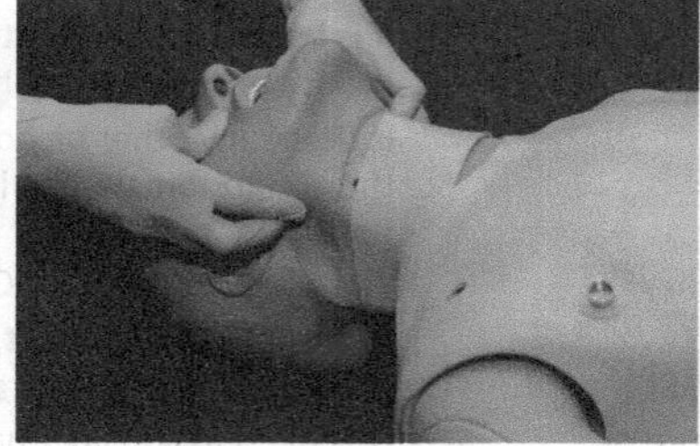

FIGURE 24.2 Jaw thrust method of opening the airway for suspected trauma patients.

TABLE 24.3 The reversible causes of cardiac arrest.

Hs and Ts	Description	Questions to ask yourself	Correction considerations
Hypoxia	Low levels of oxygen within the tissues Signs of hypoxia include: Peripheral and/or central cyanosis, poor oxygen saturation readings Are we classifying this as a cause?	Is the aetiology of the arrest due to an obstruction of the respiratory system, for example, a choking or pneumothorax?	High flow oxygen delivered by a bag, valve, mask or connected to an advanced airway Ask yourself, do you need to use an airway adjunct to ensure patency?
Hypovolaemia	Low levels of circulating blood within the circulatory system Ideally, we should be looking for blood replacements, however, most ambulances only carry fluids (sodium chloride or Hartmanns solution) therefore consider senior clinical support, who may carry blood products	Has there been a significant loss of blood either internally or externally? Does the blood volume need replacing?	Does your patient require a blood transfusion; therefore do you need clinical support? If blood products are not available does your patient need fluid resuscitation? What intravenous or intraosseous access do you have to deliver the highest flow rate of volume replacement?
Hypothermia	Body temperature below 36.5°C In hypothermia a patient of 32°C has a 50% reduction in metabolic processes	What is the temperature of your patient?	How will you rewarm your patient? Do you need blankets, foil covering, or do they need rewarming in hospital? If your patient is too hot, how will you cool them down? Do they need removing from the sun or shadowing?
Hyper and hypokalaemia and other metabolic disorders	Low levels of circulating potassium within the blood Other metabolic disorders could include hypo or hyperglycaemia or hypo and hypercalcaemia	Is there any evidence of a metabolic imbalance with your patient? This might be evident from history from a family member or medications Has your patient undergone any procedure where they may have a potassium, calcium, or glycaemic concern, for example, dialysis or diarrhoea and vomiting	Following your finding what is the most appropriate form of treatment? As an example, your patient may present with elevated T-waves on the ECG therefore suggestive of hyperkalaemia, and need calcium, insulin with glucose to rectify the problem.
Toxins	Any substance toxic to the body	Has your patient ingested any toxic substances, for example, illegal drugs or chemicals?	Do they need emergency transfer to hospital or, for example, if you suspect an opioid overdose and you carry the reversing agent could you administer it to the patient?
Tamponade (cardiac)	Bleeding into the pericardial sac that surrounds the heart, which prevents the heart from beating	Has there been any blunt or penetrating trauma to the chest?	Pericardiocentesis?
Tension pneumothorax	Air trapped in the pleural lung space, which compresses the lung	Has the patient experienced any kind of trauma to the thorax (chest) Has your patient developed or sustained a collapse of their lung caused by a build-up of air within the thorax?	Is it within your scope of practice to deliver a needle chest decompression or do you need clinical support?

(Continued)

TABLE 24.3 (*Continued*)

Hs and Ts	Description	Questions to ask yourself	Correction considerations
Thrombosis	Has your patient sustained any thrombolytic event, for example, a pulmonary embolism or a myocardial infarction. Consider risk factors such as age, gender, medical history, and pre-arrest signs and symptoms	Any history which includes dyspnoea, pleuritic or substernal chest pain, haemoptysis or unilateral calf swelling? Has the patient been immobile for an extended period of time?	Depending on the type of embolism you suspect, what is the most appropriate treatment available within your area? For example, a pulmonary embolism may be treated with anticoagulant therapies, however, some ambulance trusts do not carry this pharmacological agent so an emergency transfer is required

not be able to complete a secondary survey, this is OK, however, if your primary survey does not allude to anything requiring rapid transfer then consider completing a secondary survey.

The purpose of a secondary survey is to assess and treat non-life-threatening emergencies. On occasions the secondary survey may produce information that will assist in the understanding of why you have been requested to attend, for example, greater understanding of a patient's medical history. See Tables 24.4 and 24.5 relating to history-taking acronyms you may wish to consider to assist in a secondary survey. The secondary survey should be conducted in a conversation-style approach, it typically is only achieved with non-time critical patients so you have more time to conduct it.

TABLE 24.4 SAMPLER.

SAMPLER	Explanation
Signs or symptoms	Are there any further signs or symptoms that were not obtained during your primary survey? *A sign is something you can see, hear, or feel, for example, an audible wheeze or deformity indicating a fracture of a bone* *A symptom is something the patient tells you, for example, feeling of sickness, pain in their calf*
Allergies	Does your patient have any allergies? *An example is that they may have ingested some food and not be aware that the ingredients contain something they are allergic too*
Medications	What medications is the patient on? Is there a prescription available? *Could the reason for your attendance be because there is an interaction between two different types, or they are having a reaction to a recent addition to their prescription*
Pre-existing medication condition	What is your patient's medical history? *Have they got a chronic medical condition that has become exacerbated or had any recent surgery that could be the cause of their problem?*
Last meal	When was their last meal? *Some patients may simply forget to eat or not understand the benefits of maintaining a healthy lifestyle. In a patient presenting with nausea, if they have forgotten to eat or skipped a meal due to desire for weight loss that could be the clue*
Events	Understanding what the patient was doing prior to your attendance or leading up to your arrival could provide vital information as to the reason you are assessing them
Risks	Are there any significant risk factors you need to consider for your patient? *For example, if a patient who smokes presents with a breathing problem smoking could cause them further harm so advice on quitting smoking may be needed. Additionally, a patient who has a high-risk occupation might need to conduct a risk assessment to mitigate the exposed hazards*

TABLE 25.5 Top/head-to-toe survey.

Location	Explanation
Head	Do you notice any obvious injuries, for example, bruising or fluid omitting from the ears or peri-orbital haematomas?
Thorax	When examining the chest wall, do you notice any ipsilateral movement signifying a flail chest? As you palpate do you feel any crepitus, which indicates underlying fractures?
Abdomen	When you expose the abdomen do you observe any bruising, which could signify underlying bleeding, or any distention, which is considered abnormal?
Pelvis	Is the pelvis symmetrical, do the iliac crests look equal? Does the patient state they have pain around the pelvic area, which could cause concern for a pelvic fracture?
Long bones	Are the patient's long bones intact or do you observe or feel any gross deformities? For example, has the patient sustained an isolated or bilateral femur fracture?
Limbs	Palpate each limb looking for any hidden injuries, an open tibial and fibula fracture might not be noted under a patient who is wearing motorbike equipment unless correctly exposed
Hands and feet	It is important to note any substantial injuries to the hands and feet, it is easy to miss a fractured ankle that is causing the patient to suffer with ischaemia distal to that injury, an ischaemic limb is a cause for a time critical transfer

Understanding a patient's pain

The acronym SOCRATES is used to assist in assessing a patient's pain; but in some ambulance trusts it replaced the more traditional QTRST, both can be used and it is your decision and preference which to follow. It is important to remember that *no one size fits all;* therefore after reviewing this section it is important you use whichever method is best for you. The objective of assessing a patient's pain score is to deduce the severity and whether the response the patient provides supports your working impression or leans more towards any differential diagnosis you may be considering. Review Tables 24.6 and 24.7 to understand the different acronyms.

TABLE 24.6 SOCRATES.

SOCRATES	Explanation
Site	Where is the site of the pain?
Onset	What occurred when the pain started? How did it start?
Character	Can the patient describe the pain, does it feel like a dull ache, sharp pinpoint, or something else?
Radiates	Does the pain stay in one place or does it radiate into another area of the body? Can it be considered referred pain?
Alleviating factors	Can the patient do anything to make the pain feel easier, is there a particular position in which they feel more comfortable?
Time	What time did the pain start and how long has it been present? If the patient is no longer in pain what was the approximate duration of the pain?
Exacerbating factors	Could the patient do anything to make the pain worse, for example, movement or taking a deep breath?
Score	Can the patient provide you with a score with 0 being no pain and 10 being the worse imaginable pain the patient has ever experienced?

Application

Let us now apply the above pain acronyms to some cases studies to see if we can find out anymore pertinent information about their conditions:

Case study 5

You attend a 68-year-old male who is complaining of chest pain. He is fully alert, speaking in complete sentences, his respiratory rate is elevated to 24 rpm, and his heart rate is sitting at 55 beats per minute. The patient looks grey and ashen in complexion and appears to be sweating. You obtain a SOCRATES and listen to the following:

The pain feels like a band like pain, which started in the middle of the chest and goes all the way across. It has developed and now radiates into their left arm and jaw. They also feel sick and score the pain 8/10. Nothing the patient does makes the pain ease, and they are too scared to move as the pain was worse when they moved around their flat.

TABLE 24.7 PQRST.

OPQRST	Explanation
Onset	What was the person doing when the pain started?
Provocation	Is there anything that provokes the pain such as a movement of a joint, deep breathing, coughing, etc?
Quality	Can the patient describe the pain? Is it a dull ache, sharp, stabbing, or other description?
Radiates	Does the pain radiate into any other part of the body, or does it refer elsewhere? For example, in an ectopic pregnancy females may have referred pain in their shoulder through irritation of the phrenic nerve.
Severity	Can the patient give the pain a score? Refer to local practice for guidance A helpful guide is 0–10 (0 being no pain and 10 being the worse pain imaginable by the patient)
Time	When did the pain start? Is there a part of the day when the pain is worse, for example, morning or night?

In case study 5 we should become growingly concerned that the patient is suffering from an acute coronary syndrome (ACS) episode and therefore conduct a 12-lead ECG. Reviewing the heart tracing it shows ST-segment elevation in leads II, III, and aVF (these are the inferior leads). These leads tell us the patient is suffering from a myocardial infarction originating in the inferior part of the heart.

When reviewing Case study 6 we note there are some similarities with Case study 5, however, when we consider the mechanism of injury and the exacerbating movements that cause the sudden sharp pain increase, we begin to consider a musculoskeletal injury (MSK). Typically, MSK injuries will be worse when the patient moves them due to aggravation of the joint itself. Further examination will be required, potentially palpating the joint for symmetry, or consider an x-ray to rule out any underlying fractures or dislocations.

Working impression and differential diagnosis

The aim of any patient assessment is to ensure we conduct a thorough examination of the patient, which includes an in-depth history of the presenting complaint. Using the findings from a detailed physical examination and the history we can then formulate an appropriate treatment and follow-up plan for our patient. At all times the patient is at the centre of our assessment (person-centred care), and we must include them in any decision-making process.

As we conduct our assessments it is only a matter of time before the patient asks, 'What is wrong with me?' As you develop experience you will begin to pick up on clues as to the reason for your attendance during the initial history taking or global examination of your patient. It is important to consider 'What do I think is happening (working impression)?' At this stage you begin to consider different pathologies based on what you are seeing or hearing, and then you formulate a treatment plan.

Differential diagnosis requires the paramedic to rule out what is NOT happening to be able to work out what IS happening. For example, a person presenting with difficulty breathing but who has not sustained trauma is unlikely to be suffering from a tension pneumothorax. Therefore, that can be safely ruled out. This is known as differential diagnosis.

Case study 6

You attend a 24-year-old gender-neutral patient who was cleaning their house when they had a sudden sharp pain in their right shoulder. On global examination the patient appears well albeit panicking from the pain. They are holding their right shoulder worried about moving it. Your pain assessment deduces the following information:

The patient reports they were hovering and when the dog caused a commotion in the other room they turned suddenly, and the pain was almost instantaneous. Initially the pain radiated across from their right shoulder across their upper back and made them feel sick and they nearly collapsed. They recovered themselves, sat down and the associated sick feeling disappeared. The pain then withdrew to specifically affect the right shoulder where it is now focused. When the patient is at rest it feels most comfortable, and the pain is manageable, however, when they attempt to move it they get sharp pains and score it a 9/10.

On many occasions providing a definitive diagnosis is not possible. Many patients require further assessment in hospital such as blood tests or scans, however, by creating a working impression we can begin treating what we *think* is happening based on all our training and experience. If your treatment plan has not worked, then consider your differentials.

Our differential diagnosis also includes conditions that have similar presenting signs and symptoms to those we have found or that the patient has told us about. An example of this can be seen in Case study 6, whereby the patient is exhibiting signs of an MSK injury. However, the radiating pain has similarities to an ACS pain. Based on all the evidence provided, we could put the ACS pain into our differentials and focus on the MSK. It is important, however, to remember that not all conditions fit perfectly into one single category.

Understanding our own limitations, whether this be with our scope of practice or limit of knowledge, is important. We must be honest with ourselves and recognise that when we do our training we are only exposed to a few conditions. It is important to acknowledge that new pathologies are being discovered regularly. We should always be seeking new knowledge to ensure we are practicing safely and in line with the latest evidence.

Sometimes patients present with an array of conditions and we don't always know what is happening. This is OK, after all you are not a robot and in fact a human being with in-depth medical knowledge. Therefore, we simply know that the patient requires further assessment. Maybe they need that blood test or scan to deduce one diagnosis from the other and this is OK. The patients for whom we cannot deduce a working impression, yet we can produce an array of differentials, are sometimes those from whom we learn our new knowledge. So, remember to follow-up on their care plan and see what the outcome was.

Conclusion

In this chapter we have reviewed patient assessment, specifically the primary and secondary surveys, and applied these to cases. As out of hospital clinicians it is important we are dynamic in our approach, adapt to our surroundings, and deliver the right treatment at the right time and to the right patient. The patient is constantly providing us with information and we must give them our full attention. No patient *suddenly* goes into cardiac arrest, the clinician took their eyes off them and only noticed it when they looked back.

Activities

Now review your learning by completing the learning activities in this chapter. The answers to these appear at the end of the book. Further self-test activities can be found at **www.wileyfundamentalseries.com/paramedic/3e.**

Test your knowledge

1. Try and recite the primary survey and their associated terms?
2. What are the 4Hs and 4Ts?
3. Define and give an example of a sign and symptoms?
4. What are the two techniques used to open an unconscious patient's airway?
5. What is SAMPLER and what are the associated names for each element?
6. Define each element of SOCRATES?
7. Try and list the shockable and non-shockable cardiac arrest rhythms?
8. What do VF and VT stand for in cardiac arrest?
9. How do you define the difference between VF and VT?
10. How do you treat a patient who has sustained an airway occlusion and subsequent tension pneumothorax?

Activity 24.1

Using Case studies 3 and 4 see if you can extract the pertinent information and formulate some questions you might ask. Once you have extracted the details try and apply your taught underpinning theory and explain the patient's reason for your attendance.

When working through the case studies, ask yourself:

1. What is the main reason we are attending?
2. Conducting a primary survey, are there any concerns that need addressing?
3. What are the signs and symptoms?
4. Using your own knowledge, what is your working impression?

Glossary

ACS (acute coronary syndrome): An umbrella term used to describe conditions associated with an acute reduction of oxygen delivery to the heart.

ABCDE (airway, breathing, circulation, disability, and exposure): Patient assessment acronym.

AVPU (alert, vocal, pain, unresponsive): Rapid assessment tool used to deduce a patient's consciousness level.

CRT (capillary refill time): Clinical measurement indicating blood flow to capillaries. Either patient's finger nails (peripheral) or sternum (central) are pressed (or forehead in kids) for 5 seconds and then released. The time it takes to return to normal perfusion is calculated in seconds.

GCS (Glasgow Coma Scale): A clinical scale used to calculate a patient's consciousness level. It is a three-step tool measuring visual, verbal, and motor responses.

4Hs and 4Ts: An abbreviation used to remember the reversible causes of a cardiac arrest, hypovolaemia, hypoxia, hyper/hypokalaemia, hypothermia, cardiac tamponade, tension pneumothorax, thrombotic event, and toxins.

References

Gräsner, J-T., Herlitz, J., Tjelmeland, I B.M. et al. (2021). European Resuscitation Council Guidelines 2021: Epidemiology of cardiac arrest in Europe. *J Am Med Assoc* **161**: 61–79. doi: 10.1016/j.resuscitation.2021.02.007.

Kouwenhoven, W.B., Jude, J.R., and Knickerbocker, G.G. (1960). Closed-chest cardiac massage. *J Am Med Assoc* **173** (10): 1064–1067. doi: 10.1001/jama.1960.03020280004002.

Safar, P. and McMahon, M. (1958). Mouth-to-airway emergency artificial respiration. *J Am Med Assoc* **166** (12): 1459–1460.

Safar, P., Brown, T.C., Holtey, W.J. et al. (1961). Ventilation and circulation with closed-chest cardiac massage in man. *J Am Med Assoc* **176**: 574–576.

CHAPTER 25

Birth and the paramedic

Aimee Yarrington
Midwife and Paramedic

Jane Warland
Midwife

Contents

LEARNING OUTCOMES

On completion of this chapter the reader will be able to:

- Recognise a range of normal pregnancy-related terms.
- Recognise a range of abnormal pregnancy-related terms.
- Recognise and respond to the birth occurring in a prehospital setting.
- Triage pregnant/labouring clients appropriately.
- Contribute to the management of childbirth complications in a non-hospital setting.

Case study

You are called to attend a private address where there are reports of a birth in progress. When you arrive the woman is upstairs in the bedroom alone, stood up next to the bed. Further investigation reveals this is her first baby, and that according to recent scans the fetus has developed well, is presenting in a cephalic (head-down) position, and is engaged in the pelvis. You note that the contractions present are of an intensity that she is unable to talk through them and she is involuntary pushing with each one. The baby's head is not yet visible, but the crew decide to stay on scene as the birth appears to be imminent.

Fundamentals of Paramedic Practice: A Systems Approach, Third Edition. Edited by Sam Willis and Ian Peate.

Companion website: www.wiley.com/go/willis/paramedic3e

Introduction

Most of the many births occurring each and every day are problem free. However, there are very rare occasions when complications arise or the mother may be caught off guard, having not anticipated a rapid labour and birth or even being unaware that she is pregnant. During these circumstances an ambulance is usually called. Different women behave differently in labour, often dependent on a wide range of factors, including previous births, culture, and ability to cope with discomfort. When faced by an imminent birth, paramedics should use their existing 'assessment skills' and must be able to assist in the birth of the baby. This involves identifying if the birth is imminent, reassuring the woman, assisting with birthing the baby, and ensuring both mother and child are safe and well following the birth.

This chapter will provide an overview of the likely progress of a physiological (normal) birth and the care that the paramedic may need to provide. It outlines the complications that occasionally arise, detailing the steps the paramedic should take in such circumstances.

Physiological birth

The normal birth process involves the expulsion of the term fetus (between 37- and 42-weeks' gestation) out of the **uterus** through the vagina and into the arms of the new mother. This process of labour in the first-time mother (nulliparous) can potentially take over 24 hours of **contractions.** If labour occurs prior to 37 completed weeks' gestation, then the fetus is premature, will usually be smaller, and may therefore be born more quickly.

Sometimes paramedics are the first responders to a labouring woman who has progressed faster than anticipated. These labours are likely to progress smoothly, apart from the potential worry caused by a different birth location than had been planned. Increasing numbers of women choose to give birth outside the hospital setting. Paramedics may also attend a home birth following a request from the midwife, who may sometimes need another pair of hands to manage a situation, or assistance with moving or transporting the mother following the birth. Your role in both these circumstances is to remain calm, work with others who are present, and support and encourage the mother to give birth to her infant. You will also need to communicate with ambulance control and the receiving maternity unit, as well as remember to note significant events such as the time of birth.

No two births are the same and every person responds differently to childbirth. Knowing the phases of labour can help with understanding what is likely to occur. The process of childbirth comprises two distinct phases, known as latent and active.

Latent phase

The latent phase is the period of irregular contractions, which build in intensity and prepare the cervix to dilate and permit the passage of the fetus out of the uterus. In pregnancy the cervix is approximately two centimetres long, tubular, and firm, sitting at the back of the vagina. The cervix holds the pregnancy safe inside the uterus and helps to prevent infection ascending to the uterus and growing fetus. As labour begins, the contractions (tightening of the uterine muscles) shorten the cervix, pull it towards the front of the vagina, and press the head of the fetus down onto the cervix. This pressure causes stronger contractions under the control of hormones such as **oxytocin.** For labour to progress effectively, the woman must be relaxed and feel safe and supported (Downe and Bryrom 2019). Eventually, contractions will completely thin out the cervix, a process called **effacement,** and begin to dilate it, completing the latent phase of labour (Figure 25.1). The cervix will gradually be pulled over the head of the fetus by uterine contractions (like pulling a polo-neck jumper on).

It is common for a first-time mother to be in latent labour for 12–24 hours, during which time she will experience contractions – sometimes 2 in 10 minutes, sometimes none for an hour or so (Marshall and Raynor 2020). When a woman has not had a baby before effacement occurs before dilatation, whereas the two processes happen together once the woman has had a baby, thereby making second and subsequent labours shorter. Whilst in early labour she should remain mobile, resting, eating, and drinking when necessary. During this stage it is best for her to stay at home where she can be more relaxed. She may choose to relax by soaking in a warm bath. She might experience a bloody **show** (mucoid plug from the cervical canal that may be streaked with blood) or **ruptured membranes** (discharge of amniotic fluid in which the fetus floats, contained by membranes) during this phase of labour, but these events may not occur until the time of birth. If her waters break, she should contact her midwife, who will need to know what colour the waters are – if they are clear all is likely to be well, but if they are stained green it could indicate that the fetus is/has been distressed (meconium: the baby's first stool stains the amniotic fluid green). Similarly, any vaginal

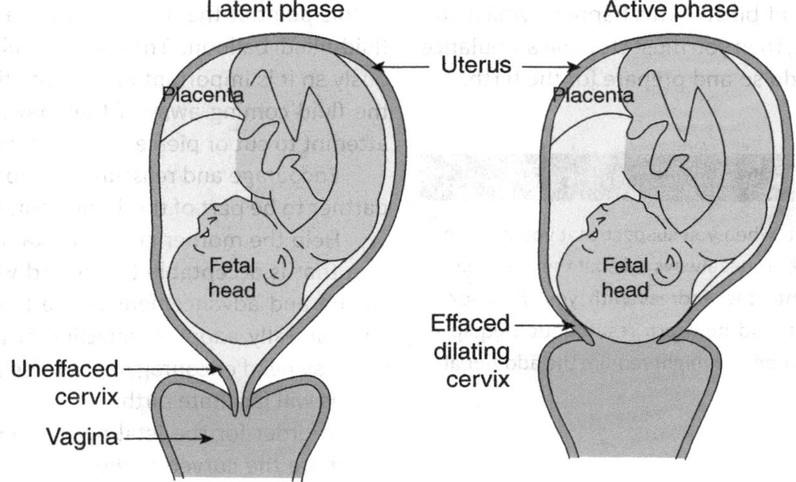

FIGURE 25.1 Effacement of cervix.

bleeding or blood-stained amniotic fluid needs checking by a midwife or obstetrician. The midwife will let the woman or her partner know the urgency of any situation and whether an ambulance should be called. Women are usually requested to plan their own transport to hospital, as birth is rarely an emergency situation. Women who have given birth before (multiparous) are likely to have much faster latent phases of labour, and some might not be aware that this is part of the process Chapman and Charles (2018).

Active phase

Once the cervix is effaced and beginning to dilate, the woman's natural oxytocin is likely to be causing contractions very regularly and of increasing strength and duration. It is common for women to start to experience contractions that are stronger and from peak to trough can last a minute or two. The woman needs calm reassurance and encouragement. It is best for her not to hold her breath during contractions, which she may do because of the strength of the sensation. Entonox may be useful to help her focus on her breathing, providing some analgesic effect. Regular contractions are powerful muscular activity of the uterus as it pushes the fetus onto the dilating cervix. Most women will prefer an upright or lateral position and should not lie supine (in pregnancy or birth), as this may interrupt the blood flow to and from the **placenta.** Limit verbal communication to the gaps between contractions, because their force may render the woman unable to answer questions. The first-time mother is likely to experience 8–12 hours of regular strong contractions during the active phase of labour, whilst a multiparous woman may be ready to push after a couple of hours. Women may experience a show or waters breaking and coming away vaginally during the active phase. As the uterus contracts, the muscles become taut and hard, which can usually be felt (gain consent prior to undertaking abdominal palpation).

Practice insight

Giving birth can be a stressful event for both the mother and other family members on scene, especially if birth was planned in hospital. Remember to remain calm yourself, and provide quiet reassurance to others who are in direct contact with the mother to help them to stay calm themselves thereby reducing stress to the mother.

Preparing for the birth

Once the birth becomes imminent, the woman's behaviour is likely to change again. She will begin to bear down at the peak of the contraction, making a guttural sound (grunting) as she exhales and pushes for several seconds or longer. She does not need to be told to push – she cannot stop; it will be involuntary, as the descending fetal head pushes the back wall of the vagina against the bowel. She may also feel as if she needs to have her bowels open and this is a sign of imminent birth. If this happens whilst you are on route to hospital, then you must stop the ambulance as soon as it is safe to do so and prepare for the birth.

Practice insight

Where resources permit, when you suspect that you may be assisting with a birth at home, always take all the maternity equipment available into the address with you. Entonox, maternity pack, towels, and newborn resuscitation equipment you never know when you might require the additional resources.

Once the woman starts pushing, external signs of imminent birth are likely to be apparent, which may include:

- The presenting part becoming visible causing bulging **perineum.**
- Gaping of the anus (and sometimes an involuntary bowel movement) as the fetal head descends lower.
- Grunting, guttural straining (sounds from the throat) as she involuntarily pushes.

In the first-time mother it may take up to an hour of pushing before these external signs are apparent, but a multiparous mother may push her baby out in only a handful of pushes. Keep visual contact with the vagina and be vigilant for the top of the fetal head.

Prepare for the arrival of the infant by ensuring the environment is warm, collecting plenty of dry towels or similar, and making sure the woman is in a safe place. Locate your neonatal resuscitation bag and mask as a precaution and put gloves on.

The fetal scalp becomes **ruched** as it passes through the vagina, so it might seem ridged and blue in colour as it appears, but hair may be visible. As the woman pushes, the fetus will advance gradually, but between contractions it is likely to retreat back into the vagina ('two steps forward, one step back') – this protects the woman's perineal tissues and also allows re-oxygenation of the fetus between contractions. Reassure the woman that this is normal. However, as she continues to push, more and more of the fetal head will show until it no longer retreats between contractions. Once the widest part of the fetal head is born, this is now known as **crowning.** At this point, the perineum, vagina, and anus will be considerably stretched and this is often distressing for the woman – let her know the likely course of events and that the stretching is normal. Usually by now the membranes will have ruptured, but they may present at this point at the maternal vagina as a cream-coloured, fluid-filled balloon. They will usually rupture spontaneously so it is important to note the time and the colour of the fluid coming away. If they have not ruptured do not attempt to cut or pierce with anything sharp.

Encourage and reassure the mother and motivate the partner to be part of this important, life-defining moment.

Help the mother get comfortable by choosing a position that is acceptable to her and where you can see the vagina and advancement of the fetus. Often the woman will naturally adopt a squatting or all-fours position, but she may need encouragement to be as upright as possible as this will facilitate birth.

In order for the fetal head to exit the pelvis, it must negotiate the curved pathway through it (curve of Carus, Figure 25.2) caused by the natural inclination of the pelvis (this contributes to the 'two steps forward, one step back' progression of the fetus).

Remember this curved route as the fetus is born – you will see the fetal head turn to face one leg or the other in order to negotiate the shoulders through the widest diameter of the pelvis. This may take one or two contractions once the head is born. The body is born in the process of lateral flexion and will follow after the next contraction after the birth of the head. If the mother is in an all-fours position the baby will still be attached to the cord and placenta so will need to be passed through the mother's legs once it has been dried and stimulated and is crying. If the woman has been squatting, the baby can be lifted by you or the mother to be placed skin to skin on her chest.

Tearing to the perineum at the point of birth unfortunately may not be avoidable. It is estimated that around 85% of women will sustain some kind of tear or graze to the vagina or perineum during birth, this percentage is reduced if women chose to give birth at home or in a midwife-led

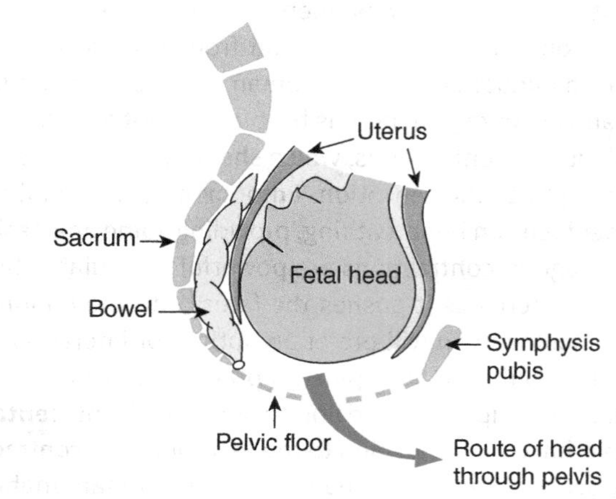

FIGURE 25.2 Curve of Carus.

unit (Chapman and Charles 2018). The midwife will assess and repair either in the woman's home or in hospital. After the head has crowned, you can assist with minimising tearing by encouraging the woman to breathe rather than push to aim for a slow, controlled birth of the fetal head.

Paramedic intervention following a normal birth

1. Once the baby has been born, use a dry towel to rub and stimulate it all over and then promptly place the naked infant on the mother's naked chest. Leave the cord intact until it has stopped pulsating.
2. Cover them both with another dry towel. This skin-to-skin contact keeps the infant at body temperature and reassures woman and child (Kahalon et al. 2022). Ensure there are no exposed parts of the baby's skin. The baby's head has the largest surface area and so should be well covered either by the towel or a beanie. The baby's toes and feet can also quickly get cold so ensure they are well covered, or booties applied.
3. Undertake an Apgar score to determine the health of the newborn (see following Practice insight).
4. Observe the infant for signs of the onset of respiration and try to note both the time of birth and of the first breath. Whilst most babies cry immediately or seconds after birth, it can sometimes take up to three minutes to establish breathing. During this time stimulation by towelling the infant dry will often cause it to gasp, as will the colder temperature it is now experiencing.
5. If there are concerns about the condition of the baby, i.e. an Apgar score less than 7, then begin neonatal resuscitation procedure. Be aware that once resuscitation has begun that the Apgar score is no longer a reliable measure of the condition of the baby. For example, the baby may be scored higher on colour because the skin is being perfused as a result of resuscitation rather than newborn breathing effort.
6. Monitor vaginal blood loss, which is typically 200–300 ml – sit the mother comfortably (with infant skin to skin) and apply a maternity or large sanitary pad between her legs so that you can see how much blood has been lost since the birth.
7. Leave the umbilical cord intact and await signs of placental separation and delivery.
8. Continue to provide pain relief to the mother as necessary and undertake a set of baseline observations on both mother and baby.

Practice insight

The Apgar score is a quick assessment undertaken at one- and five-minute intervals following birth. Virginia Apgar invented the score but her last name can also be used as an acronym to remember how to score, i.e. APGAR: appearance, pulse, grimace, activity (muscle tone), respirations. Add an Apgar cheat sheet to your current clinical guidelines to help you remember the scoring and make a note of the outcomes.

Following the birth, monitor vaginal blood loss and look and listen for cues from the mother that the placenta has separated from its site inside the uterus. When it does this, the cord lengthens at the vagina, there is a fresh trickle of blood vaginally, and the woman may report pressure in the vagina, or the need to push again. Find a receiver for the placenta, sit the woman more upright, and encourage her to push once more. The placenta will appear bluish, veiny, and shiny, covered in tough membrane and with the cord attached to it – do not pull the cord to expedite delivery. Once the cord has stopped pulsating and appears white in colour you can clamp (two clamps) and divide it (cutting between the clamps). Ensure that the placenta and membranes are kept for a midwife to inspect, either at the woman's home or once you have transferred to hospital.

Birth complications

Most births will run smoothly; however, there are occasions when things go wrong. Complications of childbirth, especially when a baby is **born before arrival** (BBA) at hospital are rare but when they happen it is important that the paramedic knows how to manage these cases:

- Antepartum haemorrhage
- Cord prolapse
- Shoulder dystocia
- Breech Birth
- Post partum haemorrhage

Antepartum haemorrhage

An antepartum haemorrhage (APH) is any frank bleeding from the genital tract after 24 completed weeks of pregnancy. APH complicates 3–5% of pregnancies and is a leading cause of perinatal and maternal mortality worldwide (RCOG 2011). The rapid assessment of the woman presenting with an APH is vital and you should ensure a timely removal to the nearest obstetric facility.

If maternal oxygen saturation falls remember to ensure oxygen therapy is used in order to prevent any further fetal compromise. Do not delay time on scene for cannulation. This should be done en route if bleeding is serious and continuous access with two large bore cannulas should be sought early as maternal shutdown often occurs quickly due to sudden onset of hypovolemic shock. The use of intravenous fluid therapy should be used in order to maintain a systolic blood pressure (BP) above 90 by giving 250 ml bolus doses of sodium chloride. But it is important to remember that during pregnancy may lose up to 50% of their circulating blood volume without a significant change in their observations. Careful assessment of fetal movements should be made in order to assess fetal viability; however, it is important to remember to be tactful in this situation, as further anxiety and alarm may cause exacerbation of the situation. It is imperative to remember the woman's pain and titrate pain relief accordingly.

A concise pre-alert to the receiving obstetric facility is important and including an estimation of blood loss is key as staff can gather the required assistance needed to deal with specific events.

Cord prolapse

This is another very rare complication of pregnancy whereby a loop of umbilical cord slips past the fetal head or bottom, through the dilating maternal cervix, and into or out of the vagina (Figure 25.3). This is more likely to occur with an ill-fitting presenting part such as in premature or breech birth but is still very rare. With maternal consent, inspect the vulva and if umbilical cord is recognised the woman needs urgent transfer to a delivery suite.

From this point, the aim is to stop the presenting part from squashing the cord against the maternal cervix, which will cut off the oxygen supply to the fetus. This is best achieved via an exaggerated recovery position with a pillow under the lower hip and a head-down tilt or the knee-to-chest position (bottom-in-the-air position) Whilst transferring, the woman must be secured into the ambulance in a exaggerated lateral position and not transferred in knee-to-chest position.

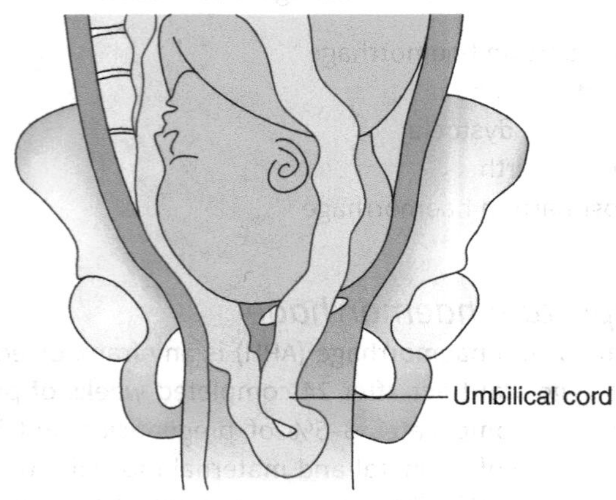

FIGURE 25.3 Umbilical cord prolapse.

This is a time-critical emergency: it requires immediate intervention and rapid removal and transfer to a consultant obstetric unit. Once in the ambulance:

- Using a dry maternity pad gently replace the cord back into the vagina this should be attempted only **ONCE** as the cord should be handled minimally to prevent spasm.
- If the loop of protruding cord is too long and not possible to replace into the vagina a dry pad should be utilised to prevent further prolapse.
- If the cord has been replaced, again a dry pad should be used. The mother should then enter the lateral position with her hips raised as much as possible to relieve pressure on the cord.
- The woman should be assisted to walk ideally to the ambulance stretcher, as sitting on a chair may cause further pressure on the already compromised cord.
- The administration of Entonox may help to prevent the woman from pushing, which would again increase the pressure on the cord.
- Do not delay time on scene to cannulate.
- Pre-alert the nearest obstetric facility.

Shoulder dystocia

This is a rare complication of the second stage of labour whereby one of the fetal shoulders gets jammed behind the maternal symphysis pubis (Figure 25.4) or against the **sacral promontory**. It can only be diagnosed following the birth of the fetal head and you see a distinctive 'turtle sign', i.e. the head extends over the perineum as it is born and then quickly recedes back such that the chin is tightly drawn up against the maternal perineum. There is no restitution of the fetal head. Do not pull on or twist the fetal head to try to encourage restitution, as the neck is already extended due to the anterior shoulder being stuck and further traction can cause significant damage. Note the time that you decide that shoulder dystocia has occurred and communicate this to colleagues at ambulance despatch or the delivery suite. *This is a time-critical complication.*

Communicate calmly with the woman and her partner – let them know their cooperation is needed to resolve this delay in the birth of the infant, and if possible be sure to have the neonatal resuscitation equipment to hand (bag-valve-mask, flat surface, and warm towels or

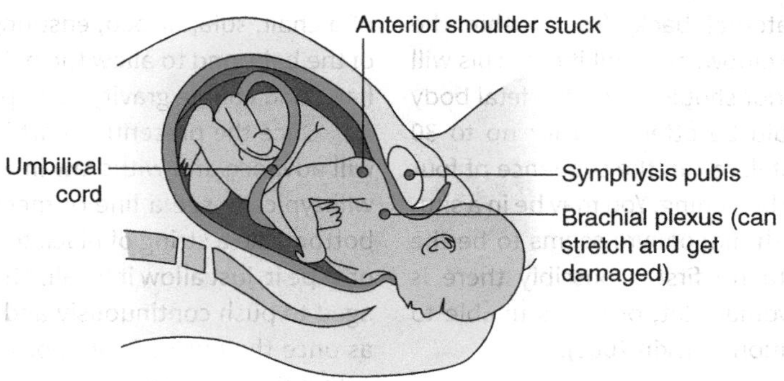

FIGURE 25.4 Shoulder dystocia.

similar). Explain to the mother that you will need to try some manoeuvres to help the baby's birth. Avoid describing the fetus as 'stuck', as this may panic the woman; rather, describe the fetus as in need of assistance to complete the birth of the rest of the baby.

The resolution of dystocia occurs by moving the fetal shoulders past the maternal symphysis pubis and this is best achieved by changing the woman's position. In the majority of cases of shoulder dystocia the anterior fetal shoulder is wedged behind the maternal symphysis pubis and a series of manoeuvres need to be executed to resolve it (Marshall and Raynor 2020). The paramedic in attendance may try the following four manoeuvres:

1. The first manoeuvre involves placing the woman supine and requires two people/paramedics/attendants. Each person helps the woman bring her bent legs towards her abdomen to achieve a 'knees-to-nipples position' without too much abduction. This is known as the McRoberts manoeuvre (Figure 25.5). When this position has been achieved, the woman should be encouraged *not* to push, whilst gentle axial traction is applied to the fetal head. Attempt to deliver the fetus for up to 30 seconds. Move on to the next manoeuvre if you see no progress of shoulders/the fetal neck (RCOG 2012).
2. The second manoeuvre involves maintenance of the McRoberts position, whilst trying to push the stuck shoulder around in the pelvis. Pressure should now be applied suprapubically by one attendant, with the intention of rotating the fetal shoulders out of the vertical axis into an oblique axis. The fetal shoulders are wedged anteroposteriorly – i.e. at 6 o'clock if you imagine a clock face. You are trying to push the shoulders to 7 o'clock to disimpact the anterior shoulder. This is usually done with the heel of the interlaced hands (similar to the technique used for cardiac massage during adult cardiopulmonary resuscitation) on the maternal abdomen just above the symphysis pubis and involves constant pressure. The second helper applies gentle axial traction to the fetal head. The woman should not push. Attempt this for up to 30 seconds before moving on to the next manoeuvre (RCOG 2012).
3. The third manoeuvre is a continuation of the second, but now the attendant who is applying suprapubic pressure changes from continuous pressure to rocking pressure, trying to move the fetal shoulders from the stuck antero-posterior position/diameter of the pelvis into an oblique and larger diameter of the pelvis. Whilst the first attendant applies this rocking pressure abdominally and suprapubically, the other attendant applies gentle axial traction on the fetal head. The woman should not push. Keep trying this manoeuvre for up to 30 seconds (RCOG 2012).
4. If no signs of advancement of the fetus are apparent, the fourth manoeuvre is to request that the woman moves into an all-fours position. It is hoped that this will recruit gravity and cause the fetus to drop towards the maternal abdomen. With maternal consent it may now be possible to grasp the posterior arm (the fetal

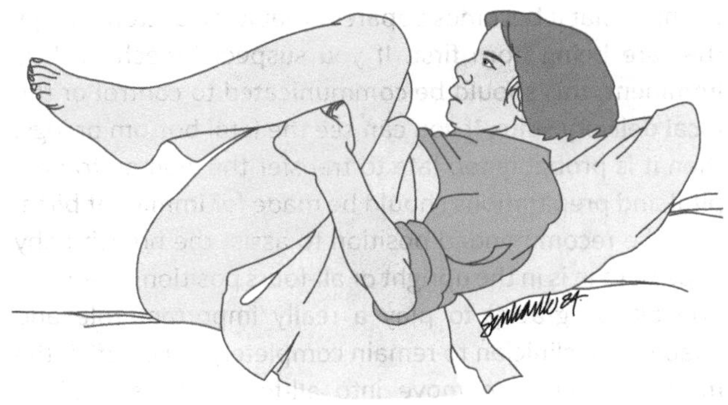

FIGURE 25.5 The McRoberts position.

arm nearest the maternal back) from within the vagina, bend it at the elbow, and pull it out. This will then release the anterior shoulder and the fetal body will follow. This should be attempted for up to 30 seconds. If unsuccessful, re-run the sequence of four manoeuvres from the beginning. You may be in a situation where this fourth manoeuvre seems to be the most practical one to try first – possibly there is nowhere to lie the woman flat, or she is unable to assume a supine position (Gaskin 2003).

If there is a midwife in attendance, they may then perform further manoeuvres in which they have been specifically trained for removing the posterior arm. The paramedic can be of assistance in this manoeuvre by helping support the woman on all-fours (as this position is best for delivering the posterior arm), as well as ensuring all equipment is ready for infant resuscitation, which will likely be needed following birth.

Once the infant is born it is likely to require resuscitation, as it may well have been deprived of oxygen during the dystocia. Note the time of birth, Apgar score, and any resuscitation interventions.

Breech birth

In some births the fetus assumes a bottom-first position, folded legs, buttocks, or knees presenting upon the cervix. This is known as a breech presentation, of which there are several types, but all mean that instead of the head being the first fetal part to be born, it becomes the last. Most women with a known breech presentation will be having a planned birth in hospital, but occasionally a fetus in the breech position is not discovered until the breech is on view during birth. The paramedic may be called by an attending midwife, or it may be that the paramedic is the first responder to a birth that is progressing rapidly at home.

Labour will progress in the same way as in a cephalic presentation and it may only be when the woman is pushing that it becomes apparent that it is a bottom or legs that are being born first. If you suspect breech birth is imminent, this should be communicated to control or the local delivery suite. If you can see the fetal bottom or legs, then it is probably too late to transfer the woman to hospital and preparations should be made for imminent birth.

The recommended position to assist the breech baby to be born in is in the upright or all-fours position. This position allows gravity to play a really important role and enables the clinician to remain completely hands off. If the mother declines to move into all-fours, she should be encouraged to move into an upright position on the edge of a chair, sofa, or bed, ensuring that there is no touching of the baby and to allow the baby's body sufficient space to hang and enable gravity to help facilitate most of the birth.

Once the presenting part is visible (i.e. the bottom) it will advance and withdraw in a similar way to a head. You will typically see a line of meconium appearing from the bottom like a string of black toothpaste. Do not touch this or wipe it, just allow it to fall. The mother should be encouraged to push continuously and not just with contractions, as once the buttocks are born birth should be completed within five minutes.

When the widest part of the bottom is born this is known as the 'rumping' like the crowning as the head is born, meaning that the 'rump' will no longer recede with contractions. Once the rumping has occurred the baby will rotate and whichever position the mother is in there should only be one back visible, i.e. you can see the mothers back if the mother is in all-fours or the baby's back if the mother is upright.

If the baby was in the frank breech position the baby's legs will typically deliver together once you see the knees. If the baby was in the complete position you will often see feet and legs emerge slightly ahead of the buttocks. This is not to be confused with a footling breech.

As the birth progresses at this point there are several points you can look out for that will tell you the health of the baby at this point:

- The baby will have good tone.
- The baby will be a good colour, i.e. usual/expected.
- The cord will be full.
- The valley of the cord will be visible (the crease that runs up the chest wall will be like a valley).
- The baby will do the characteristic 'tummy crunches' movement that is normal to encourage the birth of the arms and head.

Don't try to assist the baby during the crunches. These are the natural movements that the baby will make in order to get them into the position needed to get the arms and head born. Don't worry if the baby doesn't crunch, but this will lead to a slower descent and the baby will more likely need resuscitation.

Do not pull on the infant's trunk in an attempt to expedite the birth, as this may cause the baby to raise its arms in utero causing nuchal arms (arms that are raised over the head). Once the arms are free then again leave the baby and do not interfere with the natural physiology. This is often the most unnerving time and the point at which most clinicians want to hold the baby upward, as they fear it will damage the neck. By holding the baby at this point the head will not engage in the pelvis and it may stop the baby from being born at all.

As the head emerges and you are there to catch the baby as the head is freed from the birth canal. If slow descent is happening, there are a few key tips recommended by the breech birth network:

- Encourage movement: get the mother to rock her hips side to side to shake the baby downward.
- Get the mother to adopt the 'running start' position like a runner in the blocks of a race with one knee lifted, this will open the outlet of the pelvis.
- A gentle shoulder press when the chin is born pushing the baby backward can again facilitate the birth of the head.

Postpartum haemorrhage

This is a complication that can follow any kind of birth. It is characterised by a blood loss of 500 ml or more following the birth. The main reason is that the uterus has lost muscular tone following the birth of the infant due to prolonged labour or precipitate labour. Because of the size of the placenta (about 20 cm diameter) and the way it attaches to the inside of the uterus wall, when it detaches in the third stage it leaves a large open wound on the inside of the uterus. If the uterine muscle does not constrict these vessels, it can result in postpartum haemorrhage (PPH) that can be very heavy and rapidly lead to hypovolemic shock and even death.

As the prime reason for PPH is a loss of uterine tone, the immediate response is to stimulate (with consent) the uterus by rubbing the top (fundus) of it through the maternal abdomen (Marshall and Raynor 2020). The fundus is likely to be at a point midway between the maternal navel and the bottom of the rib cage, depending upon whether the placenta has separated or not. If the placenta has not separated, the fundus will be higher and feel wide and soft. If the placenta has separated, the fundus will be hard, muscular, at the level of the maternal navel, and about as big as an orange. If there is bleeding, the fundus will feel 'boggy' and when it is rubbed through the maternal abdomen in a firm and circular motion you should feel the muscle of the uterus contract and become hard, and the bleeding will slow and ideally stop altogether. If she is bleeding this massage of the uterus should take priority and if possible a colleague should cannulate the woman with a wide-bore cannula, monitor her for signs of hypovolemia (rising pulse, falling blood pressure, clamminess, and confusion), and provide intravenous fluids to support the circulating volume if necessary. Follow local guidelines with regard to administering a uterotonic (note the time it is given).

In order to maintain the tone of the uterus, oxytocin must be present. Natural methods of increasing oxytocin include:

- Skin-to-skin contact with baby
- Breast feeding
- Ensuring an empty bladder
- Keeping mother warm

These will all aid the natural oxytocin production and may assist with the prevention of a PPH.

Arrange urgent transfer, whilst being vigilant over uterine muscle tone; retain all blood-soaked pads and towels to enable estimation of blood loss, and the placenta if delivered; and bring the infant with the mother.

Conclusion

Childbirth is a reason for celebration for most parents and is a naturally occurring event. On the majority of occasions, childbirth occurs problem free. This chapter has outlined the progress of normal labour and birth, and the cues that the paramedic can use to decide if transfer is advisable and what to do if birth is imminent. An overview has also been provided of some of the common complications that the paramedic might encounter, with practical suggestions for their management.

Activities

Now review your learning by completing the learning activities in this chapter. The answers to these appear at the end of the book. Further self-test activities can be found at **www.wileyfundamentalseries.com/paramedic/3e.**

Test your knowledge

1. What is a normal gestation period for humans?
2. How many phases of labour are there and what are they?
3. When does the crowning occur?
4. List five complications of childbirth.

Activity 21.1

1. In pregnancy, how is the cervix structured?
2. What is the latent phase of labour?
3. At what point is the latent phase of labour considered complete?
4. How long can the latent phase last for?
5. What actions should the mother take during this period?

Activity 21.2

1. Define the term shoulder dystocia.
2. At what point will it become evident that a breech birth is present?

Activity 21.3

1. What is the main cause of postpartum haemorrhage?
2. Outline paramedic management of PPH.

Activity 21.4

What is the aim of the paramedic when presented with cord prolapse?

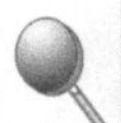

Glossary

Cervix: The tubular exit from the uterus, continuous with the vagina.

Contraction: The action of the uterine muscles that open the cervix and push the fetus out of the vagina.

Effacement: Thinning out and shortening of the cervix caused by contractions.

Meconium: Fetal bowel contents.

Oxytocin: One of the hormones that promotes labour.

Perineum: The area between anus and vagina.

Placenta: The structure that embeds in the inner wall of the uterus in early pregnancy and transfers oxygen and nutrients from woman to fetus.

Ruched: Visible pleating/folding of tissue.

Sacral promontory: The bulge of sacral vertebrae into the space of the pelvis.

Show: Loss of the blood-stained mucus plug that seals the cervix during pregnancy.

Symphysis pubis: Front bones of the pelvis palpable at the bikini line.

Uterus: The womb, in which the fetus develops before birth.

References

Chapman, V. and Charles, C. (2018). *The Midwife's Labour and Birth Handbook. 4e*. Oxford: Wiley-Blackwell.

Downe, S. (2008). *Normal Childbirth: Evidence and Debate*. 2e. Edinburgh: Churchill Livingstone.

Downe, S. and Bryrom, S. (2019). *Squaring the Circle: Normal Birth Research, Theory and Practice in a Technological Age*. London: Pinner and Martin.

Gaskin, I.M. (2003). *Ina May's Guide to Childbirth*. New York: Bantam Books.

Kahalon, R., Pries, H., and Benyamini, Y. (2022). Mother-infant contact after birth can reduce postpartum post-traumatic stress symptoms through a reduction in birth-related fear and guilt. *Journal of Psychosomatic Research* **154:** 110716. doi: 10.1016/j.jpsychores.2022.110716.

Marshall, J. and Raynor, M. (2020) *Myles Textbook for Midwives*. 17e London: Elsevier.

RCOG (Royal College of Obstetricians and Gynaecologists). (2012). *Shoulder Dystocia*. Green Top Guideline No. 42. London: Royal College of Obstetricians and Gynaecologists.

CHAPTER 26

Paediatrics: recognition of the sick child

Clare Davies

Lecturer in Nursing, Susan Wakil School of Nursing and Midwifery, Faculty of Medicine and Health, The University of Sydney, Australia

Contents

LEARNING OUTCOMES

On completion of this chapter the reader will be able to:

- **Identify the anatomical, physiological, psychosocial, and communication differences of infants and children and resulting impacts on the assessment of the sick child.**
- **Learn how to undertake an initial 'hands-off' assessment of the child using the Paediatric Assessment Tool (PAT).**
- **Gain an understanding of the systematic A–G assessment of children and the identification of 'red flags' that may indicate severity of illness and risk of deterioration.**
- **Identify common causes of severe illness in infants and children.**

Case study

You have been called to a private address to a 5-month-old infant who the parents report is having difficulty in breathing. On your arrival the parents are panicking, and the infant is lying flat on his back on the couch. On visual assessment you can see an increased respiratory rate, nasal flaring, chest retractions, and the child is cyanotic in colour.

Fundamentals of Paramedic Practice: A Systems Approach, Third Edition. Edited by Sam Willis and Ian Peate.

Companion website: www.wiley.com/go/willis/paramedic3e

Introduction

This chapter introduces students to the topic of recognising the sick infant, child, and adolescent. The need to attend paediatric emergencies is common. Sick children can present with generic symptoms and are often unable to give a clear history. It is therefore of paramount importance that the paramedic can identify red flags, that is, signs that indicate potential severe illness and risk of deterioration. The chapter begins with a consideration of the differences between adults and children. Children and young people are not just small adults and significant anatomical, physiological, psychosocial, and communication differences impact upon pathophysiology of disease, assessment, and treatment of paediatric patients. A systematic approach to assessing the sick child will then be presented, followed by an overview of some of the most common paediatric emergencies.

The difference between adults and children

Children at different ages and stages of development significantly differ from each other and from adults. As children grow, changes occur in their vital signs, cognitive ability, weight, anatomy, and physiological processes. Table 26.1 provides an overview of classifications of age groups in the paediatric population, however, be aware that these can vary in the literature.

Vital signs

Normal ranges for children's vital signs change depending on their age group. The following table provides approximate normal ranges for vital signs according to their age.

TABLE 26.1 Classification of age

Newborn	<28 days
Infancy	<1 year
Toddler	1–2 years
Pre-school	3–5 years
School age	6–12 years
Adolescence	13–18 years

TABLE 26.2 Vital sign acceptable ranges per age group.

Ages	Heart rate	Respiratory rate	Systolic blood pressure
Newborn	12–185	25–60	60–95
Infant (1 year)	105–180	20–45	70–105
Toddler (2 years)	95–175	20–40	70–105
Pre-school (4 years)	80–150	17–30	75–110
School age (8 years)	70–130	16–30	85–115
Adolescent (14 years)	60–115	14–25	90–130

Source: Paediatric Improvement Collaborative, 2023a

Anatomical and physiological differences

Airway differences in paediatrics

Anatomical differences in the child's airway can lead to increased risk of deterioration. Infants and small children have smaller airways that can lead to increased resistance in the presence of disease, injury, or foreign bodies. Infants and small children also have a relatively large tongue in a small oral cavity, which can block the airway in the event of reduced levels of consciousness, as will their proportionally larger head and poor head control. Soft cartilage in the larynx and trachea means that airways are soft and can easily collapse. During CPR, an infant's airway can be easily hyperextended during airway opening manoeuvres, leading to further airway obstruction. Infants are also preferential nose breathers. Mucus in the upper airway can quickly impact their ability to breath and feed.

Breathing differences in paediatrics

Respiratory conditions are common in infants and young children due to their smaller airways and immature immune systems. Children have less alveoli than adults, resulting in less capacity for gaseous exchange. Up to the age of 7 years, children predominantly use their diaphragm for breathing. Any abdominal distention or increased intra-abdominal pressure may therefore impact on their ability to expand

TABLE 26.3 **Summary of airway differences in paediatrics.**

Airway characteristics	Resulting impact
Smaller and narrower airways	Increased airway resistance in the presence of disease, injury, or foreign body Increased impact of oedema and mucous production Relatively large tongue in relatively small oral cavity creates increased risk of obstruction, particularly in the unconscious child
Soft, pliable airways	Infants more susceptible to airway collapse Hyperextension can lead to further obstruction
Infants are preferential nose breathers	Obstruction of nasal cavities due to secretions can quickly impact upon breathing and feeding
Large head and immature neck muscles	Inability to keep head up and maintain own airway. Large occiput will push head forward when unconscious, further compromising airway

their lungs. Poorly developed accessory muscles and a compliant chest wall with short, horizontal ribs means that chest expansion is limited. Respiratory effort is less sustainable and muscle fatigue can quickly lead to respiratory failure.

Circulation differences in paediatrics

Circulating blood volume in infants and children is higher per kg than in adults, but actual volume is smaller. What may seem like relatively small blood losses can have a significant impact in infants and small children.

Children are less able to increase stroke volume as immature myocardium limits their ability to increase contractility. Hence, increase in stroke volume is predominantly achieved by increasing heart rate. Tachycardia therefore is commonly seen in sick children. Hypotension is usually a late and pre-terminal sign of deterioration.

Unlike adults, primary cardiac events are uncommon in infants and children. Cardiac issues are congenital and coronary disease is largely absent. The origins of cardiac arrest in children are therefore predominantly respiratory and circulatory failure. A failure to recognise and respond to deterioration early will result in prolonged periods of decompensation

TABLE 26.4 **Summary of breathing differences in paediatrics.**

Breathing characteristics	Resulting impact
Less alveoli than adults	Less capacity for gaseous exchange
Infants and small children are abdominal breathers	Predominantly diaphragmatic breathing up until the age of 7 years due to immature accessory muscle development. Any abdominal distention can impact upon ability to breathe
Compliant chest wall with short, horizontal ribs	Chest expansion limited Intercostal, subcostal, and sternal recession all signs of increased work of breathing. Likelihood of chest wall collapse greater
Immature intercostal and accessory muscles	Rapid respiratory muscle fatigue Increased attempts to use accessory muscles will result in signs of respiratory distress like head bobbing
Immature respiratory control centre	Irregular breathing patterns and apnoea may occur in the presence of respiratory conditions, particularly in preterm and small infants

TABLE 26.5 **Summary of circulation differences in paediatrics.**

Circulation characteristics	Resulting impact
Circulating blood volume higher per kg but smaller total volume	Relatively small losses can have major impact, especially in infants and small children
Inability to alter stroke volume to increase cardiac output	Cardiac output is altered with increase in heart rate. Tachycardia commonly seen in sick infants and children
No early changes in blood pressure	Hypotension is a late and pre-terminal sign of deterioration
Absence of cardiac disease-primary cardiac events rare	Cardiac arrest is rare, but outcomes are poor, as it will occur following prolonged periods of decompensation

leading to cardiac arrest. Cardiac arrest in infants and children is rare but outcomes are poor. Asystole is the most common rhythm in cardiac arrest in children.

Neurological differences in paediatrics

Neurological assessment can be difficult in infants and children due to cognitive immaturity and limited communication skills. The use of standard assessment tools like the Glasgow Coma Scale (GCS) is inadequate in under 5 years old. A modified GCS should be used in this age group (Borgialli et al. 2016).

Skeletal differences in paediatrics

Infants have a thin flexible skull, which offers less protection to the brain. Following head injury, this flexibility can mean an absence of skull fractur, but damage to underlying brain tissue may still occur because of compression of the cranial bones.

At birth, sutures between the cranial bones are not fused, to allow for brain growth. There are also two open fontanelles (anterior and posterior), which close by about 18 months of age. Raised intracranial pressure (ICP) may result in increased head circumference due to this skull flexibility. Fontanelle can be useful is assessment and diagnosis (bulging may indicate raised ICP, sunken may indicate dehydration).

Incomplete calcification in infants and children means there is more flexibility in bones and cartilage that afford less protection to underlying organs. Greenstick fractures are common in young children due to the bending forces exerted on their bones as they play (Figure 26.1).

The damage to active growth plates may result in issues with bone growth. Children's underdeveloped muscles and soft bones (e.g. the skull) offer them less protection and may present issues for breathing and head control, as discussed earlier (see Table 26.6).

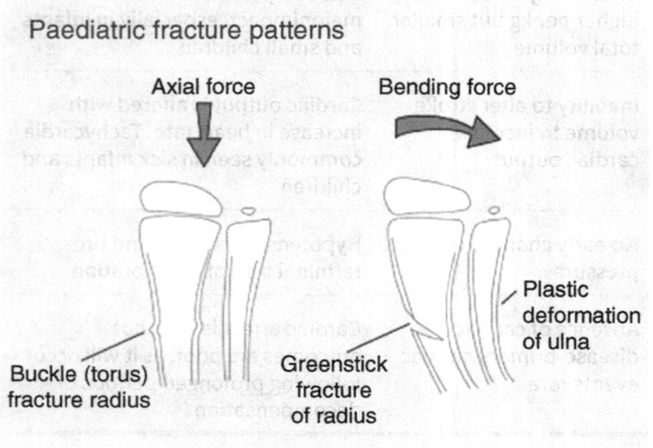

FIGURE 26.1 Greenstick fracture.

TABLE 26.6 Summary of skeletal differences in paediatrics.

Skeletal characteristics	Resulting impact
Incomplete calcification	Flexibility of bones resulting in greenstick fractures
Growth still active	Damage to growth plates may result in impaired bone growth
Soft, pliable bones and underdeveloped muscles	Less protection afforded to underlying organs
Soft, pliable skull	Less protection Danger of damage to underlying structures in the absence of fracture
Open fontanelle and unfused sutures	Increased head circumference may indicate raised ICP Skull flexibility does not protect from raised ICP

Hydration issues in paediatrics

Infants and children have a higher percentage of body water than adults and much of this is stored as extracellular fluid. Extracellular fluid is more readily lost from the body than intracellular fluid and so infants and children are more susceptible to fluid deficits and dehydration. They are also more at risk as a result of greater insensible losses (due to a higher body surface area to weight ratio and higher metabolic rates) and a reduced capacity to concentrate urine due to their immature kidney function. Depending on their age, they are often reliant on caregivers for their hydration needs. These factors all result in the vulnerability to fluid loss and dehydration.

TABLE 26.7 Summary of hydration differences in paediatrics.

Hydration characteristics	Resulting impact
Higher % body water than adults	Higher fluid requirements per kg and higher susceptibility to extracellular losses
Higher body surface area	Greater insensible losses
Immature kidney function	Inability to concentrate urine resulting in greater fluid losses

TABLE 26.8 Summary of metabolic and thermoregulation differences in paediatrics.

Metabolic and thermoregulation characteristics	Resulting impact
Larger body surface area	Greater heat losses
Higher metabolic rates	More calories per kg required especially when unwell
Poor glycogen storage capacity	Risks of hypoglycaemia when unwell, especially infants

Metabolic/thermoregulation differences in paediatrics

Infants and children have a larger body surface area to weight ratio than adults, which leads to greater heat losses. They have less insulating fat and small infants are unable to shiver, all resulting in greater risks of hypothermia. Higher metabolic rates mean that they require more calories per kg than adults. They possess a reduced capacity for glycogen storage, which can lead to hypoglycaemia, especially in the sick infant who is requiring more calories than usual.

Psychosocial and communication differences in paediatrics

Children are highly reliant on their families for psychosocial support and to assist them in communication. Children's anxiety will increase if they are separated from their parents or caregivers so parents should be encouraged to stay with their child at all times. Ensure communication with children is ongoing, reassuring, and in language that they understand to reduce anxiety. Children may not always be able to answer your questions but they should be included in all conversations. Parents know their children very well and will often be alerted to changes or deterioration earlier than health professionals. **Any parental concerns about their child's condition should be taken seriously.**

Recognition of the sick child: a systematic approach to assessment

When assessing a sick child, a methodical and structured approach can assist in prioritising health concerns. Before any

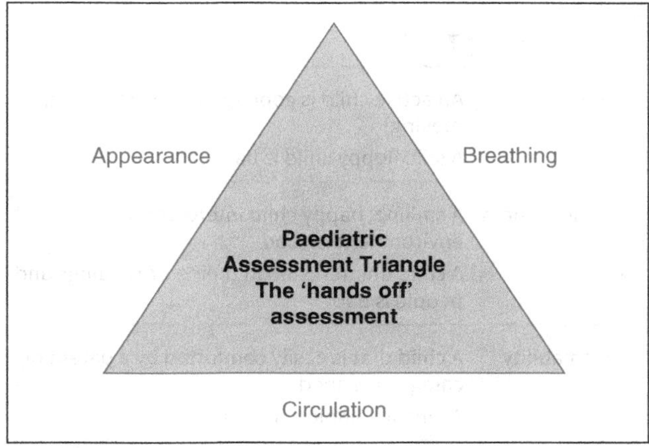

FIGURE 26.2 PAT. Source: Fernandez et al. 2017.

physical examination is undertaken, much information can be gained about the child's condition by simply observing them. The Paediatric Assessment Triangle (PAT; Figure 26.2) is one assessment approach commonly used when initially assessing a sick child (Fernandez et al. 2017).

Initial assessment – the PAT

The PAT is a framework that allows for a rapid, hands-off assessment, aimed at quickly identifying red flags and the commencement of emergency treatment. Three components are assessed: appearance, breathing, and circulation.

Visual assessment of appearance

When assessing the child's appearance, consider what is normal behaviour and activity for the child's age range or abilities. Parents will be able to assist in telling you what is normal for their child. A useful mnemonic in the assessment of appearance is TICLS (Fernandez et al. 2017) and includes the assessment of *tone* (spontaneous movement, ability to stand, floppy or hypertonia), *interactivity* (interacting and interested in the environment, parents and clinician), *consolability* (parents/caregiver ability to console and comfort them), *gaze* (ability to track and maintain eye contact), *speech/cry* (ability to use age-appropriate language/tone of cry, i.e. weak or strong, high pitched).

Visual assessment of work of breathing

Assessment of breathing starts with observing for signs of increased work of breathing. These include abnormal airway sounds (wheezing, grunting, stridor), abnormal positioning and movement (tripod position, airway maintained by sniffing

TABLE 26.9 TICLS.

Tone	An active child is good (grabbing, reaching, moving) A still, floppy child is bad
Instructiveness	A smiling, happy child interested in the environment is good A child uninterested in their surroundings and people is bad
Consolability	A child that is easily comforted by a parent or caregiver is good An inconsolable child is bad
Look/gaze	A child who maintains eye contact and looks around them in interest is good A child who stares and is unengaged in eye contact is bad
Speech/cry	A child who cries and talks is good A quiet, moaning or grunting child is bad

Source: Fernandez et al. 2017.

position, head bobbing), increased recession and retractions (subcostal, intercostal, and sternal recession, tracheal tug), nasal flaring, and respiratory rate (see Table 26.2 for normal ranges).

Visual assessment of the circulation to the skin

A hands-off assessment of circulation relates to the identification of poor perfusion to the skin and is a compensatory mechanism, as blood is shifted away from extremities to vital organs such as the heart and brain. It is identified by the presence of pallor (white or pale skin), mottling (patchy discolouration or 'marbled' appearance of skin) or cyanosis (blue tinge to skin, particularly around lips).

A–G paediatric assessment framework

Following an initial rapid assessment and the commencement of urgent treatment, the paramedic should undertake a more comprehensive assessment using the A–G assessment framework. The following section will outline this assessment in further detail. When using this framework, the primary anatomical and physiological differences discussed in the previous section should be considered.

A – Airway

The identification of partial upper airway obstruction in children is critical as it can rapidly progress to complete obstruction and respiratory arrest. Assessing airway patency in children is primarily undertaken through listening. As noted in the section above (PAT), partial obstruction of the airway can be recognised through the identification of distinct airway noises. Stridor is heard on inspiration and is often caused by swelling in the upper airway due to infection (laryngotracheobronchitis or croup) or foreign body inhalation. It is important to assess for stridor at rest as any physical activity or stress will increase the intensity. Throat examinations should not be undertaken as this can increase the intensity of the stridor. Stridor at rest is a red flag and indicative of potential deterioration.

Other indications of a partially obstructed airway include gurgling (due to difficulty in swallowing secretions) and snoring. Secondary signs of worsening obstruction include increased respiratory rate and effort, decreased oxygen saturations, increased heart rate, worsening colour, the development of agitation due to hypoxia and decreasing levels of consciousness. If partial obstruction progresses to complete obstruction, the child will quickly deteriorate, and cardiac arrest will occur if airway management is not initiated (see Table 26.10).

B – Breathing

The assessment of adequate breathing in paediatric patients is through the assessment of rate, *effort*, and *efficacy*. The assessment of rate requires counting the speed of breathing over one minute, whereas respiratory *effort* (the amount of effort that is required to maintain oxygenation) is achieved through the observation of work of breathing (recession and retractions, nasal flaring, tracheal tug, head bobbing in infants) and through the assessment of respiratory rate, symmetry of

TABLE 26.10 Severity of airway obstruction.

Mild obstruction	Moderate obstruction	Severe to complete obstruction
Able to speak/cry, may be hoarse	Tachypnoea	Hypoxia (late sign)
Intermittent stridor/ stridor on exertion	Stridor Prolonged inspiratory time	Marked tachypnoea or slow respiratory rate
Minimal or no work of breathing	Moderate work of breathing, nasal flaring, grunting	Sniffing or tripod position
Good air entry	Decreased air entry	Agitation or reduced level of consciousness

Source: Paediatric Improvement Collaborative 2023b.

chest wall movement, adventitious breath sounds (wheeze, stridor, crackles, etc), and respiratory patterns (dyspnoea, irregular breathing, apnoea, etc). Dyspnoea can be evaluated in infants with the assessment of feeding patterns, which will decline as respiratory effort increases. Tachypnoea (increased respiratory rate) is commonly seen in unwell children with respiratory conditions. Apnoea (periods of absence of breathing) can also occur in sick children and infants as they become exhausted due to increased effort of breathing and are a sign of impending deterioration. *Efficacy* of breathing, that is, how effective gaseous exchange is, is assessed through measuring oxygen saturations and observing behaviour (level of consciousness, agitation, exhaustion, muscle tone, etc) and colour (pallor, cyanosis). Normal oxygen saturations should be above 97% on room air (Samuels and Wieteska 2016). Cyanosis is not an early sign of inadequate oxygenation in children but, rather, of significantly reduced oxygen saturations and it is a pre-terminal sign. Cyanosed children are therefore at imminent risk of cardiac arrest if breathing management is not initiated. Children with ineffective oxygenation will display tachycardia, as the circulatory system attempts to compensate for hypoxia. Severe or prolonged hypoxia may lead to bradycardia, which is a pre-terminal sign in children (see Table 26.11).

There are a number of common conditions than can cause respiratory distress in children. Practitioners should be aware of 'red flags' that can indicate severity of disease and potential for rapid deterioration (Table 26.12)

C – Circulation

After the initial hands-off assessment, circulation is further assessed by taking heart rate and blood pressure. Children can maintain their blood pressure for some time even when they are seriously unwell (compensate). Changes in blood pressure therefore are not an early warning sign in children and hypotension is a pre-terminal sign. An assessment of capillary refill will give an indication of circulatory perfusion. This is measured by pressing for five seconds on the sternum, releasing, and counting how many seconds it

TABLE 26.11 Assessment of respiratory distress.

	Mild	Moderate	Severe
Behaviour	Normal Able to talk normally	Some/intermittent irritability Some limitation of ability to talk	Increasing irritability and/or lethargy Marked limitation of ability to talk or unable to talk
Tachypnoea* (at rest – i.e. not crying)	Normal or mildly increase respiratory rate *(normal values by age)*	Increased respiratory rate	Increased or markedly reduced respiratory rate as the child tires
Signs of increased work of breathing Retraction *(intercostal, suprasternal, costal margin)* *Paradoxical abdominal breathing* Accessory muscle use *Nasal flaringSternomastoid contraction (head bobbing)* *Forward posture*	None or minimal	Moderate retractions and/or accessory muscle use	Marked increase in accessory muscle use with prominent chest retraction
Oxygenation Oxygenation is only of limited utility in judging severity in many paediatric respiratory conditions. Don't just focus on the SaO_2 monitor. Look at the other signs.			O_2 saturations less than 90% (in room air) Any O_2 requirement in croup is classed as severe Cyanosis
Heart rate	Normal or slight increase	Mildly increased	Significantly increased or bradycardia
Blood pressure	Normal	Increased	Increased or decreased late

Source: RCH Melbourne 2023a.

TABLE 26.12 Common causes of respiratory distress in infants and children.

Possible cause	Red flags
Upper airway obstruction	
Croup (laryngotracheobronchitis)	Stridor at rest Signs of severe work of breathing Signs of poor perfusion Agitation/ reduced LOC
Epiglottitis	Inability to swallow secretions 'Toxic' appearance Signs of severe work of breathing Signs of poor perfusion Agitation/reduced LOC
Foreign body	Sudden onset of stridor or choking Ineffective cough Signs of severe work of breathing Signs of poor perfusion Agitation/reduced LOC
Anaphylaxis	Sudden onset (30 minutes or less from allergen exposure) Accompanied by other allergic symptoms (wheeze, urticaria) Inability to swallow Signs of severe work of breathing Signs of poor perfusion Agitation/reduced LOC
Lower airway obstruction	
Bronchiolitis	Inability to feed Signs of severe work of breathing Apnoea Signs of severe work of breathing Signs of poor perfusion Agitation/reduced LOC
Asthma	Inability to talk in full sentences Signs of severe work of breathing Signs of poor perfusion Agitation/reduced LOC
Pertussis	Infants under 6 weeks most at risk (before first vaccination) Apnoea Cyanosis during paroxysmal coughing spasms Signs of severe work of breathing Signs of poor perfusion Agitation/reduced LOC

takes for colour to return within three seconds. Poor perfusion may be indicated by slow capillary refill times, pallor or mottled skin, agitation, confusion, and loss of consciousness, all of which are red flag signs.

Tachycardia is commonly seen in unwell children, as their circulatory system attempts to increase their cardiac output. Note that anxiety, fever, crying, and some drugs such as Salbutamol, will all result in tachycardia, and this should be taken into consideration when assessing a child's heart rate. As indicated above, bradycardia is a pre-terminal sign in paediatrics. If the heart rate of a tachycardic child begins to reduce, do not assume that their condition is improving, as they may be becoming bradycardic. Always ask yourself the question: 'Does the child look like they are getting better?' Pulse volume relates to the strength of central and peripheral pulses and allows for assessment of cardiac output.

Circulatory failure or 'shock' occurs when the cardiovascular system fails to supply adequate oxygen to the cells of the body and is a leading cause of morbidity and mortality in children (Zimmerman et al. 2021). Early recognition and treatment are vital to prevent deterioration. There are a number of types of shock, but the most commonly seen in children are hypovolaemic shock (inadequate circulating blood volume) and distributive shock (dilation of blood vessels in response to inflammation). Sepsis (distributive shock) is the leading cause of shock in children (see Table 26.13 for other common causes).

TABLE 26.13 **Common causes of shock in infants and children.**

Possible Cause	Red Flags
Hypovolaemic shock	
Haemorrhage	Rapid loss of >25% circulating blood volume (see Table 26.18) Signs of poor perfusion and circulatory compromise Bradycardia Reduced level of consciousness
Intestinal obstruction (intussusception, volvulus, paralytic ileus)	Bile-stained vomiting Abdominal distension Severe colicky abdominal pain (drawing up of knees in infants) Inconsolability 'Redcurrant jelly' stools
Gastroenteritis	Less than half normal input and output in preceding 24 hours (<4 wet nappies in infants) Estimated severe dehydration (see Table 26.19) Oliguria Signs of poor perfusion and circulatory compromise Bradycardia Reduced level of consciousness
Burns	Children <12 months old at higher risk Burn or scold estimated at >10% Full thickness burns Any burn involving face, mouth, or airway (suspected smoke inhalation) Circumferential burns Chemical or electrical burns
Distributive shock	
Sepsis	Children <12 months at higher risk Non-blanching rash (petechiae or purpura) Temperature with 'toxic' signs Signs of poor perfusion and circulatory compromise Bradycardia Reduced level of consciousness
Anaphylaxis	History of previous anaphylaxis Respiratory difficulties Presence of stridor and/or wheeze Signs of poor perfusion and circulatory compromise Reduced level of consciousness

D – Disability/neurological assessment

Systematic neurological assessment of children should involve an assessment of level of consciousness, pupil reactions, and posture. AVPU (Table 26.14) is commonly used in an initial assessment of consciousness and generally corelates to GCS assessment (Janagama et al. 2022). Deterioration to P or U is a red flag and should be treated as an emergency.

A more detailed neurological assessment may be undertaken using the GCS. A modified paediatric coma scale (see Table 26.15) should be used for children under the age of 5 years (Borgialli et al. 2016).

TABLE 26.14 AVPU assessment.

A	**A**lert
V	Responding to **V**oice
P	Responding to **P**ain
U	**U**nresponsive

Source: Paediatric Improvement Collaborative 2023d.

TABLE 26.15 GCS vs modified GCS for paediatrics.

GCS		Modified GCS (<5 years)	
Eyes opening		Eyes opening	
Spontaneously	4	Spontaneously	4
To speech	3	To speech	3
To pain	2	To pain	2
No response	1	No response	1
Best verbal response		**Best verbal response**	
Orientated and converses	5	Alert: babbles, coos, words to usual ability	5
Confused and converses	4	Less than usual words, spontaneous irritable cry	4
Inappropriate words	3	Cries only to pain	3
Incomprehensible words	2	Moans to pain	2
No response to pain	1	No response to pain	1
Best motor response		**Best motor response**	
Obeys verbal commands	6	Spontaneously/obeys verbal command	6
Localises pain	5	Localises to pain/withdraws to touch	5
Withdraws from pain	4	Withdraws from pain	4
Abnormal flexion to pain (decorticate)	3	Abnormal flexion to pain (decorticate)	3
Abnormal extension to pain (decerebrate)	2	Abnormal flexion to pain (decorticate)	2
No response to pain	1	No response to pain	1
Maximum Score	15	Maximum Score	15

Source: Borgialli et al. 2016.

Pupil assessment

Assessment of pupils should include size and whether they are equal and reacting to light. Reaction to light should be brisk. Sluggish response may indicate raised intracranial pressure and fixed, dilated pupils are indicative of significant raised intracranial pressure. Unequal pupils may indicate a space occupying lesion, for example, a haemorrhage. Pinpoint pupils may indicate the ingestion of certain drugs (opioids).

Assessment of tone

Severely unwell children will often be floppy, however, involuntary abnormal posturing like decerebrate (abnormal flexion) or decorticate (abnormal extension) indicates severe brain injury. Brainstem dysfunction may result in secondary effects on the respiratory system (apnoea, irregular breathing patterns) and the cardiovascular system (hypertension, bradycardia).

There are a number of common conditions than can cause neurological deficits in childhood Practitioners should be aware of 'red flags' that can indicate potential for rapid deterioration (Table 26.12).

TABLE 26.16 Common causes of neurological deficit in infants and children.

Possible cause	Red flags
Seizures	Non-febrile Prolonged (>5 minutes) Signs of airway obstruction (see Table 26.10) Unresponsive to first line treatment
Head injury	Loss of consciousness >5 minutes Agitation/reduced GCS 3 or more vomits Seizure in non-epileptic patients Fall >3 m High-speed projectile
Infection (e.g. meningitis, encephalitis)	Signs of toxicity (see above) Fever >39°C Non-blanching rash Agitation/reduced GCS

E – Exposure

It is important to expose the child early to allow a full visual assessment of the child. This includes palpating and touching the child's skin to establish a rough temperature, identify rashes, wounds, or injury, and the assessment of pain through watching the child's posture and facial expressions.

Fever, rashes, and pain in children

Fever is common in children, and not always indicative of severe illness. However, as a general rule, febrile infants and children who have decreased alertness, arousal, and activity are at high risk of serious bacterial infection (El-Radhi 2018). Temperature should be recorded via the axilla but, in a critically unwell child, rectal temperature should be considered, as it is the gold standard for measuring accurate core temperature. Automatic use of antipyretics to reduce fever is no longer recommended. Antipyretics should be used for the treatment of symptoms and comfort rather than for reducing the temperature. The use of antipyretics to prevent febrile convulsions is unsupported (Cullen 2021).

As with fever, rashes are common in childhood, many being caused by viral illness. Rashes that should alert the practitioner are non-blanching rashes (petechial and purpuric) that may indicate septicaemia, urticaria (hives), which suggest an allergic reaction, and erythema (redness) in conjunction with fever, which may indicate toxic shock syndrome.

Assessing pain in children can be difficult, particularly in small children. Older children will be able to self-report, like adults, using numerical scales, but pre-school aged children will experience difficulties with this. A paediatric pain assessment tool like the Face Scale can be used for young children, however, an observational scale like FLACC (Table 26.17 may be useful for rapid assessment of pain (RCH Melbourne 2023b). Severe pain in children (score of >7) should be regarded as a red flag.

F – Fluids

The assessment of a child's hydration status should start with an estimation of *fluids in* and *fluids out* in the previous 24 hours. This can be established roughly by speaking with the parents, who can tell you about the child's toileting habits. Children's higher metabolic rates and greater surface area to weight ratios should be considered when estimating losses. Interruption in normal intake and output can quickly result in dehydration in children. Less than half of a child's

TABLE 26.17 FLACC pain assessment.

Category	Score 0	Score 1	Score 2
FACE	No particular expression or smile	Occasional grimace or frown, withdrawn, disinterested	Frequent to constant quivering chin, clenched jaw
LEGS	Normal position or relaxed	Uneasy, restless, tense	Kicking, or legs drawn up
ACTIVITY	Lying quietly, normal position moves easily	Squirming, shifting back and forth, tense	Arched, rigid or jerking
CRY	No cry (awake or asleep)	Moans or whimpers, occasional complaint	Crying steadily, screams or sobs, frequent complaints
CONSOLABILITY	Content, relaxed	Reassured by occasional touching, hugging, or being talked to, distractible	Difficult to console or comfort

Source: RCH Melbourne 2023b.

TABLE 26.18 Average circulating blood volume per age.

Age	ml/kg
Neonate	80–90 ml/kg
Infant	75–80 ml/kg
Toddler	70–75 ml/kg
Child	70–75 ml/kg
Adolescent	65–70 ml/kg

Source: Davis and Cladis 2022.

normal input and/or output (less than four wet nappies for infants and small children) in the preceding 24 hours is a red flag. Blood loss, even when small, may represent a relatively significant proportion of the child's circulating volume, particularly in infants (see Table 26.18).

The degree of dehydration can be estimated through observable signs and symptoms (see Table 26.19), which, accumulatively, can provide a reasonable estimate of fluid losses. Estimation of percentage of losses is important for the calculation of fluid replacements.

G – Glucose

Hypoglycaemia may be the reason for reduced levels of consciousness in infants and children. As outlined previously in this chapter, small children are unable to convert glucose to glycogen storage in the same way as adults and will use up their blood glucose rapidly when unwell, especially if they are not feeding normally. Normal blood glucose levels (BGL) for children are 3–5 mmol/l. A BGL <3 mmol/l is a red flag. In a conscious child, hypoglycaemia should be considered if a child presents with sweating, pallor, 'jitteryness', and slurred speech.

Other considerations

Certain children are at higher risk of severe illness than others and this should be considered when assessing for risk of deterioration. These groups include infants and young children; those with chronic and complex illness; and those with pre-existing medical conditions (Borensztajn et al. 2022). Immediate transfer to hospital should be considered for these children.

Timely assessment and the identification of 'red flags' is essential for early intervention to prevent deterioration in the paediatric population. Children can often present with generic symptoms such as fever. A general rule for identifying whether a feverish child is 'toxic' (at risk of sepsis) is with the consideration of the following:

- 'A' is for arousal, alertness, or activity decreased.
- 'B' is for breathing difficulties (tachypnoea, increased work of breathing).

TABLE 26.19 Assessment of dehydration in paediatrics.

Description of dehydration	Dehydration % body weight	Signs and symptoms
Mild	<5%	Moist mucous membranes Mild tachycardia Reduced urine output Thirsty
Moderate	5–9%	Above signs plus: Dry mucous membranes Lethargy Reduced skin turgor Sunken eyes/fontanelle Moderate tachycardia Prolonged capillary refill time
Severe/shock	10%	Above signs plus: Poor perfusion (pale, mottled, slow capillary refill) Deeply sunken eyes/ fontanelle Reduced level of consciousness Thready or absent peripheral pulses Marked tachycardia Hypotension Markedly prolonged capillary refill time

Source: Paediatric Improvement Collaborative 2023c.

- 'C' is for poor colour (pale or mottled), poor circulation (cold peripheries, increased capillary refill time) ,or cry (weak, high pitched) .
- 'D' is for decreased fluid intake (less than half normal) and/or decreased urine output (fewer than four wet nappies a day).

The presence of any of these signs may indicate serious illness. The presence of more than one sign indicates severe illness and the risk of imminent deterioration.

Conclusion

This chapter has provided an overview of the differences between adults and children and the impact that this has on the assessment and recognition of the sick child. The student was introduced to the assessment of the sick child with the initial hands-off assessment (PAT) followed by the more comprehensive and systematic A–G assessment. Common causes of severe illness in infants and children were presented and red flags that indicate potential deterioration in these conditions were outlined. The paramedic must be able to rapidly assess the sick child and recognise the potential for deterioration, as early intervention and management is key to optimal outcomes. Working with and listening to parents is essential for accurate assessment and calm, clear communication vital in what can often be extremely stressful situations.

Activities

Now review your learning by completing the learning activities in this chapter. The answers to these appear at the end of the book. Further self-test activities can be found at **www.wileyfundamentalseries.com/paramedic/3e.**

Test your knowledge

1. Name three anatomical differences in an infant or child's respiratory system.
2. How do these differences impact upon the pathophysiology of respiratory disease?
3. Name one common condition that may lead to circulatory failure in infants. What are the red flags that may indicate severe illness or deterioration?
4. What are the signs of severe dehydration in a child?

Glossary

Stridor: Abnormal, high-pitched inspiratory sound that indicates partial airway obstruction.

Dyspnoea: Shortness of breath.

Cyanosis: A bluish colour to skin caused by depleted of oxygen to blood haemoglobin.

Tachycardia: Abnormally rapid heart rate.

Tachypnoea: Abnormally rapid respiratory rate.

Axilla: Underarm.

Intra-abdominal pressure: Pressure in the abdominal cavity.

Primary cardiac event: A medical event caused by cardiac insufficiency.

Greenstick fracture: A break in only one part of the bones thickness.

Growth plate: Areas of new bone growth at the end of long bones in children and teenagers.

References

Borensztajn, D.M., Hagedoorn, N.N., Carrol, E.D. et al. (2022). Febrile children with comorbidities at the emergency department – a multicentre observational study. *European Journal of Pediatrics* **181**(9): 3491–3500.

Borgialli, D.A., Mahajan, P., Hoyle, J.D. et al. (2016). Performance of the paediatric Glasgow Coma Scale score in the evaluation of children with blunt head trauma. *Acad Emerg Med* **23** (8): 878–884. doi: 10.1111/acem.13014.

Cullen, C. (2021). Febrile and first-time seizures. *Pediatric Emergency Medicine Reports* **26**(3).

Davis, P.J. and Cladis, F.P. (2022). *Smith's Anesthesia for Infants and Children*. Philadelphia, PA: Elsevier.

El-Radhi, A.S. (2018). Fever. In: *Clinical Manual of Fever in Children* (ed. A.S. El-Radhi), pp. 1–28). Cham: Springer International Publishing.

Fernandez, A., Benito, J., and Mintegi, S. (2017). Is this child sick? Usefulness of the Pediatric Assessment Triangle in emergency settings. *J Pediatr (Rio J)* **93** (suppl 1): 60–67. doi: 10.1016/j.jped.2017.07.002.

Janagama, S.R., Newberry, J.A., Kohn, M.A. et al. (2022). Is AVPU comparable to GCS in critical prehospital decisions? – A cross-sectional study. *The American Journal of Emergency Medicine* **59**: 106–110. doi: 10.1016/j.ajem.2022.06.042.

Paediatric Improvement Collaborative (2023a). Acceptable ranges for physiological variables. The Royal Children's Hospital Melbourne. Available at: https://www.rch.org.au/clinicalguide/guideline_index/Acceptable_ranges_for_physiological_variables (accessed 13 January 2023).

Paediatric Improvement Collaborative (2023b). Acute upper airway obstruction. The Royal Children's Hospital Melbourne. Available at: https://www.rch.org.au/clinicalguide/guideline_index/Acute_Upper_Airway_Obstruction (accessed 13 January 2023).

Paediatric Improvement Collaborative (2023c). Dehydration. The Royal Children's Hospital Melbourne. Available at: https://www.rch.org.au/clinicalguide/guideline_index/Dehydration (accessed 13 January 2023).

Paediatric Improvement Collaborative (2023d). Altered conscious state. The Royal Children's Hospital Melbourne. Available at: https://www.rch.org.au/clinicalguide/guideline_index/Altered_conscious_state (accessed 13 January 2023).

The Royal Children's Hospital Melbourne. (2023a). Assessment of severity of respiratory conditions. The Royal Children's Hospital Melbourne. Available at: https://www.rch.org.au/clinicalguide/guideline_index/Assessment_of_severity_of_respiratory_conditions (accessed 13 January 2023).

The Royal Children's Hospital Melbourne. (2023b). Pain assessment and management. The Royal Children's Hospital Melbourne. Available at: https://www.rch.org.au/rchcpg/hospital_clinical_guideline_index/Pain_assessment_and_measurement/#Pain%20Assessment%20Tool (accessed 28 March 2023).

Samuels, M. and Wieteska, S. (2016). *Advanced Paediatric Life Support: A Practical Approach to Emergencies*. John Wiley & Sons, Inc.

Zimmerman, J.J., Clark, R.S.B., Fuhrman, B.P. et al. (2021). *Fuhrman and Zimmerman's Pediatric Critical Care*. 6e. Philadelphia, PA: Elsevier.

CHAPTER 27

Medical emergencies

Jennie McGowan
Paramedic St John Ambulance, Western Australia, Australia and Registered Nurse

Jane Jennings
Paramedic St John Ambulance, Western Australia, Australia

Marco Scarvaci
Paramedic St John Ambulance, Western Australia, Australia

Contents

Case study

You have been called to a 20-year-old female who has a raised itchy rash over her face and torso after eating at a restaurant, she tells you she is allergic to peanuts. Your initial assessment finds that her observations are all within normal ranges, she does not have a wheeze and denies any shortness of breath or tightness in her throat. During transport to hospital, you notice her respiratory rate has increased, her most recent blood pressure is 90/50 mmHg and she has begun to have a dry persistent cough.

Introduction

Paramedics respond to a wide range of medical emergencies in the line of their duties. This chapter highlights the medical emergencies paramedics are likely to experience and provides clinical assessment considerations from an out-of-hospital (OOH) management perspective. This chapter will discuss the importance of early recognition and response to a deteriorating person; and will cover neurological emergencies, metabolic emergencies, sepsis, and anaphylaxis.

Fundamentals of Paramedic Practice: A Systems Approach, Third Edition. Edited by Sam Willis and Ian Peate.

Companion website: www.wiley.com/go/willis/paramedic3e

Early recognition and response to a deteriorating person

Paramedics must be able to recognise a deteriorating person. Early recognition of deterioration allows paramedics to proactively respond to the situation and reduce the severity and occurrence of adverse outcomes related to deterioration (Bourke-Matas et al. 2022). Clinical deterioration is observable by the paramedic and is often preceded by an acute change in the patient's observations, including their vital signs (Patel et al. 2018; Silcock et al. 2018). The changing vital signs can be placed into an early warning scores (EWS) system to help paramedics identify a deteriorating person.

EWS systems require the paramedic to allocate a numerical value to a patient's physiological observations, providing the clinician with a score (Silcock et al. 2018). Patients with a higher score are more at risk of clinical deterioration than those with a lower score (Patel et al. 2018; Silcock et al. 2018). These tools are helpful for promoting the paramedic's critical thinking and awareness of deterioration in their patient and implementing appropriate escalation and management of the patient's condition (Patel et al. 2018; Silcock et al. 2018; Gill et al. 2021).

It is important for paramedics to document clinical observations whilst being critical and assessing for changes in the patient's observations during all patient interactions. Age-appropriate EWS should be used where available to assist with the recognition, response, escalation, and communication of clinical deterioration throughout the patient's care and during handover to hospital staff.

Paramedics should have a higher index of suspicion for deterioration in patients with (Bourke-Matas et al. 2022):

- Nonspecific complaints such as those who are generally unwell or have experienced a functional decline.
- Multiple comorbidities such chronic illnesses including diabetes, hypertension, and COPD.
- Lifestyle factors including obesity, malnutrition, and smoking.
- Age dependency (young and elderly).
- Unresponsiveness to clinical interventions.

Neurological emergencies

Paramedics will routinely attend patients with neurological emergencies. Typical neurological emergencies include seizures and cerebrovascular events (stroke). Autonomic dysreflexia is another less common but potentially fatal condition that may present in patients with spinal cord injuries (SCI) (Thomas et al. 2022). These three conditions can mimic many other medical presentations (Aaron et al. 2020; Lehn et al. 2021; Jankovic 2022) therefore the elimination of mimics will facilitate accurate diagnosis, directing treatment to avoid iatrogenic harm and ensuring a favourable outcome for the patient (Lehn et al. 2021; Stack and Cole 2021).

Seizures

Seizures are caused by an imbalance in the brain's normal electrical activity (see Figure 27.1). Rapid bursts of electrical energy disrupt the normal brain processes resulting in transient motor, sensory, visual, and autonomic symptoms (AANS 2019). Seizures may be the result of a known epileptic condition or due to a specific trigger (AANS 2019). Approximately 10% of people will experience at least one seizure in their lifetime (WHO 2022).

Clinical assessment of seizures

The clinical presentation of seizures is diverse and dependent on which area of the brain is affected (Leibetseder et al. 2020). When abnormal electrical activity affects both sides of the brain this is classified as a generalised seizure (Rowland and Lambert 2022). These seizures can have numerous symptoms, including loss of awareness, as several brain processes have been affected (Rowland and Lambert 2022). If the seizure commences in one area of the brain it is classified as a focal seizure. These seizures are less obvious and patient symptoms can be mistaken for intoxication or daydreaming (Rowland and Lambert 2022) (Figure 27.1).

Tongue biting, witnessed posturing, head-turning, and postictal events are common signs of a seizure (Abrams et al. 2019). Urinary incontinence is also common but frequently accompanies syncope, stroke, and other medical events (Stroke Foundation 2022; Tasdelen and Ekici 2022). Careful history taking covering events before, during, and after the seizure, from bystanders and patients, is crucial (Leibetseder et al. 2020). Pertinent history may identify potential triggers. These include pregnancy, diabetes, dementia, migraines, lesions, recreational drug use, new or poor adherence of medications, persistent fevers, and alcohol withdrawal (Leibetseder et al. 2020). A secondary survey should be completed to identify indications for

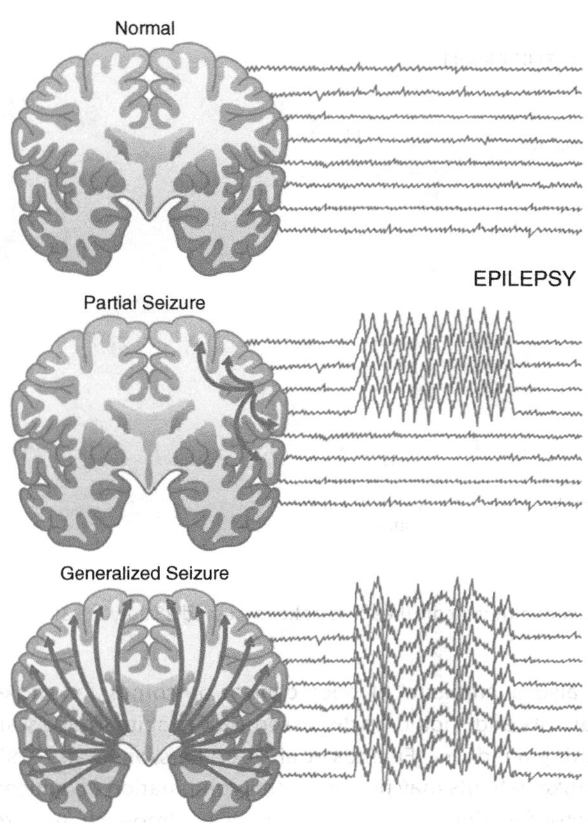

FIGURE 27.1 Electrical activity in the brain during a seizure. Source: Drugs.com. https://www.drugs.com/health-guide/seizure.html (accessed 28 July 2023).

potential triggers of the seizure (Leibetseder et al. 2020). When completing the secondary survey, look for signs of drug use or trauma. Head trauma may be the cause of the seizure or subsequent injury post-seizure (Hart 2020; Tan et al. 2019). Posterior shoulder dislocation caused by forceful, imbalanced, and unopposed contractions is a common, often missed seizure-related injury (Langenbruch et al. 2019). Used in conjunction with pertinent history, this can distinguish a seizure from syncope (Abrams et al. 2019).

OOH management of the seizing patient

Many seizures attended by paramedics are brief and self-limiting (Hart 2020). OOH management for these patients will include making the environment safe (for example, removing tables and hard objects and putting pillows under them), positioning them onto their side to allow the airway to be maintained (when safe to do so), suctioning of the airway, providing supplemental oxygen, assisted ventilations post-seizure (in the presence of respiratory insufficiency), and the use of early airway adjuncts and airway manoeuvres (Hart 2020). Prompt blood glucose testing and checking the patient's temperature will allow the paramedic to quickly rule out and reverse potential causes relating to low blood sugar and fever (Hart 2020). Continual monitoring of the patient's oxygen saturation, cardiac monitoring, and end-tidal carbon dioxide ($ETCO_2$) is essential for safe patient management (Hart 2020).

Seizure management plans may be in place for a patient with a known seizure condition (Epilepsy Action Australia 2020). Paramedics may be able to source essential medical history and treatment regimens from these plans (Epilepsy Action Australia 2020). It is important to acknowledge and encourage the use of these plans, empowering caregivers and in turn potentially lessening the impact of the seizure for both the patient and caregivers (Epilepsy Action Australia 2020).

If the seizure does not end by itself (is not self-limiting), paramedics will need to administer seizure suppressing drugs to terminate the seizure activity (Kanner and Bicchi 2022). Benzodiazepines are effective emergency medications commonly used to abort seizure activity (Kanner and Bicchi 2022). Intranasal drug administration is rapid, painless, reduces infection risk, lowers the cognitive load for paramedics, and reduces stressors for patients, maximising the opportunity for a favourable patient outcome (Chhabra et al. 2021).

Patients with a known seizure disorder, who have made a full recovery – for example, returned to their baseline GCS, has no apparent injuries, and may have an adequate plan for treatment and monitoring – might decline transportation to a hospital (Hart 2020). Patients outside of these criteria should be referred to definitive care, which might include a local emergency department (ED) (Hart 2020).

Cerebrovascular events (stroke)

Strokes occur when the blood supply to the brain is interrupted (Stroke Foundation 2022). This is caused by a blocked (ischaemic stroke) or a rupture of a weakened artery (haemorrhagic stroke) (Stroke Foundation 2022) (see Figure 27.2). Ischaemic strokes are the most common accounting for 87% of all strokes (Stroke Foundation 2022). The impairment of blood supply to the brain leads to a lack of essential oxygen and nutrients resulting in damaged

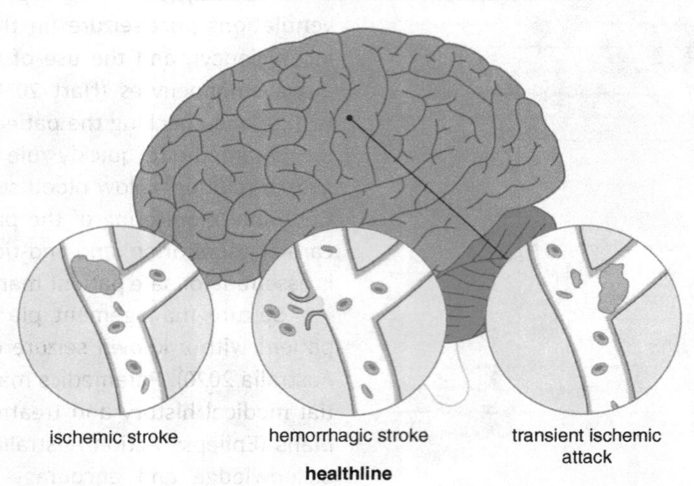

FIGURE 27.2 Types of strokes. Source: Healthline Media. https://www.healthline.com/health/stroke (accessed 28 July 2023).

brain cells (Stroke Foundation 2022). A transient ischaemic attack (TIA) is known as a temporary or mini stroke, as the patient experiences full cerebrovascular events (CVE) symptoms but the situation fully reverses itself within a 24-hour period. Stroke is one of the most common diseases affecting one in four people during their lifetime, affecting all ages, from newborns to the elderly (Buck et al. 2021; Stack and Cole, 2021).

Clinical assessment of the CVE patient

There has been great advancement in OOH assessment and management of stroke patients, leading to improved patient outcomes (Rehani et al. 2019). Recent evidence suggests that some patients may benefit from extended treatment windows (up to 24 hours) (Rehani et al. 2019). The onset of symptoms outside of what used to be a four-hour window, including patients with unknown onset time or symptoms upon waking, were previously considered as outside of the intervention window (Lindsay 2018; Rehani et al. 2019).

Half of hospital admissions for suspected stroke end up being common medical conditions that mimic stroke (Buck et al. 2021). Comprehensive history taking and detailed clinical assessment will assist paramedics in providing the appropriate care for each patient presentation (Buck et al. 2021). A capillary blood glucose test should be performed for all patients with focal neurological symptoms to rule out hypoglycaemia (Singh et al. 2020). Hyperglycaemia is also a predictor of poor clinical outcomes for stroke patients and should be discussed with hospital triage staff during handover (Fuentes et al. 2017; Larsson et al. 2019). Stroke patients may present with a combination of reduced motor function and coordination, facial droop, changes to speech, difficulty swallowing, cognitive impairment, and visual disturbances (Stroke Foundation 2022).

It is vital for paramedics to be able to identify when the patient was last known to be well (Buck et al. 2021). Table 27.1 identifies some focused questions that will assist paramedics with identifying symptom onset and severity (Micieli et al. 2020). Detection of treatable patients, timely transportation, and selection of primary or comprehensive stroke centre will minimise damage to the patient's brain tissue (Buck et al. 2021). To accomplish this goal, OOH dispatch and stroke scales such as the National Institute of Health Stroke Scale, FAST test, and RACE score have been developed (Fu et al. 2018; Buck et al. 2021). Patients with persistent neurological symptoms, screening positive with a validated stroke scale, should be transported as priority one (Fu et al. 2018). Receiving hospitals should be pre-alerted to allow activation of hospital stroke protocol (Fu et al. 2018).

OOH management of the CVE patient

OOH care is focused on early recognition and primary survey symptom management prioritising safety of the airway, breathing, and circulation (Alexander 2020). Managing a CVE patient who presents with a reduced GCS will likely require

TABLE 27.1 CVE-focused questions

CVE history-gathering questions
What time did the symptoms start?
What were you doing at the time?
Have the symptoms improved or got worse?
Have you experienced these symptoms before?
Do you have any new weaknesses?
Have you noticed any change in sensation?
Have you noticed any changes in vision?
Have you experienced any balance or coordination changes?
Has your speech changed?
Have you been treated for high blood pressure, atrial fibrillation, or diabetes?

Source: Adapted from Micieli et al. 2020.

airway adjuncts; airway suctioning; and considerate patient positioning such as elevating the patient's head end of the bed or placing the patient in the recovery positioning on the non-affected side (Alexander 2020). Extrication may prove more difficult if the patient has reduced motor function leading to a patient who cannot position themselves upright or walk. Additional resources should be activated early to avoid unnecessary delays (Fu et al. 2018).

With an understanding of how a stroke patient is managed once in the hospital, paramedics can facilitate and expedite the global management of their patient (Alexander 2020). The patient may require intravenous (IV) cannulation, for example, to provide fluids for dehydration. If IV access is required, an 18 G cannula should be sited in the patient's antecubital vein as a preferred site (Alexander 2020). The patient should also remain nil by mouth until assessed at hospital. These considerations can prevent crucial time delays in subsequent treatment once in the hospital setting (Alexander 2020).

Early identification of a CVE is crucial for positive patient outcomes. Mobile Stroke Units (MSUs) were initially introduced in Germany and the US and are now available for the assessment of acute stroke patients in at least 30 stroke centres around the world (Buck et al. 2021). MSUs allow specialists to expedite evaluation with access to neuroimaging equipment and treatment in the prehospital field (Fu et al. 2018).

Autonomic dysreflexia

Autonomic dysreflexia (AD) is an exaggerated response from the autonomic nervous system (ANS) resulting from a noxious stimulus below the level of SCI (Wahl 2015). When assessing patients with a SCI at the T6 level or above, paramedics need to maintain a high index of suspicion for AD. The disconnection of the ANS feedback loop, caused by the SCI, leads to a disruption of the body's ability to maintain homeostasis (Wahl 2015). AD can lead to life-threatening, acute, uncontrolled hypertension (Allen and Leslie 2022). SCI patients are 90% susceptible to this condition and are at a 300–400% increased risk of having a stroke (Allen and Lesilie 2022).

Clinical assessment of the AD patient

Alongside a thorough history, paramedics need to understand the potential triggers of AD, allowing early detection and potential correction in the OOH environment (Stephenson 2019). The patient presentation will vary amongst individuals but some signs that should alert paramedics to consider AD are bradycardia, high blood pressure (BP), diaphoresis above the level of injury, pallor skin below the injury level, and severe headache (Thomas et al. 2022). Paramedics should confirm the patient's baseline BP with the patient or carer, to identify relative elevated systolic BP greater than 20 mmHg above the base level. Upon recognition of potential AD symptoms paramedics need to act quickly and complete an assessment focusing on known triggers to eliminate noxious stimuli (Thomas et al. 2022). Potential triggers may include blocked catheters, urinary retention, bowel impaction, constipation, boils, pressure sores, ingrown toenails, and unidentified injuries or fractures below a SCI.

OOH care for the AD patient

Upright positioning of the patient to promote orthostatic drop and removal of tight clothing, shoes, and dressings may eliminate stimulus (Thomas et al. 2022). Paramedics should also be receptive to management and treatment plans from patients regarding their care (Wahl 2015). If the patient's symptoms persist antihypertensives, analgesia, and prompt transportation to the hospital should be prioritised until the cause of symptoms can be determined (Thomas et al. 2022).

Metabolic emergencies

Metabolic emergencies occur when organs of metabolism (also known as endocrine organs) malfunction and are injured. Metabolic injuries include hyperglycaemia, hypoglycaemia, and adrenal crisis.

Hyperglycaemia

Diabetes is a major health problem that affects 1 in 20 Australians, amounting to around 1.1 million people (Davis et al. 2018). The body's blood glucose level (BGL) is regulated by the pancreas and its ability to produce and release insulin (Higginson et al. 2019). Insulin causes cells to utilise glucose from the bloodstream as energy or to store glucose for later use (Higginson et al. 2019). In diabetes, insulin deficiency causes the BGL to rise, resulting in hyperglycaemia and potential complications (Higginson et al. 2019). Two common complications that can arise from relative or absolute insulin deficiency are diabetes ketoacidosis (DKA) and hyperglycaemic hyperosmolar state (HHS), both of which are diabetic emergencies (Higginson et al. 2019). DKA is an acute life-threatening hyperglycaemic condition commonly occurring in patients with type 1 diabetes. Patients with type 1 diabetes have an absence of insulin as the pancreas produces small amounts of or no insulin, which results in an inability of cells to utilise glucose from the bloodstream (Bonner 2019). The body then breaks down fat cells for energy and ketones are produced as a by-product of fat metabolism; these ketones cause acidaemia, which is life-threatening (Bonner 2019). Hyperglycaemia is dangerous when serum glucose levels are significantly elevated, causing the renal threshold to be reached; in this case, glucose is secreted in the urine, which depletes the body of sodium, potassium and water and results in dehydration and electrolyte deficiency (Bonner 2019).

HHS is characterised by hyperglycaemia and severe dehydration without significant ketoacidosis; it is more common in patients with type 2 diabetes (Lenahan and Holloway 2015). Unlike DKA patients, those with HHS have some insulin, which avoids the occurrence of lipolysis and the resulting ketoacidosis (Fajardo 2017). In HHS, the kidneys are unable to filter the large amount of glucose in the body, which leads to the release of glucose into the urine; this results in progressive polyuria and polydipsia over several days (Fajardo 2017). The osmotic diuresis causes severe dehydration and hypovolemia due to the loss of water in the urine (Fajardo 2017). Electrolyte abnormalities may be severe, and as a result, the bloodstream becomes dehydrated and there is a higher concentration of solutes, making the patient hyperosmolar (Wolfsdorf et al. 2014). As a result, the patient will require large amounts of fluids and electrolytes during treatment.

Clinical assessment of the hyperglycaemic patient

Paramedics should investigate and assess for the signs and symptoms listed in Table 27.2.

OOH management of the hyperglycaemic patient

Management of DKA and HHS extends much further than OOH interventions to achieve a return to normal blood sugar levels (Wolfsdorf et al. 2014). OOH management should focus on the following principles:

- Reassurance.
- A detailed history from family of how the patient responds to insulin.

TABLE 27.2 **Diabetic ketoacidosis (DKA) and HHS signs, symptoms, and clinical findings.**

Body system	DKA	HHS
Neurological	Lethargy, malaise, fatigue, confusion, coma	Lethargy, confusion, altered conscious state, coma
Respiratory		Tachypnoea
Cardiovascular	Tachycardia, hypotension, dysrhythmias	Tachycardia, pronounced hypotension, dysrhythmias
Integumentary	Flushed skin, dry mucous membranes, poor skin turgor	Flushed skin, severely dry mucosal membranes, poor skin turgor
Renal	Polydipsia, polyuria, ketonuria	
Gastrointestinal	Nausea, vomiting, abdominal cramps	Less severe symptoms than DKA
Scrum levels		

Source: Adapted from Wolfsdorf et al. 2014.

- Airway management where required.
- Oxygen management to correct hypoxia.
- Correct rehydration and dilute sugar levels through IV fluid therapy.
- Symptom management of nausea, vomiting, pain, and cardiac dysrhythmias.
- Monitoring for response to fluid therapy.
- Patient comfort by including family members when appropriate.

Hypoglycaemia

Hypoglycaemia is defined as a BGL of 3.9 mmol/L or lower (Keller-Senn et al. 2017). Hypoglycaemia is a common medical emergency among patients with diabetes and is potentially caused by:

- Incorrect administration of glucose-lowering medications
- Unexpected exercise expenditure
- Stress
- Poor diet
- Poor management of diabetes (Keller-Senn et al. 2017; Bonner 2019)

Hypoglycaemia symptoms can also occur from rapid BGL drops such as 15.5 mmol/L to 8 mmol/L (Bonner 2019).

Clinical assessment of hypoglycaemic patients

Paramedics should consider hypoglycaemia in all unresponsive patients, as insufficient glucose stores will affect all vital organs and tissues, causing cardiovascular symptoms (Bonner 2019; Liu et al. 2021). A lack of glucose affects the nervous system, resulting in neurological symptoms such as confusion, slurred speech, and lack of coordination (Hubert and Vanmeter 2018). Secondary symptoms occur from stimulation of the sympathetic nervous system, resulting in diaphoresis, pallor, anxiety, and tremors (Hubert and Vanmeter 2018). If hypoglycaemia remains unmanaged, then unconsciousness, seizures, and death can occur (Hubert and Vanmeter 2018). Paramedics should focus on identifying the above signs and symptoms whilst gathering the patient's vital signs and prioritising the BGL in unconscious diabetics (Hubert and Vanmeter 2018). This will allow the paramedic to detect and correct the BGL urgently in hypoglycaemia events. A detailed history will also aid in the patient's diagnosis, and if hypoglycaemic events are not common, it is important to determine why the event has occurred.

OOH management of the hypoglycaemic patient

Principles for managing hypoglycaemia include:

- Managing the airway using airway adjuncts and positioning when the patient has a compromised airway.
- Administering oral glucose agents if the patient can swallow (Sinclair et al. 2019).
- If it is unsafe to administer oral glucose agents due to an altered level of consciousness or difficulty swallowing, IV access can be obtained for IV glucose administration (Sinclair et al. 2019).
- Hyperglycaemic agents like glucagon can also be administered intramuscularly. These agents may be preferred in patients who are difficult to cannulate or where there is likely to be a delay in cannulating (Sinclair et al. 2019).
- The paramedic should also be aware that the patient might have a seizure and must be prepared for this.
- If the patient has had a period of semi or unconsciousness, plenty of reassurance will be required as the patient recovers.
- A thorough history is also important and should be obtained once the patient has been stabilised, as this will be useful when deciding where to refer the patient and for ongoing care purposes.
- Reassuring the family as the patient may be unconscious which can be distressing to see.

Adrenal crisis

Adrenal insufficiency is a common precursor to adrenal crisis, where glucocorticoid production is inadequate (Courtney 2021). Adrenal crisis is an acute physiological disturbance in patients with known hypoadrenalism due to the inadequate production of glucocorticoids and corticoid hormones (Rushworth et al. 2019; Courtney 2021). The patient may exhibit symptoms of adrenal insufficiency, but these are not severe enough to consider adrenal crisis (Courtney 2021). This is because the symptoms of adrenal insufficiency and adrenal crisis are similar, with the main difference being that cardiovascular function is unable to be maintained in adrenal crisis due to adrenal insufficiency (Courtney 2021). Adrenal insufficiency can be classified as primary, secondary, congenital, or acquired (Baines 2015). In primary adrenal insufficiency, the adrenal glands cannot produce cortisol, aldosterone, or both due to the destruction of adrenal gland tissue (Baines 2015). In secondary adrenal insufficiency, there is a lack of corticotropin hormone from the hypothalamus and/or adrenocorticotropic hormone secretion from the pituitary gland, causing adrenal cortex malfunction (Baines 2015). Cortisol is a glucocorticoid that assists in the regulation of the BGL and is released in response to stress (Baines 2015). If corticosteroids are not produced, stress causes hypotension, shock, and potential death (Baines 2015). Decreases in aldosterone exacerbate adrenal crisis through sodium and water loss and potassium retention, which exacerbates hypotension and causes electrolyte imbalances (Courtney 2021).

Clinical assessment of the adrenal crisis patient

The greatest challenge for paramedics is recognising an adrenal crisis event, as the signs and symptoms are very nonspecific, making diagnosis difficult (Courtney 2021). Common clinical signs and symptoms can include acute abdominal pain, hyponatraemia, hypoglycaemia and pyrexia, nausea, vomiting, headaches, generalised body aches, fatigue, and postural hypotension (Baines, 2015; Rushworth et al. 2019). Adrenal crisis is defined in adults as an acute deterioration in health status with a systolic BP <100 mmHg or a decrease in systolic BP equal to or greater than 20 mmHg with clinical symptoms that resolve with corticoid treatment (Rushworth et al. 2019).

OOH management of the adrenal crisis patient

Hydrocortisone is the main lifesaving intervention that paramedics can use in the OOH environment (Courtney, 2021). It is important to note that it is better to administer hydrocortisone if adrenal crisis is suspected, as an increased dose of this steroid is not harmful over an acute period, but an adrenal crisis event can be (Courtney, 2021; Baines, 2015). Intravenous fluid therapy may also be required to maintain the patient's BP.

Sepsis

Sepsis is a life-threatening organ dysfunction as a result of a heightened host response to an infection. The global incidence of sepsis is difficult to know as it is likely underreported especially in developing regions, although it is thought to affect over 30 million people globally each year (Huang et al. 2019) and is the leading cause of mortality in children (Weiss et al. 2020).

During sepsis the body reacts to a pathogen such as bacteria through the activation of innate immune cells: primarily macrophages, monocytes, neutrophils, and natural killer cells (Gyawali et al. 2019; Huang et al. 2019). The reaction between these immune cells and the pathogen leads to the release of proinflammatory cytokines (Gyawali et al. 2019) and it is these cytokines that cause the vasodilation and increased vascular permeability leading to hypovolaemic shock, as well as activation of the clotting cascade leading to disseminated intravascular coagulopathy (Gyawali et al. 2019).

Clinical assessment of the septic patient

Beyond taking a full set of vital signs, paramedics must conduct a thorough assessment of the patient to identify the potential source of their sepsis including a full respiratory assessment, abdominal assessment, and exposing the patient's skin to look for skin rashes or wounds (Australian Commission on Safety and Quality in Health Care 2022). Patients who have indwelling medical devices, are immunocompromised, immunosuppressed, or undertaking cancer treatments are at an increased risk or sepsis (Australian Commission on Safety and Quality in Health Care 2022). Although an elevated temperature can identify patients with an infection, the presence of an abnormal mental state, hypotension, and an abnormal respiration rate are more indicative of a patient with sepsis (Lane et al. 2020). Patients with sepsis may experience many nonspecific symptoms such as nausea, fatigue, breathlessness, reduced urine output, and pain; patients may even present in a hypothermic state (Australian Commission on Safety and Quality in Health Care 2022). EWS have been found to be effective in predicting poor patient outcomes in sepsis due to clinical deterioration (Silcock et al. 2018).

Measuring venous lactate level is beneficial in the detection and assessment of sepsis (Wardi et al. 2020). Lactate levels are raised due to either anaerobic metabolism secondary cellular hypoperfusion or the increased production of lactate in the presence of increased metabolic activity in an aerobic state secondary to the release of proinflammatory cytokines (Wardi et al. 2020).

Paediatric considerations during sepsis

Parental concern or multiple interactions with general practitioners, ED, or the ambulance for the same or similar presentation within 48 hours should act as a red flag to paramedics that a child is at risk of having sepsis (Harley et al. 2021). Paediatric patients can present as floppy, have mottled or discoloured skin, non-blanching rash, and may even have long pauses in their breathing (Australian Commission on Safety and Quality in Health Care 2022). Hypotension is a late and fatal sign; normal BPs can provide false reassurance (Harley et al. 2021).

OOH management of the septic patient

The key to improving sepsis survival is early recognition and early goal-directed care (Floer et al. 2021). Beyond recognition, sepsis management includes antibiotics, optimising haemodynamics, and supportive care.

In some services paramedics may start broad-spectrum antibiotic therapies to begin treatment prior to arrival at hospital. Antibiotics are used to treat the bacterial infection that has caused the infection leading the sepsis (Evans et al. 2021).

In patients with sepsis and hypotension (a systolic BP below 100mmHg), intravenous fluid administration is vital in reducing morbidity and mortality (Lane et al. 2018). Fluid resuscitation aids by reducing end organ dysfunction in septic shock. The surviving sepsis campaign 2021 suggests that 30 ml/kg (calculated using ideal body weight) within the first three hours of sepsis is associated with a lower mortality rate (Evans et al. 2021). The use of inotropes such as adrenaline or vasopressors may be required to support the patient's BP if adequate response to fluids is not seen; often this requires a higher skilled clinician. Further to this, supportive management includes airway management, providing supplemental oxygen to manage hypoxia, and the management of other comorbid symptoms such as pain and nausea or vomiting.

Anaphylaxis

Anaphylaxis is a severe rapid systemic hypersensitivity reaction, which can be fatal (Cardona et al. 2020). Anaphylaxis is triggered by a re-exposure to an allergen such as a bee sting, resulting in the release of inflammatory mediators including histamine, cytokines, and prostaglandins (Wilkinson-Stokes et al. 2021). The inflammatory cascade leads to increased vascular permeability and vasodilation causing distributive and hypovolaemic shock; as well as bronchoconstriction, bronchial oedema, mucous plugging, angioedema, and laryngeal oedema reducing the adequate movement of air via respiration leading to eventual hypoxia and respiratory arrest (Wilkinson-Stokes et al. 2021).

Clinical assessment of the anaphylactic patient

Rapid assessment and diagnosis of anaphylaxis are important (Muraro et al. 2021). Paramedics should identify the potential allergen and remove it as quickly as possible, although paramedics should not induce vomiting as this poses a significant airway risk via aspiration of vomit. The 2020 World Allergy Organization Anaphylaxis Guidance outlines that anaphylaxis is highly likely when one of the below criteria is fulfilled (Cardona et al. 2020; Dodd et al. 2021).

1. Rapid onset of illness (minutes to several hours) involving the skin and/or mucosal tissue with at least one of the following:
   - **(a)** Respiratory compromise (dyspnoea, wheeze, stridor, hypoxaemia).
   - **(b)** Reduced BP or signs associated with end organ dysfunction (collapse, syncope, incontinence).
   - **(c)** Severe gastrointestinal symptoms (severe cramping abdominal pain, repetitive vomiting), especially when exposure was to a non-food allergen.
2. Rapid onset illness (minutes to several hours) without skin or mucosal involvement, after exposure to a known or highly probable allergen with any of the following:
   - **(a)** Acute hypotension (SBP reduction greater than 30% of pts baseline or SBP <90 mmHg in adults).
   - **(b)** Bronchospasm (wheeze, persistent cough).
   - **(c)** Laryngeal involvement (stridor, vocal changes, painful swallow).

Paramedics should also be mindful that a biphasic reaction might occur after the initial reaction has resolved, these reactions may happen despite no further exposure to a trigger and often occur within 12 hours but may be a delayed reaction of up to 72 hours (Wilkinson-Stokes et al. 2021).

OOH management of the anaphylactic patient

Prompt administration of intramuscular (IM) adrenaline is required (Muraro et al. 2021). Community use of auto injectors is recommended if they are available, as they are quick and safe to administer (Muraro et al. 2021). Adrenaline stabilises the mast cell wall, reversing symptoms quickly and most importantly inducing peripheral vasoconstriction and bronchodilation, further to this it reduces the ongoing release of inflammatory mediators (Wilkinson-Stokes et al. 2021). Oxygen maybe required to maintain normoxia, high flow oxygen is preferential where there are signs of hypoxaemia (Muraro et al. 2021; Wilkinson-Stokes et al. 2021). Beta 2 agonists, such as salbutamol should be administered if a wheeze is present (Muraro et al. 2021) to further support bronchodilation. The use of Ipratropium Bromide concurrently with a beta 2 agonist leads to greater relaxation of bronchial smooth muscle enhancing bronchodilation (Wilkinson-Stokes et al. 2021). IV fluid administration is particularly important when cardiovascular compromise is present. Fluid administration should be carefully considered to avoid associated risks such as acidosis and fluid overload (Wilkinson-Stokes et al. 2021). Consider nebulised adrenaline if laryngeal/pharyngeal oedema is suspected with the presence of a stridor; IM adrenaline is still required as minimal adrenaline will be absorbed systemically when inhaled (Muraro et al. 2021).

Conclusion

Paramedics care for patients across their lifespan experiencing a vast array of medical emergencies and therefore require a broad knowledge base to be able to diagnose and manage patients' conditions. This chapter provides an overview of the assessment and management of a selection of common medical emergencies likely to present to paramedics. Students should use this chapter as a starting block for a basic understanding to facilitate ongoing learning.

Activities

Now review your learning by completing the learning activities in this chapter. The answers to these appear at the end of the book. Further self-test activities can be found at **http://www.wileyfundamentalseries.com/paramedic/3e.**

Test your knowledge

1. What are the management priorities for a patient experiencing a hypoglycaemic episode?
2. What factors should the paramedic consider as potential causes leading to an episode of AD?
3. In your own words describe sepsis.
4. Describe the difference between an ischaemic and haemorrhagic stroke.
5. What are some specific considerations when looking after a paediatric patient with suspected sepsis?
6. What are some causes of a seizure?
7. Outline the symptoms required to meet the criteria for anaphylaxis and how would you manage a patient with anaphylaxis?
8. How would a person experiencing an adrenal crisis present?

Glossary

Absolute insulin deficiency: The body is unable to produce any insulin.

Aerobic metabolism: Metabolism in an oxygenated environment.

Anaerobic metabolism: Metabolism in an oxygen-poor environment.

Biphasic reaction: The recurrence of anaphylaxis symptoms without further exposure to the allergen, usually within 72 hours of the initial event.

Extrication: The process of assisting a patient to get from the scene such as their house, public place, care facility, or from being entrapped in a vehicle into the ambulance or simply out of the starting location.

Hyponatraemia: When the sodium (Na) concentration in blood is abnormally low.

Hypoperfusion: Reduced blood flow, this may lead to tissue ischaemia.

Disseminated intravascular coagulopathy: The abnormal formation of multiple clots throughout the vascular system of the body. This process uses up the body's clotting factors which can lead to uncontrolled bleeding elsewhere in the body.

Lipolysis: The breakdown of lipids into glycerol and free fatty acids to mobilise stored energy.

Normoxia: SpO2 reading of above 94%, or 88–92% in those with COPD.

Orthostatic drop: A sudden drop in BP related to a change in the person's position. Most frequently when moving from sitting or lying to a standing position.

Pathogen: Any organism or agent that causes disease such as bacteria or a virus.

Relative insulin deficiency: The body doesn't produce enough insulin or the cells of the body have an insulin resistance requiring more insulin.

Vascular permeability: The ability for molecules and cells to move through vessel walls.

References

Aaron, S., Prabhakar, A.T, Mathew, V. et al. (2020). Acute stroke mimics: etiological spectrum and efficacy of FAST, BE FAST, and the ROSIER scores. *Journal of Stroke Medicine* **3** (2): 151–158. doi: 10.1177/2516608520973520

Abrams, M., Magee, M.A., Risler, Z. et al. (2019). Unorthodox use of point-of-care ultrasound to evaluate seizures. *Cureus* **11** (1): e3960. doi: 10.7759/cureus.3960.

Alexander, J. (2020). Enhancing stroke management. *JEMS* (14 July). Available at: https://www.jems.com/patient-care/enhancing-stroke-management (accessed 17 October 2023).

Allen, K.J. and Leslie, S.W. (2019). Autonomic dysreflexia (8 April). Nih.gov/ StatPearls Publishing. Available at: https://www.ncbi.nlm.nih.gov/books/NBK482434 (accessed 25 January 2023).

American Association of Neurological Surgeons (AANS). (2019). Epilepsy – seizure types, symptoms and treatment options. American Association of Neurological Surgeons. Available at: https://www.aans.org/en/Patients/Neurosurgical-Conditions-and-Treatments/Epilepsy (accessed 25 January 2023).

Australian Commission on Safety and Quality in Health Care. (2022). Sepsis clinical care standard. Available at: https://www.safetyandquality.gov.au/sites/default/files/2022-06/sepsis_clinical_care_standard_2022.pdf (accessed 25 January 2023).

Baines, A. (2015). Adrenal insufficiency: improving paramedic practice. *Journal of Paramedic Practice* **7** (4): 192–200. doi: 10.12968/jpar.2015.7.4.192.

Bonner, A. (2019). Renal and genitourinary emergencies. In: *Emergency and Trauma Care for Nurses and Paramedics*. 3e (ed. K. Curtis and C. Ramsden). Elsevier Australia.

Bourke-Matas, E., Bosley, E., Smith, K. et al. (2022). Challenges to recognising patients at risk of out-of-hospital clinical deterioration. *Australasian Emergency Care* **26** (1): 24–29. doi: 10.1016/j.auec.2022.07.003.

Buck, B., Akhtar, N., Alrohimi, A. et al. (2021). Stroke mimics: incidence, aetiology, clinical features and treatment. *Annals of Medicine* **53** (1): 420–436. doi: 10.1080/07853890.2021.1890205.

Cardona, V., Ansotegui, I.J., Ebisawa, M. et al. (2020). World Allergy Organization Anaphylaxis Guidance 2020. *World Allergy Organization Journal* **13** (10). doi: 10.1016/j.waojou.2020.100472.

Chhabra, R., Gupta, R., and Gupta, L.K. (2021). Intranasal midazolam versus intravenous/rectal benzodiazepines for acute seizure control in children: A systematic review and meta-analysis. *Epilepsy & Behavior* **125:** 108390. doi: 10.1016/j.yebeh.2021.108390.

Courtney, C. (2021). Adrenal insufficiency: a review. *Emergency and Urgent Care* **13** (11): 460–465. doi: 10.12968/jpar.2021.13.11.460.

Davis, W.A., Peters, K.E., Makepeace, A. et al. (2018). Prevalence of diabetes in Australia: insights from the Fremantle Diabetes Study Phase II. *Internal Medicine Journal* **48** (7): 803–809. doi: 10.1111/imj.13792.

Dodd, A., Hughes, A., Sargant, N. et al. (2021). Evidence update for the treatment of anaphylaxis. *Resuscitation* **163:** 86–92. doi: 10.1016/j.resuscitation.2021.04.010.

Epilepsy Action Australia. (2020). Home. Epilepsy Action Australia. Available at: https://www.epilepsy.org.au (accessed 25 January 2023).

Evans, L., Rhodes, A., Alhazzani, W. et al. (2021). Surviving sepsis campaign: international guidelines for management of sepsis and septic shock 2021. *Critical Care Medicine* **49** (11): e1063–e1143. doi: 10.1097/ccm.0000000000005337.

Fajardo, E.C. (2017). Management of hyperglycemic hyperosmolar syndrome. In: *Evidence-Based Critical Care* (ed. P.E. Marik), pp. 441–445. Springer International Publishing.

Floer, M., Ziegler, M., Lenkewitz, B. et al. (2021). Out-of-hospital sepsis recognition by paramedics improves the course of disease and mortality: a single center retrospective study. *Advances in Clinical and Experimental Medicine* **30** (11): 1115–1125. doi: 10.17219/acem/140357.

Fu, P., Wang, Z., and Ding, Y. (2018). Prehospital stroke care, a narrative review. *Brain Circulation* **4** (4): 160. doi: 10.4103/bc.bc_31_18.

Fuentes, B., Ntaios, G., Putaala, J. et al. (2017). European Stroke Organisation (ESO) guidelines on glycaemia management in acute stroke. *European Stroke Journal* **3** (1): 5–21. doi: 10.1177/2396987317742065.

Gill, F.J., Cooper, A., Falconer, P. et al. (2021). Development of an evidence-based ESCALATION system for recognition and response to paediatric clinical deterioration. *Australian Critical Care* **35** (6): 668–676. doi: 10.1016/j.aucc.2021.09.004.

Gyawali, B., Ramakrishna, K., and Dhamoon, A.S. (2019). Sepsis: the evolution in definition, pathophysiology, and management. *SAGE Open Medicine* **7** (7). doi: 10.1177/2050312119835043.

Harley, A., Schlapbach, L.J., Johnston, A.N.B. et al. (2021). Challenges in the recognition and management of paediatric sepsis – the journey. *Australasian Emergency Care* **25** (1): 23–29. doi: 10.1016/j.auec.2021.03.006.

Hart, L. (2020). Prehospital treatment of the adult patient whose seizure has stopped. *JEMS: EMS, Emergency Medical Services – Training, Paramedic, EMT News*. Available at: https://www.jems.com/patient-care/prehospital-treatment-of-the-adult-patient-whose-seizure-has-stopped (accessed 25 January 2023).

Higginson, R., Burrows, P., and Jones, B. (2019). Continuing professional development: diabetes and associated diabetic emergencies. *Journal of Paramedic Practice* **11** (6): 1–5. doi: 10.12968/jpar.2019.11.6.cpd1.

Huang, M., Cai, S., and Su, J. (2019). The pathogenesis of sepsis and potential therapeutic targets. *International Journal of Molecular Sciences* **20** (21): 5376. doi: 10.3390/ijms20215376.

Hubert, R.J. and Vanmeter, K.C. (2018). *Gould's Pathophysiology for the Health Professions. 6e*. Elsevier.

Jankovic, J. (2022). Spinal cord trauma. In: *Bradley and Daroff's Neurology in Clinical Practice* (ed. J. Jankovic, J. Mazziotta, S. Pomeroy et al.), pp. 929–949. Elsevier.

Kanner, A.M. and Bicchi, M.M. (2022). Antiseizure medications for adults with epilepsy. *JAMA* **327** (13): 1269–1281. doi: 10.1001/jama.2022.3880.

Keller-Senn, A., Lee, G., Imhof, L. et al. (2017). Hypoglycaemia and brief interventions in the emergency department – a systematic review. *International Emergency Nursing* **34:** 43–50. doi: 10.1016/j.ienj.2017.02.006.

Lane, D.J., Wunsch, H., Saskin, R. et al. (2020). Epidemiology and patient predictors of infection and sepsis in the prehospital setting. *Intensive Care Medicine* **46** (7): 1394–1403. doi: 10.1007/s00134-020-06093-4.

Lane, D.J., Wunsch, H., Saskin, R. et al. (2018). Association between early intravenous fluids provided by paramedics and subsequent in-hospital mortality among patients with sepsis. *JAMA Network Open* **1** (8): e185845. doi: 10.1001/jamanetworkopen.2018.5845.

Langenbruch, L., Rickert, C., Gosheger, G. et al. (2019). Seizure-induced shoulder dislocations – case series and review of the literature. *Seizure* **70** (70): 38–42. doi: 10.1016/j.seizure.2019.06.025.

Larsson, M., Castrén, M., Lindström, V. et al. (2019). Prehospital exenatide in hyperglycemic stroke – a randomized trial. *Acta Neurologica Scandinavica* **140** (6): 443–448. doi: 10.1111/ane.13166.

Lehn, A., Watson, E., Ryan, E.G. et al. (2021). Psychogenic nonepileptic seizures treated as epileptic seizures in the emergency department. *Epilepsia* **62** (10): 2416–2425. doi: 10.1111/epi.17038.

Leibetseder, A., Eisermann, M., LaFrance Jr, W.C. et al. (2020). How to distinguish seizures from non-epileptic manifestations. *Epileptic Disorders* **22** (6): 716–738. doi: 10.1684/epd.2020.1234.

Lenahan, C.M. and Holloway, B. (2015). Differentiating between DKA and HHS. *Journal of Emergency Nursing* **41** (3): 201–207. doi: 10.1016/j.jen.2014.08.015.

Lindsay, E. (2018). Thrombectomy 6 to 24 hours after stroke with a mismatch between deficit and infarct. *The Journal of Emergency Medicine* **54** (4): 583–584. doi: 10.1016/j.jemermed.2018.02.029.

Liu, S.L., Columbus, M.P., Peddle, M. et al. (2021). Hypoglycemia requiring paramedic assistance among adults in southwestern Ontario, Canada: a population-based retrospective cohort study. *CMAJ Open* **9** (4): E1260–E1268. doi: 10.9778/cmajo.20200184.

Micieli, A., Joundi, R., Khosravani, H. et al. (2020). History taking. *The Code Stroke Handbook* (ed. J. Gladstone, R. Joundi, and J. Hopyan), pp. 1–13. doi: 10.1016/b978-0-12-820522-8.00001-6.

Muraro, A., Worm, M., Alviani, C. et al. (2021). EAACI guideline: anaphylaxis (2021 update). *Allergy* **77** (2): 357–377. doi: 10.1111/all.15032.

Patel, R., Nugawela, M.D., Edwards, H.B. et al. (2018). Can early warning scores identify deteriorating patients in pre-hospital settings? A systematic review. *Resuscitation* **132:** 101–111. doi: 10.1016/j.resuscitation.2018.08.028.

Rehani, B., Ammanuel, S.G., Zhang, Y. et al. (2019). A new era of extended time window acute stroke interventions guided by imaging. *The Neurohospitalist* **10** (1): 29–37. doi: 10.1177/1941874419870701.

Rowland, K. and Lambert, C. (2022). *Evaluation after a first seizure in adults. American Family Physician* **105** *(5): 507–513. Proquest.*

Rushworth, L.R., Torpy, D.J., and Falhammar, H. (2019). Adrenal crisis. *The New England Journal of Medicine* **381** (9): 852–861. doi: 10.1056/NEJMra1807486.

Silcock, D.J., Corfield, A.R., Rooney, K.D. et al. (2018). Superior performance of National Early Warning Score compared with quick Sepsis-related Organ Failure Assessment Score in predicting adverse outcomes. *European Journal of Emergency Medicine* **26** (6): 433–439. doi: 10.1097/mej.0000000000000589.

Sinclair, J.E., Austin, M., Froats, M. et al. (2019). Characteristics, prehospital management, and outcomes in patients assessed for hypoglycemia: repeat access to prehospital or emergency care. *Prehospital Emergency Care* **23** (3): 364–376. doi: 10.1080/10903127.2018.1504150.

Singh, R.-J., Doshi, D., and Barber, P.A. (2020). Hypoglycemia causing focal cerebral hypoperfusion and acute stroke symptoms.

Canadian Journal of Neurological Sciences/Journal Canadien Des Sciences Neurologiques **48** (4): 550–552. doi: 10.1017/cjn.2020.246.

Cole, J. and Stack, C. (2021). The clinical approach to stroke in young adults. In: *Stroke* (ed. S. Dehkharghani), pp. 53–78. Exon Publications.

Stephenson, R. (2019). Autonomic dysreflexia in spinal cord injury: overview, pathophysiology, causes of autonomic dysreflexia (12 November). *Medscape.* Available at: https://emedicine.medscape.com/article/322809-overview (accessed 25 January 2023).

Stroke Foundation. (2022). Home – Stroke Foundation Australia. Available at: https://strokefoundation.org.au (accessed 25 January 2023).

Tan, M., Boston, R., Cook, M.J. et al. (2019). Risk factors for injury in a community-treated cohort of patients with epilepsy in Australia. *Epilepsia* **60** (3): 518–526. doi: 10.1111/epi.14659.

Tasdelen, A. and Ekici, A. (2022). Transient loss of consciousness in children: syncope or epileptic seizure? *Neurology Asia* **27** (2): 309–315. doi: 10.54029/2022nfr.

Thomas, A., Riviello, J., Davila-Williams, D. et al. (2022). Pharmacologic and acute management of spinal cord injury in adults and children. *Curr Treat Options Neurol* **24** (7): 285–304. doi: 10.1007/s11940-022-00720-9.

Todd, V.F., Moylan, M., Howie, G. et al. (2022). Predictive value of the New Zealand Early Warning Score for early mortality in low-acuity patients discharged at scene by paramedics: an observational study. *BMJ Open* **12** (7): e058462. doi: 10.1136/bmjopen-2021-058462.

Wahl, J. (2015). Autonomic dysreflexia: an educational intervention for first responders to recognize this medical emergency (pp. 1–82). Thesis. Regis University.

Wardi, G., Brice, J., Correia, M. et al. (2020). Demystifying lactate in the emergency department. *Annals of Emergency Medicine* **75** (2): 287–298. doi: 10.1016/j.annemergmed.2019.06.027.

Weiss, S.L., Peters, M.J., Alhazzani, W. et al. (2020). Surviving sepsis campaign international guidelines for the management of septic shock and sepsis-associated organ dysfunction in children. *Intensive Care Medicine* **46** (S1): 10–67. doi: 10.1007/s00134-019-05878-6.

Wilkinson-Stokes, M., Rowland, D., Spencer, M. et al. (2021). Care in the field: adult anaphylaxis for paramedics. *Australasian Journal of Paramedicine* **18:** 1–6. doi: 10.33151/ajp.18.916.

Wolfsdorf, J., Allgrove, J., Craig, M. et al. (2014). Diabetic ketoacidosis and hyperglycemic hyperosmolar state. *Pediatric Diabetes* **15** (S20): 154–179. doi: 10.1111/pedo.12165.

World Health Organization (WHO). (2022). Epilepsy (9 February). WHO. Available at: https://www.who.int/news-room/fact-sheets/detail/epilepsy (accessed 25 January 2023).

CHAPTER 28

Caring for older adults

Melinda (Dolly) McPherson

Advanced Clinical Practitioner, University Hospital Southampton Emergency Department, UK
Specialist Paramedic (critical care), Hampshire and Ilse of Wight Air Ambulance, UK

Contents

LEARNING OUTCOMES

On competition of this chapter the reader will be able to:

- Understand the anatomical and physiological changes associated with ageing.
- Describe additional factors to consider when assessing the older patient.
- Weigh up the options of treatment locations and referrals for older persons.
- Understand the special circumstances associated with older persons conditions and presentations.

Introduction

Care of the older person in the pre-hospital environment forms a significant part of the paramedic workload (Forsgärde et al. 2020). It is internationally recognised that the population is ageing with a subsequent impact on healthcare resources (WHO 2022). Understanding and acting on the intricacies of ageing and complexities of managing the older person is vital to the outcomes of these patients (BGS 2019). This chapter identifies and discusses key concepts when caring for the elderly in the prehospital context.

The elderly population

In your work as a paramedic, many of your patients will be elderly. The elderly are not a **homogeneous** mass and are amongst the most interesting people you will ever meet. If you are lucky, your older patients will share with you some of their many and varied life experiences. Remember that you are in a privileged position to care for this patient group.

The WHO reports that between 2015 and 2050 the proportion of the world's population aged over 60 years will go

Fundamentals of Paramedic Practice: A Systems Approach, Third Edition. Edited by Sam Willis and Ian Peate.

Companion website: www.wiley.com/go/willis/paramedic3e

from 12% to 22% with a significant proportion of these living in low- and middle-income countries. In 2020, the number of people over the age of 60 outnumbered children younger than 5 years (WHO 2022). The range of health and well-being amongst this large cohort is significantly broad with multiple factors impacting on individual state (BGS 2019). Socioeconomic factors, health in younger life, social support, and sense of purpose have a high impact on healthy ageing (Office for Health Improvement and Disparities 2022). There is a recognised gap in life expectancy between those who live in the most and least deprived areas of their countries with a gap of six to nine years in the UK and seven to nine years in Australia (with the large proportion of these being from the indigenous community).

A number of physiological, psychological, and socioemotional changes occur as part of the normal ageing process. Such changes have impact on an individual's feeling of wellness and must be considered when we seek to treat their illnesses. With an ageing population, access to high-quality assessment, treatment, and care should not be restricted by age (Office for Health Improvement and Disparities 2022). The care provided by ambulance services must fit the needs of older patients, which are different from those of the younger adult population due to their differing physiology, capabilities, and responses to illness and injury.

It is recognised that the role of the ambulance service has moved away from simple conveyance, towards being a mobile healthcare provider tailored to individual needs. As such, the skill of the paramedic is in deciding when to convey to hospital and when to refer on to an appropriate care pathway. Alternative care pathways such as falls referral teams and specialist paramedics are becoming increasingly available to help manage a variety of conditions and prevent hospital attendance (Lofthouse-Jones 2021; Ambulance Victoria 2023).

Anatomy and physiology

A good understanding of the anatomical and physiological changes that occur during normal ageing is key to the assessment and management of the older person (GBS 2019). This knowledge will form the basis of your decision-making and has an impact on treatment options and modalities.

Physiology of ageing

Physiological changes during the ageing process occur in every body system, including the cardiovascular system, respiratory system, musculoskeletal system, skin, special senses, immunity, thermoregulation (temperature), and brain.

Changes to the cardiovascular system due to ageing

A combination of factors results in a decrease in cardiac output after the age of 40 years. Changes in the blood vessels make it harder for blood to flow: the arteries stiffen due to arteriosclerosis and atherosclerosis develops. The heart wall also stiffens and response to inotropic hormones decreases. Systolic blood pressure increases more markedly than diastolic pressure (RACGP 2019). The pressure receptors that detect blood pressure become less responsive, which means that it takes longer for the blood pressure to change when required (Dani et al. 2021). This explains why **orthostatic hypotension** and orthostatic syncope are more common in elderly people. Orthostatic hypotension is a fall in systolic pressure of at least 20 mmHg or a fall in diastolic pressure of at least 10 mmHg within three minutes of standing. This may be due to age-related cardiovascular changes or may be medicine induced (RACGP 2019; Dani et al. 2021).

Changes to the respiratory system due to ageing

Although overall lung capacity remains constant, vital capacity decreases and residual volume increases. This is because the chest wall becomes more rigid, the effects of the respiratory muscles lessen, and there is less elastic recoil of the lung (Arif and Pisani 2020). Many protective mechanisms weaken. As less saliva is produced and the mucociliary escalator becomes less efficient, colonisation of bacteria becomes more likely, resulting in a higher frequency of infections (RACGP 2019). Many patients lived in a time when awareness of the impact of smoking and asbestos was limited so have a higher incidence of lung disease than that of the younger population (RACGP 2019).

Changes to the musculoskeletal system due to ageing

There is a progressive decrease in muscle mass with advancing age. This is due to **atrophy** and loss of muscle cells. The strength of muscle contraction decreases, as does innervation of muscles (Dopsaj et al. 2020). Bone mass also decreases with the prevalence of osteoporosis rising from 2% at 50 years old to nearly 50% at 80 years old (NICE 2021). Degenerative joint disease is extremely common, with many of the over-70s suffering some degree of pain and movement restriction.

Skin

The epidermis becomes thinner through atrophy. Sagging and wrinkling become evident as the skin loses elasticity, particularly in exposed areas such as the face and hands. The number of blood vessels serving the skin also decreases with age (RACGP 2019). This means that the skin has a reduced ability to heal and hence its protective function is reduced if the barrier is breached.

Special senses

There is a functional decline in all the senses as we age. The implications of a less sensitive sense of smell may range from the benign overuse of perfume to the potentially dangerous inability to smell a smoke from a fire. The sense of taste also declines, with flavours having to be at least twice as strong at age 70 years as at age 20 years. This is potentially problematic since an individual may not recognise when food is dangerously inedible.

Hearing loss is a common occurrence and tends to be greater in men than in women. This may make conversation difficult or embarrassing, which could lead to a lower desire for social interaction, including accessing emergency care.

Reduced visual acuity may render furniture an obstacle course. However, most people become expert at navigating the furniture in their own house. Bear this in mind if you need to move any furniture during your encounter with an elderly patient. It is very important that it is returned to the exact spot from which it was taken. Glare becomes a problem too. Try to make sure you are well lit and do not have a window or other bright light directly behind you when interacting with your older patients. Colour discrimination also reduces, which may have implications for self-administration of medication.

Finally, appetite lessens as taste and smell decrease and the antrum of the stomach fills more quickly. This leads to weight loss, which can in turn lead to pressure ulcers, hip fractures, and cognitive impairment (RACGP 2019).

Immune function

Immune function deteriorates, meaning that the elderly are more at risk from infection. There is also an increased prevalence of autoimmune illness and **neoplasms.** The older persons response to vaccines is decreased with some vaccines such as influenza, pneumococcal, and herpes sometimes requiring higher doses, and the requirement for more frequent doses of the Covid-19 vaccine to maintain protection (Haag and Religa 2022). The elderly may also be unable to access vaccines easily due to reduced mobility or lack of social support.

Thermoregulation

The response to cold diminishes as vasoconstriction decreases. The body is also less able to respond to heat, as sweating becomes impaired due to decreased output from each sweat gland and reduced skin blood flow (Meade et al. 2020).

Multimorbidity

Multimorbidity is the term used to describe the state where an individual is experiencing an accumulation of problems due to the coexistence of two or more long-term conditions, with complex multimorbidity defined as three or more chronic conditions affecting three or more body systems (RACGP 2019). Multimorbidity is known to be more common with increased age. The prevalence of multimorbidity in patients over 85 years is as high as 90% (Beil et al. 2021). It impacts all aspects of a patient's well-being: as well as the physical effects, it can threaten a patient's mental health, their financial status, and their emotional well-being.

Multimorbidity is associated with increased demand on healthcare services, not only because patients require more assessment and treatment for their conditions but also due to some of the consequences of multiple treatments. The concurrent use of five or more medications on a long-term basis, known as polypharmacy, can lead to problems. The more medications a person takes, the greater their chance of experiencing an adverse drug reaction. Some medications interact with other medications, which may lead to undertreatment of a condition at one end of the spectrum, and to hospitalisation or death at the other (Nickel et al. 2021). When attending patients who take a long list of medications, ask them when they last had a medication review. This information may be pertinent in the handover either to hospital staff or to the general practitioner (GP).

Not all older people with multiple conditions will encounter such problems. Those with low social support and low self-efficacy are more likely to feel burdened by multiple treatments, which places them at greater risk of a reduced quality of life. For these patients, it is even more important to find solutions that not only relieve their symptoms but also allow them a degree of control over their choices and encourage social support and interaction (RACGP 2019). GPs are often thought of as the gatekeepers to other health and social care services, but as a paramedic you may be the only healthcare worker who sees the patient in their home environment. You may recognise signs that the patient is overburdened and discuss with them the possibility of GP referral for review. Some systems encourage 'GP triage', whereby the paramedic speaks directly to the GP. This shared decision-making between patient, paramedic, and GP ideally leads to the most appropriate care and follow-up, leaving all parties feeling empowered.

Assessing older adults

As well as conducting your usual patient assessment, there are additional factors to consider when assessing the older adult. In this patient group it is useful to your clinical reasoning if the patient's 'normal' parameters can be identified. This might be done through the location of old patient notes, discharge letters, care folders, or obtaining collateral history from the patient's GP. Many of these might be available on electronic data bases such as electronic shared patient records. Some key areas of assessment are:

- Pain assessment.
- Diagnostic tests.
- Social assessment and falls risk assessment.
- Cognitive assessment.

Pain assessment

Many people believe that pain must simply be accepted as an unavoidable consequence of ageing. Although often associated with degenerative conditions of older age, pain should not be considered a normal state (Hosseini et al. 2022)

Chronic pain in older people is often multidimensional. It is influenced by more than mere tissue damage. Social isolation, depression, fear, and co-morbidities are all likely to have an impact on the experience of pain (Chan and Chan 2022). Conversely, experiencing pain may lead to or exacerbate these problems.

Where a patient has cognitive impairment, pain may be expressed in terms of increased confusion, aggression, or social withdrawal. Such changes are only possible to detect for those who know the patient such as a carer or relative. Other non-verbal cues such as grimacing, guarding, and crying are more universal and should be considered as possible pain indicators. The Abbey pain scale and Wong-Baker faces pain scale can be used for the assessment of pain in patients with cognitive impairment (Nickel et al. 2021).

Where possible, assess the multidimensional aspects of pain:

- Sensory: nature, location, and intensity (using a recognised pain score).
- Affective: emotional response to pain.
- Impact: on function.

Cognitive assessment

If you have concerns about your patient's cognitive function, a quick and simple tool that can help in your assessment is the Abbreviated Mental Test score (AMT-4). This involves asking about place, age, date of birth, and year, and is a quick and easy assessment of cognitive impairment (Locke et al. 2013). This can be combined with the 4AT if you suspect delirium in your patient. The 4AT score uses the AMT-4 score plus tests alertness, attention, and the rapidity of change (De et al. 2017). If this identifies impairment, a more in-depth assessment is required. For this onward assessment the National Institute for Health and Care Excellence (NICE 2022) and the Australian Commission on Safety and Quality in Health Care (2022) recommend the use of the abbreviated mental test score (AMTS) as a validated tool to assess for cognitive impairment. Remember to document and hand over your findings to the hospital or GP.

Social assessment and falls risk assessment

When assessing older adults, a social assessment is as important as a physical assessment. The older body has a reduced ability to heal, and the location of a patient's recovery is likely to be determined by the level of social support to which they have access. It can be much easier for hospital staff to start planning for discharge if they have a good assessment from the person who saw the patient in their home context. A full comprehensive **geriatric** assessment (CGA) (BGS 2019) is beyond the scope of the paramedic and takes around 90 minutes to complete, so is not appropriate, but taking a good social history from the patient and from any relatives or carers on scene is important. Handing this over to any teams that the patient is referred to (both verbal and written handover) can be invaluable in their ongoing care, treatment escalation decisions, and future discharge plans.

As a part of your social assessment, it is vital to perform a falls risk assessment. Falls are nearly always multifactorial and as such require a comprehensive understanding of the numerous potential contributing factors (NICE 2019). Paramedics are in the privileged position to assess patients in their home environment and as such are perfectly placed to gather the information required for a falls risk assessment. A history of falls is one of the greatest risk factors for another fall so assessment of the older adult should routinely ask about previous recent falls and the circumstances surrounding this (NICE 2019). Other risk factors to explore are outlined in Table 28.1.

Patients who are at risk of falls, especially those who present with a fall and are discharged on scene, should be referred to a community falls service for ongoing assessment if locally available.

Diagnostic tests

Some diagnostic tools are of less use in the frail and/or older patient (Abbot and Dykes 2017). Whilst it is tempting to use every diagnostic tool available, it is important not to over investigate. Any investigations must be done with a specific question in mind to guide management or decision-making (Abbot and Dykes 2017).

A controversial diagnostic test in the older person is Urinalysis. Urinalysis has extremely poor specificity for identification of urinary tract infection (UTI) and will most likely diagnose an asymptomatic bacteraemia (Abbot and Dykes 2017). It should not be used to routinely investigate patients presenting with acute frailty syndromes as it can lead to over-prescription of antibiotics and delayed treatment for the true underlying cause (Givler 2022). The diagnosis of UTI is in the history but beware that confusion is not a sufficient symptom – constipation is a more common cause of confusion than UTI in this patient group (Abbot and Dykes 2017).

Electrocardiogram (ECG) abnormalities commonly exist in this patient group and should be interpreted in the context of the presenting complaint. Consider if the patient's ECG warrants further investigation in a secondary care setting or whether primary care referral is sufficient. For example, an incidental finding of new atrial fibrillation without adverse features might be suitable for GP follow up, whilst a new bundle branch block in the context of possible collapse might warrant follow up in the emergency department.

TABLE 28.1 Other risk factors to explore.

Conditions that affect balance: e.g. Parkinson's, previous strokes, diabetic neuropathy, arthritis
Polypharmacy and medications known to result in postural hypotension or psychoactive changes. See the STOP/START medications (Nickel et al. 2021)
Other conditions such as visual impairment, substance misuse, muscle weakness, cognitive impairment, or urinary incontinence
Home environment hazards: e.g. uneven floor surfaces, steps, loose carpets or rugs, poor lighting, soft bed edges, etc

Source: NICE 2019.

Disposition decisions

Hospital admission for the frail older person has a long-term and sometimes irreversible detrimental effect on functionality and physical health (Abbot and Dykes 2017). A week-long admission for a frail older person can result in deconditioning of muscles by up to 10% (Abbot and Dykes 2017). Not only does a stay in hospital result in poor outcomes for these patients but transport to the emergency department even without onward admission can also result in adverse events. The frail older person can develop a pressure sore within only a short time in the emergency department (ED) on a trolley (RCEM 2018; Nickel et al. 2021). In addition, it is recognised that in increasingly busy ED environments important time-critical medications such as Parkinson's medications, insulin, and anti-epileptic medication commonly taken by older patients are missed (RCEM 2017).

The decision as to whether the patient would benefit from hospital admission or community pathways can be supported by emerging evidence suggesting that combining the National Early Warning Score (NEWS) and Clinical Frailty Scale could help to inform your management and referral of these patients (Table 28.2) (Davey and Cole 2015; Abbot and Dykes 2017). This concept weighs up the frailty of the patient against their clinical acuity. Community pathways might include social services, outpatient clinics, community hospitals, GP home visits, or specialist community services such as community respiratory or heart

TABLE 28.2 **Frailty decision matrix.**

		National early warning score (NEWS)	
		0–4	5+
Clinical frailty score	**0–4**	Aim to keep out of hospital. Look at ambulatory care options instead of admission	Consider admission
	5+	NEWS = 0, CFS = 5+: consider if social services might resolve the problem without need for admission. With higher NEWS than 0 consider ambulatory care options for medical management	Discuss the options and look at care plans. Is this patient end of life? (remember 'Do not attempt resuscitation (DNAR)' does not mean do not treat.) What will admission achieve? 'What matters' to this patient?

Source: Davey and Cole 2015 and Abbot and Dykes 2017.

failure teams, older persons mental health teams, charitable societies, and many more.

If your patient does require transport to an ED, it is worth considering their discharge planning early. This can be done by documenting the patient's home situation along with social support, lining up family to collect the patient or to be at home for discharge, having a key safe code documented, packing patient's clothes to help prevent 'pyjama paralysis' (Oliver 2017), or bringing key medications with the patient so that patient does not have to wait for the hospital pharmacy prior to departure.

Special circumstances

Falls

Falls are a common occurrence across the world. The WHO (2021) state that approximately 37.3 million falls severe enough to require medical attention occur each year. Besides the obvious risk of injury, there are often unseen consequences of falling such as a loss of self-confidence (NICE 2019). This can produce a downward spiral of reduced mobility leading to reduced strength, increasing the risk of further falls.

It is important to assess thoroughly any patient who has sustained a fall. On approaching the patient, in addition to your patient assessment triangle, consider the environment in which they have fallen. Perhaps they were sitting on the side of the bed and have merely slipped onto a carpeted floor, or maybe they have fallen from standing onto a hardwood floor, their head striking the mantelpiece as they fell. Obtain a good history if possible. The patient themselves may have no memory of falling, so question any witnesses for confirmation of what happened. It is important to distinguish between **intrinsic and extrinsic** causes of the fall, and to consider any red flags.

Change in level of consciousness

Falls in the older person are usually multifactorial. It is recognised that clinicians in the emergency setting should assess for the possibility of syncopal falls (Nickel et al. 2021). It is especially useful to question a witness if present, who may be able to describe what happened. Ask about what they saw, including the patient's position when they collapsed, any skin pallor, whether they were shaking/jerking, and how long the episode lasted. If the patient has no memory of falling, and there are no witnesses to suggest otherwise, investigate the patient as though they had experienced a syncopal event (Royal College of General Practitioners 2023).

There may not have been a total loss of consciousness, but a reduced level of consciousness or new-onset confusion may be present. In either case, the patient will need further investigation at hospital.

Major trauma from falls

It has become increasingly recognised that mechanism of injury for an older person's major trauma can be much lower than their younger counterparts. Up to 50% of patients admitted to major trauma centres (MTCs) across the UK have had a fall from standing (Barker 2022). Whilst the UK Trauma Audit and Research Network (TARN) define the age of 60 years as the point that the age–outcome relationship changes (TARN 2017), much of the literature cites ages 65 or older as older persons trauma (Mater 2020; Barker 2022). The majority of injuries associated with major trauma in the older person are to the head and chest (TARN 2017) with falls in the elderly being a leading cause of traumatic brain injury (Lafiatoglou et al. 2021). Older people are more susceptible to brain injury, as the blood vessels in the brain weaken as we age, making them more likely to rupture during head trauma. Anti-coagulant medications commonly used by older patients such as warfarin, rivaroxaban, apixaban, dabigatran, etc also increase the likelihood of intracranial bleeding following trauma.

There is currently no universally accepted trauma triage tool for the older patient. Several local tools are being used nationally and internationally and the following common themes can be gleaned from these.

The common features to many of these trauma triage tools are:

1. The patient is anticoagulated.
2. Blood pressure <110 systolic.
3. More than two body systems injured.
4. Heart rate >90 beats per minute.

OR

High mechanism of injury even without the above criteria (McPherson 2023).

It is important to identify older patients with major trauma so that they can be conveyed to an appropriate trauma centre. Whilst it is accepted that these patients have higher morbidity and mortality than their younger counterparts, those patients – particularly with traumatic brain injury – who do survive often return to a life free of disability (RCEM 2019).

Long lie

In some cases, your patient may have been unable to alert anyone to the fact that they had fallen. When a patient has been immobile on the floor for an extended period (a 'long lie') they may start to develop a condition called **rhabdomyolysis,** which may lead to potentially life-threatening kidney injury. Prolonged contact with a hard surface places the underlying muscle tissue under sustained pressure, which can result in permanent damage. When striated muscle is damaged through trauma, muscle cells die and release their contents into the circulation. In mild cases the patient may be **asymptomatic,** but in severe cases large quantities of **myoglobin** are released, which may lead to acute renal failure (Knott 2021).

The length of time it takes to develop rhabdomyolysis will vary for different people depending on factors such as the type of surface, whether they have been able to move around, existing co-morbidities, and hydration status. You should recognise the potential for the development of this condition, which can only be identified and managed in hospital.

Safeguarding

Safeguarding seeks to protect those with care needs who are at risk of or are experiencing abuse or neglect and are unable to protect themselves due to their care or support needs (Age UK 2022). Due to the natural care needs that commonly arise with ageing older adults are at risk of falling into this category. Paramedics are well placed in the community to identify abuse and neglect in the older adult and may be the first to suspect it (Cannell et al. 2020). Perpetrators of abuse in the older person are often people who are known and trusted by the victim and, when compared to other age groups, patients >85 years are much more likely to be the subject of safeguarding. Some of the ways in which abuse may occur in the older person are highlighted in Table 28.3.

TABLE 28.3 Some ways in which abuse may occur in the older person.

Financial abuse	Trusted persons attempting to gain control of finances Coercion to alter financial wills or financial power of attorney Theft from the patient's property by contractors or carers, for example Online scams
Physical abuse	With increasing costs of living, adult children are living back with older parents. This can on occasion result in physical abuse Physical abuse from a partner suffering from dementia or other cognitive impairment Physical abuse from other care home residents
Neglect	Organisational abuse from care homes or carers through neglect Unintended neglect by loved ones struggling to manage care needs Self-neglect (see below)
Psychological abuse	Threats of harm or abandonment Deliberate isolation Withdrawal or withholding of medication, services, or support networks

Source: Age UK 2022.

Self-neglect is a complex area of safeguarding due to the importance of allowing people with capacity to make decisions about how they choose to live their own life. Each case of self-neglect should be evaluated on an individual basis taking into consideration the person's capacity, the impact of their neglect on their health and well-being, and their ability to protect themselves from harm. If in doubt, a safeguarding report/referral to adult social services should be made as this may facilitate additional assistance for the patient (Age UK 2022). Always notify your patient that you intend to do a referral and your reasons why (AACE 2017).

End-of-life care

'End of life' refers to the period leading to anticipated death, a situation that is increasingly planned for. Paramedics are called usually to provide transport to another facility or to manage an unexpected crisis. In some cases you will be called to manage reversible emergencies. These are situations that require time-critical transfer to the emergency department in order to improve quality of life. They include metastatic spinal cord compression, superior vena cava compression, and neutropenic sepsis (AACE 2016).

Just as paramedics have a role throughout the life course in facilitating a good quality of life, the aim at the end of life is to help the patient achieve a good death. A 'good death' may mean different things to different people, but it has been suggested that the ability to make their own decisions, to be comfortable, to retain dignity, and to be with family members are likely priorities for most (National Institute for Health and Care Research 2022).

NICE (2019a) lists a number of priorities for clinicians supporting patients at the end of life. These include:

- Recognising when a person is in the last days of life.
- Good communication (with the patient, their family, and carers to support shared decision-making).
- Maintaining good hydration (although this is likely to be managed by the community nursing team, you should monitor for signs of dehydration and may be required to help a patient take sips of fluid).
- Pharmacological intervention (paramedics may administer prescribed JIC medications).

Recognising when a patient is at the end of their life can be challenging, as the patient is likely to be unknown to the paramedic. Some of the signs in Table 28.4 may be evident. Whatever situation you are presented with, you have a small window of opportunity to get to know the patient and their wishes in dealing with whatever crisis has presented.

TABLE 28.4 End-of-life signs and symptoms.

Abnormal clinical observations
Irregular breathing, possibly with apnoeic periods
Reduced level of consciousness
Impaired vision/fixed stare
Restlessness
Confusion
Loss of appetite
Loss of bowel/bladder function
'Rattling' respiratory secretions
Cool peripheries

Source: Adapted from AACE 2016.

You may find that you need to manage pain, especially 'breakthrough' pain, as well as other symptoms such as breathlessness and noisy secretions, nausea and vomiting, anxiety and agitation. As with many symptoms, nonpharmacological treatments such as patient positioning and reassurance should be your first-line treatment. Should you require medication, these may be provided in a JIC box. Paramedics can administer these medications as long as they are competent in the method of delivery, have access to information about the medications, and a signed and authorised patient-specific medication chart is present (HCPC 2021).

The paramedic also has a role in supporting people's grief. Whether this is the anticipatory grief of the patient (or their relatives) or the post-death grief of the relatives, it is important to allow individuals to share their memories and anxieties. You can support people with empathic listening and reassurance that these feelings are normal. You may be able to relieve distress from various causes. If the patient is becoming confused, gently remind them of the place, the time, and who is present. If the patient is incontinent, replace soiled pads so that they feel dry. Keep their lips moist with lip balm and keep them warm with extra blankets (Nickel et al. 2021)

When death comes, tactfully and unobtrusively establish that life is extinct and explain this to the family. The usual protocols for expected death should be followed. Ensure you maintain communication with family and carers throughout, giving as much information as possible about the next steps and support available (Blackmore 2022).

Chapter 33 in this volume discusses in more detail issues surrounding end of life and end-of-life care.

Frailty

Frailty can be thought of as the opposite of resilience. It is indicative of a person's vulnerability. Normally we can call on our body's reserves to battle through illness and injury and restore health to previous levels. The frail person is already employing their reserves just to keep them at their normal level of health. Thus, any further insult presents a major challenge to their body. Patients with frailty may not be able to recover to their prior levels of activity and health following illness or injury (RACGP 2019).

Most commonly associated with older age, around 10% of the over-65s have frailty and 25–50% of those are over 85 years (Age UK 2023). With both absolute and relative numbers of elderly persons increasing, the paramedic is increasingly likely to encounter frail patients as their career progresses.

Often people can cope with additional stressors if they have the protective effects of a social network to support them. Without that boost to their reserves, they become vulnerable to the effects of further demands.

Recognition of frailty

Although those with frailty often have multiple long-term conditions, that is not necessarily the case: some patients may have frailty but no long-term conditions. This latter group of patients may not be known to the GP (RACGP 2019; Nickel et al. 2021). The paramedic may be the first person to recognise frailty and is therefore well placed to refer the patient for a fuller assessment. The validated method for assessing frailty in older people is by undertaking a CGA. This takes account of all aspects of the person and their situation, not only their physical condition. However, this is impractical in the emergency situation, since it takes around 90 minutes to complete, as mentioned earlier. Ambulance services are using alternative methods of identifying frailty that may be applied quickly and easily. The Rockwood Clinical Frailty Scale (Rockwood et al. 2020) is such a frailty scoring scale. It does not take full account of the patient's situation as in the CGA, but the score may be useful when referring a patient on from your care. Remember this scale is calculated based on the patients' baseline state, not as they present when they are acutely unwell (Rockwood et al. 2020) (see Figure 28.1)

Implications of frailty

Paramedics should be especially mindful of the five frailty syndromes, the presence of any of which should alert the paramedic to look beyond the obvious signs and symptoms. A patient with frailty may express a serious underlying condition via one or more of these syndromes, shown in Table 28.5.

Paramedics are frequently called to attend a patient who has a 'collapse in the home' or to a patient who is less mobile than usual. Sometimes the cause is not obvious. But frail patients may be expressing non classic symptoms of a serious underlying illness such as sepsis, stroke, or myocardial infarction, which would present in more predictable ways in younger patients (Nickel et al. 2021). Be mindful that these frailty syndromes may be masking something more sinister.

In each case, assessment of the patient's clinical condition should take priority. If there are no red flags for conveyance to hospital, consider the person's ability to undertake their activities of daily living. Many older people with frailty will have developed their own coping mechanisms for retaining control over their day-to-day living, but when challenged by illness or social circumstance they may lose some of this control (Nickel et al. 2021). For example, can they get out of bed and get to the toilet? Is there a significant decline in their ability to perform these functions? Consider their mental status: is this worse than usual?

When the frail person suffers a crisis, it is the paramedic's job to help restore this control. If the patient is not unwell but there is a change in their care needs, there may be a community-based solution that is more appropriate than hospital admission (Melady and Hogan 2021). They may require referral to the GP or local community geriatric services for a CGA and development of a care and support plan. This will depend on the alternative care pathways available in your locality. Older people with frailty will tend to do better in their home environment, but only with appropriate support (Melady and Hogan 2021).

Dementia

Dementia is a condition caused by structural changes in the brain. It is not a normal consequence of ageing, although it is more prevalent in older people. Currently 1 in 23 people aged 65 years and above in the UK has dementia

Clinical Frailty Scale

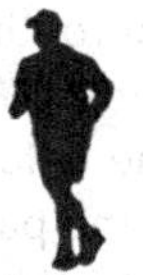

1 Very Fit - People who are robust, active, energetic and motivated. These people commonly exercise regularly. They are among the fittest for their age.

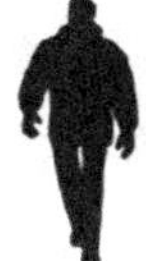

2 Well - People who have no active disease symptoms but are less fit than category 1. Often, they exercise or are very active occasionally, e.g. seasonally.

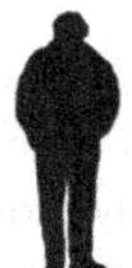

3 Managing Well - People whose medical problems are well controlled, bur are not regularly active beyond routine walking.

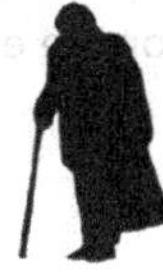

4 Vulnerable - While not dependent on others for daily help, often symptoms limit activities. A common complaint is being "slowed up", and/or being tired during the day.

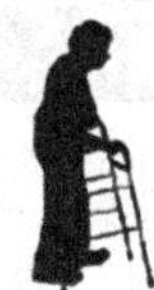

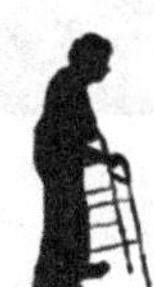

5 Mildly Frail - These people often have more evident slowing, and need help in high order IADLs (finances. transportation, heavy housework, medications). Typically, mild frailty progressively impairs shopping and walking outside alone, meal preparation and housework.

6 Moderately Frail - People need help with all outside activities and with keeping house. Inside, they often have problems with stairs and need help with bathing and might need minimal assistance (cuing, standby) with dressing.

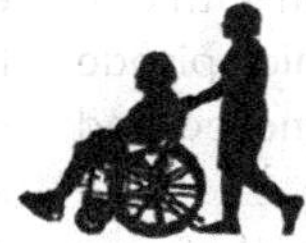

7 Severely Frail - Completely dependent for personal care, from whatever cause (physical or cognitive). Even so, they seem stable and not at high risk of dying (within ~ 6 months).

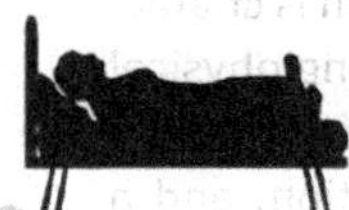

8 Very Severely Frail - Completely dependent, approaching the end of life. Typically, they could not recover even from a minor illness.

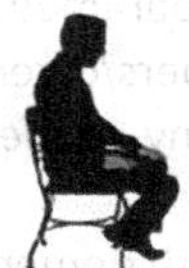

9 Terminally Ill - Approaching the end of life. This category applies to people with a life expectancy <6 months, who are not otherwise evidently frail.

Scoring frailty in people with dementia

The degree of frailty corresponds to the degree of dementia. Common **symptoms in mild dementia** include forgetting the details of a recent event, though still remembering the event itself, repeating the same question/story and social withdrawal.

In **moderate dementia,** recent memory is very impaired, even though they seemingly can remember their past life events well. They can do personal care with prompting.

In **severe dementia,** they cannot do personal care without help.

FIGURE 28.1 The Rockwood Clinical Frailty Scale. Source: Rockwood et al. 2020.

TABLE 28.5 Frailty syndrome presentations.

Falls
Immobility
Delirium
Incontinence
Susceptibility to side effects of medication

Source: Adapted from Nickel et al. 2021.

(www.alzheimers.org.uk) and there are 1 in 15 people >65 years in Australia with dementia (Health Direct 2023).

Common symptoms of the condition include:

- Problems with memory (especially short-term memory)
- Changes in mood
- Difficulty concentrating
- Difficulty communicating

People with dementia can display some of or all these; but be mindful that such symptoms can also be caused by other medical conditions. For example, a person with diabetes mellitus who experiences a hypoglycaemic episode may appear confused but once correctly diagnosed and treated will quickly recover.

It is important to also consider the possibility that your patient is displaying delirium. Whilst there are some behavioural features common with dementia, delirium is characterised by an acute onset linked to an underlying physical condition. Typically, the patient will present with clouded consciousness, poor attention and concentration, and a fluctuating pattern of symptoms (Nickel et al. 2021). Where a patient is presenting with confusion, the paramedic should take a good history from family members/carers and should suspect delirium where there is any *sudden* change in mental state or behaviour.

Usually, when you are called to a patient with dementia, the presenting condition will not be the dementia but something more acute. In these cases, your decision on whether to convey the patient to hospital will be guided not only by that presenting condition but also by the presence of dementia. A change of environment or routine can have a negative impact on a patient with dementia (Nickel et al. 2021). Consider whether transfer to the unfamiliar, and often noisy, ED is necessary or whether the patient's current condition would be better managed by the GP or district nurse.

Conclusion

Paramedics will spend a large amount of their time caring for the elderly population. To do so effectively requires a sound understanding of how ageing affects the whole person. This chapter provides a summary of key issues that will influence paramedic care whilst caring for the elderly population.

Glossary

Asymptomatic: An individual who presents with no symptoms.

Atrophy: Wasting away.

Frailty: A state of increased vulnerability.

Geriatric: Term used to describe an elderly person.

Gerontology: The scientific study of the ageing process and problems that occur in older age.

Homogeneous: An object or substance that is uniform in composition.

Intrinsic vs extrinsic causes: Causes internal to the person (e.g. dizziness) vs those that are external (e.g. tripping over a loose rug).

Myoglobin: An iron-/oxygen-binding protein located in muscle cells.

Neoplasms: Abnormal growth of tissue on the body.

Orthostatic hypotension: A fall in systolic pressure of at least 20 mmHg or a fall in diastolic pressure of at least 10 mmHg within three minutes of standing.

Rhabdomyolysis: A breakdown of muscle tissue that can lead to acute kidney injury.

References

AACE (Association of Ambulance Chief Executives). (2017). Safeguarding adults at risk 2017 guideline. JRCALC. Available at: https://aace.org.uk/jrcalc-updates-2016/safeguarding-adults-at-risk-2017-guideline (accessed 9 February 2023).

Abbot, C. and Dykes, L. (2017). Geriatric medicine: A selection of Top Tips to get you started. [cited 8 Feb 2023]. Available at: https://docs.wixstatic.com/ugd/bbd630_9068591ed32045ef9e10c04cdf3086a2.pdf?index=true.

Age UK. (2022). Safeguarding older people from abuse and neglect. Available at: https://www.ageuk.org.uk/globalassets/age-uk/documents/factsheets/fs78_safeguarding_older_people_from_abuse_fcs.pdf (accessed 9 February 2023).

Age UK. (2023). Understanding frailty. Available at: https://www.ageuk.org.uk/our-impact/policy-research/frailty-in-older-people/understanding-frailty (accessed 10 February 2023).

Ambulance Victoria. (2023). RACER for aged care residents [Internet]. Available at: https://www.ambulance.vic.gov.au/community/racer (accessed 8 February 2023).

Arif, S. and Pisani, M. (2020). Ageing and respiratory diseases. *US Respiratory and Pulmonary Diseases* **5** (1): 33–37. doi: 10.17925/USPRD.2020.5.1.33.

Australian Commission on Safety and Quality in Healthcare. (2022). Early identification of risk. Available at: https://www.safetyandquality.gov.au/our-work/clinical-care-standards/delirium-clinical-care-standard/quality-statements/early-identification-risk (accessed 9 February 2023).

Barker, J. (2022). Silver trauma. Available at: https://www.generalbroadcast.org.uk/blog/silver-trauma (accessed 11 August 2022).

Beil, M., Flaatten, H., Guidet, B. et al. (2021). The management of multi-morbidity in elderly patients: ready yet for precision medicine in intensive care? *Critical Care* **25:** 330–337. Available at:https://www.ncbi.nlm.nih.gov/pmc/articles/PMC8431262 (accessed 13 February 2023).

BGS (British Geriatrics Society). (2019). Comprehensive geriatric assessment toolkit for primary care practitioners. Available at: https://www.bgs.org.uk/sites/default/files/content/resources/files/2019-02-08/BGS%20Toolkit%20-%20FINAL%20FOR%20WEB_0.pdf (accessed 8 February 2023).

Blackmore, T. (2022). *Palliative and End of Life Care for Paramedics*. Brightwater: Class professional publishing

Cannell, B., Weitlauf, J., Livingston, M.D., et al. (2020). Validation of the detection of elder abuse through emergency care technicians (DETECT) screening tool: a study protocol BMJ Open. *British Medical Journal* **10**: e037170. doi: 10.1136/bmjopen-2020-037170.

Chan, H. and Chan, C. (2022). Managing chronic pain in older people. *Clinical Medical Journal* **22** (4): 292–294. doi: 10.7861/clinmed.2022-0274.

Dani, M., Dirksen, A., Taraborrelli, P. et al. (2021). Orthostatic hypotension in older people: considerations, diagnosis and management *Clinical Medical Journal* **21** (3): e275–e282. [Cited 14 Feb 2023] doi: 10.7861/clinmed.2020-1044. PMID: 34001585; PMCID: PMC8140709.

Davey, N. and Cole, A. (2015). Design, implement and measure: A guide to improving transfers of care and handover. [cited 2018 *May 8]*. Available at: https://www.england.nhs.uk/signuptosafety/wp-content/uploads/sites/16/2015/09/safe-comms-design-implmnt-meas.pdf.

De, J., Wand, A.P.F., Smerdely, P.I. et al. (2017). Validating the 4A's test in screening for delirium in a culturally diverse geriatric inpatient population. *Int J Geriatr Psychiatry* **32** (12): 1322–1329.

Dopsaj, M., Kukic, F., Đorđević-Nikic, M. et al. (2020). Indicators of absolute and relative changes in skeletal muscle mass during adulthood and ageing. *Int J Environ Res Public Health* **17** (16): 5977–5990. doi:10.3390/ijerph17165977.

Forsgärde, E., Elmqvist, C., Fridlund, B, et al. (2020). Patients aged ≥65 years dispositions during ambulance assignments, including factors associated with non-conveyance to hospital: a longitudinal and comparative study. *BMJ Open* **10**: e038885. doi: 10.1136/bmjopen-2020-038885.

Givler, D.N. and Givler, A. (2022) Asymptomatic bacteriuria. StatPearls. Available at: https://www.ncbi.nlm.nih.gov/books/NBK441848 (accessed 14 February 2023).

Haag, S. and Religa, D. (2022). COVID vaccination in older adults. *Nature Microbiology* **7** (8): 1106–1107.

HCPC (Health and Care Professionals Council). (2021). Medicines and prescribing rights: sale, supply and administration. Available at: https://www.hcpc-uk.org/standards/meeting-our-standards/scope-of-practice/medicines-and-prescribing-rights/sale-supply-and-administration (accessed 14 February 2023).

Health Direct. (2023). *Dementia statistics*. Available at: https://www.healthdirect.gov.au/dementia-statistics (accessed 9 Feb 2023).

Hosseini, F., Mullins, S., Gibson, W. et al. (2022). Pain management for older adults. *Clinical Medicine* **22** (4): 302–306. doi: 10.7861/clinmed.22.4.ac-p.

Knott, L. (2021) *Rhabdomyolysis and myoglobinuria*. Available at: https://patient.info/doctor/rhabdomyolysis-and-other-causes-of-myoglobinuria (accessed 13 February 2023).

Lafiatoglou, P., Ellis-Hill, C., Gouva, M. et al. (2021). A systematic review of the qualitative literature on older individuals' experiences of care and well-being during physical rehabilitation for acquired brain injury. *Journal of Advanced Nursing* **78** (2): 377–394. doi: 10.1111/jan.15016.

Locke, T., Keat, S., Tate, M. et al. (2013). Assessing the performance of the four question abbreviated mental test in the acute geriatric setting. *Acute Med* **12** (1): 13–17. PMID: 23539371.

Lofthouse-Jones, C., King, P., Pocock, H. et al. (2021). Reducing ambulance conveyance for older people with and without dementia: evidence of the role of social care from a regional, year-long service evaluation using retrospective routine data. *Br Paramed J* **1;6 (3)**: 58–69. doi: 10.29045/14784726.2021.12.6.3.58.

Mater, E.D. (2020). What is silver trauma? Available at: https://www.materem.org/silver-trauma (accessed 1 August 2022).

McPherson, D. (2023). Slip, slop, 2SPLAT: major trauma in the older person. *Standby CPD* Volume 13, issue 2. Class Publishing.

Meade, R.D., Akerman, A.P., Notley, S.R. et al. (2020). Physiological factors characterizing heat-vulnerable older adults: a narrative review. *Environment International* **144:** 105909. doi: 10.1016/j.envint.2020.105909.

Melady, D. and Hogan, T. (2021). Silver book II: training and development. Available at: https://www.bgs.org.uk/resources/silver-book-ii-training-and-development (accessed 10 February 2023).

National Institute for Health and Care Research. (2022) End of life care: research highlights the importance of conversations and need for equal access. doi: 10.3310/collection_49245

NICE (National Institute for Health and Care Excellence). (2019) Falls-risk assessment. Available at: https://cks.nice.org.uk/topics/falls-risk-assessment/background-information/complications (accessed 13 February 2023).

NICE. (2019a). *End of Life Care for Adults: Service Delivery. NICE Guideline 142*. London: NICE.

NICE. (2021). Osteoporosis – prevention of fragility fractures. Available at: https://cks.nice.org.uk/topics/osteoporosis-prevention-of-fragility-fractures/background-information/prevalence (accessed 14 February 2023).

NICE. (2022). Dementia. Available at: https://cks.nice.org.uk/topics/dementia (accessed 9 February 2023).

Nickel, C., Arendts, G., Lucke, J. et al. (2021). Silver book II: geriatric syndromes. Available at: https://www.bgs.org.uk/resources/silver-book-ii-geriatric-syndromes (accessed 10 February 2023).

Office for Health Improvement and Disparities. (2022). Healthy ageing: applying all our health. Available at: https://www.gov.uk/government/publications/healthy-ageing/healthy-ageing-applying-all-our-health (accessed 9 February 2023).

Oliver, D. (2017). David Oliver: fighting pyjama paralysis in hospital wards. *BMJ* **357:** j2096. Available at: https://www.bmj.com/content/357/bmj.j2096 (accessed 9 February 2023).

RCEM (Royal College of Emergency Medicine). (2017). Safety newsflash: time critical medicines. Available at: http://www.rcem.ac.uk/docs/Safety/Time%20critical%20meds%20-%20Nov%202017_Final%20Version.pdf (accessed 8 May 2018).

RCEM. (2018). Safety alert: early to bed. Available at: http://www.rcem.ac.uk/docs/Safety/RCEM%20Safety%20Alert%20-%20Pressure%20Ulcers%20FINAL.pdf (accessed 8 May 2018).

RACGP. (2019). RACGP aged care clinical guide (silver book): Part A. Frailty. Available at: https://www.racgp.org.au/getattachment/f5d92839-e553-45d4-a779-fd08184054b1/Frailty.aspx (accessed 10 February 2023).

RACGP. (2019). RACGP aged care clinical guide (silver book). 5e. Part B. Physiology of ageing. Available at: https://www.racgp.org.au/getattachment/d22bd61f-816a-45b1-b6b0-64e58f77f6ab/Physiology-of-ageing.aspx (accessed 8 February 2023).

RACGP. (2019). RACGP aged care clinical guide (silver book). 5e. Part A. Multimorbidity. Available at: https://www.racgp.org.au/clinical-resources/clinical-guidelines/key-racgp-guidelines/view-all-racgp-guidelines/silver-book/part-a/multimorbidity (accessed 13 February 2023).

RCGP (Royal Collage of General Practitioners). (2023). Syncope toolkit. Available at: https://elearning.rcgp.org.uk/mod/book/view.php?id=12386&chapterid=260 (accessed 13 February 2023).

Rockwood, K., Fay, S., Theou, O. et al. (2020). Top tips to help you use the clinical frailty scale. Available at: https://cdn.dal.ca/content/dam/dalhousie/pdf/sites/gmr/CFS-Top-Tips_2020Jun05_EN_Letter.pdf (accessed 9 February 2023).

Royal College of Emergency Medicine. (2019). Safety alert: silver trauma. Available at: https://rcem.ac.uk/wp-content/uploads/2021/10/RCEM_safety_alert_Silver_Trauma_Sept_2019.pdf (accessed 9 February 2023).

Trauma Audit and Research Network (TARN). (2017). Major trauma in the older person. Available at: https://www.tarn.ac.uk/content/downloads/3793/Major%20Trauma%20in%20Older%20People%202017.pdf (accessed 20 July 2022).

Wallace, J. and Raven, D. (2018). RCEM learning: silver trauma. Available at: https://www.rcemlearning.co.uk/foamed/silver-trauma (accessed 11 August 2022).

WHO (World Health Organization). (2020). Ageing and health. Available at: https://www.who.int/news-room/fact-sheets/detail/ageing-and-health (accessed (accessed 9 February 2023).

WHO (2021). Falls. Available at: https://www.who.int/news-room/fact-sheets/detail/falls (accessed 13 February 2023).

CHAPTER 29

Managing minor injuries in the out-of-hospital setting

Craig Barlow

Consultant Paramedic, St Georges University Hospital NHS

Clinical Director, EMFS Group, UK

Contents

LEARNING OUTCOMES

On completion of this chapter the reader will be able to:

- Discuss the term 'minor injury'.
- Identify the importance of history taking when managing a patient with a minor injury.
- Define the structured systematic approach to clinical assessment in patients with minor injuries (Look, Feel, Move).
- Discuss documentation and the medical model history-taking process.
- Identify and discuss a range of minor medical conditions and how to manage them.

Fundamentals of Paramedic Practice: A Systems Approach, Third Edition. Edited by Sam Willis and Ian Peate.

Companion website: www.wiley.com/go/willis/paramedic3e

Case study

You have received a call to an 85-year-old female who has fallen in the garden. As she fell, she put her left hand out in front of her to stop the fall, but sustained a deep laceration to her hand, a 10 cm laceration to her forehead, and injured her left ankle.

Introduction

This chapter will equip you with the knowledge and skills required to assess, treat, and refer minor injury patients within your everyday practice. Recognising the challenges of assessment and treatment in the out-of-hospital (OOH) environment, the chapter will allow you to consider the different referral pathways available, giving you the confidence to make sound clinical decisions.

What is a 'minor injury'? The question is more complex than it might first appear, since there is no universally accepted definition locally, nationally, and internationally with variations existing between each care provider. A minor injury is whatever has been agreed within your local area: this will have been decided at a senior level (for example, at the **clinical governance board** or within the **integrated care board**), based on local population needs, other services available within the local system and the skills and competences of the practitioner(s) within these units. Within Oxfordshire (UK), for example, the practitioners working within minor injury units (MIU) comprise **emergency practitioners** (EPs), **specialist practitioners** (SPs), and **advanced clinical practitioners** (ACPs); the skill sets between paramedics and other healthcare professionals within these settings are almost identical. Following the publication of 'The NHS Long Term Plan' (NHS England 2019), we will soon see MIUs integrating to form part of new **urgent treatment centres** (UTCs). These centres offer a combination of minor injury/illness and acute rapid assessment, operated by a wider team of multidisciplinary professionals, thus offering an extensive range of patient-centred care and assessment within primary care.

The best advice in terms of establishing what an MIU or UTC might cover in your own region or service is to find out exactly what your local agreement is regarding the type of injuries that such an establishment will routinely see (Box 29.1).

Background

It is suggested that the number of patients attending UK emergency departments (EDs) has risen by 40% over the last 15 years, with 12.5 million 'unheralded' attendances of patients self-presenting to urgent and emergency care services (NHS England 2020) and a 6.9% increase of attendances across Australian EDs between 20192020 and 2020–2021 (ABS 2022). Over the course of a year, there are typically around 16 million attendances at major UK hospital EDs and 9 million at alternative urgent care facilities such as walk-in-centres (WIC), UTCs, and MIUs (Baker 2023). Of those ED attendances, between 10% and 90% are classified as 'inappropriate' (Parkinson et al. 2021) and could have been assessed and/or managed appropriately within an alternative urgent care service. Due to the differing healthcare models between Australia and the UK, the like for like data is not available for comparison.

With the ever-growing need and demand for urgent and same day emergency care (SDEC) services, the need for NHS ambulance services to provide urgent and ambulatory care to service users within the community is high (NHS England 2019). NHS ambulance services are already working with system partners (primary care, community care, acute hospitals, and independent ambulance services) to ensure that patients receive the 'Right care, First time' and where applicable these are at alternative facilities to EDs, such as urgent community response (UCR),

BOX 29.1 **Common ground between MIUs and UTCs**

- **Musculoskeletal** and **ligamentous** Injury
- Mild head injury (Glasgow coma score 15)
- Eye injury
- Burns
- Foreign body removal
- Bites and stings
- Wound care
- Limb fractures
- X-ray facility

UTCs, MIUs, and SDEC services. By doing so, we will see an improvement in patient care/outcomes and satisfaction, as well as a reduction in the increasing demand on EDs and the wider NHS economy (NHS England 2019).

Although some national ambulance services have slowly started to change their strategy and working practice, it is felt that to adequately meet the ever-growing urgent care needs of the population, further improvements are required across national ambulance services. For example, investment and commitment into career development beyond that on a paramedic, educational opportunities/ pathways, development and progression opportunities in advanced clinical practice roles, adequate supervision and support, collaborative working opportunities, alternative care pathways, review of utilisation and mobilisation processes (Right Skill/Person; First Time), to name a few.

It is evident from this shift that knowledge and education in regard to minor injuries/illnesses, as well as advanced patient assessment are now an essential element of the role of a contemporary paramedic. This education and learning will form a solid grounding for future career development opportunities, within specialist and advanced practice (College of Paramedics 2018).

The importance of history taking

As with every clinical assessment, history taking (Box 29.2) is an important aspect of the assessment process, allowing clear understanding of the **mechanism of injury,** direction, magnitude, and duration of force and progress.

Before starting any physical assessment it is important that you listen to and observe the patient to establish the full mechanism of injury. There are a number of 'consultation models' available to clinicians, allowing a structure to the consultation 'Pendleton, Calgary-Cambridge, Neighbour and Silverman', to name but a few (Denness 2013). These models are effective in undertaking a consultation safely and in a timely manner; as well as an opportunity to discuss and consider the 'ideas, concerns and expectations' (ICE) of the patient.

Obtaining and considering the patient's motives for the consultation, ICE will help to assist with a safe, effective, and accurate assessment and diagnosis, and it should form part of the history-taking process (Rickenbach 2019).

Only once you have obtained a full history can a systematic approach commence.

Practice insight

Be sure to get into the habit of asking *what*, *when*, *where*, *how*, and *why* early on in your practice and for every patient, in order to establish a baseline of questioning that you can then build on throughout your career.

Consent to treatment

Before any physical assessment takes place, it is important to obtain informed consent from your patient(s), unless 'assumed consent' is appointed in an emergency situation. The Health and Care Professions Council (HCPC) describes consent as:

> *[P]ermission for a student or registrant to provide any care, treatment or other services, given by a service user, or someone acting on their behalf, after receiving all the information they reasonably need to make that decision. (HCPC 2016)*

BOX 29.2 **History taking: the medical model (related to injury)**

PC = Presenting complaint
What is wrong with your patient, i.e. leg injury (specific)?

HPC = History of presenting complaint
What actually happened (specific)? ***When*** did it happen? ***How*** did it happen (inversion versus eversion)? ***Why*** did it happen (tripped on kerb)? ***Who*** was the history obtained from (patient, bystander, relative)?

OLDCART:

Onset
Location
Duration
Characteristics
Attributing factors
Relieving factors
Treatment already given

Shx = Social history
Demographics – age, gender, occupation, leisure and hobbies, social circumstances, e.g. do they live alone, occupation, hand dominance (in arm/shoulder-related injury)

Dhx = Drug history
What medication/dosage?
Any self-administration of analgesia? Time/dose?
Any known allergies, e.g. medicines, dressings?
Tetanus status

Pmhx = Past medical history
Relevant medical history, previous injury/surgery

It is therefore important to ensure that you have gained consent before any procedures (care, treatment, or other services) are carried out, taking into consideration the differing backgrounds of your patient(s), including age, communicative ability, any learning disabilities, intoxication, language barriers, and religious beliefs. The patient is also entitled to have a chaperone present during any examination; it is always good practice to have one (where practicable). During the documentation process, ensure you accurately record how and when consent was obtained, along with the full details of the chaperone present as applicable. If a chaperone was declined, this should also be fully documented.

Clinical examination

The examination of a patient with an acute injury can often be difficult due to bleeding, swelling, pain, and anxiety; however, a systematic approach is required with every clinical examination. Before the examination takes place, it is important to understand the anatomy in detail (cartilage, ligaments, tendons, joints, muscles, bones) and to be aware of common injury patterns. Ensure that both you and the patient are comfortable and that you are able to examine the patient easily.

Examination of limbs

During examination of limbs, it is important to expose both limbs to allow for comparison, as well as to expose and examine the joint above and below the injury site, as commonly there are associated injuries within these areas (Purcell 2022). Checking the joint proximal to the injury first is good practice; usually the joint above is unaffected and this helps to make contact with the patient without causing too much discomfort or pain. During examination you should establish what is 'normal' for your patient. For example, do they normally walk with a particular gait; how flexible are they normally; is their right ankle always more swollen than the left?

When carrying out your examination, follow the standard orthopaedic practice of Look, Feel, Move.

Look

- Compare with the unaffected side.
- Bleeding, swelling, bruising (Figure 29.1).
- Wounds/scars (Figure 29.1).
- Look from all angles/aspects.
- Foreign bodies.
- Deformity, wasting.
- Colour – cyanosis, pallor, **erythema.**
- **Tracking**, **lymphangitis.**

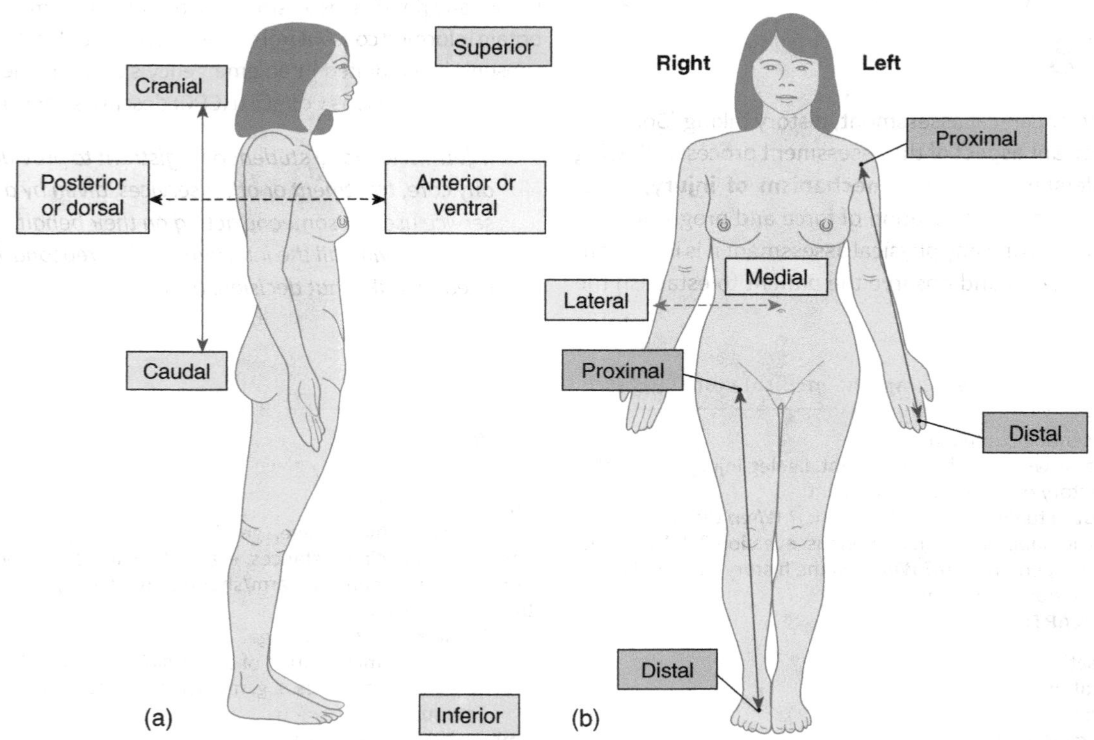

FIGURE 29.1 Anatomical positions – knowing your anatomical positions/landmarks will make for a smoother and more professional handover.

Feel

- Start palpating in the proximal joint away from the site of pain.
- Feel one area at a time, using a single finger.
- Identify the anatomical landmarks in a systemic manner.
- Relate surface anatomy to underlying structures and try to identify specific areas of tenderness.
- Observe for facial expressions and gestures, as well as verbal expressions of pain.
- Skin temperature.
- Crepitus.
- Check sensation (**two-point discrimination**).
- Feel for distal pulses/**capillary refill time.**

Any patient presenting with tenderness to any bony structures must be appropriately referred for an x-ray and further assessment.

Move

- Know how the joint is supposed to move.
- Compare the range of movement to the unaffected side.
- *Active movement* – the patient performs the movement without assistance and using their own power.
- *Passive movement* – movement of the limb is performed on the patient by the clinician.
- *Resisted movement* – in testing resisted movement, the joints do not move and the integrity of the musculotendon is tested, e.g. a straight leg raise testing the extensor mechanism in the knee.

Any patient presenting with reduced movement should be referred for further assessment and possible physiotherapy review, using the most appropriate and suitable pathway.

Your clinical assessment must indicate what injuries are possible and the urgency of diagnosis; this will help with decision-making and your referral process.

Practice insight

Be sure to protect the patient's dignity. For example, undertaking a 'Look, Feel, Move' assessment in the street might require blankets to be placed around the patient with assistance from police or other reliable bystanders.

Remember – in the presence of any bony involvement or bony tenderness, x-ray imaging and review is required.

Clinical documentation

Documentation is an important part of the examination process, allowing for clear and factual accounts of events, continuity of care, audit/research, and a legal record that can be used in a court of law. In court, any account of events in which you have played a professional role will be taken from your notes made at the time of your assessment, thus the need for completeness and accuracy is paramount.

Over the past few years, electronic patient records (EPRs) have been introduced across healthcare sectors, these are well established within many UTC, ED, MIU, and primary care settings. EPRs have a number of benefits to patient care; safer care, computer-aided monitoring, data sharing, audit, increase in operational performance, to name a few (NHS England 2019).

It is important to note and document exactly what your positive and negative findings are, following the Look, Feel, Move assessment method. Clearly document where these findings are situated anatomically (Figure 29.2). The use of diagrams to support your documentation is an excellent way to label and indicate where the injury is on the body. Most EPRs now have anatomical diagrams allowing the clinician to annotate the site of injury or take and upload pictures of the injury site; it is important to note that these images should only be used through approved clinical applications and must not be distributed or shared through any unapproved applications or platforms such as social media. However, if you do not have access to EPRs you do not need to be an expert artist to produce diagrams, as they will still prove to be a valuable aid and reference

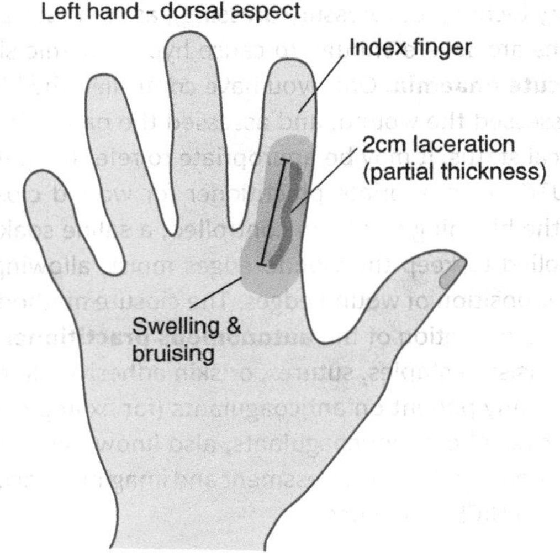

FIGURE 29.2 Assessment and measurement of a wound.

point, proving the value of the saying 'A picture is worth a thousand words'. Also remember to label the diagram or picture, even if it is clear to you at the time; this includes labelling the body part, specifying whether it is right or left, back or front, and drawing and labelling the injury, specifying what the injury is and its size and depth. Again, most EPRs will do this automatically for you, but it is always worth checking.

Be sure to document your findings (both positive and negative) clearly and legibly, with the correct date, time, and patient details.

Minor head injuries

A significant number of emergency calls will require you to attend patients affected by falls, road traffic collisions, collapses, and assaults where patients or bystanders will state a history of a head injury. The severity of head injury can vary from patient to patient, depending on their perception of events, clinical observations, and the mechanism of injury. For example, haematoma, laceration to scalp/eyebrow, or no visible injury to the head can all be classed as a head injury. All head injury patients need to be assessed neurologically in accordance with the UK's National Institute for Health and Care Excellence (NICE) Clinical Guideline 176 (2019) and the Joint Royal Colleges Ambulance Liaison Committee (JRCALC) Clinical Practice Guidelines (2023).

As the scalp has a complex vascular supply, when assessing head injuries, it is important to establish the location of the wound and the source of the bleeding. The smallest of wounds in this area can cause extreme bleeding; it is important that the bleeding is controlled with primary techniques (pressure dressing), as some scalp lacerations are severe enough to cause hypovolaemic shock and **acute anaemia.** Once you have controlled the bleeding, assessed the wound, and assessed the patient's neurological status, it may be appropriate to refer the patient to a UTC or appropriate practitioner for wound closure. Once the bleeding has been controlled, a saline soak can be applied to keep the wound edges moist, allowing for good opposition of wound edges. The closure method will be at the discretion of the **autonomous practitioner** and may consist of staples, sutures, or skin adhesive. Remember that any patient on anticoagulants (for example, warfarin or novel oral anticoagulants, also known as NOACs) should undergo further assessment and imaging, in accordance with NICE guidelines.

Nasal injuries

Where a patient presents with a nose injury, a formal neurological head injury assessment must also be carried out. Remember to consider the mechanism of injury: was there any loss of consciousness, are there other associated facial or head injuries, and can you exclude a cervical spinal injury?

Management of an epistaxis:

- Ensure that you sit the patient with their upper body tilted forward and their mouth open; avoid lying them down unless they are feeling faint.
- Leaning forward decreases blood flow through the nasopharynx, allows spitting out of blood, and minimises swallowing blood that drains into the pharynx.
- Pinch the cartilaginous (soft) part of the nose firmly and hold it for 10–15 minutes without releasing the pressure, whilst breathing through their mouth.

A common misconception is that compression of the nasal bones will help stop bleeding, which is not the case (NICE 2022).

If bleeding does not stop after 10–15 minutes following the above treatment, then nasal packing/cautery should be considered; this may need to be undertaking in a clinical setting such as a UTC/ED.

Once you have controlled any bleeding, carried out these assessments, and ruled out any neurological deficits, an assessment of the nose itself can be carried out.

At this initial stage of the injury, there are some important areas that need to be assessed:

- Is the airway compromised?
- Is there a **septal haematoma?**
- Is there a severe **epistaxis?**
- Is there severe displacement?
- Are there associated fractures to the face?

If the answer to any of these questions is 'yes', then the patient needs to be transferred to the nearest ED for further assessment by ear, nose, and throat (ENT) specialists.

If a patient presents with a mild epistaxis (that has ceased) and/or mild displacement to the nose, then an urgent ENT referral and follow up (usually 7–10 days after the initial injury) would be an appropriate pathway. This allows for the initial swelling to subside and for easier manipulation to take place (Razavi et al. 2014; Basheeth et al. 2015).

Practice insight

When treating a nosebleed by pinching the cartilaginous aspect of the nose, do not be tempted to release or reassess the bleeding for at least five minutes, as this may allow bleeding to resume. Also have a vomit bowl handy, as blood can sometimes find its way to the back of the patient's throat, and they may need to expectorate excess blood.

Wound assessment and care

When it comes to wound care assessment, it is important to distinguish between the different types of wounds you are likely to assess (Box 29.3). This will assist in assessment, treatment, and documentation.

Assess and explore the wound fully to establish what type of wound you are dealing with – as well as assessing for underlying structural damage and possible foreign bodies – and establish the approximate size of the wound (<XFREFF>Figure 29.1). Before you start to explore the wound, it is important that you explain the process to your patient and obtain verbal consent. It is also beneficial at this point to offer the patient simple analgesia, to allow for a comfortable examination where possible.

Areas of assessment for wounds include:

- History and mechanism. (Is this an open fracture?)
- Location and underlying structures.
- Time of injury.
- Size (accurate measurement) (Figure 29.1).
- Colour and type of tissue bed (erythema, **exudate**, tracking).
- Visible foreign body or underlying structures.
- Neurological deficit or compromise to the area.
- Description of wound edges and surrounding tissue.
- Temperature (hot to touch) (Baranoski and Ayello 2020).

It is inherently difficult for healthcare professionals to identifying common skin conditions (including localised skin/wound infections) in skin of colour, owing to the lack of inclusivity and representation in medical textbooks and practical training, which have historically focused on Caucasian/light skin tones (Perlman et al. 2021). For this reason, it is important that you undertake a thorough clinical assessment and history of your patient; if there is any doubt of infection you should seek further senior support and advice from a practitioner.

Special considerations

Foreign bodies

Ensure that the wound is clear from debris and foreign bodies (FBs) before wound closure or dressing. If you are unable to clean the wound thoroughly or unsure if there is a FB, refer the patient on for further assessment and review (local UTC or ED).

Fractures/bony involvement

Where a wound is present over a bony tender site, an open fracture should be considered until proven otherwise with radiological examination. If able, administration of antibiotics is best practice; follow local policies and antimicrobial guidelines in your area of practice.

Range of movement

If you are able to see underlying visible structures (tendon or ligaments) or there is reduced range of movement (flexion/extension) at the joint of a wound, further investigation and therefore referral will be required.

BOX 29.3 Definitions of common wounds

- Cut (incised wound, incisional wound) – these involve a breach in the skin caused by a sharp edge such as a kitchen knife or glass. The wound edges are well defined and are often straight, with little soft tissue bruising.
- Laceration (Latin *lacerare,* to tear) – a breach in the skin as a result of a fall, a blow from a blunt object, or crushing force. The wound is irregular, with tearing of the tissues.
- Contused wound – a breach in the skin with surrounding bruising.
- Contusion – an area of bruising due to a blunt force, without a break in the skin.
- Haematoma – a subcutaneous collection of blood giving rise to a fluctuant swelling.
- Penetrating wound – a wound with a fine path made by a pointed object, for example, railing spike, knife, or rusty nail.
- Burn – a wound caused by wet heat, dry heat, radiation, electricity, or chemicals.

Tetanus status

All wounds should be thoroughly cleaned and debrided to assist with the prevention of tetanus. Provided that the patient has had a full course of human tetanus immunoglobulin (five doses), it is considered sufficient to give lifetime immunity (Parry 2022). Certain wounds are considered to be tetanus prone:

- Infected wounds
- Puncture wounds
- Wounds contaminated by soil or manure
- Wounds untreated >6 hours

People with these wounds may require passive immunisation with a human tetanus immunoglobulin; if there is any doubt, consult your local UTC or ED for further guidance.

Bite wounds

Any patient who describes a human or animal bite (in particular from a cat or dog) should be assessed further by a practitioner who is able to review the wound and prescribe antibiotics, where appropriate, as these patients are usually commenced on prophylactic antibiotics due to the nature of the wound and the increased risks associated with infection.

Time of injury

A wound that requires suture closure >6 hours is assumed to be infected and therefore it is not always possible or appropriate for a practitioner to commence closure without further discussion with the specialist colleagues such as plastic surgeons. Again, you will need to review your local pathways for further guidance, as some practitioners may close a wound >6 hours old.

Lip wound

If a facial wound crosses the boundaries of the lip, known as the 'vermilion border', these patients should be referred to a plastic surgeon for assessment. This is due to cosmetic implications, as the vermilion boarder must be aligned so that the lip line is smooth. This referral can be made by an autonomous practitioner.

Wound care

Once you have assessed the wound, you should clean it thoroughly with either running drinking water or saline solution (Fernandez et al. 2022). It is important that the wound is cleaned as soon as possible to reduce the risk of infection and to remove any debris or FBs, to allow for adequate healing or wound closure.

Following your assessment of the wound, you may have decided that further assessment or wound closure is required. If the wound is open and requires closure, a non-absorbent dressing soaked in saline or drinking water is preferable. This will allow the wound to be covered, reduce infection, control bleeding, prevent the dressing adhering to the wound, and allow the wound edges to remain moist, permitting good opposition of wound edges by the preferred method of closure (Wilkins 2014). Wound closure can be achieved by many different methods:

- Sutures
- Staples
- Tissue adhesive (glue)
- Steristrips
- SkinLink

Following further assessment by the autonomous practitioner, a decision will be made as to which method of wound closure would be appropriate, based on the information already discussed. All methods of wound closure can be carried out with ease by a practitioner within the community environment, who is trained and competent to do so. If closure of the wound is not required, the patient may benefit from a further assessment at the local UTC, where they would be able to apply the appropriate dressing and refer the patient to another healthcare professional in a few days for further assessment and review (as required).

Ankle injuries

Ankle sprains are one of the most common musculoskeletal injuries and account for up to 5% of all ED visits in the UK annually, which is approximately 5,600 injuries per day (Bestwick-Stevenson et al. 2021). They are regularly reported as one of the most common sports-related injuries, with around a quarter of injuries across all sports being ankle sprains (Palmer-Green et al. 2016). However, there is very little in the way of specific education in their treatment offered to paramedics. As discussed earlier in this chapter, it is important to obtain a clear history and mechanism of injury from the patient and any bystanders. Doing so will help with diagnosis, treatment plan, and referral options to best meet the patient's clinical needs (Delahunt 2018).

An x-ray image of the ankle is required only if the patient presents with tenderness in either the posterior edge or tip of the malleolus (a and b) or is unable to put weight on the ankle. An x-ray image of the foot is required only if the

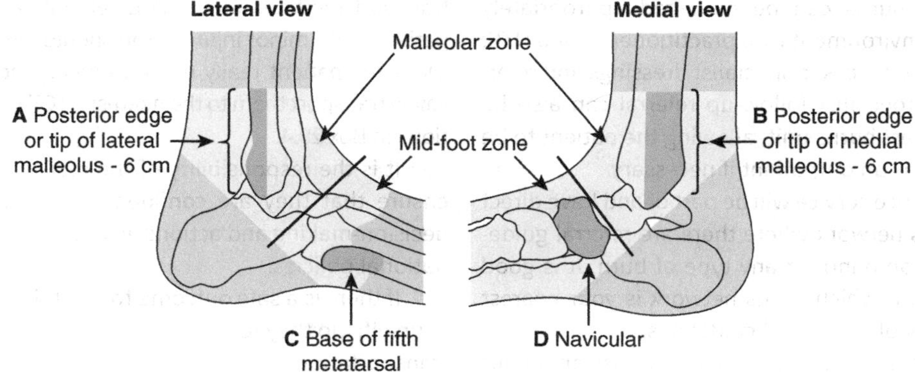

FIGURE 29.3 The Ottawa Ankle Rules.

patient presents with tenderness in either the base of fifth metatarsal (c) or the navicular (d) or is unable to bear weight.

Once you have established a clear history and mechanism of injury, you will need to undertake a thorough clinical assessment using the Look, Feel, Move approach. Before you start your examination, it is important to explain the process to your patient, obtain verbal consent, and offer simple analgesia.

Assessment of an ankle injury should be guided by the Ottawa Ankle Rules (Figure 29.3), guidelines developed to aid EPs in deciding when to use radiography for patients with injuries to the ankle. Stiell et al. (1994) showed that these rules led to a decrease in the use of ankle radiography, waiting times, and costs, without patient dissatisfaction or missed fractures. The rules can be used by paramedics within the OOH environment as an aid to clinical decision-making.

Using the Ottawa Ankle Rules as an aid to examination will allow for safe diagnosis and appropriate treatment of ankle injury. If, following your examination, you have excluded a bony injury and the need for ankle radiography, a referral to your local UTC or GP for further advice and physiotherapy (as required) would be appropriate. It is important to understand that although your patient may not have a bony injury, they could be experiencing ligamentous injury. These are graded according to the severity of the injury, and such patients should still be reviewed by your local UTC or ED.

Minor burns

Minor burns and scalds particularly in children are a common occurrence in the OOH setting. It is important to assess each burn individually and commence rapid treatment to minimise the risks of complications such as scarring, blistering, and infection. Consider the six-stage treatment plan for minor burns shown in Table 29.1.

TABLE 29.1 Six-stage treatment plan for minor burns.

Stage	Treatment	
1	**Cooling**	Cool the affected body area for a minimum of 20 minutes, ideally with cool running water. Remove any non-adherent clothing and jewellery
2	**Analgesia**	Burns are very painful, and it is important to **administer appropriate analgesics** as soon as possible
3	**Assessment**	Assess the burn thoroughly. Does the burn require further assessment or treatment? If so, be guided by your local referral guidelines Elevate any effected limbs to reduce any swelling
4	**Cover**	Cover the burn with loose, longitudinal strips of plastic wrap (i.e. Cling Film) and cover the plastic wrap with a wet dressing to keep the affected area cool. You may have to continue cooling on route to hospital using 0.9% sodium chloride Remember **do not** cover facial areas with plastic wrap
5	**Consideration**	Consider complications such as ABCs (airway, breathing, circulation), hypothermia, intravenous fluid challenge, nonaccidental injury. A full primary and secondary assessment must be carried out on all burn patients, to establish any potential complications
6	**Review**	Continually review and assess

Source: Adapted from London and South East Burns Network (LSEBN) 2018.

Most minor burns can be managed appropriately within the OOH environment by a practitioner or at a UTC, where there will be access to specialist dressings and referral pathways. A specialist follow-up referral can also be made to the nearest burns unit, allowing the patient to be assessed further as an outpatient if necessary.

Each ambulance service will be part of and have direct access to a burns network where there are referral guidelines and advice on hand for any type of burn. It is good practice to find out which burns network is your nearest and obtain a copy of its referral guidelines.

There has been a good deal of discussion about whether blisters should be removed. The London and South East Burns Network (LSEBN 2018) recommends that burn blisters over the size of the patient's little fingernail should be 'de-roofed'. This is not generally a skill performed by an ambulance paramedic and therefore should not be performed unless the individual has the knowledge, skill, competency, and governance to support this procedure. This skill can, however, be performed by a practitioner within your local UTC or ED.

Transporting minor injury patients

Paramedics must possess the confidence, knowledge, and competence to make decisions regarding suitable alternative transport methods for onward referrals and treatment for patients with minor injuries. You should always ask yourself: 'Does my patient really need an emergency ambulance to safely transport them to the nearest UTC?' Consider the questions in Box 29.4.

It is the responsibility of the registered paramedic to ensure that they are confident and competent in their decision-making and actions, in accordance with local and national policies.

If there is a safe outcome to all of these questions, ask yourself: 'Do they really need an emergency ambulance for transportation?'

Conclusion

This chapter has outlined methods of minor injury assessment and treatment in everyday paramedic practice and has indicated the different referral pathways available to paramedics, supported by their UTC or practitioners, to make sound clinical and patient-focused decisions in order to achieve the best outcomes.

BOX 29.4 Transport considerations for minor injury patients

Question	Response	Safe outcome
Is the patient clinically stable? Have you ruled out all 'red flags'?	Yes	✓
Does the patient have capacity?	Yes	✓
Do they require any ongoing treatment en route?	No	✓
Are they likely to deteriorate en route following their current injury?	No	✓
Have they been administered any analgesia such as intravenous morphine to manage their pain?	No	✓
Have you given the patient verbal and written 'safety netting' advise?	Yes	✓
Will they be safe via another method of transport? (relative, patient transport service, car, taxi)?	Yes	✓
Does your local policy/guidance support non-ambulance transport?	Yes	✓

Activities

Now review your learning by completing the learning activities in this chapter. The answers to these appear at the end of the book. Futher self-test activities can be found at **www.wileyfunrdamentalseries.com/paramedic/3e.**

Test your knowledge

1. Define 'mechanism of injury'.
2. List the characteristics of a Look, Feel, Move assessment.
3. Define the Ottawa Ankle Rules.
4. List the six-stage treatment plan for a minor burn.
5. Identify the referral criteria for an UTCs in relation to minor injuries.
6. What are the five wound-closure methods available in the OOH setting?
7. What are the five considerations during a nose injury assessment?

Activity 29.1

Based on your prior experiences, write a detailed history using the 'medical model' approach to history taking. This should be based on a patient where you have been involved in the assessment or treatment process of an injury.

Activity 29.2

1. What is a haematoma?
2. What is a penetrating injury?
3. What is a contused wound?

Activity 29.3

Describe the different characteristics of the types of wounds you could encounter in your role as a paramedic and the considerations for these wounds.

Activity 29.4

1. Ankle injuries are commonly caused by which mechanism?
2. Do you need to gain verbal consent from your patient before assessing the limb?
3. What guidelines should guide the paramedic when treating an ankle injury?

Activity 29.5

Reflect on a variety of patients you have attended recently. Could any of them have been managed at home or by an alternative care pathway?

Contact your local UTCs and practitioner(s) and find out what their referral criteria are for minor injuries. You may be surprised by what they can do to help!

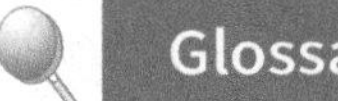

Glossary

Acute anaemia: Anaemia caused by internal bleeding resulting from the rupture of a blood vessel.

Advanced clinical practitioner (ACP): An experienced practitioner (paramedic, nurse, physiotherapist) who has undertaken a master's degree or approved equivalent in a subject relevant to their practice. They will have acquired and continue to demonstrate an expert knowledge base, complex decision-making skills, competence, and judgement in their area of advanced practice.

Autonomous practitioner: A practitioner with the authority to make decisions and the freedom to act in accordance with their professional knowledge and competence.

Capillary refill time: The time taken for a distal capillary bed to regain its colour after pressure has been applied to cause blanching. On a healthy person/limb this should be <2 seconds.

Integrated care board (ICB): A statutory NHS organisation that is responsible for developing a plan for meeting the health needs of the population, managing the NHS budget, and arranging for the provision of health services in a geographical area.

Clinical governance board: A multidisciplinary team of senior clinicians and managers who ensure patients receive the highest possible quality of care.

Emergency practitioner (EP): A paramedic or nurse who has studied at a higher academic level and works to a medical model, with the attitude, skills, and knowledge to deliver holistic care and treatment within the OOH, primary, and acute care settings with a level of autonomy for minor injuries/illness.

Epistaxis: A nosebleed or haemorrhage from the nose, usually due to the rupture of small vessels overlying the anterior part of the cartilaginous nasal septum.

Erythema: Redness of the skin caused by dilatation and congestion of the capillaries, often a sign of inflammation or infection.

Exudate: A fluid that has exuded out of a tissue or its capillaries due to injury or inflammation.

Ligamentous: Referring to a sheet or band of tough, fibrous tissue connecting bones or cartilages at a joint or supporting an organ.

Lymphangitis: Inflammation of a lymphatic vessel.

Mechanism of injury: The circumstance in which an injury occurs, for example, sudden deceleration, wounding by a projectile, or crushing by a heavy object.

Musculoskeletal: Referring to the system of muscles and tendons and ligaments and bones and joints and associated tissues that move the body and maintain its form.

Septal haematoma: A mass of extravasated blood that is confined within the nasal septum.

Specialist practitioner (SP): A paramedic or nurse who has undertaken, or is working towards, a postgraduate diploma in a subject relevant to their practice. They will have acquired and continue to demonstrate an enhanced knowledge base, complex decision-making skills, competence, and judgement in their area of specialist practice.

Tracking: Line of least resistance taken by pus from abscess cavity to exterior surface/internal cavity/remote site.

Two-point discrimination: Ability to discern that two nearby objects touching the skin are two distinct points, not one.

Urgent treatment centres (UTC): Operating a minimum of 12 hours a day, 7 days a week, integrated with local urgent care services and offering urgent and emergency care to patients who do not need hospital treatment by a wider range of multidisciplinary clinicians, with access to diagnostic facilities.

References

Australian Bureau of Statistics (ABS). (2022) National, state and territory population. ABS. Available at: https://www.abs.gov.au/statistics/people/population/national-state-and-territory-population/mar-2022#data-download (accessed April 2023).

Baranoski, S. and Ayello, E. (2020). *Wound Care Essentials: Practice Principles. 5e*. Philadelphia, PA: Lippincott Williams & Wilkins.

Baker, C. (2023). NHS key statistics: England. House of Commons Library. Available at: https://commonslibrary.parliament.uk/research-briefings/cbp-7281 (accessed 18 October 2023).

Basheeth, N., Donnelly, M., Smyth, D. et al. (2015). Acute nasal fracture management: a prospective study and literature review. *The Laryngoscope* **125:** 2677–2684.

Bestwick-Stevenson, T., Wyatt, L.A., Palmer, D. et al. (2021). Incidence and risk factors for poor ankle functional recovery, and the development and progression of posttraumatic ankle osteoarthritis after significant ankle ligament injury (SALI): the SALI cohort study protocol. *BMC Musculoskeletal Disorders* **22** (1): 362.

College of Paramedics (2018). *Paramedic Post Registration – Career Framework., 4e*. Bridgewater: College of Paramedics.

Denness, C. (2013). What are consultation models for? *InnovAiT* **6** (9): 592–599.

Delahunt, E., Bleakley, C., Bossard, D. et al. (2018) Clinical assessment of acute lateral ankle sprain injuries (ROAST): 2019 consensus statement and recommendations of the International Ankle Consortium. *British Journal Sports Medicine* **52** (20): 1304–1310.

Fernandez, R., Green, H.L., Griffiths, R. et al (2022). The effects of water compared with other solutions for wound cleansing. *Cochrane Database of Systematic Reviews* **9**: CD003861. doi: 10.1002/14651858.CD003861.pub4

Ghaye, T. (2011). *Teaching and Learning Through Reflective Practice: A Practical Guide for Positive Action. 2e*. London: Routledge.

HCPC (Health Care Professions Council) (2016). Standards of conduct, performance and ethics. Available at: https://www.hcpc-uk.org/standards/standards-of-conduct-performance-and-ethics/ (accessed 23 March 2023).

Joint Royal Colleges Ambulance Liaison Committee (2023). *UK Ambulance Services Clinical Practice Guidelines*. Bridgewater: Class Professional Publishing.

London and South East Burns Network (LSEBU). (2018). Health Care Professional – downloads. Available at: https://www.mysurgerywebsite.co.uk (accessed 23 March 2023).

National Institute for Health and Care Excellence (NICE). (2019). Head injury: assessment and early management. Available at: https://www.nice.org.uk/guidance/cg176 (accessed March 2023).

National Institute for Health and Care Excellence (NICE). (2022). Management of an acute epistaxis. Available at: https://cks.nice.org.uk/topics/epistaxis-nosebleeds/management/acute-epistaxis/ (accessed March 2023).

NHS England. (2019). The NHS Long Term Plan. Available at: https://www.longtermplan.nhs.uk/publication/nhs-long-term-plan/ (accessed March 2023).

NHS England. (2020). Transformation of urgent and emergency care: models of care and measurement. Available at: https://www.england.nhs.uk/wp-content/uploads/2020/12/transformation-of-urgent-and-emergency-care-models-of-care-and-measurement.pdf (accessed March 2023).

Palmer-Green, D.S., Batt, M.E., and Scammell, B.E. (2016). Simple advice for a simple ankle sprain? The not so benign ankle injury. *Osteoarthritis Research Society International* **24** (6): 947–948.

Parkinson. B., Meacock, R., Checkland, K. et al. (2021). Clarifying the concept of avoidable emergency department attendance. *Journal of Health Services Research & Policy* **26** (1): 68–73.

Parry, C. (2022) Tetanus. *British Medical Journal* best practice. Available at: https://bestpractice.bmj.com/topics/en-gb/220 (accessed March 2023).

Perlman, K.L., Williams, N.M., Egbeto, I.A. et al. (2021) Skin of colour lacks representation in medical student resources: a cross-sectional study. *International Journal of Women's Dermatology* **7:** 195–196.

Purcell, D. (2022). *Minor Injuries: A Clinical Guide*. 4e. Oxford: Churchill Livingstone.

Razavi, A., Farboud, A., Skinner, R. et al. (2014). Acute nasal injury. *British Medical Journal* **349** (18): g6537.

Rickenbach, M. (2019). Enhancing the medical consultation with prior questions including ideas, concerns and expectations. *Future Healthcare Journal* **6** (1): s181.

Stiell, I., McKnight, R., Greenberg, G. et al. (1994). Implementation of the Ottawa Ankle Rules. *Journal of the American Medical Association* **271** (16): 827–832.

CHAPTER 30

Major incident management

Brian J. Sengstock

Charles Sturt University, Port Macquarie, New South Wales, Australia

Contents

LEARNING OUTCOMES

On completion of this chapter the reader will be able to:

- Define what constitutes a major incident in a paramedic context.
- Discuss the approach to declaring a major incident.
- Apply the adult triage process in a paramedic context.
- Recognise approaches to paramedic scene management at a major incident.
- Discuss the different tiers of incident management employed in response to a major incident.

Case study

On 20 January 2017, a vehicle was observed doing burnouts at the intersection of Swanston and Flinders Streets in the Melbourne CBD, sending pedestrians running. The vehicle then drove north along Swanston Street, turning left into the Bourke Street pedestrian mall, continuing west at high speed along Bourke Street for three blocks, before being stopped on Bourke Street just west of William Street. Initial emergency calls suggest there are as many as 50 people injured, with reports of gunshots being heard. Subsequent reports indicated that the vehicle killed 6 people and led to 37 others being hospitalised for their injuries. The youngest victim was only 3 months old (*DPP v Gargasoulas* [2019] VSC 87).

Within six minutes the first ambulance arrived on scene. If you and your partner were this crew, would you know what to do?

Fundamentals of Paramedic Practice: A Systems Approach, Third Edition. Edited by Sam Willis and Ian Peate.

Companion website: www.wiley.com/go/willis/paramedic3e

Introduction

As emergency health professionals, paramedics have a responsibility to ensure their preparedness to respond to a major incident. Whilst major incidents are a rare occurrence, when they do occur, they can place significant stress on the resources available for the response. In defining a major incident, this chapter adopts the definition proposed by Gleeson and Mackway-Jones (2023a, p. 3), which defines a major incident as being 'any incident where the location, number, severity, or type of live casualties requires *extraordinary resources*'. Gleeson and Mackway-Jones' (2023a) inclusion of 'extraordinary resources' is significant to the definition of a major incident as this qualifier effectively removes any specific threshold beyond which an incident is deemed to be a major incident. Using this definition allows for consideration of the resources that are normally available in the area where the incident has occurred. The resources available to respond to an incident in a large urban or metropolitan centre will be far different to those available in a small rural town. This definition also allows for a distinction between the definition of a major incident for the responding agencies as depending on the nature of the incident, it may not require 'extraordinary resources' from all of the responding agencies.

This chapter will consider the techniques that paramedics can use for the safe management of a major incident scene, including the requirement for effective on-scene command of resources and the need for communication within the organisation and beyond in relation to the incident. Approaches to casualty management through the use of triage, treatment, and transport are considered. The use of incident management systems and the tiers of incident command are then discussed. The chapter concludes with a brief consideration of emergency management arrangements surrounding the elements of preparedness, planning response, and recovery as applicable to a major incident.

The nature of a major incident

The causes of major incidents are classified under two broad categories: natural and generated (Table 30.1). No-notice incidents occur with little or no warning, whilst rising-tide incidents have a slow onset, producing a surge in the number of casualties over time.

TABLE 30.1 **Classification of disasters.**

Natural disasters	Human-generated disasters
No-notice incidents	
Earthquakes	Transport/vehicular crashes
Landslides	Structural fires
Floods	Structural collapse
Cyclones/hurricanes/tornadoes	Mining accidents
Heatwaves	Hazardous materials release
Bushfires	Radiation accidents
Volcanic eruptions	Terrorism
Pandemics/epidemics	War/complex humanitarian emergencies
Rising-tide incidents	
Pandemics/epidemics	Hazardous materials release Radiation accidents

Source: Adapted from Conlon et al. 2019.

As a major incident escalates, the available resources of the responding agencies can be rapidly exhausted. If the ambulance response capability is overwhelmed, paramedics may be faced with a situation where they are unable to provide the level of patient care that would normally be provided to patients. The management of a major incident response should therefore focus on two key elements in the response phase: the efficient management of available resources to minimise the reduction in patient care and, when this is not possible, ensuring that the limited resources are applied to ensure the greatest benefit for the greatest number of people. Paramedic approaches to ensuring this goal is achieved are discussed later in this chapter.

The nature of major incidents is such that they can occur anywhere, at any time, with all available resources required to manage the event. Despite major incident management being a specialist field, requiring specialist training and practice to maintain competency, paramedics at all levels should understand the principles of major incident management and their role within the major incident plans that operate in their jurisdiction.

First ambulance arriving on scene: managing the incident site

The first ambulance crew to arrive on site at a major incident adopts the command and triage responsibilities for the incident. The most senior paramedic on the crew will adopt the command responsibilities, whilst the second paramedic on the crew will take on the triage responsibilities, commencing the **Sieve** and **Sort processes.** Information gained during the initial Sieve of the casualties – casualty numbers, priorities, and mechanisms of injury – needs to be communicated to the paramedic who has adopted the command responsibilities. They will communicate information about the incident to the ambulance communications centre through a preliminary assessment of the incident. The use of the mnemonic METHANE is recommended to ensure a clear, concise communication. This initial communication is vital in activating predetermined emergency response plans to ensure that an appropriate major incident response from ambulance services, emergency services, hospitals, and other key emergency management stakeholders occurs in a timely manner.

Major incident declaration: METHANE

The mnemonic METHANE is widely used across ambulance services in Australia, New Zealand, and the UK, allowing for the use of a common communication model to pass information between the incident scene, major incident management centres, and other organisations involved in the response to the incident (JESIP 2016; Gleeson and Mackway-Jones 2023b). Figure 30.1 demonstrates the structure of METHANE with guidance on each element.

The ambulance command role assumes responsibility for the provision of the METHANE report as well as operational command. Consideration needs to be given to overall scene management along with the establishment of a forward control point, ambulance command post, ambulance parking and access point, triage, and transport areas, as well as a body holding area. As no two incidents are the same, the specific requirements for each incident will vary. This requires a high level of situational awareness and a constant reassessment of the incident scene to ensure that the scene layout can be managed according to the requirements of the specific incident. Major incident scenes are dynamic in nature and the requirements for and location of each key location will vary based on the specific requirements of a scene. The ambulance commander for the incident should engage and liaise with the commander/s from the other agencies responding to the incident, with the nature of the incident determining the lead agency, and potentially requiring reassessment of key locations at an incident.

Practice insight

Maintaining situational awareness of an incident scene (and of the general environment) is imperative as the situation can change rapidly, particularly in the initial stages of a major incident. Regularly assessing the HANE (the second half of METHANE) elements ensures that commanders are continually evaluating the situation and reporting this information to the control centre. This ensures that the higher-level commanders (and other agencies) have sufficient information for continued decision-making. Early and frequent communication is often more effective than waiting to confirm exact details.

The transport area at a major incident also serves as a secondary triage (Sort) and treatment area ahead of casualties being transported from the scene. It is important that

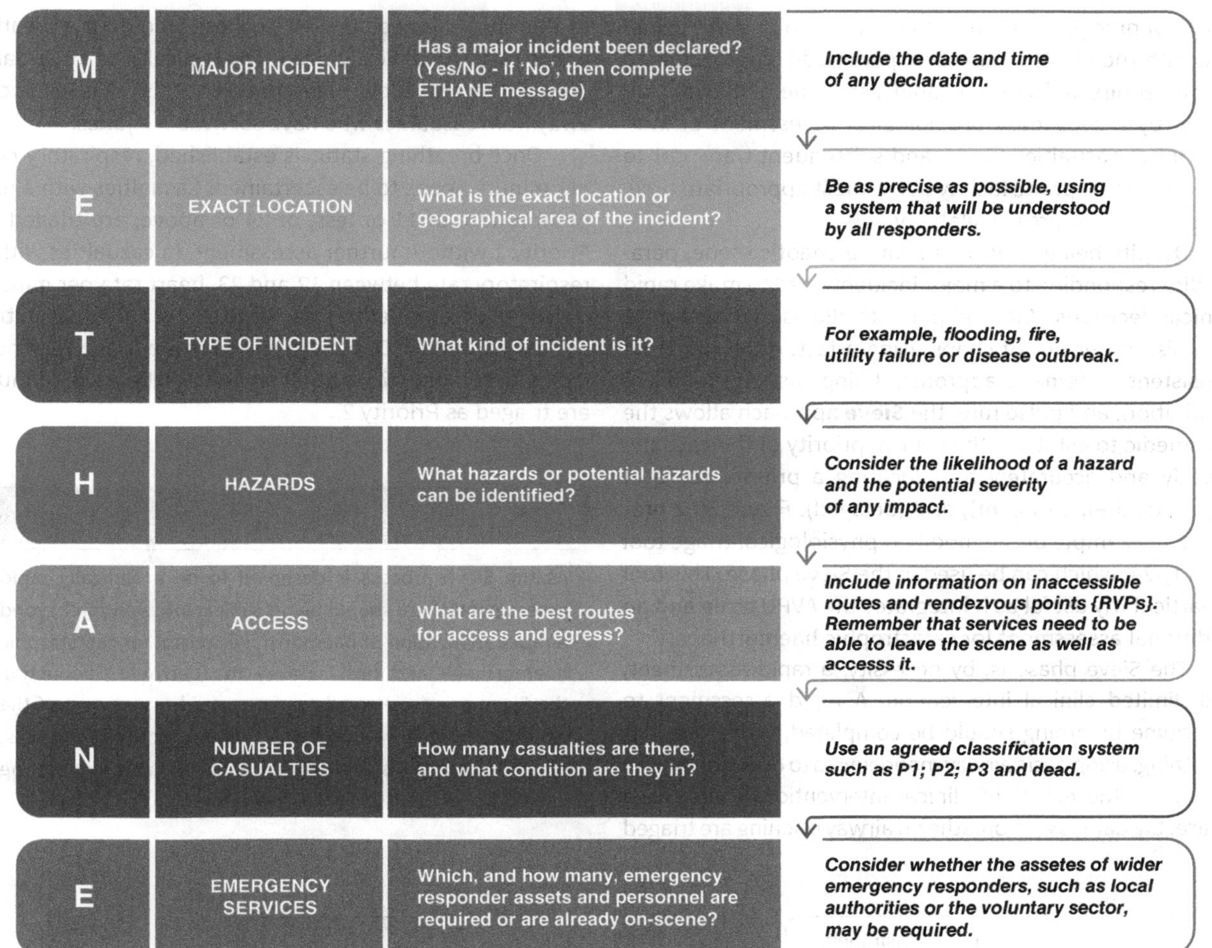

M
MAJOR INCIDENT
Has a major incident been declared? (Yes/No - If 'No', then complete ETHANE message)
Include the date and time of any declaration.
E
EXACT LOCATION
What is the exact location or geographical area of the incident?
Be as precise as possible, using a system that will be understood by all responders.
T
TYPE OF INCIDENT
What kind of incident is it?
For example, flooding, fire, utility failure or disease outbreak.
H
HAZARDS
What hazards or potential hazards can be identified?
Consider the likelihood of a hazard and the potential severity of any impact.
A
ACCESS
What are the best routes for access and egress?
Include information on inaccessible routes and rendezvous points {RVPs}. Remember that services need to be able to leave the scene as well as accesss it.
N
NUMBER OF CASUALTIES
How many casualties are there, and what condition are they in?
Use an agreed classification system such as P1; P2; P3 and dead.
E
EMERGENCY SERVICES
Which, and how many, emergency responder assets and personnel are required or are already on-scene?
Consider whether the assetes of wider emergency responders, such as local authorities or the voluntary sector, may be required.

FIGURE 30.1 Joint Emergency Service Interoperability Principles (JESIP) METHANE model. Source: Reproduced with permission of JESIP 2016.

the transport area is safe, well-lit, and has adequate access and egress to/from the triage area or scene and to/from the ambulance loading point. Once established, the transport area should have different zones for the various priorities (red/yellow/green), with these areas clearly identified and marked.

Practice insight

The commander needs to continually review workloads and resource allocation as an incident evolves. Systematic allocation of resources is essential to prevent duplication of effort and to ensure that no tasks are missed as the response escalates. As the incident response scales down, the commander continues reviewing resourcing and stands down crews as appropriate to reduce the logistical burden.

Casualty management

Triage

Originating in the military, the goal of triage was the treatment of the less severely wounded, and returning them to battle, before engaging in the treatment of severely wounded individuals. This approach assisted with maintaining a battle-capable force, whilst minimising the use of valuable resources on non-survivable injuries. In a contemporary civilian context, the use of triage at a major incident is aimed at achieving the greatest good for the greatest number of casualties. This contrasts with routine incidents where the most critical casualties receive the highest level of care and the most resources.

Mass casualty incident management systems, based on major incident medical management and support

(MIMMS) practices, are utilised in Australia and the UK. In line with the MIMMS approach, paramedic approaches to triage require a focus on rapid assessment (Sieve), followed by a secondary physiological assessment of individual live casualties (Sort), and subsequent transport to the most appropriate facility at the most appropriate time, considering resource availability.

Despite being confronted with a chaotic scene, paramedics responding to a major incident need to make rapid clinical decisions. 'Sieving' patients allows paramedics to establish order out of chaos using a fast, easy, safe, and consistent systematic approach. Using casualty mobility, respiration, and pulse rate, the **Sieve** approach allows the paramedic to establish the clinical priority of the casualty quickly and accurately by allocating a priority score of 1 (immediate), 2 (urgent), or 3 (delayed). Figure 30.2 provides an example of the modified physiological triage tool (MPTT)-24, which can be used in the Sieve phase. This tool is particularly useful as it integrates the AVPU scale and an additional assessment for catastrophic haemorrhage.

The Sieve phase is, by necessity, a rapid assessment, with limited clinical intervention. A rapid assessment to determine breathing should be completed, if they are not breathing, using basic airway manoeuvres to open the airway should be the extent of clinical intervention in the Sieve phase. Casualties who breathe on airway opening are triaged as Priority 1 (immediate), whilst those who do not breathe are considered clinically dead. The clinically dead casualty does not receive active resuscitation as this takes resources away from casualties who have survivable injuries.

Once breathing status is established, respiratory rate per minute needs to be ascertained. Casualties with a respiratory rate of 11 or less, or 24 or above, are triaged as Priority 1 without further assessment. In casualties with a respiratory rate between 12 and 23, heart rate per minute is used to determine the final Sieve score. Those casualties with a heart rate >100 beats per minute are triaged as Priority 1, whilst those with a heart rate of <100 beats per minute are triaged as Priority 2.

Practice insight

As the Sieve process is designed to be a clinically rapid assessment, there should be no clinical intervention beyond a rapid application of haemorrhage control for catastrophic haemorrhage and basic airway manoeuvres. Conducting the Sieve process also allows for a rapid assessment of the situation to assist with determining appropriate resources, emergency response from other agencies, and informs the development of an initial METHANE report.

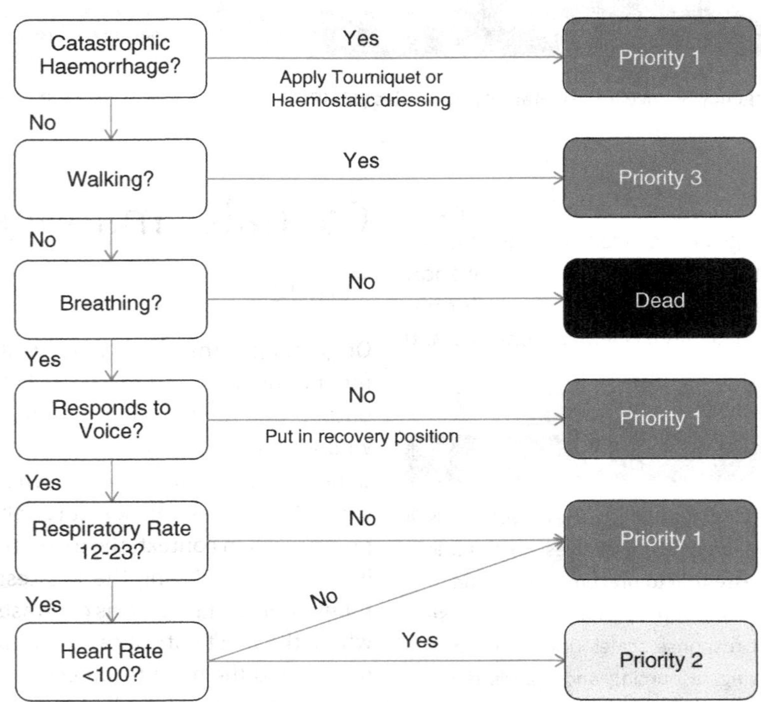

FIGURE 30.2 Modified physiological triage tool (MPTT)-24. Source: Vassallo, Smith, and Wallis 2018/CC BY 4.0.

Sort

The Sieve transitions into the Sort phase, which provides for a comprehensive physiological assessment of casualties using a modified Triage Revised Trauma Score (TRTS) (Champion et al. 1989; Mohammed et al. 2022). The TRTS assesses Glascow Coma Scale (GCS), respiratory rate, and systolic blood pressure to assign a numerical score to each casualty (Table 30.2). The TRTS has undergone rigorous validation for use as an independent predictor of survivability and mortality of trauma casualties over more than 30 years (Lichtveld et. al. 2008; Mohammed et al. 2022). Using the TRTS in the initial Sort, and subsequent reassessments of casualties, allows for a reprioritisation of casualties. Furthermore, the TRTS also provides paramedics with a tool for making evidence-based decisions around the appropriateness of the destination facility, based on injury severity. Lichtveld et al. (2008) and Mohammed et al. (2022) indicate that the survival rate of critically injured casualties is significantly improved when they are sorted to a multidisciplinary trauma centre, following the use of the modified TRTS in the Sort process.

Paramedics can calculate the TRTS for a casualty by adding the score for each clinical measurement to obtain a number between 0 and 12, allowing for a revision of the casualties' priority score assigned during the Sieve. Casualties with a score of 10 or less are allocated a Priority 1; a score of 11, Priority 2; and those receiving a score of 12 are allocated to Priority 3hree. A fourth, expectant priority (expectation of death) for casualties who receive a TRTS score of between 1 and 3 is proposed by Carley and Mackway-Jones (2018). At this time, the expectant priority is not widely used in Australia or the UK in the out-of-hospital setting.

TABLE 30.2 **Modified TRTS.**

Clinical Measurement	Parameter	Score
GCS	13–15	4
	9–12	3
	6–8	2
	4–5	1
	3	0
Respiratory rate (breaths/minute)	10–29	4
	>29	3
	6–9	2
	1–5	1
	0	0
Systolic blood pressure (mmHg)	>90	4
	76–89	3
	50–75	2
	1–49	1
	0	0

Source: Adapted from Gleeson and Mackway-Jones 2023d and Champion et al. 1989.

Paediatric patients

Paramedics must be consciously aware of not being distracted by paediatric casualties at a major incident. A focus on paediatric casualties, at the expense of adults who may be survivable with minimal clinical interventions during the Sieve, can result in higher adult mortality rates. By design, triage Sieve and Sort processes are based on adult physiological parameters. Applying these parameters to paediatric casualties results in a 'false high' triage priority. 'False high' triage of paediatric casualties can adversely impact the availability of specialist paediatric resources due to over triaging, leading to a reduction in the capacity of these specialist facilities to deal with genuine, high priority paediatric casualties (Gleeson and Mackway-Jones 2023d). The over-prioritisation of paediatric casualties also reduces the resources available to provide care to adult casualties at the scene and during transport, thus resulting in increased adult mortality rates.

In response to concerns about the probable over-prioritisation of paediatric casualties, MIMMS best practice is now considered to be the use of a paediatric triage tape. Paediatric triage tapes are based on an assertion that a paediatric casualty's length is proportional to age, weight, and vital signs (Gleeson and Mackway-Jones 2023d). Placing the triage tape directly beside the paediatric casualty allows the paramedic to determine a modified triage score by correlating the casualty's length against the predetermined vital signs displayed on the paediatric triage tape. This ensures an accurate, paediatric-specific triage priority is allocated minimising the risk of over-prioritisation of paediatric casualties.

Triage tags

Individual casualty priority needs to be clearly displayed to ensure the triage assessment is communicated to all rescue and medical personnel. Triage labelling generally uses highly visible triage tags, whilst also allowing for any alteration of priority to be easily reflected. Tags must be adequately secured to the casualty so as to not be lost during subsequent movement of the casualty, or during transport.

Triage tags provide 'trending' information from the time of the initial Sieve to when the casualty arrives at the receiving facility and beyond.

Treatment on scene

Resource availability and casualty priority are key considerations in the clinical management of casualties, with treatment at the scene being aimed at the provision of life-saving clinical interventions and stabilisation to allow for safe transportation, whilst minimising the risk of exacerbating the casualty's injury profile. Optimal medical management occurs when the treatment is kept at this level – if not enough is done, there is a risk of unnecessary death; if too much is done, then the time spent with that casualty could lead to the needless death of other casualties (Gleeson and Mackway-Jones 2023e).

Transport

Whilst triage and treatment are both important considerations, decisions regarding transport and destination facilities are also key considerations in casualty management. Early consideration needs to be given to transport, along with possible receiving facilities for casualties, to provide as much advance warning as possible to allow the facilities to activate surge capacity. Transporting the right casualty, at the right time, to the right facility is a critical consideration. Transport decisions are complex and intertwined, there is no one single influencing factor that directs the decision-making process in this type of incident. Considering the casualty injury profile, age, gender, triage priority, stabilisation required for transport, and the number of each triage priority that a facility can manage is essential when making transport decisions. An awareness of the surge capacity available at a facility can assist in decision-making; for instance, a facility may have rapid surge capacity to accept Priority 2 or Priority 3 casualties but limited rapid surge capacity to accommodate an influx of Priority 1 casualties due to the staffing mix available at the facility.

Where possible, it is generally preferable to select a specialist paediatric facility for paediatric casualties, although the severity of the injuries, or a lack of specialist paediatric facilities, will influence transport decisions in these cases. Casualties with significant head injuries are best transported to a tertiary neurological trauma centre or regional trauma centre, whilst patients with severe burns will benefit from transport to a burns centre. Paramedics should have a sound operational knowledge of the facilities in their area and the capabilities of the local facilities. Priority 3 casualties may not necessarily need to be transported to a hospital in the first instance and consideration should be given to directing these lower priority casualties to local medical facilities in the community such as GP clinics. This assists with minimising the impact of a surge of lower priority casualties on the receiving hospital's capacity to manage the higher priority casualties that will be transported. Selecting the right facility for the right casualty at the right time assists with significantly reducing mortality rates.

Practice insight

Transport priority and timing should be aligned with triage and treatment priority. The reality of clinical practice, however, is that treatment and stabilisation together with the complexities of transport decision-making may permit those with less urgent priority to be transported from the scene first. Priority 3 casualties can generally walk and are often able to be stabilised for transport quickly. Taxis and buses can be used to clear these casualties quickly and effectively from the scene to local medical centres or other health providers with no impact on the transport of higher priority casualties.

Incident management system

From a single crew response, through to a major incident involving a large and complex multi-agency response the principles and processes underpinning the response form an incident management system. Incident management systems ensure a consistent approach, allowing a response to be scaled up, and down, both efficiently and effectively. A key consideration in any incident management system is the division of management responsibility, with a clear delineation of the three key functions of command, control, and co-ordination.

Command refers to the way directions are issued within an organisation. The ambulance commander role will usually be adopted by the highest-ranking paramedic at the incident scene. Responsible for issuing instructions, through the chain of command, the ambulance commander is responsible for paramedic crews on the scene. In a multi-agency response, each agency will have its own chain of command, resulting in a number of commanders in place for any particular incident.

Control is different to command and refers to the overall management of an incident. The authority associated with the control role may be founded in legislation or established by agreement in emergency plans. Police have legislated authority for public safety and a senior police officer will generally assume control of a major incident.

Co-ordination involves the management of resources and information in support of the incident. In the initial stages of an incident, co-ordination may be conducted using routine management systems, with paramedics being allocated across several concurrent emergencies. In mass casualty, or disaster, incidents which are likely to be more significant and protracted in nature, co-ordination is often managed by a co-ordinating group or committee who will meet to consider strategic co-ordination issues.

Larger or more complex incidents require the availability of more management personnel, with the incident controller assuming responsibility for ensuring sufficient command personnel are in place, and the scale-up process is effectively managed. Too many, or too few, staff reporting to a single commander will impact their ability to manage their role, resulting in inefficiencies and poor or miscommunication, both up and down the chain of command. The Australasian Inter-service Incident Management System (AIIMS), the leading incident management system in Australia, suggests a span of control of one supervisor to between three and seven subordinates (AFAC 2017). Managing this 'span of control' is one of the key considerations in the AIIMS approach. AIIMS also implements the principle of 'unity of command', which is underpinned by the principle that each person should report to a single superior. Ensuring a single reporting line eliminates dual reporting relationships, simplifies communication, and provides clarity in the allocation of key tasks.

Decision-making processes

Incident management systems should inform the decision-making process of agencies responding to a major incident. The Joint Decision Model (JDM), which has been adopted in the UK (JESIP 2016), is an example of a tool that can be applied to decision-making processes, regardless of the scale of an incident. A commander at a small incident can use the JDM as a mental checklist in the development of a management plan for an incident. In a multi-agency response, agency commanders can use the JDM to allocate specific components of the decision-making process to command personnel to effectively manage the decision-making process.

A key aspect of the JDM is the development of a working strategy that allows the commander to articulate their intentions for the management of the incident to resolution. This allows for the communication of a clear vision of what needs to be achieved, with the ability to incorporate additional contingencies as required. Figure 30.3 demonstrates the components of the JDM. The AIIMS model adopts a similar approach, referring to 'management by objectives' (AFAC 2017). Commanders using the 'management by objectives' approach should ensure objectives are clearly articulated, and then assess operational progress and performance against these objectives.

Practice insight

It is important to remember that an incident management system is a *tool* to support an effective incident response, and that it should be applied flexibly based on the specific requirements of each incident. As no two incidents are ever the same, incident managers need to consider their actions and decisions in the context of the effect that these will have on the ground, and the overall incident, and then adapt management practices to achieve the desired outcome.

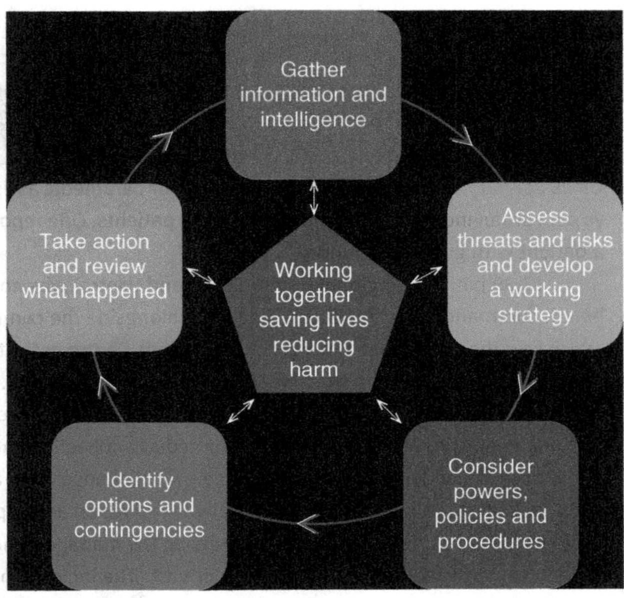

FIGURE 30.3 JDM. Source: Reproduced with permission of JESIP 2016.

Tiers of incident command

Management responsibilities at a major incident are often separated into several tiers as the incident response scales up. Doing so ensures a clear definition of responsibilities, whilst also preventing confusion and duplication of effort. Terminology used to define the tiers varies between jurisdictions, however, the responsibilities are generally the same. The overall response strategy and the allocation of resources to an incident are set at the top-level tier. This strategic level tier is removed from the scene and will usually operate from the organisation's headquarters, or a joint emergency service centre. The next tier is tactical in nature and has direct responsibility for resolving the incident and managing responding personnel. Command at this level is generally performed at the incident scene. If the event is a large scale or protracted incident the command may be performed from a nearby emergency services facility. The final tier is essentially operational, located at the incident scene, with responsibility for the implementation of the response plan. Multiple commanders may be present at this level, with responsibility for different 'sectors' or response functions on scene.

Emergency management

Major incident management occurs within the context of a broader emergency management approach founded in legislative and management arrangements. These legislative and management arrangements provide the basis for how major incidents or disasters are managed, outlining how government, non-government, and private sector entities may work together to manage emergencies, before, during, and after the event. In the Australian context, emergency management is the responsibility of the individual state or territory government, resulting in different approaches to emergency management across the various jurisdictions (Australian Institute for Disaster Resilience 2019). Despite the differences, the legislative arrangements tend to be similar, with most jurisdictions operating on a three-tier management structure involving co-ordination at the local, district, and state/territory level. In responding to large or protracted incidents, there will likely be a co-ordinated response involving all three tiers in order to co-ordinate a multi-agency response to manage strategic issues. The Commonwealth may also become involved following a request for assistance from state/territory governments.

In the UK, emergency management is governed by the Civil Contingencies Act 2004 (Walker and Broderick 2006). Pursuant to the provisions of this Act, organisations with emergency management responsibilities participate in local resilience forums. These groups are focused on the co-ordination of risk assessment, planning, and preparedness and have no operational role in the response and recovery phase of an incident. In an operational context, emergency management is managed through co-ordinating groups operating at the strategic, tactical, and operational levels.

Case study: Bourke Street incident

On 20 January 2017, at 1.34 p.m. the first call for paramedic assistance was received by Ambulance Victoria to respond to a vehicle vs pedestrian incident with approximately 20 patients. One report had as many as 50 patients, with some reports of gun shots and a patient with gunshot wounds.

At 1.39 p.m. the Regional Health Command (Metro) was notified, and an Emergency Response Plan was escalated. The state health commander was briefed at 1.40 p.m., alongside the commencement of a Red escalation of the Emergency Response Plan, which saw the Ambulance Emergency Operations Centre activated and staff allocated to AIIMS roles. The first paramedics arrived on scene at 1.40 p.m., with the first SITREP received at 1.42 p.m. It should be noted that the scaling up of the ambulance response commenced based on initial reports from the scene, with a decision to commence a Red escalation of the Emergency Response Plan made prior to arrival of the first paramedics and well ahead of the first SITREP.

The post-incident review identified several challenges that are typical of major incidents. For example, it was noted that there was a lack of situational awareness, initially there was an assumption that there were two separate incidents as opposed to a single incident spread over several blocks. Identifying the management structure on scene was challenging, as all the managers on scene were wearing the same health commander vest. The incident health commander at the scene also noted that people across the organisation were bypassing the Ambulance Emergency Operations Centre and attempting direct contact to the scene, creating challenges in the management of information and resources.

Conclusion

Major incident management is a complex process that extends the role of the paramedic far beyond the clinical requirements of routine paramedic responses, having implications for on-scene clinical care and the challenges associated with incident command, control, and co-ordination. One of the greatest challenges to paramedics arriving at a major incident is the requirement to abstain from the provision of traditional clinical interventions, which detract from the ideology of 'doing the most good for the greatest number'. This requirement to abstain from the provision of clinical care challenges the paramedics' own ethical principles of non-maleficence and clinical judgement. The use of early reporting through METHANE is crucial in ensuring a strategic and tactical response to a major incident, whilst also maintaining responses to the routine day-to-day operational requirements. Regular engagement with inter-agency responses to simulated incidents, risk assessments and mitigation, and emergency planning are critical elements in ensuring that a robust response is available when a major incident inevitably occurs.

Activities

Now review your learning by completing the learning activities in this chapter. The answers to these appear at the end of the book. Further self-test activities can be found at **www.wileyfundamentalseries.com/paramedic/3e.**

Test your knowledge

1. What is the definition of a major incident?
2. Why is 'extraordinary resources' a key consideration in the definition of a major incident?
3. Apply the Sieve phase of triage to a patient with the following: inability to walk, respiratory rate of 6 breaths per minute, pulse of 130 beats per minute.
4. Apply the Sort phase of triage to a patient with the following: GCS of 12, respiratory rate 34 per/min, systolic blood pressure 80 mmHg.
5. In clinical practice, all patients must be transported in order of their triage priority – true or false?
6. What are the phases of emergency management?
7. Consider the Bourke Street Case study and construct a METHANE situation report based on the information available on arrival at the scene.
8. Command relates to overall control of an incident, and is established in plans or legislation – true or false?
9. Multiple operational commanders can report to a single incident co-ordinator at a major incident – true or false?
10. What is the recommended ratio of operational paramedics to each ambulance commander on scene?

Glossary

Commander:	A member of a responding agency with authority to assume command or control of an incident.
Mass casualty:	An incident that involves multiple injured individuals.
METHANE:	An accepted model for communicating information in relation to a major incident.
Mitigation:	Reducing the severity of something.
Pathophysiology:	Disordered physiological processes associated with injury.
Sieve process:	The initial phase of triage to prioritise individuals involved in a major incident.
Sort process:	The secondary phase of triage involving a formal assessment of everyone to arrive at a revised priority score.
Triage:	Prioritising the degree of urgency based on an individual's injuries in order to determine treatment priority.
Triage Revised Trauma Score (TRTS):	A physiological scoring system to triage patients.

References

AFAC (Australian Fire and Emergency Service Authorities Council). (2017). *The Australasian Inter-Service Incident Management System for any Emergency.* 5e. Melbourne: Australasian Fire and Emergency Service Authorities Council.

Australian Institute for Disaster Resilience (2019). *Australian Disaster Resilience Handbook: Australian Emergency Management Arrangements*. Melbourne: Commonwealth of Australia.

Carley, S. and Mackway-Jones, K. (2018). *Major Incident Medical Management and Support: The Practical Approach in the Hospital.* 2e. *Oxford: Blackwell.*

Champion, H., Sacco, W., Copes, W. et al. (1989). A revision of the trauma score. *Journal of Trauma: Injury, Infection and Critical Care* **29** (5): 623–629. doi: 10.1097/00005373-198905000-00017.

Conlon, L., Clements, A., and Wills, S. (2019). *Major incident preparedness and management*. In: *Emergency and Trauma Care for Nurses and Paramedics* 3e (ed. K. Curtis, C. Ramsden, R.Z. Shaban et al.), pp. 201–242. Elsevier.

DPP v Gargasoulas [2019] *VSC* 87.

Gleeson, T. and Mackway-Jones, K. (2023a). Introduction. In: *Major Incident Medical Management and Support: The Practical Approach at the Scene* 4e (ed. T. Gleeson and K. Mackway-Jones), pp. 3–12. Chichester: Wiley-Blackwell.

Gleeson, T. and Mackway-Jones, K. (2023d). The structured approach to major incidents. In: *Major Incident Medical Management and Support: The Practical Approach at the Scene* 3e (ed. T. Gleeson and K. Mackway-Jones), pp. 13–18. Chichester: Wiley-Blackwell.

Gleeson, T. and Mackway-Jones, K. (2023c). Assessment. In: *Major Incident Medical Management and Support: The Practical Approach at the Scene* 3e (ed. T. Gleeson and K. Mackway-Jones), pp. 89–92. Chichester: Wiley-Blackwell.

Gleeson, T. and Mackway-Jones, K. (2023d). Triage. In: *Major Incident Medical Management and Support: The Practical Approach at the Scene* 4e (ed. T. Gleeson and K. Mackway-Jones), pp. 95–108. Chichester: Wiley-Blackwell.

Gleeson, T. and Mackway-Jones, K. (2023e). Treatment. In: *Major Incident Medical Management and Support: The Practical Approach at the Scene* 4e (ed. T. Gleeson and K. Mackway-Jones), pp. 109–114. Chichester: Wiley-Blackwell.

JESIP (Joint Emergency Services Interoperability Programme) (2016a). *Joint Doctrine: The Interoperability Framework.* 2e. London: Joint Emergency Services Interoperability Programme.

JESIP (2016b). JESIP graphics. Available at: https://www.jesip.org.uk/jesip-graphics (accessed 10 December 2022).

Lichtveld, R., Spijkers, A., Hoogendoorn, J. et al. (2008). Triage revised trauma score change between first assessment and arrival at hospital to predict mortality. *International Journal of Emergency Medicine* **1** (1): 21–26. doi: 10.1007/s12245-008-0013-7.

Linton, N. (2021). The PPRR model in emergencies and disasters: is it relevant today? Available at: https://nlinton.net/pprr-model-emergencies-disasters (accessed 10 December 2022).

Mohammed, Z., Sakleh, Y., AbdselSalam, E.M. et al. (2022). Evaluation of the Revised Trauma Score, MGAP, and GAP scoring systems in predicting mortality of adult trauma patients in low-resource setting. *BMC Emergency Medicine* **22** (90). doi: 10.1186/s12873-022-00653-1.

Vassallo, J., Smith, J.E., and Wallis, L.A. (2018). Major incident triage and the implementation of a new triage tool, the MPTT-24, *Journal of the Royal Army Medical Corps* **164** (2): 103–106. doi: 10.1136/jramc-2017-000819.

Walker, C. and Broderick, J. (2006). *The Civil Contingencies Act 2004: Risk, Resilience, and the Law in the United Kingdom*. Oxford: Oxford University Press.

CHAPTER 31

Low acuity care

Seán Bolger

Registered Nurse and Clinical Educator, St John of God Healthcare, Western Australia, Australia

Contents

LEARNING OUTCOMES

On completion of this chapter the reader will be able to:

- Discuss the term 'low acuity'.
- Understand how to provide low acuity care.
- Identify equipment and technology that can assist in the assessment.
- Gain an understanding of community services available to patients with low-acuity complaints.

Case study

A 32-year-old woman called the ambulance service with a report of urinating more frequently, pain with urination, and feeling lethargic. Upon your arrival, you find her alert and preparing dinner for her children. A comprehensive history is undertaken in which she denies blood in her urine, fevers, chills, flank pain, or vaginal discharge. She reports having experienced similar symptoms a few years ago and that they went away after a course of antibiotics. She has no other co-morbidities. Pertinent history reveals she has been sexually active with her boyfriend for the past four years and uses condoms for contraception. She reports two previous partners and two pregnancies with both live births. She denies any sexually transmitted diseases and her last menstrual period was one week ago. Your physical assessment does not uncover any red flags and you determine the patient is suffering from a urinary tract infection. You contact the patient's doctor and provide a handover of your findings. The doctor organises a prescription for antibiotics to be sent to the local pharmacy. You provide the patient with self-care and safety netting advice before leaving for your next call.

Fundamentals of Paramedic Practice: A Systems Approach, Third Edition. Edited by Sam Willis and Ian Peate.

Companion website: www.wiley.com/go/willis/paramedic3e

Introduction

The purpose of this chapter is to distinguish alternative pathways for those patients that call an ambulance for non-emergency complaints. Reviewing three common non-emergency presentations, we will review the assessment and treatment options available. With increased pressure on emergency departments (EDs), ambulance crews are spending longer at hospitals waiting to handover. When paramedics are unable to handover quickly, it can lead to delays in responding to other emergencies, as well as a shortage of ambulances on the road. Additionally, patients may be left waiting in ambulances for extended periods, which can result in a worsening of their condition. This issue can be compounded by the arrival of additional patients who do not need ED levels of care. Within the UK, it is estimated that more than 1 in 10 ambulances waited over an hour to handover in July 2022. This changed the average dispatch time from 4 minutes to 36 minutes (Alarilla et al. 2022)

What is low acuity care?

Low acuity care in the paramedicine sense refers to care that is designed to treat patients with non-life-threatening illnesses or injuries. This includes conditions such as minor cuts, sprains, colds, and flu-like symptoms. These patients typically do not need hospitalisation or emergency medical attention but still require assessment and treatment.

The aim of low acuity care is to provide treatment in out-of-hospital (OOH) settings such as primary care clinics, urgent care centres, or patients' homes. These settings are typically less expensive and more accessible to patients who do not have a primary care physician or cannot afford to visit an ED in countries that charge for medical treatment such as the US. They often offer flexible appointment hours and shorter wait times, which can be particularly important for patients who require medical attention but have busy schedules due to work or childcare commitments.

One of the key benefits of low acuity care is that it allows for more efficient use of healthcare resources. When patients with non-life-threatening conditions are treated in OOH settings, hospitals can focus on treating more severe cases that require more resources and attention. This can help to reduce the strain on hospital EDs, which are often overcrowded and have long wait times, as well as free up ambulance crews to attend other calls.

Another benefit of low acuity care is that it can help to improve patient outcomes. By providing timely and appropriate care for patients with non-life-threatening conditions, low acuity care can prevent these conditions from worsening and requiring more intensive medical interventions in the future. This can lead to better health outcomes for patients, as well as lower healthcare costs over time.

There are several types of low acuity care providers such as primary care physicians, urgent care centres, retail centres, and specialist paramedics. Primary care physicians are typically the first point of contact for patients seeking medical care and can provide ongoing care for patients with chronic conditions or complex medical needs. Urgent care centres are designed to provide immediate medical attention for patients with non-life-threatening conditions that require prompt attention. Retail clinics are typically located in pharmacies and offer basic medical services such as flu vaccinations, blood pressure checks, and treatment for minor illnesses and injuries. Specialist paramedics or paramedic practitioners are seen in a variety of settings, including general practitioner (GP) surgeries, urgent care centres, out-of-hours services, and ambulance services. They have expertise in health promotion, disease prevention and early identification, lifestyle advice and modification, assessment, treatment, and, where necessary, onwards referrals for acute or chronic health conditions.

History taking

History taking is a vital aspect of the assessment process. It is important to ask clarifying questions during the history taking aspect of your assessment. This allows the paramedic to understand what is meant by each symptom. For example, 'spitting up blood' may be blood arising from the gastrointestinal tract but might also mean blood arising from the respiratory system. Qualify each symptom by learning about the acuity of onset, triggering events, quality, progression, and exacerbating and relieving factors. As you progress through your career you will be able to modify your questioning to more focused questions relevant to the presenting complaint. Combining a thorough history-taking process with a comprehensive clinical examination is central to sound clinical reasoning and establishing an astute differential diagnosis. Reviewing three common non-emergency presentations we will review the assessment and treatment options available.

Urinary tract infection

The term urinary tract infection (UTI) refers to an infection that can occur in any part of the urinary tract, which includes the kidneys, ureters, bladder, and urethra. The urinary tract can be further divided into two parts: the upper tract, which consists of the kidneys and ureters, and the lower tract, which includes the bladder and urethra. A UTI is the most common infection seen in primary care. Infection of the kidney is called pyelonephritis (Medina and Castillo-Pino 2019).

Urological history taking

Some urinary symptom questions that you may ask whilst taking a history include:

- Do you experience any difficulty when trying to urinate?
- How frequently do you urinate?
- Do you wake up during the night to urinate? If so, how often?
- What is the volume of urine you pass each time?
- Do you feel any pain or burning sensations when urinating?
- Do you ever feel the need to rush to the bathroom to urinate?
- Do you ever involuntarily leak urine?
- Can you sense when your bladder is full and when you are urinating?

In the case of female patients, they may be asked if they experience urine loss when coughing, sneezing, or laughing. This is a common experience for around 50% of young women, even before having children. It is important to note that occasional urine leakage may not be significant. For male patients, they may be asked if they have trouble starting their stream, if they need to stand close to the toilet to urinate, if they experience changes in the force or size of their stream, if they need to strain to urinate, if they hesitate or stop in the middle of urination, or if they experience dribbling at the end of urination.

Common symptoms of a UTI include:

- Passing very small amounts of urine.
- Feeling the need or 'urge' to pass urine frequently.
- Feeling that the bladder is still full after passing urine.
- Feeling unwell with nausea and fever.

Pain

Disorders of the urinary tract can cause pain in the abdomen or back, with bladder disorders causing suprapubic pain. Dysuria is pain on urination, often described as a burning sensation caused by irritation or infection of the bladder.

Urgency

Described as the intense and immediate desire to void. UTI can be the cause of urge incontinence and the increased frequency of urination.

Haematuria

Blood in the urine is a major cause for concern among patients. When visible to the naked eye it is called gross haematuria. Blood may be detected only during microscopic urinalysis, known as microscopic haematuria. In women, it is important to distinguish menstrual blood from haematuria. There are also some medications that will turn urine a reddish colour such as Senna or Levodopa, as well as certain foods. The use of a urine dipstick can help differentiate between discolouration and haematuria.

Physical examination

A full set of observations should be undertaken on all patients and should include:

- Respiratory rate
- Oxygen saturation
- Pulse
- Blood pressure
- Temperature
- Pain score
- Blood sugar level

This basic assessment of vital signs can highlight indications of sepsis. A focused assessment of the urinary system includes an abdominal assessment. During this assessment, percussion of the kidney is undertaken to assess for costovertebral angle (CVA) tenderness. This is done by first explaining the procedure to the patient. They then lie down on their side or sit upright with their back straight. The paramedic places the palm of one hand on their flank area just below the lower rib cage and above the hip bone, on the side of the kidney being assessed. The paramedic makes a fist with the other hand and gently strikes the hand that is already on the flank area with the ulnar surface of the fist. This should cause a perceptible but painless jar or thud on the area. If the patient experiences pain or tenderness with pressure or fist percussion, it could indicate inflammation of the renal capsule due to conditions such as pyelonephritis. However, it is important to note that CVA tenderness can also be musculoskeletal in origin, this is why history taking is important in diagnosis. If the patient has associated symptoms such as fever and dysuria, it may increase the likelihood of pyelonephritis as the cause of the CVA tenderness.

Urine dipstick

The urine dipstick test is a simple and quick diagnostic tool that is commonly used in healthcare settings to assess the composition of a patient's urine. The test involves dipping a small plastic strip with several reagent pads into a urine sample and observing the colour changes that occur. The benefits of urine dipstick testing by paramedics include:

Quick results: The dipstick test can provide results within minutes, which allows for prompt diagnosis and treatment.

Non-invasive: The test only requires a small urine sample, which makes it easy to perform and more comfortable for the patient.

Cost-effective: The dipstick test is relatively inexpensive and does not require specialised equipment or training, which makes it a cost-effective diagnostic tool.

Accuracy: A totally negative dipstick test is associated with negative microscopy in 90–95% of cases (Rehmani 2004).

When interpreting the urine dipstick for the presence of UTI, leucocytes and nitrites are examined. Leucocytes detect the presence of whole or broken white cells in the urine. This is an indication of infection; however, there are some foods and drugs that turn urine red and can give a false positive. Nitrites in the urine are found in the presence of Gram-negative bacteria. The presence of nitrites strongly suggests infection (Cadogan and Rogers 2020). Paramedics who are colourblind will have difficulty interrupting the results.

Treatment

Self-care

D-mannose is a kind of sugar that is available in health food shops or pharmacies and is thought to prevent certain kinds of bacteria from sticking to the walls of the urinary tract and preventing colonisation. Advise paracetamol for pain or, if preferred and suitable, ibuprofen. Advise drinking enough fluid to avoid dehydration. There is no evidence found for cranberry products or urine alkalinising agents lowering UTI.

Antibiotics

It is important to adjust antibiotic treatment based on local susceptibility patterns, especially given the increasing prevalence of multi-drug resistant infections. This complexity makes it crucial for clinicians to be aware of the antimicrobial resistance trends among urinary isolates in their region. This knowledge can help guide the appropriate use of antibiotics and inform evidence-based recommendations for empirical treatment of UTIs. This information can be gained from local clinical guidelines. Paramedics who do not have prescribing rights or are not backed by clinical practice guidelines can seek guidance from GP surgeries and urgent care centres. A comprehensive handover to a clinician over the phone or via telehealth may enable the prescribing clinician to organise antibiotics without the patient leaving the house.

Patients may need assessment in the hospital for further investigation if they are displaying the following red flags, due to the risk of further deterioration:

- Are pregnant.
- Older than 65 years or younger than 16 years.
- Have symptoms that are persistent or do not resolve with antibiotic treatment.
- Have recurrent UTI (2 episodes in 6 months or 3 in 12 months).
- Have a urinary catheter in situ or have recently been catheterised.
- Have risk factors for resistance or complicated UTI such as abnormalities of the genitourinary tract, renal impairment, residence in a long-term care facility, hospitalisation for more than seven days in the last six months, recent travel to a country with increased resistance, or previous resistant UTI.
- Have atypical symptoms.

Safety netting advice

It is important the paramedic provides the patient with information on when to seek further review if they do not improve or begin to feel more unwell. This is called safety netting advice and should be given to the patient on when to seek further help. This may include seeking a medical review if patient presents with the following symptoms:

- Have shivering, chills and muscle pain.
- Feel confused or are drowsy.
- Have not passed urine all day.
- Are vomiting.
- Have blood in their urine.
- Have a temperature above 38°C.
- Have kidney pain.
- Symptoms get worse.
- Symptoms are not starting to improve within 48 hours of taking antibiotics.

Falls

The definition of a fall, provided by Public Health England (2018), is when an individual lands on a lower level unintentionally without experiencing any major intrinsic events such as a stroke. Falls in older people are cases regularly seen by paramedics with approximately 8% of emergency ambulances in London UK attending fall-related calls. Of those aged 65 and over, 30% will have one fall per year with this increasing to 50% in those aged over 80 years old. Those that have fallen have a high mortality, morbidity, and immobility rate, and recovery is often delayed especially in older people (Snooks et al. 2017). With the ageing population and associated disease progression, the likelihood of falling increases due to a multitude of risk factors. These include frailty, conditions affecting balance or mobility like diabetes or arthritis, and impairments in cognition or vision. Additionally, the presence of fear of falling or having fallen within the past 12 months, as well as the use of certain medications such as benzodiazepines and antihypertensives or the regular use of more than four medications regardless of their type, are also included as risk factors for falls (NICE 2019).

History taking for the falls patient

Detailed history taking is an essential component in finding the cause of the fall. Thorough history provides insights into red flags that may indicate a patient's need for hospitalisation. Speaking to witnesses to the fall can also give insight as to the cause. If there aren't any, the interview skills of the paramedic come to the forefront of the assessment. When the patient fell in relation to when the call for help was made is important. A patient who has spent a long time on the floor is at risk of Rhabdomyolysis. If the patient is unsure of when they fell, questions such as 'What were you doing at the time?' and 'Was it day or night?' can help estimate the length of time on the floor. The activity the patient was doing when they fell can also indicate the cause, e.g. getting out of a chair and falling could be a sign of postural hypotension.

Where the patient fell, inside or outside, can lead paramedics to investigate other conditions. A patient who falls on the road in Australia may suffer burns from a hot pavement, whilst a patient falling on ice in the UK may become hypothermic. Investigating what happened before, during, and after the fall is important. Some patients may have had symptoms prior to the fall such as palpitations. During the fall, was there any incontinence or tongue biting indicating a seizure? Did the patient lose consciousness indicating a head injury? A patient who was pale or flushed prior to the fall could have suffered a hypoglycaemic or vasovagal event. Did the patient injure themselves?

Chapter 29 in this volume can assist the paramedic in the treatment and assessment of minor injuries sustained from a fall. Addressing the post-fall period allows the paramedic to determine the severity of any injuries. Patients that were able to return to normal activities are unlikely to have any injuries. Those who spent long periods on the floor, struggled to get up, or required assistance to get up may have injuries related to the fall or from crawling to reach furniture to assist themselves. Patients who had any weakness or speech difficulty post-fall may have suffered a stroke or transient ischaemic attack (TIA). Any recent change in medications should be explored to see if this has contributed to the fall.

Physical assessment of the falls patient

A systems approach to the physical examination can help the paramedic gain a better understanding of the cause of the fall.

Cardiovascular assessment

Palpation of the radial pulse can identify arrhythmias such as atrial fibrillation, and a weak pulse may be related to the underfilling of the heart due to dehydration. Postural blood pressure should be taken from a lying to a standing position and should be taken three times to gain an accurate measurement. Patients should lie rather than sit for five minutes prior to testing. When standing, blood pressure should be taken at one and three minutes, if the blood pressure continues to fall it should be taken again until no further fall is noted. A fall of greater than 20 mmHg or a systolic of below 90 mmHg is considered significant (Royal College of Physicians 2017). A cardiac murmur may be found in patients with aortic stenosis or congestive heart failure leading to the fall, and an electrocardiogram (ECG) should be taken, as this can highlight predisposes to syncope such as a heart block.

Respiratory assessment

When assessing a patient who has fallen, it is important to assess for evidence of infections such as pneumonia, as a fall can be the first notable sign of infection in the elderly (Kelly 2019). The presence of shortness of breath on exertion may be caused by fluid overload or anaemia. Any evidence of chronic respiratory problems such as chronic obstructive pulmonary disease (COPD) may suggest to the paramedic there might be increased shortness of breath and frailty, contributing to the fall. The patient should be assessed for equal pain-free air entry on auscultation of the lungs. Fractured ribs from a fall can cause hypoventilation, a risk factor for pneumonia and difficulty attending to activities of daily living (ADLs). The availability of point-of-care testing for full blood count can assist the paramedic in excluding infection or anaemia as a cause of a fall, which may require assessment in the hospital.

Abdominal assessment

Constipation in the elderly can lead to delirium, a cause of falls. The paramedic can assess for constipation whilst obtaining a history and also through an abdominal examination. Patients who are constipated may have a distended abdomen. Percussion may be dull due to the presence of faeces. Urinary retention can also cause delirium. Palpation of the bladder is over the symphysis pubis; however, it is not normally palpable unless it is distended, presenting as tender if in retention. If percussion is dull there is a volume of 400–600 ml present. By performing a urine dipstick the paramedic can exclude UTI as a cause.

Neurological assessment

A full neurological examination as explained in Chapter 21 can help the paramedic ascertain a stroke or a disability from a previous stroke as a factor. Symptoms of cerebellar degeneration can affect balance and are highlighted in the assessment of cranial nerves. Peripheral neuropathy secondary to diabetes and alcohol abuse affects sensation, which may have caused the fall. Blood sugar levels should be checked as this may cause weakness or confusion. When assessing gait the paramedic should ensure the patient uses their mobility aids as usual to gain a true comparison of their mobility. A cognitive assessment can help the paramedic identify the risk of future falls, as poor performance on these tests is associated with an increased likelihood of falling. These cognition tests can be Abbreviated Mental Test Score, mini-mental state examinations, or other recognised exams.

Integumentary (skin) assessment

Performing a comprehensive skin inspection can uncover wounds that may need attention in a hospital or on scene. It also highlights any swelling or bruising indicating injured areas. Performing a skin inspection can also help identify other disease processes that can contribute to falls such as lower limb oedema, caused by fluid overload in congestive cardiac failure.

Managing the falls patient

Any wounds found as a result of the patient's fall need to be treated appropriately. This may be on scene by the attending paramedic, calling for a specialist paramedic, transferring to an urgent care centre, or if required to the ED. It is important to remember if treating wounds in an elderly patient's home that they are likely to need follow-up care given the compromised properties of their skin due to age and diseases such as diabetes. This can be organised through their GP surgery or by contacting a local visiting nursing service. A referral to a falls prevention service can assist in reducing the incidence of falls and providing strategies for patients to use within their own homes to prevent future falls (Ganz and Latham 2020). Some ambulance services provide falls teams, which consist of an allied health professional such as a physiotherapist or occupational therapist and a specialist paramedic. These teams can be called to assess patients in their home environment, care for injuries sustained, provide ADL equipment such as walking frames or commodes, and referral for follow up in a falls clinic.

There are several assessment tools available – depending on the geographical area of practice – the paramedic can use to assess if a patient is safe to be left at home following a fall. Within Western Australia, for example, the FROP-Com screening tool is used to score a patient's risk of falling. A more comprehensive tool used in the UK is the SAFER 2 clinical decision flow chart (Figure 31.1), which, based on a comprehensive assessment, assists the paramedic in clinical decision-making should a patient require transport to the ED (Snooks et al. 2017; Mascarenhas et al. 2019). Regardless of the assessment tool used, paramedics should look out for the following red flags:

- Headache: A headache that gets worse and/or is not relieved with simple pain medication.
- Blurred vision: Problems focusing or diplopia.
- Drowsiness: Fainting, drowsiness, feeling more tired than usual.
- Nausea and/or vomiting: Feeling sick or vomiting and symptoms do not settle within two to three hours.
- Dizziness and/or weakness.
- Confusion.
- Seizures.
- Continual clear fluid or bleeding from the ear or nose.
- Increased pain affecting ADLs.

Safety netting advice

The paramedic should ensure the patient understands that they should seek a medication review from their GP to see what may have contributed to the fall. It is important that the paramedic follows up with a referral to the local falls service. Hazards within the home, e.g. rugs, clutter, or pets, should be discussed with the patient and the paramedic must tell them to seek medical review if further falls occur.

Chronic obstructive pulmonary disease

Chronic obstructive pulmonary disease (COPD) is a progressive disease of the respiratory system and is characterised by chronic airway inflammation. It is the umbrella term for emphysema, chronic bronchitis, and chronic asthma. Approx 10% of the world's population is diagnosed with the condition and this continues to rise. COPD is associated with significant personal, social, and economic costs (Agusti et al. 2020). A high percentage of cases of COPD exacerbations seen by the ambulance service are transferred to emergency departments, but over 30% of those patients are discharged several hours later without admission to a medical ward (Sneath et al. 2022). In light of this, can the paramedic provide treatment at home without requiring the patient to be transferred?

History taking for the COPD patient

In the context of COPD, patients will generally have an element of shortness of breath, however, the paramedic should ascertain when this became worse. Ask the patient to gauge the severity of this. This may be done through a dyspnoea score or asking how it affects their ADLs or exercise tolerance. The paramedic should ask about worsening and relieving factors, if they require more pillows when sleeping, or if bronchodilators help. Patients may describe an increase in wheeze, especially on exertion, this is likely upper airway sounds. The patient may describe feeling tight chested and having chest pain when coughing. Has the patient developed a new cough or has their cough become worse? Is it productive and if so, what colour is the sputum?

Examining the COPD patient

The paramedic should observe the patient's face. Central cyanosis may be seen on the oral membranes or tongue and can indicate severe hypoxia. Candidiasis or oral thrush may be present in patients on long-term inhaled steroids. Raised supraclavicular nodes might indicate a pulmonary infection. Tracheal deviation or raised jugular veins are signs of a tensioning pneumothorax, and those with chronic respiratory disease are at risk of developing a pneumothorax.

Observation of the chest can indicate asymmetrical movements or flail segments, red flags for a critically unwell patient. The paramedic can also assess the use of accessory muscles through observation. Palpation of the chest allows the paramedic to assess symmetrical chest expansion. Hyperinflation of the chest is found in patients with long-standing COPD. Chest crepitus felt on palpation can indicate a pneumothorax. Percussion of the chest can identify areas of consolidation or collapse if dullness is heard, or emphysema if hyper-resonance is heard. Auscultation of the chest in COPD may reveal a wheeze related to the narrowing of airways from disease, mucus, or crackles from fluid in the lung.

Observations should be taken to exclude sepsis and severe infection, which require transport to the ED. Work of breathing and ability to speak in full sentences should be assessed. A point-of-care ultrasound undertaken by a paramedic allows the identification of life-threatening conditions such as pneumothorax or large pulmonary effusions. A point-of-care C-reactive protein (CRP) test allows

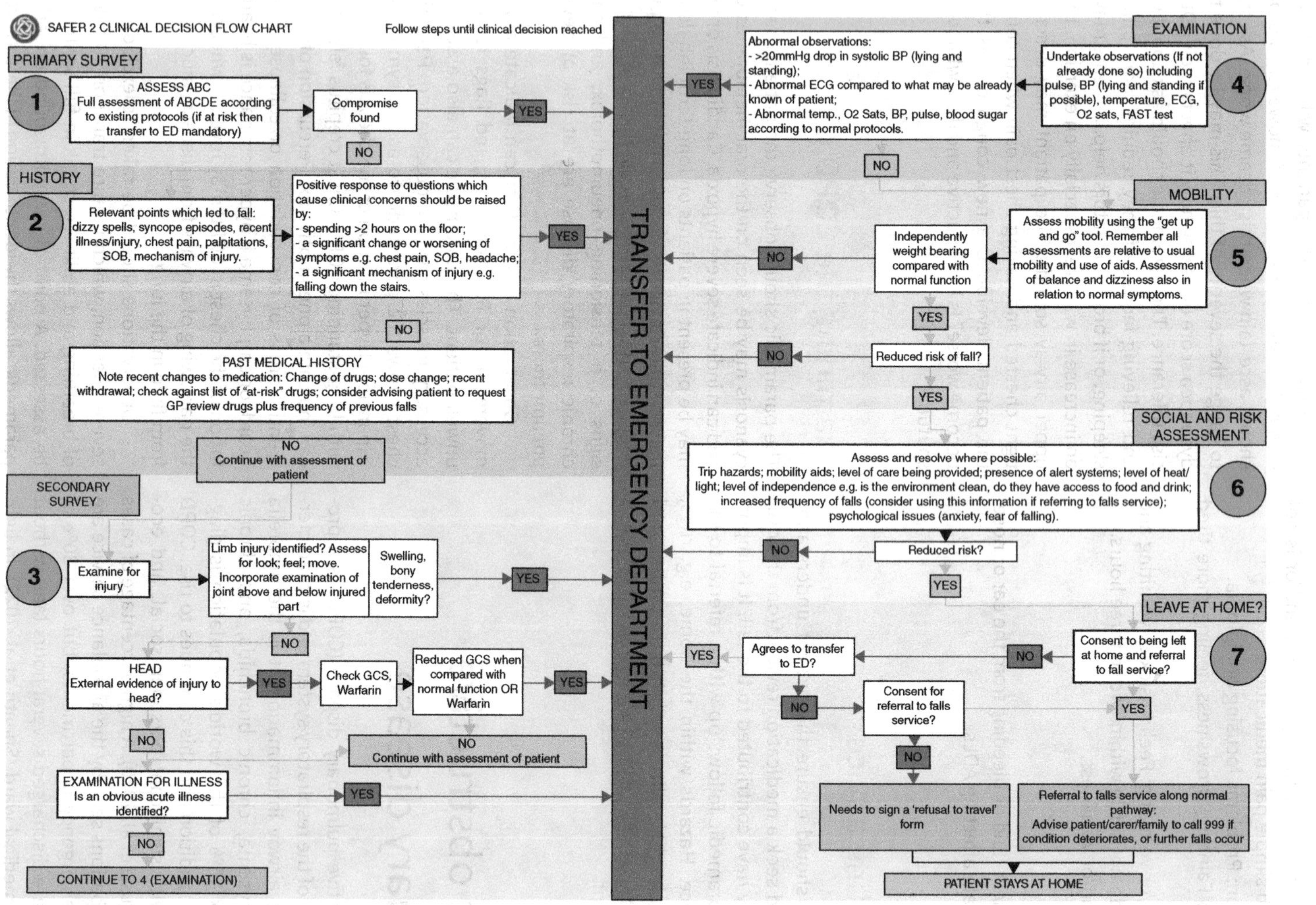

FIGURE 31.1 Clinical decision-making tool. Source: Snooks et al. 2017.

the paramedic to differentiate between a viral and bacterial infection. Point-of-care blood gas analysis enables the paramedic to consider the severity of the illness and ventilation of the patient, indicating if the patient needs transport to an ED for non-invasive ventilation (Nadim et al. 2021).

Managing the COPD patient

Treatment of exacerbation of COPD in the community depends on the severity of symptoms. Exacerbation symptoms include:

- Increase in dyspnoea
- Change in sputum volume
- Change in sputum purulence
- Cough new or increased

In patients with one symptom present, the exacerbation is considered mild and increasing the use of their bronchodilator, i.e. Ventolin, will improve symptoms. A spacer is recommended. This also gives the paramedic a chance to review the patient's inhaler technique to ensure inhaler administration is effective. Moderate exacerbation is considered in those with two symptoms. These patients require corticosteroids and/or antibiotics. The use of a point-of-care CRP test will inform the paramedic if the patient requires antibiotics. If a CRP test is not available, both steroids and antibiotics should be started. These may be available in the patient's home if they are on a COPD management plan. The paramedic can also contact the patient's primary physician or urgent care centre for a prescription to be sent out. A severe exacerbation of three or more symptoms will need assessment at the ED. The paramedic should explain to the patient that they need to contact their primary physician for review to document the exacerbation and for a possible medication review to see if any changes need to be made for ongoing disease management.

The paramedic should look out for the following red flags:

- Frequent episodes – may require medication review with GP or in hospital.
- Diagnostic uncertainty – cause of shortness of breath is unclear.
- Advanced age – likely to deteriorate due to reduced physiological reserve.
- Change in mental status.
- Symptoms that are poorly responsive to current treatment.
- Advanced or end-stage COPD.
- Little or no psychosocial support.

Safety netting advice

The paramedic must advise the patient to seek medical review from their GP if not improving despite increasing their Ventolin and starting steroids and/or antibiotics. They should contact the ambulance service again if they experience sudden or worsening shortness of breath which does not respond to Ventolin or if they are unusually confused, drowsy, or are having chest pains. The patient should be given a home action plan such as the one in Figure 31.2.

Conclusion

The issue of a significant proportion of ambulance service calls being categorised as low acuity is compounded by the fact that the elderly population is expected to continue to grow, exacerbating the problem. Transporting all of these low-acuity patients to the ED increases strain on the hospital system, leading to longer delays, increased ambulance wait times, and a negative impact on patients' healthcare experiences. This issue can be addressed by utilising comprehensive history taking and examinations, technology, and community services to effectively treat patients with low-acuity conditions in their homes. By doing so, paramedics can help to alleviate the strain on the hospital system and ensure that patients receive the appropriate care in the right location.

This chapter has delved into three common conditions that can be effectively managed at home with the right support and experience. By applying the principles outlined in this chapter to other low-acuity conditions, paramedics can identify the most appropriate treatment for each patient and provide the necessary care in a timely manner. By doing so, patients can avoid the inconvenience and potential risks associated with hospitalisation and receive high-quality care in the comfort of their own homes. Overall, effective management of low-acuity conditions by paramedics can improve healthcare experiences for patients and alleviate pressure on the hospital system.

Home Action Plan
For adults with COPD

AsthmaWA

When you feel well

You are doing your usual activities. You have usual levels of breathlessness and phelgm. Perform these actions, and **take** these medications for your COPD.

- Follow our tips for things you can do to keep well on the other side of this plan

Medicine	Dose	When

O2 at home? ☐ Resting ____ L/min Exertion ____ L/min Sleeping ____ L/min

Keep taking all your regular medicines.

When you feel unwell

You are coughing more. You have more phlegm. You are finding it hard to breathe. Perform these actions, and **increase** your reliever medicine.

- Tell your emergency contact person, prepare to contact your GP

Medicine	Dose	When

If increasing your reliever medicine isn't helping

Perform these actions, and **start** your **steroid**.

- Contact your GP and make an appointment **ASAP**

Prednisolone ________ ________

If you also have fever or changes in phlegm

Start your **antibiotic**.

________ ________ ________

When you feel horrible or very worried

You are very short of breath. You are very wheezy. You have a high fever or confusion. You have chest pain or slurred speech.

Perform these actions, and **increase** your reliever medicine

- Go to your nearest Emergency Department

or

- Call 000 for an ambulance

Government of Western Australia
WA Country Health Service

FIGURE 31.2 Home action plan for patient with COPD. Source: Asthma WA 2022.

Activities

Now review your learning by completing the learning activities in this chapter. The answers to these appear at the end of the book. Further self-test activities can be found at **www.wileyfundamentalseries.com/paramedic/3e.**

Test your knowledge

1. List three low-acuity cases a paramedic may be called to that can be managed at home?
2. What does the presence of leukocytes in the urine indicate?

3. What red flags indicate a patient with a UTI may require a medical assessment?
4. What is a definition of a fall?
5. List four causes of a fall?
6. What services can patients be referred to post-fall?
7. What treatments can a paramedic offer for exacerbation of COPD?
8. What point-of-care testing is available to paramedics?
9. With consenting peers or family, undertake a history taking and physical assessment exercise.
10. Practise chest palpation, auscultation, and percussion with consenting peers and family.

Glossary

Candidiasis: Any of a variety of infections caused by fungi of the genus Candida, occurring most often in the mouth, respiratory tract, or vagina.

Pyelonephritis: Inflammation of the kidney and its pelvis, caused by a bacterial infection.

Suprapubic: Above the pubic bone.

Microscopic urinalysis: This test looks at a sample of your urine under a microscope. It can see cells from your urinary tract, blood cells, crystals, bacteria, parasites, and cells from tumours.

Antibiotic: A drug that kills or stops the growth of bacteria.

Frailty: An ageing-related syndrome of physiological decline, characterised by marked vulnerability to adverse health outcomes.

Pneumonia: Inflammation of lung alveoli, the tiny air sacs deep within the lungs where carbon dioxide and oxygen are exchanged.

Pneumothorax: An abnormal collection of air in the space between the thin layer of tissue that covers the lungs and the chest cavity.

Delirium: A mental state in which a person is confused and has reduced awareness of their surroundings.

Cyanosis: A pathologic condition that is characterised by a bluish discoloration of the skin or mucous membrane.

Hyperinflation: Air gets trapped in the lungs and causes them to overinflate resulting in a barrel shaped chest.

Chest Crepitus: Palpable or audible popping, crackling, grating, or crunching sensation that can occur when air is pushed through the soft tissue in the chest.

Point-of-care testing: a form of testing in which the analysis is performed where healthcare is provided close to or near the patient.

CRP: C-reactive protein is a protein that is made by the liver when there is inflammation or tissue damage in the body.

References

Agusti, A., Vogelmeier, C., and Faner, R. (2020). COPD 2020: changes and challenges. *American Journal of Physiology-Lung Cellular and Molecular Physiology* **319** (5): 879–883. doi: 10.1152/ajplung.00429.2020.

Alarilla, A., Stafford, M., Coughlan, E. et al. (2022). Why have ambulance waiting times been getting worse? The Health Foundation (4 November). Available at: https://www.health.org.uk/publications/long-reads/why-have-ambulance-waiting-times-been-getting-worse (accessed 17 March 2023).

Asthma, W.A. (2022). Home action plan for adults with COPD. Available at: https://asthmawa.org.au/new-resources-for-adults-with-copd (accessed 1 April 2023).

Cadogan, M. and Rogers, J. (2020). Dipstick urinalysis. Life in the Fast Lane. Available at: https://litfl.com/dipstick-urinalysis (accessed 25 March 2023).

Ganz, D.A. and Latham, N.K. (2020). Prevention of falls in community-dwelling older adults. *New England Journal of Medicine* **382** (8): 734–743. doi: 10.1056/nejmcp1903252.

Kelly, K. (2019). Infection masquerading as a fall in the elderly. *Journal of Urgent Care Medicine* **13** (6): 17–19

Mascarenhas, M., Hill, K.D., Barker, A. et al. (2019). Validity of the falls risk for older people in the community (FROP-Com) tool to predict falls and fall injuries for older people presenting to the emergency department after falling. *European Journal of Ageing* **16** (3): 377–386. doi: 10.1007/s10433-018-0496-x.

Medina, M. and Castillo-Pino, E. (2019). An introduction to the epidemiology and burden of urinary tract infections. *Therapeutic Advances in Urology* **11**: 175628721983217. doi: 10.1177/1756287219832172.

Nadim, G., Laursen, C.B., Pietersen, P.I. et al. (2021). Prehospital emergency medical technicians can perform ultrasonography and blood analysis in prehospital evaluation of patients with chronic obstructive pulmonary disease: a feasibility study. *BMC Health Services Research* **21** (1): 1–12 doi: 10.1186/s12913-021-06305-7.

NICE (National Institute for Health and Care Excellence). (2019). Falls – risk assessment. Available at: https://cks.nice.org.uk/topics/falls-risk-assessment (accessed 27 March 2023).

NICE. (2022). Urinary tract infection (lower) – women: assessment. Clinical Knowledge Summaries. Available at: https://cks.nice.org.uk/topics/urinary-tract-infection-lower-women/diagnosis/assessment/#:~:text=Red%20flags%20such%20as%20haematuria,such%20as%20polycystic%20kidney%20disease (accessed 27 March 2023).

Public Health England. (2018). *Falls: applying all our health. Available at:* https://www.gov.uk/government/publications/falls-applying-all-our-health/falls-applying-all-our-health (accessed 23 October 2023).

Rehmani, R. (2004). Accuracy of urine dipstick to predict urinary tract infections in an emergency department. *Journal of Ayub Medical College Abbottabad* **16** (1): 4–7.

Royal College of Physicians. (2017). Measurement of lying and standing blood pressure: a brief guide for clinical staff. (3 January). Available at: https://www.rcplondon.ac.uk/projects/outputs/measurement-lying-and-standing-blood-pressure-brief-guide-clinical-staff (accessed 21 March 2023).

Sneath, E., Tippett, V., Bowman, R.V. et al. (2022). The clinical journey of patients with a severe exacerbation of chronic obstructive pulmonary disease (COPD): from the ambulance to the emergency department to the hospital ward. *Journal of Thoracic Disease* **14** (12): 4601–4613. doi: 10.21037/jtd-22-328.

Snooks, H.A., Anthony, R., Chatters, R. et al. (2017). Paramedic assessment of older adults after falls, including community care referral pathway: cluster randomized trial. *Annals of Emergency Medicine* **70** (4): 495–505.e28. doi: 10.1016/j.annemergmed.2017.01.006.

CHAPTER 32

Family and domestic violence

Simon Sawyer

Director of Education, Australian Paramedical College
Adjunct Senior Lecturer, Griffith University, Australia

Contents

LEARNING OUTCOMES

On completion of this chapter the reader will be able to:

- Define family and domestic violence (FDV) and its common manifestations.
- Understand the prevalence of FDV in Australia.
- Explain why FDV occurs and its impact on individuals.
- Understand the role of PPP in responding to patients experiencing FDV.

Case study

You are dispatched to a 35-year-old female, who requested an ambulance due to shortness of breath.

You arrive to find the patient, Grace, sitting and breathing heavily. Grace states she is having an asthma attack and her salbutamol isn't working. You perform a full assessment of Grace. She has a history of asthma and hypertension and is on medication for depression and anxiety.

You treat Grace for asthma and her breathing slowly returns to normal. After a repeat assessment you are satisfied that her symptoms have resolved. Grace thanks you and states that she is sorry to have bothered you, and that she feels like an 'idiot' for not being able to make her salbutamol work.

(Continued)

Fundamentals of Paramedic Practice: A Systems Approach, Third Edition. Edited by Sam Willis and Ian Peate.

Companion website: www.wiley.com/go/willis/paramedic3e

Looking around you see that Grace's home is mostly clean and tidy, but there is a broken window that has been boarded over and damage to a number of walls.

You offer to take Grace into the emergency department (ED) to be seen by a doctor, but Grace refuses saying she 'doesn't want to waste anyone else's time'.

At this stage you decide there is nothing further you can do for Grace's asthma but you have a feeling there might be something more to Grace's presentation, though you can't put your finger on what's giving you this feeling.

Before reading on consider this scene:

- Do you see any indicators of the potential for FDV? What are they?
- If you did suspect that Grace may be experiencing FDV, what would you do?

Take a moment to consider both these questions and write down some thoughts before reading on.

Introduction

Paramedics encounter patients experiencing family and domestic violence (FDV) frequently in their practice. However, due to a lack of education and training it often goes undetected, meaning opportunities to connect patients with the right care and support are frequently missed (Sawyer, Parekh et al. 2014; Sawyer, Coles et al. 2015; Sawyer et al. 2018b).[1] It is important that paramedics have a sound understanding of FDV, as they have a role to play in identifying persons at risk of violence, neglect or abuse, and connecting them with the right care and support to reduce the harm patients are exposed to (WHO 2013b).

To do this, paramedics need to understand what constitutes FDV, why it occurs, who it can impact, and what to do when they encounter a patient experiencing FDV. This chapter will aim to provide the necessary knowledge for a paramedic to respond appropriately when encountering a patient experiencing FDV.

Defining and understanding FDV

FDV is a common occurrence worldwide. The term refers to all forms of actual or threatened physical violence, emotional abuse, neglect, or other controlling behaviours occurring between members of a family or in a domestic setting (Krug et al. 2002). This can include violence, abuse, or neglect arising from or between children, siblings, parents, extended family, or any other person within a domestic or residential setting.

As distinct from other forms of interpersonal violence, FDV often occurs between people who know each other, and frequently they live closely with one another. Because of this ongoing relationship between the patient and the perpetrator, the violence, abuse, or neglect has a much higher potential to occur over an extended period of time, which results in more overall harm than might occur with a single random act of violence or abuse from a stranger.

It is not always easy to clearly define behaviours that would be considered violent, abusive, or neglectful. For example, parents and children often argue, and arguments might contain a level of physical contact or emotionally charged exchanges, but they wouldn't always be considered FDV. What generally makes FDV distinct is that it contains a *power imbalance* in the relationship, one person will be exerting unreasonable control over another through coercive means. What this means is that, in the setting of FDV, generally one person will use physical or psychological abuse or intimidation to control another. Table 32.1 provides some further guidance on specific behaviours which may be considered violent, abusive, or neglectful.

The challenge to determine if a behaviour is considered as FDV is somewhat easier to understand when considering neglect. Neglect can happen because of a wilful action designed to harm or coerce, or it may occur due to a lack of resources or education. For example, a person might threaten to withhold medication as a means to frighten and control another, which would meet the definition of FDV. Conversely, they may not have adequate resources to obtain or pay for medication, resulting in the same outcome, but in this case it would not usually be

[1]A note on nomenclature: throughout this chapter we will refer to a person who may be experiencing FDV as a 'patient', rather than use a term such as 'victim' or 'survivor'. This is done to emphasise a patient-centric model of care, and to avoid causing distress by referring to a patient by terms such as a 'victim of domestic violence' or an 'abused child', which may cause offence. Likewise, a person who uses violence, abuse, or neglect within the context of FDV will be referred to as a 'perpetrator'. This should not be read to mean that person is acting wilfully but only that their behaviour meets the accepted definition.

TABLE 32.1 Defining family violence

Physical violence and abuse	Behaviours that may inflict pain or injury, e.g. pushing, slapping, hitting, kicking, beating, strangulation, or attempts to murder or cause serious harm Also includes the use of threats or weapons to intimidate, destruction of property, or the killing or harming of property, pets, other family members, or children
Emotional or psychological abuse	Behaviours that may cause psychological or emotional harm, e.g. verbal intimidation, belittling, or humiliating, or threats of suicide or self-harm from the perpetrator This may be subtle or overt but is usually designed to frighten the patient, who may in turn lose confidence, self-esteem, or self-determination
Sexual assault or abuse	Adult sexual assault refers to any type of non-consensual sexual activity. This includes physical contact, exposing the patient, the perpetrator exposing themselves, or penetration of the victim. It is important to note that certain individuals may be unable to consent, such as patients with dementia Child sexual assault may include forcing or enticing a child to take part in sexual activities, regardless of whether the child is aware of what is happening, as well as non-contact activities such as allowing a child to view or be involved in the production of pornographic material, watching sexual activities, or encouraging children to behave in sexually inappropriate ways
Controlling behaviours	Behaviours that attempt to prevent a person from following their desired course of action. This might include preventing freedom of movement, access to social contact, or freedom to express oneself (e.g. culturally or religiously). This may also include monitoring movements or restricting access to information, assistance, money, or resources
Neglect	A failure to provide basic health or well-being, social, educational, or medical needs of a person in your care. For children this also includes a failure to protect them from violence or harm, or exposing them to FDV

Source: Adapted from Krug E et al. 2002 and The Royal Australian College of General Practitioners 2014.

considered FDV. In these examples, we can see that it is not necessarily the action but often the intention behind the action that defines FDV.

Therefore, when considering violence, abuse, and neglect, it is important to understand that it can be very difficult even for experts to determine why the behaviours are occurring, and if they are intentional or not. Because of this, paramedics should focus on the impact of behaviours, rather than attempting to assign blame. For example, it is less helpful to focus on labelling a perpetrator as 'abusive' than to recognise the presence of abuse and help connect patients with the proper care and support.

Common types of FDV

FDV can manifest in a number of different ways. Four common presentations that paramedics would expect to encounter include:

- **Child abuse and neglect (CAN):** This refers to any type of threatened or actual physical violence, emotional abuse, sexual abuse, neglect, negligence, or exploitation of a child, which results in actual or potential harm to the child's health, survival, development, or dignity in the context of a relationship of responsibility, trust, or power (Renner and Slack 2006).

  In addition, allowing a child to be exposed to FDV is considered a form of CAN, due to the impact this can have on a child's well-being (Butchart et al. 2006).
- **Intimate partner violence (IPV):** This refers to any type of threatened or actual physical or emotional harm, sexual abuse, or other controlling behaviours transpiring between people who are, or were formally, in an intimate relationship, which can include married, de-facto, or dating couples (Krug et al. 2002).
- **Elder abuse and neglect:** This refers to any type of threatened or actual physical or emotional harm, sexual abuse, neglect, or use of controlling behaviours of a person aged 65 years or over. This can occur in a residential aged-care facility, in private care, or with elderly people living independently and it can be a single or repeated act, or lack of appropriate action, occurring within any relationship where there is an expectation of trust, which causes harm or distress to an older person. Both family members and carers can perpetrate elder abuse or neglect (WHO 2008).
- **Sexual violence:** This refers to any sexual act, attempt to obtain a sexual act, or other act directed against a person's sexuality using coercion by any person regardless of their relationship to the victim, in any setting.

This includes rape, which is defined as the physically forced or otherwise coerced penetration of the mouth, vulva, or anus with a penis, other body part, or object (WHO 2013b).

Within Australia, every person has the right to consent, or not to consent, to sexual activity. Sexual assault is most commonly perpetrated by a known person, such as a family member or friend (Australian Institute of Criminology 2013).

Key groups at risk of FDV

While FDV is known to occur across all levels of society and within all population groups, there are some individuals who may be more at risk of experiencing FDV. First Nations peoples such as Aboriginal and Torres Strait Islander, Māori, and Pacific Islander women are many times more likely to experience FDV and more likely to be murdered by a current or past partner than non-indigenous people (Marie et al. 2008; Australian Productivity Commission 2014). Likewise, Indigenous children have been shown to be more likely to receive child protection services than non-Indigenous children (Australian Institute of Health and Welfare 2017; Kōkiri 2017). FDV is not a part of the culture of First Nations people, it is rather the disadvantages this population faces that lead to a higher risk of FDV occurring (Al-Yaman et al. 2006).

It is not clear if culturally and linguistically diverse (CALD) and migrant peoples have a higher or lower risk of experiencing FDV, but it is known that they do have high barriers to disclose violence, abuse, and neglect (Ghafournia 2011). Barriers include language difficulties, accessing culturally specific services, and knowledge of their rights (Vaughan et al. 2016).

The LGBTQIA+ community appears to show similar rates of FDV to heterosexual couples (Blosnich and Bossarte 2009), however, victims may be less likely to seek support due to discrimination and other barriers, meaning rates may be underreported (Inwin 2008).

Disabled people commonly report higher rates of violence, abuse, and neglect (Hughes et al. 2011), particularly from family members or carers who they depend on for care and support. In particular these people may experience withdrawal of accessibility devices (such as walking frames, hearing or communication devices) or withholding of medication, medical care, or socialisation, as well as the threat of institutionalisation. When a disabled patient is reliant on their abuser for care, or where their disability prevents or impacts communication, they can have little opportunity to access help and support.

Why does FDV happen?

There is no single reason that can be used to explain the presence of violence, abuse, or neglect. The Ecological Model can be used to describe the factors that are known to make FDV more or less likely to occur. For example, factors such as endorsement of gendered roles and male entitlement, lower education or socio-economic status, and the lack of robust legislation holding perpetrators to account all increase the likelihood of FDV occurring (Krug et al. 2002).

FDV is often labelled a *gendered issue*. This means that gender is a contributing factor to the presence of FDV. To unpack this we can explore two key statistics:

1. The primary victims of family violence are female, and the primary perpetrators are male (Krug et al. 2002).
2. Not all males are violent, and not all women experience violence. In fact most males aren't violent, and most women don't experience violence in relationships (Krug et al. 2002; WHO 2013a).

Extrapolating from these two statistics we can see that while women can perpetrate FDV, and men can be the victims, the evidence consistently demonstrates that the majority of the most damaging violence is perpetrated by males against women. Yet most men aren't violent. So, what sets those who use violence in their relationships apart from those who don't? The answer is most likely that it's the attitudes we hold that lead to violence. For example, beliefs that are predominantly held by males – such as 'men can't control their impulse for sex' or 'women should be subservient' – are attitudes that are associated with the use of FDV. What this tells us is that it's not someone's *gender* that causes FDV, it's more likely to be the attitudes that are predominantly held by that gender. One might say that the root cause of FDV is simply violence supportive attitudes.

Given this association, the cure to violence becomes changing attitudes that encourage or excuse violence and embracing attitudes that support non-violent approaches to relationships.

Prevalence and impacts of FDV

CAN

CAN is most frequently perpetrated by someone known to the child, particularly members of their family (Hanson et al. 2003). CAN may lead to acute and chronic health and behavioural problems, which continue into adulthood. In the majority of children, physical injuries generally do less harm than the long-term impacts of violence and abuse on behavioural and emotional development (Norman et al. 2012). Because of this, a key focus should be on early identification and access to support to reduce the overall harm experienced by a child.

Within Australia, between 2020 and 2021, there were over 178,000 children (aged <18) receiving child protection services, with over 49,000 substantiated reports of CAN and over 46,000 children in out-of-home care (Australian Institute of Health and Welfare 2021). Emotional abuse is most commonly reported (55%), followed by neglect (21%), physical abuse (14%) and sexual abuse (10%).

CAN can have significant impacts, including increasing the chances of developing mental health disorders like depression, anxiety, and eating disorders, and increased incidence of suicide attempts and drug use (Norman et al. 2012). There is limited evidence that allergies, malnutrition, asthma, headaches, type 2 diabetes, and obesity can be related to experiencing CAN (Norman et al. 2012). In Australia, it is estimated that 25 children die each year from CAN attributed causes (Australian Institute of Health and Welfare 2017). Importantly, the evidence shows that up to a third of children who died from CAN-related incidents were previously assessed by healthcare practitioners who did not recognise the potential for CAN (King et al. 2006).

IPV

IPV occurs across all cultures and communities, and it is the most common form of violence against women in Australia (Australian Bureau of Statistics 2012). In Australia, 17% of women over the age of 15 have experienced at least one incident of violence from an intimate partner (6.1% for men) (Australian Bureau of Statistics 2016). Additionally, around 25% of women experience emotional abuse from a current or past partner (14% for men).

IPV is the leading preventable contributor to death, disability, and illness in young Australian women (VicHealth 2004), more than double any other risk factor. Injuries to the eyes, ears, head, neck, breasts, and abdomen are frequently associated with IPV (Campbell 2002), and IPV has been linked to traumatic brain injury (Black 2011). More than one woman is killed each week in Australia by a current or past male partner for 'domestic motives', which accounts for 66% of all domestic homicides in Australia (Dearden et al. 2008). IPV has also been associated with an increased risk of varied stress-mediated conditions such as asthma, irritable bowel syndrome, diabetes, headaches, chronic pain, sleeping difficulties, and poor general physical health (Black et al. 2011).

IPV is associated with a higher risk for depression, anxiety, post-traumatic stress disorder and other mood and sleep disorders (Black 2011). Additionally, IPV has been linked with self-harm (Roberts et al. 1997) and substance abuse (WHO 2000). One Australian study estimating that 25% of children and young people have witnessed IPV (Office of Women's Policy 2002), demonstrating that IPV can also lead to CAN.

Elder abuse and neglect

The prevalence of elder abuse in Australia is reported as being 14.8%, with rates slightly higher for women than men (Qu et al. 2021). Psychological abuse is the most common manifestation and most elderly people only report one type of abuse. It is expected that incidence of elder abuse and neglect will increase as the average population age is increasing around the world (WHO 2011).

The presence of elder abuse and neglect is associated with injuries from trauma, depression and anxiety, and even premature death (WHO 2011). The consequences of abuse directed towards the elderly can be disproportionately high, due to their lowered capacity to cope with even minor injuries (WHO 2011).

Sexual assault

In 2021, it was reported that 23% of women and 8% of men in Australia aged over 18 had experienced sexual violence at least once in their lifetime (Australian Bureau of Statistics 2016). These figures are expected to be underreported due to high barriers to reporting. Sexual assault is most common in children aged 10–14, and then declines with increasing age. Women experience sexual assault at greater rates than men in all age groups (Australian Institute of Criminology 2013).

Sexual assault is known to be traumatising, and reporting the assault can result in even more trauma. It is associated with depression, anxiety, and PTSD (Tjaden and Thoennes 2000; Jozkowski and Sanders 2012), with one study finding that almost a third of people sexually assaulted will develop PTSD and are three times as likely to experience major depressive disorder (Green 1993). Sexual assault is also associated with self-harm and suicidality, substance abuse, chronic gastrointestinal problems, and unexplained pain, particularly in the pelvic or genital region (Tjaden and Thoennes 2000; Jozkowski and Sanders 2012).

The role of paramedics and ambulance services

The role of pre-hospital practitioners when encountering patients experiencing FDV is relatively straight forward; however, it does require training. Research with paramedics and paramedic students has shown that they are supportive of learning about FDV and want to respond properly but they are fearful of responding inappropriately and therefore desire formalised training.

It is beyond the scope of any book chapter to provide comprehensive training, at present the evidence indicates that this is best done in a face-to-face setting. Therefore, the remainder of this chapter will describe the theoretical response. Paramedics wishing to undertake face-to-face training can usually access this through FDV training services, which are widely available across Australia and other countries.

When discussing the response of paramedics to FDV, a simple four-step method is used: recognise, respond, refer, and record (Sawyer, Coles et al. 2018a). We will discuss each aspect below and continually return to the case study from the start of this chapter to aid us in our discussion about these four steps.

Recognise

At present, there is no published data that has attempted to describe exactly how a patient experiencing FDV would present to an ambulance service or to a paramedic. Because of this, we need to look at data from other emergency and health services such as EDs and general practitioner (GP) clinics. What this data tells us are scene findings, patient symptoms, or other situational factors that are commonly associated with a person who is experiencing FDV. This data can then be distilled to describe potential indicators of FDV (Table 32.2). Note that the presence of any or all of the following indicators does not mean that a person is *definitely* experiencing FDV but, rather, that presence of indicators should increase the paramedic's index of suspicion.

Consideration of the presence of FDV should be part of every paramedic's standard clinical approach. It is recommended that paramedics take a risk-based approach to FDV identification, which means that you should use things like the presence of indicators to inform your opinion of the risk to a patient. The higher the risk, the greater your suspicion, which should in turn result in an increased level of response.

Because we can see the *potential* for FDV, we would conclude that it would be in the patient's best interests to ask about FDV.

TABLE 32.2 Known indicators of FDV in healthcare settings.

Feelings	The patient appears depressed, withdrawn, anxious, or distressed The patient or the patient's children or dependants appear fearful, particularly of a specific person
Behaviours	Suicidality or self-harm Alcohol or other drug abuse Repeated or suspicious callouts with no clear diagnosis Inconsistent or implausible explanations for injuries or symptoms Scene findings or behaviours of those on scene that indicate an unsafe environment, which may be particularly relevant for children, elderly, or the disabled
Medical signs	Unexplained chronic symptoms, especially pain, gastrointestinal, or genitourinary symptoms Pregnancy-related complications or trauma, or delays in care
Controlling people	Intrusive or controlling people on the scene The patient (or their children or dependants) is unwilling to respond without approval from a controlling person A controlling person who minimises or explains away injuries or symptoms, or who states the patient is not to be believed Communication or mobility devices are being withheld, over/under medication (especially for elderly or disabled patients), or other evidence on unreasonable control
Trauma	A presentation related to an assault or suspicion of assault (e.g. presence of weapons or signs of violence) The patient has suspicious bruises or injuries, especially to the neck, face, breasts, or genitals The patient states or indicates someone has threatened to kill or harm them, their children/dependants, or their pets Evidence of sexual assault (actual or attempted)
Neglect	Evidence of malnutrition or neglect, particularly in children, elderly, or disabled patients Unsanitary or unsafe living conditions Evidence of untreated or uncontrolled medical conditions Lack of supervision (especially in children or disabled patients)

Source: Black 2011; Norman et al. 2012; The Royal Australian College of General Practitioners 2014; and Sawyer, Coles et al. 2018b).

Case study

When considering Grace's presentation, we can now see that there are several indicators that might raise our suspicion of FDV.

- Risk factors: Grace is young (35 years old) and female, and we know that young females disproportionately experience FDV.
- Feelings: Grace is continually talking down to herself, referring to herself as an 'idiot' and saying she was wasting people's time. Such comments could be linked to having a controlling or abusive person in her life, which is negatively impacting her self-esteem and self-worth.
- Medical conditions: We know that asthma can be associated with experiencing IPV, likewise Grace is young to be experiencing hypertension, which might indicate she lives with high stress. Grace is also experiencing depression and anxiety, which is also associated with IPV.
- Trauma: We can also see evidence of damage to the house, which may be unrelated but again may raise our index of suspicion that Grace is living with a violent person, though at this stage we haven't seen any evidence that Grace is being physically assaulted.

Respond

It will rarely be possible for a paramedic to be certain of the presence of FDV. Importantly you do not need any definitive evidence, or even any specific indicators of FDV, to progress to the response stage.

The response stage is about talking about FDV with your patient and providing them space to disclose anything they wish to you. This can be nuanced and requires care, skill, and practice, which is why training is so important. In general, a good response will be to ask *fear and safety* questions. These questions focus on the patient's experiences and feelings, rather than requesting specific details (WHO 2014).

Responding can be done in many different ways. As long as it is done in a supportive, non-judgemental, and empathetic manner, it is ok to use your own unique approach. This aspect is what most healthcare practitioners request formal training for, and so whilst we will describe an exemplar response below, it is not expected that you would be properly prepared to undertake this process by only reading this chapter.

Generally, it is advised to gently broach the subject by asking lead-in questions, which help build rapport and trust. You might start by asking general questions about your patient's work or well-being, and then slowly build towards questions about their home life and relationships. It's also important to move slow and make space for the patient to answer in their own time and on their own terms. When they do respond, you can show you are listening, you understand, and you aren't judging them by validating what they are saying. We can explore this process though an example conversation with Grace.

Case study

You decide that you'd like to ask Grace about FDV. An example conversation is provided in Figure 1.

Broaching the subject

You would usually start by building rapport with Grace, by asking about her general well-being. You might also let Grace know that you just wanted to check in with her and make sure everything is ok before you leave. For example, the conversation might go like this:

'Now we have your asthma under control Grace, is there anything else that I can do for you at the moment?'

Usually the patient would reply with any other medical issues if any were present; or would say 'no' if they felt their issue was dealt with. You might then ask about general well-being. For example, you might say:

'So apart from the asthma today, you're otherwise well and happy?'

(*Continued*)

Again it's common for patients to respond by saying they are fine to questions like this. Allow space for the patient to respond however they wish and then you can gently probe further, slowly moving towards the topic of FDV. For example, you might ask:

'How are things at work? Not too stressful?'

And maybe

'And you work with some good people, boss treating you well?'

As the patient becomes comfortable with your questions, and as you demonstrate your genuine concern for the patient's well-being, you might gently ask more direct FDV questions?

'And how's everything at home? Things going well?'
'You're able to get enough good food, and have everything you need at home?'

If the patient has children, you might ask:

'How are the kids at the moment, are they all doing well?'

If you've built enough rapport and your questioning is going well, you might then ask about their partner:

'And your partner, you have a good relationship with them?'

It is possible that at this stage, if Grace is willing to trust you, she might disclose something. This may be a very small disclosure, as she tests for your reaction. For example, Grace might say something like:

'Oh you know how it is, my partner is under a lot of stress.'

Such a response can be viewed as an invitation to ask further questions.
Depending on the situation, you might consider a formal statement before asking further questions such as:

'I'd like to ask a question but before I do, I just want you to you know that your answers will be confidential, and we won't be overheard' (obviously you need to make sure that you won't be overheard).

Fear and safety questions

Questions such as 'Is someone abusing you?' or 'Did your husband do this?' are generally considered the wrong approach, as they focus on trying to make the patient assign blame. Instead, preferred questions ask about fear and safety such as:

'Grace, I'm wondering if you feel safe at home, is there anyone that's making you afraid?'

Or:

'Grace, I wonder if your asthma attack today might have happened because you were feeling unsafe?'

Again it's important to remember that this can be an incredibly confrontational question for the patient, take your time and give them space to respond. You might have to allow a few seconds for them to formulate their response. If they don't respond you might add a statement to show you're concerned about them such as:

'I'm asking because I'm feeling concerned about your safety.'

Or:

'I'm asking because I just want to make sure you are feeling safe.'

If the patient discloses anything related to FDV, or requests help, before anything else it can be very beneficial to validate and reassure them. To do this let them know you have heard them, and you believe what they've told you, for example:

'Grace, thank you for telling me this, I know that would have been hard.'

And/or:

'I believe everyone has the right to feel safe at home and I will do what I can to support you.'

Once this happens you can move towards asking the patient about their needs, which we will discuss in the refer section.

The conversation may go in a very different way, and it's important that you access the right training before attempting such conversations with you patients. Remember, however the conversation goes, getting a disclosure is not the goal. The goal is to make space for your patient to disclose anything they would like to in a safe way. Just because your patient doesn't disclose anything doesn't mean you've made a mistake. Potentially there is no FDV issue, potentially the patient isn't ready to disclose to you (or anyone else), or potentially the patient doesn't recognise their situation is linked to FDV.

The more people that enquire about someone's safety and express genuine concern, the more opportunities the patient will have to access care and support. Even if they don't disclose to you, they may disclose to the next person who asks, because you have contributed to their feeling safe to seek help.

Refer

The needs of a person experiencing FDV can be quite broad, and as such there is no single right referral option. What is most important is that you take the time to discuss your patient's needs and find an option that is right for them. For example, patients might require general or legal advice, counselling, protection, or refuge accommodation. Options may vary based on the availability of resources in the patient's location, so it's a good idea for paramedics to know what is available in their area.

The best way to understand what a patient's needs might be is simply to ask them. They may be unsure, so you might offer some different options. Referrals are generally made by providing contact details directly to the patient so that they can make contact when they are ready. It is not advised that paramedics contact referral agencies without the patient's consent, except in cases of mandatory reporting.

Record

Recording of encounters with patient's experiencing FDV is important but must be done with care. Confidentiality of medical records is paramount, as the patient may not be safe if the perpetrator was to discover that the patient had disclosed anything to you.

Generally, documentation should include:

- A description of anything you observed on the scene that you felt could be indicative of FDV. This might include a description of any injuries, symptoms, or behaviours, or statements made by the patient. It can be useful to write direct quotes where appropriate.

Case study

In Grace's case, you may find that she has a specific service or need in mind, such as general advice or counselling. She may be looking for a way to escape the violent situation and therefore want to speak to police or crisis accommodation services. Grace may also be interested in legal advice.

In Grace's situation, it would be best to allow Grace to discuss her experiences and needs, and together find the most suitable referral service.

If Grace wanted counselling, you might consider offering her a helpline such as the 1800RESPECT phone number, which offers phone counselling for patients experiencing FDV in Australia.

Case study

Documentation for a case such as Grace's might look like this:

35yo F, called ambulance due to SOB. o/a presented with mild asthma symptoms, resolved with salbutamol. Hx of asthma, hypertension, and depression/anxiety. Grace appeared embarrassed about calling the ambulance. Evidence of physical damage to house (broken window and 4 x visible holes in walls).

Grace asked about personal safety, declined any support, provided referral to 1800RESPECT.

- A note of if there were any children or other witnesses present and if they were involved at all.
- If you discussed the potential for FDV with the patient and if any referral option was provided.
- Any other relevant scene findings or statements made by the patient or potential perpetrators.

A note on specialist responses

While the above method can be considered a general response to FDV, there are some situations where you may need to engage an expert. For example, in cases of suspected CAN (including sexual abuse) it may not be appropriate for you to directly question the patient. You can certainly listen to anything the patient wishes to tell you, however, rather than questioning further, you may consider it best to contact the appropriate services for advice or a referral. Mandatory reporting legislation may be relevant, however, this changes with location and so paramedics should refer to their employer for local advice.

Conclusion

FDV is common in society and paramedics are likely to encounter patients experiencing violence, abuse, or neglect in their practice. It is important that paramedics understand FDV, and how to respond appropriately, to ensure opportunities to reduce the harm to patients are not missed. There are several things that paramedics can do to support patients experiencing FDV, and learning this process will ensure you are providing the best practice to your patients.

Activities

Now review your learning by completing the learning activities in this chapter. The answers to these appear at the end of the book. Further self-test activities can be found at **www.wileyfundamentalseries.com/paramedic/3e.**

Test your knowledge

1. A failure to provide basic healthcare to someone under your care is known as?
   (a) Physical abuse.
   (b) Controlling behaviours.
   (c) Neglect.
   (d) Emotional abuse.
2. Which of the following statements is correct with regards to CAN?
   (a) CAN is the most frequently occurring form of FVD.
   (b) Allowing a child to be exposed to FDV is considered a form of CAN.
   (c) CAN is most commonly perpetrated by a stranger.
   (d) Experiencing CAN as a child is directly linked to perpetrating FDV as an adult.
3. Which of the following statements is correct with regards to FDV?
   (a) The primary victims of FDV are male and the primary perpetrators are female.
   (b) The majority of males perpetrate FDV.
   (c) The majority of women experience FDV.
   (d) The majority of the most damaging FDV is perpetrated by males against women.
4. Experiencing CAN increases the likelihood a child will attempt suicide – true or false? True
5. The most prevalent form of FDV is?
   (a) Intimate partner violence.
   (b) Child abuse and neglect.
   (c) Sexual violence.
   (d) Elder abuse and neglect.

6. What do the 4 Rs stand for, with respect to the response of paramedics to FDV?
   Recognise, Respond, Refer, Record
7. Which of the following is not a known indicator that a patient may be experiencing FDV?
   (a) Alcohol or other drug use.
   (b) Depression symptoms.
   (c) Mobility devices being withheld.
   (d) The patient has more than four children.
8. A good example of a question you can ask a patient you suspect might be experiencing FDV would be:
   (a) Are you a victim of family violence?
   (b) Did you do something to upset your partner?
   (c) Do you feel safe at home?
   (d) You were hit by your partner, weren't you?
9. When recording a patient encounter, which of the following should be included if you suspected FDV?
   (a) A description of scene finding you feel indicate the potential for FDV.
   (b) A note of if there were children present on the scene.
   (c) If you discussed FDV with the patient.
   (d) All of the above

References

Al-Yaman, F., Van Doeland M., and Wallis, M. (2006). *Family violence among Aboriginal and Torres Strait Islander Peoples*. Australian Institute of Health and Welfare Canberra.

Australian Bureau of Statistics. (2012). Personal safety survey. Cat. No. 4906.0.

Australian Bureau of Statistics. (2016). Personal safety survey. Cat. No. 4906.0.

Australian Institute of Criminology. (2013). Australian crimes: facts and figures. Available at: https://www.aic.gov.au/publications/facts/facts-14 (accessed 3 August 2023).

Australian Institute of Health and Welfare. (2017). Child protection Australia 2015–16. Child Welfare series No. 66. Cat. No. CWS 60.

Australian Institute of Health and Welfare. (2021). Child protection Australia 2020–21.

Australian Productivity Commission. (2014). Overcoming indigenous disadvantage-key indicators. Available at: https://www.pc.gov.au/ongoing/overcoming-indigenous-disadvantage/2014 (accessed 3 August 2023).

Black, M.C. (2011). Intimate partner violence and adverse health consequences implications for clinicians. *American Journal of Lifestyle Medicine* **5** (5): 428–439.

Black, M.C., Basile, K.C., Breiding, M.J. et al. National intimate partner and sexual violence survey. Atlanta, GA: Centers for Disease Control and Prevention. Available at: chrome-extension://efaidnbmnnnibpcajpcglclefindmkaj/https://www.cdc.gov/violenceprevention/pdf/2015data-brief508.pdf (accessed 3 August 2023).

Blosnich, J.R. and Bossarte, R.M. (2009). Comparisons of intimate partner violence among partners in same-sex and opposite-sex relationships in the United States. *Am J Public Health* **99** (12): 2182–2184.

Butchart, A., Phinney Harvey, A., Mian, M. et al. (2006). Preventing child maltreatment: a guide to taking action and generating evidence. Available at: https://iris.who.int/handle/10665/43499 (accessed 19 October 2023).

Campbell, J.C. (2002). Health consequences of intimate partner violence. *The Lancet* **359** (9314): 1331–1336.

Dearden, J. and Jones, W. (2008). Homicide in Australia: 2006–07. National homicide monitoring program annual report. Australian Institute of Criminology. Available at: https://www.aic.gov.au/sites/default/files/2020-05/mc32.pdf (accessed 3 August 2023).

Ghafournia, N. (2011). Battered at home, played down in policy: Migrant women and domestic violence in Australia. *Aggression and Violent Behavior* **16** (3): 207–213.

Green, A.H. (1993). Child sexual abuse: Immediate and long-term effects and intervention. *J Am Acad Child Adolesc Psychiatry* **32** (5): 890–902.

Hanson, R.F., Kievit, L.W., Saunders, B.E. et al. Correlates of adolescent reports of sexual assault: Findings from the National Survey of Adolescents. *Child Maltreatment* **8** (4): 261–272.

Hughes, R.B., Lund, E.M., Gabrielli, J. et al. Prevalence of interpersonal violence against community-living adults with disabilities: A literature review. *Rehabilitation Psychology* **56** (4): 302–307.

Irwin, J. (2008). Counted stories: domestic violence and lesbians. *Qualitative Social Work* **7**(2) :199–215.

Jozkowski, K.N. and Sanders, S.A. (2012). Health and sexual outcomes of women who have experienced forced or coercive sex. *Women Health* **52** (2): 101–118.

King, W.K., Kiesel, E.L., and Simon, H.K. (2006). Child abuse fatalities: are we missing opportunities for intervention? *Pediatr Emerg Care* **22** (4): 211–214.

Kōkiri, T.P. (2017). Māori Family Violence Infographic. Available at: https://www.tpk.govt.nz/en/o-matou-mohiotanga/health/maori-family-violence-infographic (accessed 3 August 2023).

Krug, E., Dahlberg, J., Mercy, J. et al. (2002). *World Report on Violence and Health*. Geneva: World Health Organization.

Marie, D., Fergusson, D.M., Boden, and J.M. (2008). Ethnic identity and intimate partner violence in a New Zealand birth cohort. *Social Policy Journal of New Zealand* **33:** 126–145.

Norman, R.E., Byambaa, M., De, R. et al. (2012). The long-term health consequences of child physical abuse, emotional abuse, and neglect: a systematic review and meta-analysis. *PLoS medicine* **9** (11): e1001349.

Office of Women's Policy. (2002). *A* policy framework: a co-ordinated approach to reducing violence against women, women's safety strategy. Melbourne, Victoria: Office of Women's Policy. Available at: https://catalogue.nla.gov.au/catalog/681334 (accessed 3 August 2023).

Qu, L., Kaspiew, R., Carson, R. et al. (2021). National elder abuse prevalence study: final report. (Research Report). Melbourne: Australian Institute of Family Studies. Available at: https://aifs.gov.au/sites/default/files/publication-documents/2021_national_elder_abuse_prevalence_study_final_report_0.pdf (accessed 3 August 2023).

Renner, L.M. and Slack, K.S. (2006). Intimate partner violence and child maltreatment: Understanding intra-and intergenerational connections. *Child Abuse Negl* **30** (6): 599–617.

Roberts, G.L., Lawrence, J.M., O'Toole, B.I. et al. (1997). Domestic violence in the emergency department: I: two case-control studies of victims. *Gen Hosp Psychiatry* **19** (1): 5–11.

Royal Australian College of General Practitioners. (2014). *Abuse and Violence: Working with Our Patients in General Practice.* 4e. Melbourne: The Royal Australian College of General Practitioners.

Sawyer, S., Parekh, V., Williams, A. et al. (2014). Are Australian paramedics adequately trained and prepared for intimate partner violence? A pilot study. *Journal of Forensic and Legal Medicine* **28** (1): 32–35.

Sawyer, S., Coles, J., Williams, A. et al. (2015). Preventing and reducing the impacts of intimate partner violence: Opportunities for Australian ambulance services. *Emerg Med Australas* **27** (4): 307–311.

Sawyer, S., Coles, J., Williams, A. et al. (2018a). Paramedics as a New Resource for Women Experiencing Intimate Partner Violence. Journal of Interpersonal Violence. 2018:0886260518769363.

Sawyer, S., Coles, J., Williams, A. et al. (2018b). The knowledge, attitudes and preparedness to manage intimate partner violence patients of Australian paramedics – a pilot study (unpublished).

Tjaden, P. and Thoennes, N. (2000). Full report of the prevalence, incidence, and consequences of violence against women (NCJ 183781). National Institute of Justice, Office of Justice Programs, Washington, DC. Available at: https://www.ojp.gov/pdffiles1/nij/183781.pdf (accessed 3 August 2023).

Vaughan, C., Davis, E., Murdolo, A. et al. (2016). Promoting community-led responses to violence against immigrant and refugee women in metropolitan and regional Australia: the ASPIRE Project: Key findings and future directions. Available at: https://anrowsdev.wpenginepowered.com/wp-content/uploads/2019/02/12_1.2-Landscapes-ASPIRE-web.pdf (accessed 3 August 2023).

VicHealth. (2004). The health costs of violence: measuring the burden of disease caused by intimate partner violence: a summary of findings. Carlton: VicHealth. Available at: https://www.mujereslibresdeviolencia.usmp.edu.pe/wp-content/uploads/2015/03/The-health-costs-of-violence.pdf (accessed 3 August 2023).

WHO (World Health Organization). (2008). A global response to elder abuse and neglect: building primary health care capacity to deal with the problem worldwide: main report. Geneva: WHO.

WHO. (2011). Elder maltreatment fact sheet. Geneva: WHO. Available at: https://www.who.int/news-room/fact-sheets/detail/abuse-of-older-people (accessed 3 August 2023).

WHO. (2013a). Responding to intimate partner violence and sexual violence against women: WHO clinical and policy guidelines. Geneva: WHO

WHO. (2013b). Global and regional estimates of violence against women: prevalence and health effects of intimate partner violence and non-partner sexual violence. In: Department of Reproductive Health and Research LSoHaTM, South African Medical Research Council, editor. Geneva: WHO. Available at: https://gsdrc.org/document-library/global-and-regional-estimates-of-violence-against-women-prevalence-and-health-effects-of-intimate-partner-violence-and-non-partner-sexual-violence (accessed 3 August 2023).

WHO. (2014). *Health Care for Women Subjected to Intimate Partner Violence or Sexual Violence: A Clinical Handbook*. Geneva: WHO.

WHO. (2000). *Women's Mental Health: An Evidence Based Review*. Geneva: WHO.

CHAPTER 33

End-of-life care

Justin Honey-Jones
Specialist Lecturer Practitioner (Paramedic)

Alexander Palmer
Clinical Paramedic Specialist – Palliative Care

Contents

LEARNING OUTCOMES

On completion of this chapter the reader will be able to:

1. Describe the differences in the mind set of paramedics attending palliative and end-of-life care patients in the prehospital setting.
2. Identify key terminology used in palliative and end-of-life care.
3. Describe the approaches and tools available to aid a paramedic's decision-making.
4. Describe the signs, symptoms, and supportive approaches to the palliative and of end-of-life patient.
5. Describe the legal considerations that are specific to paramedics supporting people receiving palliative and end-of-life care.

Fundamentals of Paramedic Practice: A Systems Approach, Third Edition. Edited by Sam Willis and Ian Peate.

Companion website: www.wiley.com/go/willis/paramedic3e

Case study

George is a paramedic and is working with Guthrie, an emergency medical technician. They are working together on a double crewed ambulance in a busy urban city.

They are dispatched to a category 1 emergency call for a 52-year-old male patient who is in cardiac arrest. CPR is in progress. The crew are 7 minutes away from the address.

Whilst en route, they are running through the advanced life support algorithm and George has allocated Guthrie specific tasks to do.

On arrival, the crew are first on scene and are confronted by family members who are distraught. CPR is being administered by the patient's partner.

The crew observe the CPR being administered on a hospital bed in the living room and there is a syringe driver attached to the patient.

What are the crew's priorities?

Introduction

The role of a paramedic has been shaped over time and the public can see and hear ambulances with their blue lights and sirens throughout their day. As McCann (2022) notes, 'there is a mystique, even a romance to the work: speeding vehicles, experts functioning under sometimes extreme pressure, caring professionals providing a compassionate service to the public, the exhilaration of rescue and the tragedy of loss'.

This perception is generated through public interactions with paramedics and popular reality TV programmes such as *Ambulance* on the BBC or *Ambulance Australia,* which follow the work of paramedics attending emergencies. These programmes not only show case the knowledge, skills, and behaviours of those professionals on scene but also the variety of specialist equipment and people that can be called upon to help such as helicopters and hazardous area response teams.

The reality TV is echoed by paramedics who demonstrate their profession via social media, online blogs, and the authoring of books. All of this gives insight into the role and it is reading about and watching the traumatic and challenging incidents that give the public perception that the role of a paramedic is an emergency one.

Ingrained in the paramedicine curriculum in various forms over the last few decades are the three principles of ambulance work:

- Preserve life
- Promote recovery
- Prevent deterioration

Returning to the Case study, George and Guthrie were expecting to attend a patient in cardiac arrest with a reversible cause that they could treat and contribute to the preservation of life. There was a shift in mind set when they saw the patient was in a hospital bed in their living room and they were receiving end-of-life care drugs via a syringe driver.

It is recognised that anxious loved ones and carers often call the emergency services because they are worried about the unexpected symptoms of the disease as it has progressed or the possibility of death (Blackmore 2022). Another reason is that they want someone to help them in their time of need.

Paramedics are increasingly becoming involved in community and primary care practice. Therefore, they have become more involved in palliative and end-of-life care, which involves the supporting of patients who are considered to be at the end of their lives (Patterson et al. 2019).

Palliative and end-of-life care in paramedicine requires a different approach and it frequently goes against the nature of a paramedic's core education, which is about saving life. The principles of palliative and end-of-life care are comparable to the words of William Osler, who famously said 'to cure sometimes, to relieve often, to comfort always'. The paramedic has transferable clinical and people skills, including communication, empathy, patient-centred care, leadership, and collaborative working. All of these are invaluable in the provision of palliative and end-of-life care in the community.

This chapter explores the fundamentals of palliative and end-of-life care in paramedic practice.

Principles of palliative and end-of-life care

In its original medieval Latin meaning, the term 'palliative' means 'to cloak'. The most widely accepted definition of palliative care is that of the World Health Organization (WHO 2022):

> *Palliative care is an approach that improves the quality of life of patients (adults and children) and their families who are facing problems associated with life-threatening illness.*
>
> *It prevents and relieves suffering through the early identification, correct assessment and treatment of pain and other problems, whether physical, psychosocial or spiritual.*

Within England, the term 'end-of-life care' refers to the last year of life (NHS England 2023). The typical journey of a palliative care patient to end of life is illustrated in Figure 33.1.

The provision of palliative care worldwide is inconsistent. It is estimated that 56.8 million people worldwide need this care, including 25.7 million who are in the last year of their life (WHO 2020).

The provision of palliative care is delivered by a range of healthcare professionals, including all grades of ambulance clinicians, doctors, nurses, healthcare assistants, nursing associates, occupational therapists, and physiotherapists. All healthcare professionals are duty bound and must work together to provide person-centred care. They should always remember a patient's legal human right to health.

To be person-centred, all clinicians must ensure that the care being provided is respectful, responsive, and meets the needs of the person concerned. This includes their preferences, needs, and values (Health Education England 2023). Clinicians need to empower each and every patient to know their rights.

According to Graves (2020), human rights are based on our shared values, including:

- Fairness
- Respect
- Equality
- Dignity
- Autonomy

Dame Cicely Saunders sums up the meaning of human rights and person-centred care with her famous words: 'You matter because you are you. You matter to the last moment of your life, and we will do all we can, not only to help you die peacefully, but also to live until you die.'

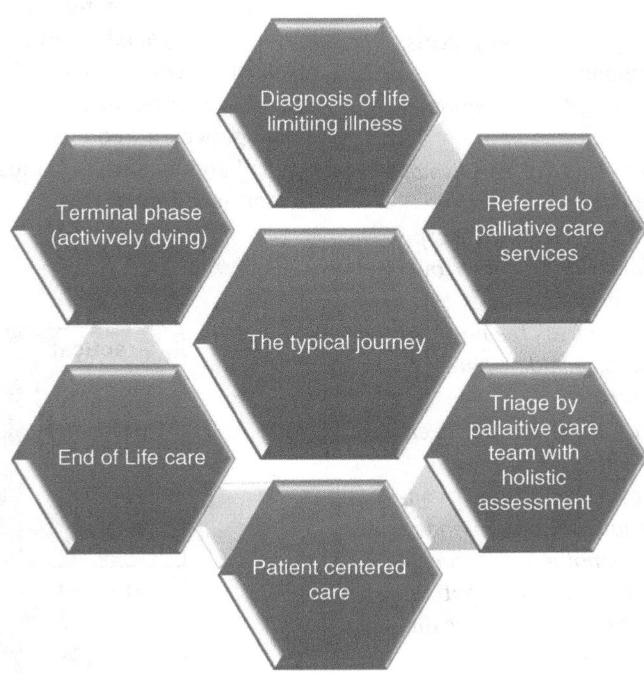

FIGURE 33.1 The journey of a palliative care patient to end of life.

Practice insight

The provision of person-centred care and the Human Rights Act 1998 are inextricably linked.

The relevant human rights include:

- Article 2: Right to life.
- Article 3: Right to be free from inhuman or degrading treatment.
- Article 5: Right to liberty.
- Article 8: Right to private and family life, home, and correspondence.
- Article 9: Right to freedom of thought, conscience, and religion.
- Article 14: Right to enjoy all these human rights without discrimination.

Aims of palliative and end-of-life care

The WHO (2019) states the aim of palliative care is to:

- *Provide relief from pain and other distressing symptoms*
- *Affirm life and regard dying as a normal process*
- *Neither hasten nor postpone death*
- *Integrate the psychological and spiritual aspects of patient care*
- *Offer a support system to help patients live as actively as possible until death*
- *Offer a support system to help the family cope during the patient's illness and in their own bereavement*
- *Use a team approach to address the needs of patients and their families, including bereavement counselling, if indicated*
- *Enhance quality of life, and may also positively influence the course of illness*
- *Be applied early in the course of illness, in conjunction with other therapies that are intended to prolong life, such as chemotherapy or radiation therapy, and includes those investigations needed to better understand and manage distressing clinical complications.*

The overall aim of end-of-life care is to:

- Manage the patient's physical symptoms including nausea, vomiting, and pain.
- Offer emotional support to the patient and their family.
- Support the patient to talk about their needs and wishes.

It is important to recognise the role of the paramedic and ambulance clinicians is not isolated but that the approach taken must be holistic and work in conjunction with the wishes of the patient and the decisions made by other healthcare professionals involved in their direct care. These wishes may be expressed by the patient or outlined in care planning documentation, which may be accessed via the patient's clinical notes on scene or electronically.

History of palliative care

Palliative care was recognised as a speciality within medicine in the 1980s, as a result of the work of the modern hospice movement in the UK lead by Dame Cicely Saunders in the 1960s.

Saunders begun caring for patients with terminal illness in 1948 and made a significant contribution to the field by lecturing and authoring articles and books. This led to St Christopher's Hospice being founded in 1967. The hospice was the first to link pain and symptom control, compassionate care, teaching, and research and has been a pioneer for palliative medicine around the world. It has established what is recognised as 'holistic care' today. Saunders used her experience and understood that care for a dying person requires more than symptom control. Medical and nursing care must be combined with holistic support (see Figure 33.2).

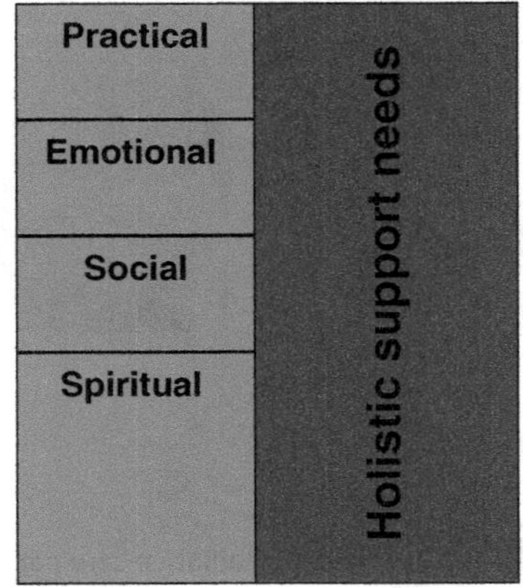

FIGURE 33.2 Holistic support needs of patients.
Source: St Christopher's Hospice 2023.

Biopsychosocial model of health and illness

The traditional approach to medicine for health and disease has been to use the medical model and/or biological models, which treat patients' conditions exclusively by medical means (Inerney 2002). These approaches have been challenged over the decades. George Engel (1977) suggested that to understand a person's medical condition, we must not be limited to considering just the biological factors but should also consider the psychological and social factors. Engel implied that behaviours, thoughts, and feelings may influence the physical state of a person (Inerney 2002), and his model has influenced the training of medical professionals to ensure other factors are also considered in the management and treatment of patients (see Figure 33.3).

These factors include:

- **Biological** – physiological pathology of the patient.
- **Psychological** – thoughts, emotions, and behaviours.
- **Social** – socio-economic, the environment, and cultural factors.

This biopsychosocial model is inextricably linked to the holistic approach Saunders introduced with the hospice movement and this has influenced the approach to care and management of palliative and end-of-life patients. This approach is relevant to the principles of palliative and end-of-life care that will be introduced throughout this chapter.

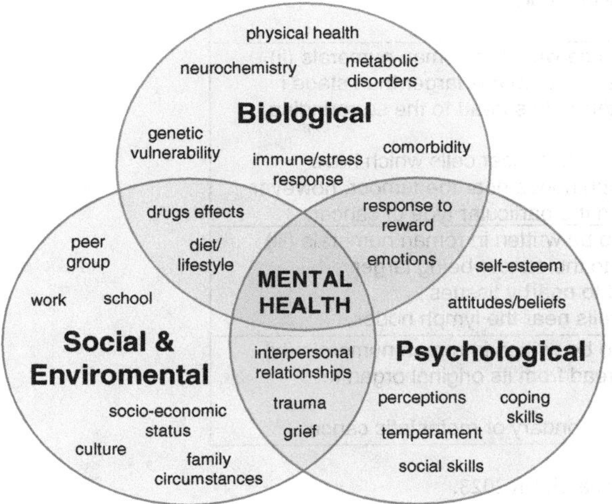

FIGURE 33.3 Engel's biopsychosocial model.

Opportunities and challenges for paramedics

Patient's receiving palliative and end-of-life care often specify when they reach the end stage of their illness that their preferred place of death is their home (Blackmore 2022). For the patient, this offers the comfort of being surrounded by their memories, loved ones, pets, and belongings but for paramedics the home environment poses possible challenges.

Patterson et al. (2019) identified the following challenges for paramedics:

- Uncertainty about how to care for end-of-life patients who are dying.
- Due to limited information on scene to make an informed clinical decision, paramedics may adopt a 'default' approach and convey patients to the emergency department (ED).
- Paramedics are reliant on advanced care planning documents to aid their clinical decision-making but often struggle to understand it if it is available.
- Due to inconsistencies and poor access to advanced care planning information, paramedics feel ill prepared to provide the right level of care.

The ambulance service is available 24/7, however, not all parts of the health and care services have the same level of availability. This poses challenges with seeking advice and support from palliative care professionals when the patient calls outside of normal working hours.

It is accepted that paramedics report being fearful about the care of a dying patient. This is associated with the issues surrounding the Do Not Attempt Cardiopulmonary Resuscitation (DNACPR) recommendations due to:

- Difficulties locating the document.
- Not understanding the legal requirements associated with the recommendations.
- Uncertainty about whose responsibility it is to discuss this with the patient, their families, and carers,

In addition, there are challenges associated with documentation at the patient's home including:

- It is often out of date.
- Inconsistency across the country.
- Limited information is available.

These challenges can contribute both to the lack of confidence in this area of paramedicine and to the 'defensive clinical practice culture rather than a person-centred culture, resulting in the dying patient's conveyance to hospital' (Blackmore 2022). They may hinder the actioning of a patient's specific wishes and ultimately affect their final days, hours, and minutes with their loved ones. As professionals, we have to be conscious of the impact our clinical decisions can have and remember 'how someone dies lives on in the memory of those left behind' (Dame Cicely Saunders).

Practice insight

DNACPR recommendations are sometimes also referred to as:

- Do Not Attempt Resuscitation (DNAR).
- Do Not Resuscitate (DNR).

Common terminal illnesses

Terminal illness (sometimes referred to as a life-limiting illness) is a term used to describe a medical condition that is incurable because the treatment is no longer effective and will therefore limit a person's life. Examples of life-limiting illnesses include:

- Advanced cancer.
- Dementia (including Alzheimer's).
- Motor neurone disease (MND).
- Lung disease, e.g. Chronic Obstructive Pulmonary Disease (COPD.)
- Neurological diseases such as Parkinson's.
- Advanced heart disease, e.g. heart failure.

The stages of cancer

When attending palliative and end-of-life patients with cancer, the paramedic may hear reference to the stage of the cancer by the patient or read it in their clinical records (see Figure 33.4).

Communication in palliative care

Like all forms of patient care, effective communication is paramount in palliative and end-of-life care. Communication is important to connect with the patient, develop a rapport, and be able to provide compassionate care. The paramedic may experience difficulties in effective communication due to emotions from the patient and/or loved ones. Potential barriers to communication include patients with illnesses that specifically affect their communication such as:

- Cerebrovascular Accident (CVA)
- Dementia
- Brain tumours
- Parkinson's disease
- Multiple sclerosis
- Motor Neurone Disease (MND)

Stage	
Stage 1	▪ The stage may also be written in Roman numerals (i) ▪ Usually contained within the organ where the cancer started and is small in nature.
Stage 2	▪ This stage may also be written in roman numerals (ii) ▪ This usually means the tumour is larger than stage i however has not started to spread to the surrounding tissues ▪ Sometimes this refers to cancer cells which have spread into the lymph nodes near the tumour, however this is dependent on the particular type of cancer.
Stage 3	▪ This stage may also be written in roman numerals (iii) ▪ This usually refers to the cancer being larger ▪ It may have spread to nearby tissues ▪ There are cancer cells near the lymph nodes.
Stage 4	▪ This stage may also be written in roman numerals (iv) ▪ The cancer has spread from its original organ to another ▪ This is also called secondary or metastatic cancer.

FIGURE 33.4 The stages of cancer. Source: Adapted from Cancer Research UK 2023.

TABLE 33.1 Communication tips.

Getting to know the patient and their families/carers	• Take time to get to know the patient and how they like to communicate. • Establish a relationship with people close to the patient such as family members, friends, and carers. • Find out what the patient already knows.
Making the patient feel comfortable	• Introduce yourself with your name and role when you meet a new patient. If someone has confusion or memory problems, you may need to do this each time you see them. • If possible, have important discussions in an environment that makes communication easier. This should be a private place that is quiet, calm and without distractions. • Make sure you have enough time for the conversation but be aware the person might need a break if they get tired.
Sharing information	• Share information in a way the patient can understand. For example, you may need to write words down, use objects or pictures. Check they have understood important information by asking them to repeat what you said, in their own words if possible. • Provide written information such as booklets or websites. This means patients can find information in their own time and have support when you are not there. • Tell them why you are there, for example, to give medicines, personal care, or have a conversation.
Your language and communication skills	• Ask open-ended questions, like 'How are you feeling?' instead of 'Are you feeling better?' • Be aware of your body language. Good eye contact and an open posture with arms and legs uncrossed can make patients feel more at ease. • Use plain language instead of medical jargon. • Avoid unclear language – for example, say 'dying' instead of 'passing away'. • Actively listen to what they are saying, concentrating on what they're telling you, rather than what you might respond with. • Check you have understood what the person has told you. Be honest if you do not understand something. • Consider ways to make communication easier whilst wearing personal protective equipment (PPE).

- Head and neck cancer
- Severe head injury

The communication tips in Table 33.1 are recommended for all healthcare professionals by Marie Curie (2022).

Due to the nature of the role of the paramedic and ambulance clinicians who are often called to palliative and end-of-life care patients, some patients may have specific communication needs and these can add complexity to an emergency call. These include:

- Sensory loss or impairment including deafness/hearing loss and blindness/sight loss.
- Learning disabilities.
- Language.
- Emotional distress.
- Drowsy or unconscious patients.

Marie Curie (2022) offer the tips outlined in Table 33.2 to all healthcare professionals.

Practice insight

Learning British Sign Language is available through courses at local colleges and training providers.

The British Sign Language website has a useful dictionary and has video demonstrations for a host of common words. BSL Dictionary – British Sign Language (BSL) Dictionary & Resources

The Auslan Sign Bank (Australia) includes similar resources. Signbank (auslan.org.au)

The multi-disciplinary team involved in holistic care

The provision of palliative care and end-of-life care involves a multi-disciplinary team (MDT) working together for the

TABLE 33.2 Specific communication needs.

Specific communication needs	Tips to communicate
Deafness/hearing loss May communicate by: lipreading, sign language (British Sign Language is usually preferred), fingerspelling, reading written information	• Find out how the person prefers to communicate. • Make sure the person can see your face clearly – where possible use clear face masks or visors when using PPE. • Speak clearly but try not to exaggerate your mouth movement. • Speak at a normal volume – shouting can be uncomfortable for patients wearing hearing aids. • Check the person understands. • Learn some key words and phrases in British Sign Language.
Blindness/sight loss May be blind or partially sighted and may communicate in different ways	• Ask how they prefer to communicate. • Offer information in other formats, like large print, Braille, or audio. • Let them know you are there, and who you are, each time you start a conversation. • Check they understand and repeat yourself if needed. • Make sure equipment they need is nearby, like magnifiers or tablets/assistive devices.
Learning disabilities There are different types of learning disability and include mild, moderate, severe, or profound (Mencap 2023) They may have difficulty understanding new or complicated information.	• Learn how they like to communicate, for example, they may use a communication aid such as a picture board or app. • Find out if they need support to communicate and include people who know them well. • Avoid jargon and unclear language – for example, say 'dying' instead of 'passing away' • Find out how they express discomfort or pain. • Allow enough time for conversations – be patient and ready to repeat yourself if needed. • Check they understand by asking them to repeat what you said, using their own words if possible. • Ask open-ended questions. For example, ask 'What questions do you have?' or 'Which parts shall I repeat?' instead of 'Do you understand?' • Learn some symbols and signs in Makaton – a language programme that uses symbols, signs, and speech to help people communicate.
Language	• There are things you can do to support patients who speak a different language to you: • Learn key words and phrases in the patient's first language – like food, water, toilet, or pain – depending on what's most important to them. • Use free apps or websites such as Google Translate – be aware these are not always accurate. • Find information booklets or support line services in the patient's native language. Ask your employer for access to a translation or interpreter service such as language line.
Emotional distress	• Encourage them to talk about their fears and worries in a calm, private, and safe environment. Listening without judgement and being patient is important for this. • It is important not to try and fix emotional problems. Asking open questions and allowing them to talk freely about how they're feeling is likely to be more helpful. • Help them to feel relaxed. Find out what helps them to relax and try to arrange this – you could speak to people close to the patient for help with this. • If someone is too distressed or too tired to talk, let them know you can talk at another time (if not an emergency). Try not to give too much information at once. Highlight the most important information and arrange another time to talk.
Drowsy or unconscious patients	• You may be able to reassure them by: • Talking to them. • Encouraging family and friends to talk to them – it is important to sensitively prepare them not to expect a response. • Playing their favourite music. • Using touch such as holding hands, when appropriate. • Being careful what conversations you have around the patient – avoid upsetting topics.

patient's specific needs and can include the following healthcare professionals:

- Paramedic
- District nurse (DN)
- Clinical nurse specialist (CNS)
- Clinical paramedic specialist (CPS)
- General practitioner (GP)
- Consultant in palliative medicine
- Speciality doctor in palliative medicine
- Pharmacist
- Physiotherapist
- Occupational therapist
- Counsellor
- Psychologist

The MDT collectively work together to provide holistic and patient-centred care that is in accordance with the patient's wishes. When making decisions, the MDT have a wide range of expertise to call upon and this will form the care the patient receives.

Paramedics and ambulance clinicians can access advice about their patients by utilising the expertise of the healthcare professionals overseeing their care.

Practice insight

Isabel Hospice in Welwyn Garden City, Hertfordshire (UK) provide a 24-hour telephone clinical advice line, which can be accessed by patients, carers, family members, and healthcare professionals who need guidance and support on delivering palliative care.

Find out about the hospices in your local area and support they can offer you.

Common reasons for paramedic attendance

An emergency ambulance is usually called by family members and/or carers due to a sudden deterioration in the patient. The symptoms they experience often include:

- Pain
- Nausea
- Agitation
- Secretions
- Difficulty in breathing
- Fatigue

Associated symptoms are:

- Anxiety
- Depression
- Constipation
- Fatigue
- Difficulty sleeping

Introduction to pain

Pain is different for everyone and some patients are afraid of being in pain. Some patients with a terminal illness will not experience any pain, whereas for others it can be very common. It is important to remember that 'pain is whatever the experiencing person says it is, and exists whenever he says it does' McCaffery (1968, in Campbell 2012, p. 30).

Pain can be caused by the illness itself, by side effects of medications, by the treatment being received, e.g. a surgical procedure, or other co-morbidities such as osteoporosis. Physical pain experienced by patients is caused by the disease and the severity will vary from patient to patient. Forty per cent of pain seen in cancer patients is neuropathic and this is caused by the pathological changes within the nervous system (Charles and Nicholls 2012).

The overall pain of a patient, sometimes referred to as the 'total pain', is not limited to just the physical pain but can also include other types of pain (Morris and Collier 2012), including:

Emotional pain: The emotional pain most often experienced by patients is the stress associated with the prospect of their own death and it can lead to depression, anxiety, and even guilt.

Social pain: The development of the condition can significantly impact patients socially and they may lose their social contacts. This can lead to loneliness, missed opportunities, and the feeling of isolation.

Spiritual pain: The patient may lose hope and their purpose in life. Some patients may not be able to make sense of their condition and its impact on their life and of those around them and therefore create the patient pain.

Religious pain: Patients can feel they have been deserted by their God or even being punished. Some patients may feel pain because they are not well enough to attend religious services, and this can be linked to social pain.

Cultural pain: English may be the patient's second language or they may not speak English at all. This can prevent their culture and wishes from being considered in terms of their care. Patients may feel isolation from their community, country, or culture and this can cause distress and fear. It is important that culture – including rituals, customs, traditions, and dietary requirements – is taken into account when healthcare professionals support patients.

Causes of cancer pain

Research shows us that cancer pain is usually caused by the tumour pressing on organs, nerves, and bones. However, other types of pain can be the result of chemotherapy drugs, which can cause numbness and a tingling sensation in the hands and feet, and the routes of injection (both subcutaneous and intramuscular) can cause a burning sensation. Radiotherapy can also cause irritation of the skin (Cancer Research UK 2020).

The types of cancer pain

Cancer pain can be acute or chronic in nature. Acute pain typically lasts a short period of time as a result of damage caused by an injury and is usually managed with pain relief. Chronic pain can range from being mild to severe in nature and can be the result of changes to the nerves, the chemicals produced by the tumour, and the tumour pressing onto bones, organs, and nerves.

The types of cancer pain include:

Nerve pain: This is referred to as neuropathic pain and is a result of the tumour pressing on nerves. Patients often describe it as a burning, shooting, or tingling feeling under the skin.

Bone pain: This is sometimes referred to as somatic pain and is often described by patients as a dull, aching, or throbbing pain in a specific area of the body. Cancer can spread into the bones, which damages bone tissue, causing pain.

Soft tissue pain: This is sometimes referred to as visceral pain and is often described as a pain that is not easy to pin point. It is usually sharp in nature or can be a cramping, aching, or throbbing. Soft tissue pain refers to pain that is caused by an organ or muscle.

Phantom pain: This is often described as unbearable pain and is associated with a part of the body that has been removed, e.g. a mastectomy (the removal of the breast). About one in three women experience phantom pain in the breast following their mastectomy.

Referred pain: This is the feeling of pain from an organ in the body that is referred to a different part of the body. For example, a swollen liver may cause pain in the right shoulder due to the pressing of associated nerves (see Figure 33.5).

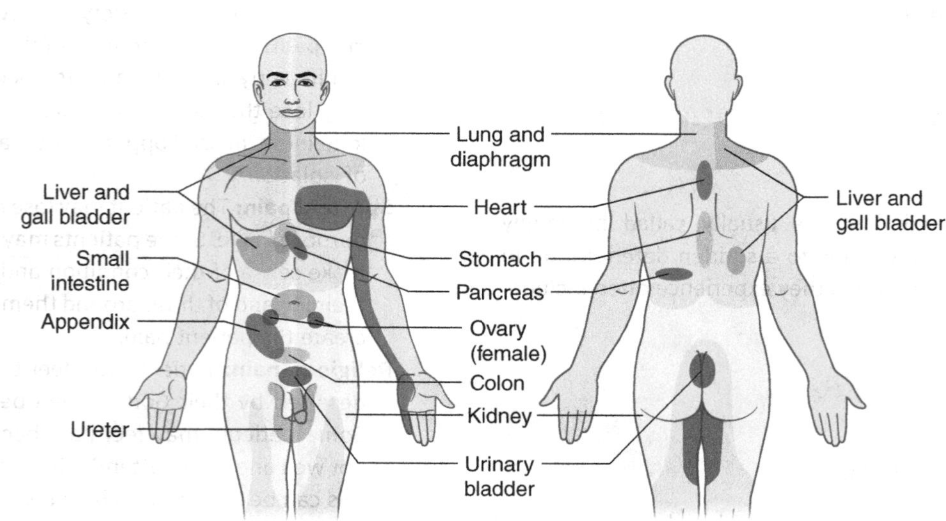

FIGURE 33.5 Common sites of referred pain. Source: Cancer Research UK 2020.

Pain tolerance factors

Pain is different in everyone, and pain tolerance can be increased or lowered depending on a range of factors. Morris and Collier (2012, p. 44) indicate that these various factors are:

Factors that lower pain tolerance, including:
- Discomfort
- Insomnia
- Fatigue
- Anxiety
- Fear
- Anger
- Boredom
- Sadness
- Depression
- Introversion
- Social abandonment
- Mental isolation

Factors that increase pain tolerance, including:
- Relief of symptoms
- Sleep
- Rest
- Physiotherapy
- Relaxation therapy
- Explanation/support
- Understanding/empathy
- Diversion
- Listening
- Elevation of mood
- Finding meaning and significance
- Social inclusion
- Support to express emotions

Approaches to pain

Pain can be managed using both pharmacological and non-pharmacological means.

Pharmacological approaches

The management of pain is not wholly specific to pharmacological means but must be assessed and managed with a holistic approach. In 1986, the WHO proposed the 'WHO analgesic ladder' as an approach to provide the adequate pain relief for cancer patients (Ventafridda et al. 1985). The WHO analgesic ladder has become a standard of care across the world for cancer patients because of its approach in reducing and managing pain whilst minimising the side effects experienced by patients (Anekar et al. 2023).

The WHO analgesic ladder guides the approach to pain management outlined in Table 33.3.

TABLE 33.3 WHO analgesic ladder and JRCALC pain scoring.

WHO analgesic ladder step	Type of pain	Pain score	Examples of pharmacological management
Step 1	Mild	<3/10	Paracetamol Aspirin Ibuprofen
Step 2	Mild to moderate	3–6/10	Codeine Tramadol
Step 3	Moderate to severe	>6/10	Morphine Oxycodone Fentanyl Buprenorphine

Source: Adapted from JRCALC 2022 and Marie Curie 2022.

The WHO analgesic ladder refers to 'adjuvants'. An adjuvant is a medicine that has been designed for other medical conditions but is also effective for certain types of pain (NHS 2020). Adjuvants can be prescribed to compliment other pain medication such as opioids.

Marie Curie (2022) provide the following examples of adjuvants:

- Anticonvulsants for nerve pain.
- Antidepressants for nerve pain.
- Antispasmodics such as hyoscine butylbromide for crampy pain (colic).
- Bisphosphonates for bone pain.
- Steroids which reduce inflammation.

Non-pharmacological approaches

Cancer charities and hospices use a range of non-pharmacological methods including:

- Complementary therapies
- Distraction
- Heat and cold therapy
- Kindness
- Listening
- Maximising comfort
- Occupational therapy
- Physiotherapy
- Positioning
- Talking therapies
- Thoughtfulness
- Transcutaneous electrical nerve simulation (TENS)

(Adapted from Morris and Collier 2012; Marie Curie 2022).

Routes of medication administration

Palliative and end-of-life care patients are usually given medications in the least invasive way, with the method of administration selected to cause the least amount of discomfort, pain, or distress (NHS 2020). Medication can be administered via the following routes (see Figure 33.6):

- Oral
- Subcutaneous
- Intravenous
- Transdermal patch
- Syringe driver

Just in case medications

Just in case (JIC) medications (see Table 33.4) are prescribed in advance to patients in anticipation of their needs changing in the future. Advanced prescription ensures there is no delay in the patient receiving the treatment for their changing needs. This is often the most useful if the patient is living in their own home or being cared for in the community. The medications are often stored in a box labelled JIC medications (NICE 2015).

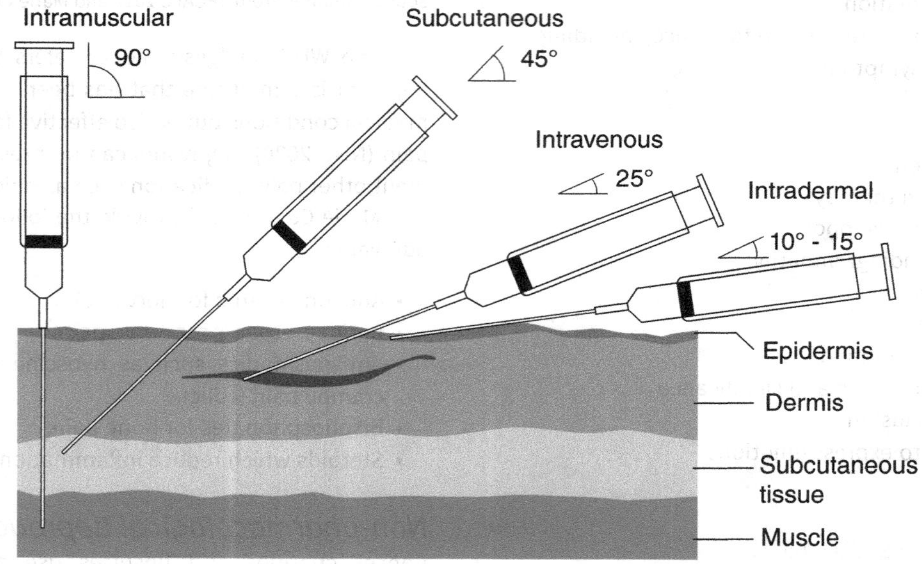

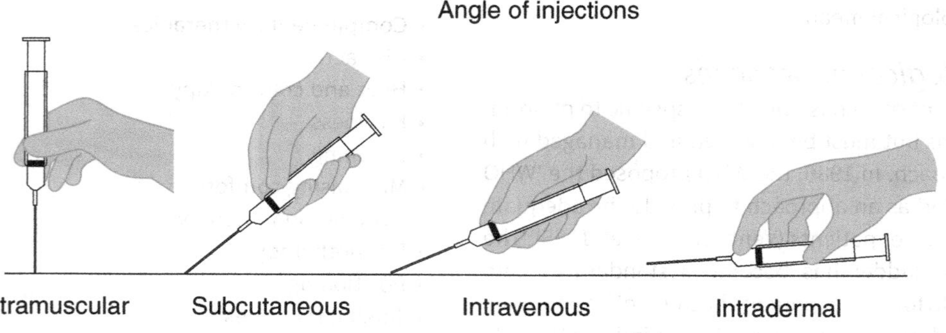

FIGURE 33.6 The needle insertion angles for IM, SC, and IV

TABLE 33.4 JIC medications commonly prescribed.

Sign/symptom	Medication
Pain/breathlessness	Morphine sulphate Oxycodone
Nausea/vomiting	Cyclizine Metoclopramide Ondansetron Antiemetic
Agitation	Midazolam Anxiolytic sedative Lorazepam
Secretions	Glycopyrronium Hyoscine butylbromide
Patient-specific: Heart failure/pulmonary oedema Seizures	Furosemide (antidiuretic) Midazolam

Syringe driver

A syringe driver (also referred to as a syringe pump) is a small battery powered pump that delivers specific medications to a patient subcutaneously at a constant rate. The syringe driver is often set up in the few weeks and days of a patient's life, however it can be used at all stages of treatment, depending upon the needs of the patient. The medications administered via this method are used to help make patients comfortable by:

- Managing pain
- Managing nausea
- Managing vomiting
- Managing agitation
- Helping with excessive respiratory secretions

A healthcare professional working as part of an MDT may decide to set up a syringe driver for a number of clinical reasons, including:

- The patient has nausea and/or vomiting.
- The patient has difficulty swallowing oral medicines.
- Symptoms can't be managed well with oral medicine.
- To avoid having to give injected medicines frequently.
- The patient can't absorb medicines through their gut effectively.

(Marie Curie 2022)

Practice insight

Paramedics and ambulance clinicians may be called out of hours to a person who is at the end of their life and is deteriorating.

The patient's notes may indicate that the JIC medications have been prescribed and are to be administered in specific situations, e.g. pain, nausea, vomiting, excessive respiratory secretions. Some of these drugs might be outside of the paramedic's scope of practice, however, they may be competent in the specific route of administration, e.g. subcutaneous injection.

Seek advice from the patient's clinicians or seek advice from other healthcare professionals and follow local protocol.

If any JIC medications are administered, ensure that your own documentation and the medication administration record in the patient's notes are completed.

Pain assessment tools

Assessing pain is the key to understanding the amount of discomfort the patient is in. However, it must be recognised that, according to Mallinson (2022, p. 125), assessing pain can be challenging.

Gangaram et al. (2021) identify that pain is often poorly assessed in the prehospital setting, which can result in the patient receiving inappropriate care. Paramedics and ambulance clinicians can use assessment tools to aid and structure their assessment. The common tools used are:

- SOCRATES (see Table 33.5).
- The Abbey Pain Scale (a tool used to measure pain in patients who cannot verbalise).

TABLE 33.5 SOCRATES.

SOCRATES	**Site** **Onset** **Character** **Radiation** **Associated symptoms** **Time** **Exacerbation** **Severity**

Paramedics and ambulance clinicians can also use specific questions. Marie Curie (2022) suggest the following:

- Where is the pain? Is there more than one area of pain?
- Can you describe the pain? For example, is it an ache or a sharp, stabbing pain?
- On a scale of 1 to 10, how bad is the pain?
- How long have you had it?
- When did it start?
- How long does it last for?
- Is it new or have you had it before?
- What makes the pain better or worse?
- Did it start gradually or come on quickly?
- Does it start in one place and move to somewhere else?
- Do you have any other symptoms like vomiting, finding it hard to look at light, needing to empty your bowels, or breathlessness?
- Are you having any homeopathic treatment?
- How is it affecting your daily activities?

There are a number of indicators of pain in patients who are not able to communicate. Marie Curie (2022) suggest the following:

- Agitation or increased temper.
- Being reluctant to move.
- Bending over or favouring one side when walking.
- Changes in breathing.
- Changes in mood.
- Frowning or grimacing.
- Groaning or crying.
- Lack of concentration.
- Massaging, rubbing, or guarding the painful area.
- Refusing care.
- Refusing food.
- Withdrawal or refusal to make eye contact.

The last year of life

Palliative care healthcare professionals use a variety of tools to help identify patients who are approaching the end of life. Examples of these tools include:

Gold standards framework (GSF) proactive indicator guidance (PIG): The national GSF is designed to provide a 'gold standard of care' for all patients nearing the end of their lives. The framework supports local healthcare systems to develop and integrate cross boundary care. GSF meetings are held regularly and focus on the patient's clinical and holistic care needs. People who attend these meetings typically include clinicians involved in the patient's care. Working together facilitates better-quality care and decision-making for patients during the final months of their lives.

Palliative care outcome scale (POS): The POS is a family of tools designed to capture patients' physical symptoms, psychological state, emotional and spiritual needs, and other support requirements. This is a validated instrument used to collect information. Patients will be asked to complete a POS and the results help medical staff to understand the individual patient's overall holistic and clinical picture.

Outcome Assessment and Complexity Collaborative (OACC): A group of measures designed to help measure and improve care for patients.

Indications of last year of life

If death is likely to occur within the next 12 months, then the patient could be considered as 'approaching end of life'. This includes patients with advanced life-limiting illnesses such as cancer or motor neurone disease, or patients with frailty due to advancing age. The dying process may come into view about one to three months before death. Although this can vary from person to person (see Table 33.6 for examples of indications).

Some people have existing conditions that mean they are at risk of dying from a sudden crisis in their condition such as a ruptured aortic aneurism. Some have a life-threatening acute condition caused by a sudden catastrophic event such as an accident or stroke.

There may be different health and social care professionals involved in an end-of-life care journey. Including GPs,

TABLE 33.6 General indications of the last year of life.

- Decreasing levels of activity
- Different co-morbidities
- A decline in physical health
- An increased need for support
- Choosing to no longer receive treatment
- Progressive weight loss over a 6-month period (>10%)
- Complex symptom management from advanced progression of the disease
- A physiological decreasing response to treatment
- Repeated crisis admissions
- A serious fall
- Being transferred to a nursing home due to the type of care needed

Source: Adapted from JRCALC 2022, p. 14.

community care teams, district nurses, physiotherapists, occupational therapists, as well as hospital doctors and nurses.

Care in the last few days of life

As the patient's condition progresses, the words of Dame Cicely Saunders must never be forgotten by paramedic's and ambulance clinicians: 'How someone dies lives on in the memory of those left behind.'

Palliative care teams will aim to facilitate the person's preferred place of care and death. Care in the last few days of life is vitally important to the patient's and relatives' well-being. There may be specialist teams involved such as clinical nurse specialists or paramedic specialists, hospice at home, or other community-based help. These teams can address complex care needs and provide enhanced care and symptom control. Family and friends may also be closely involved in the person's care and healthcare professionals should work together with them to ensure patient-centred care is provided.

Signs of the very end of life

It can be difficult to know exactly when someone is reaching the very end of life. The dying process can last for months, but the very end of life is sometimes referred to as the 'terminal phase' or 'actively dying'. This will typically be the last days or hours of life.

Everyone's experience and presentation of dying is different and even experienced clinicians sometimes struggle to give an exact timeframe. However, there are common signs and symptoms that can help the paramedic and ambulance clinicians recognise when someone is in the last days or hours of life. Typically, there will be changes happening to the person's condition day by day or hour by hour. The following signs may indicate the very end of life is approaching (JRCALC 2022, p. 14):

- Abnormal clinical observations.
- Changes in breathing, e.g. irregular (shallow with deep signs), pauses (apnoeic episodes).
- Reduced levels of consciousness.
- Sleeping more and difficult to arouse.
- Confusion.
- Agitation.
- Loss of appetite.
- Restlessness.
- Incontinence.
- Following death, a 'last sigh' may be heard.
- Respiratory secretions that can make a rattle noise in the throat.
- The legs, arms, and hands feel cool to touch.
- A purple-blue colour may be seen on the feet and legs (mottled).
- The face may become pale.

The paramedic and ambulance clinicians may be called to scene shortly before or following death.

On arriving at the scene, if the patient is in the final stages of dying and all reversible causes of death have been considered, the approach must be on the provision of supportive care to the patient and their families/carers (JRCALC 2022, p. 15)

After death

Deaths are classified as expected or unexpected.

If the death is expected, the paramedic is required to follow their own organisation's protocol and contact the patient's GP to arrange for the death to be certified. Expected deaths is when the death is anticipated. The patient would have been approaching end of life due to ill health or frailty/ old age. In good practice, patients should have been given the chance to partake in advanced care planning, with palliative care teams, GPs, hospital doctors, and clinical specialists who will try to facilitate this. Although it is important to note this is not always successful.

Unexpected deaths will involve the police and the local corners' office. This is when a death happens suddenly such as a result of a road traffic collision or fall. Police are required to attend the scene of unexpected deaths to complete an initial investigation on behalf of the coroner and establish that the death is not suspicious and has no third-party involvement.

Verifying and certifying the death

Following a death in the community, a trained healthcare professional can verify death by completing a set of checks according to their local policy to confirm the person has died. A doctor will need to certify the death and complete a medical certificate. This will outline the cause if it was expected, and they believe it was from natural causes.

After a doctor has certified the death, the next stage usually involves the funeral director or other arrangements the patient or family have made.

Advance care planning

Advance care planning is a term used in England, Wales, Northern Ireland, and Australia. In Scotland, this is referred to as 'anticipatory care planning'.

Advance care planning offers patients a way to express their wishes about how they would like to be cared for as their illness progresses, including what treatment they want or may not want. This considers their values, goals, and preferences (JRCALC 2022, p. 132). These wishes come into effect when the patient has been assessed as no longer having mental capacity to make their own decisions. This process is not legally required and is entirely voluntary.

Healthcare professionals proactively discuss advanced care planning with their patients, although not all patients are receptive to making these decisions. The benefits of advance care planning according to Marie Curie (2022) include:

- Allowing the person to have more choice and control over what happens to them.
- Improving the quality of the end-of-life care that someone receives.
- Reducing the chance that someone receives care or treatment they don't want at end of life.
- Making it more likely that someone's wishes are known and carried out – for example, they may be more likely to die in their preferred place of death.
- Lessening the burden on family and friends who would otherwise have to be involved in decisions without knowing what the person wanted.
- Reducing anxiety and depression in family and friends after the person dies.
- Allowing the person to think about who's important to them, which can help to heal relationships.
- Allowing the person to reflect on their life and think about spiritual issues, resulting in them feeling more hopeful.

Murphy-Jones and Timmons (2016) express concern for the inappropriateness and the potentially negative consequences of the transfer of nursing home patients to the ED by paramedics in end-of-life patients who are nearing the end of their lives.

For paramedics and ambulance clinicians, the advance care plan is an invaluable tool because it can provide them with the necessary information to make informed decisions on scene, which can be emotional and challenging. Table 33.7

TABLE 33.7 Types of advance decision-making.

Type of advance care plan	Summary	Criteria	Law
Advance decision to refuse treatment (ADRT)	An ADRT is a decision to refuse a specific type of treatment in the future; when they no longer have mental capacity to make their own decisions	It is legally binding if: • It complies with the Mental Capacity Act • Is valid • Applies to the situation An ADRT is only valid if: • The person is aged 18 or over • They had the mental capacity at the time and were able to communicate the decision • The treatments being refused are clearly stated • The circumstances in which they are to be refused is explained • It is signed by the patient • A statement that the patient has made the decision on their own accord, and they have not been harassed by anyone else • Nothing has been said (e.g. they have changed their mind) or done (e.g. appointed a Lasting Power of Attorney for Health) since the decision was made	**Mental Capacity Act 2005**
Advance decision to refuse life-sustaining treatment	This is a decision by the patient to refuse life-sustaining treatment such as resuscitation and antibiotics This decision comes into effect when they no longer have mental capacity to make their own decision	It Is legally binding if: • It is written down • It is signed by the patient • Signed by an independent witness (must be over 18 years old) • It specifies the circumstances it applies too • It includes the statement 'even if life is at risk'.	

TABLE 33.7 (*Continued*)

Advance directive (Scotland only)	As per ADRT and advance decision to refuse life-sustaining treatment, however, the Mental Capacity Act 2005 does not apply to Scotland and is therefore not subject to the same criteria It is sometimes referred to as a living will	It has not been tested in the Scottish courts; however, Macmillan (2019) recommend the following: • Have the legal capacity to make the decision at the time • Aged 16 or over • The treatment chosen to be refused applies to their specific circumstances • Ideally the directive is in writing	**Common law**
Do not attempt cardiopulmonary resuscitation (DNACPR)	RCUK (2023) state the purpose of a DNACPR recommendation is to provide immediate guidance to those present (mostly healthcare professionals) on the best action to take (or not take) should the person suffer a cardiac arrest or die suddenly It is part of advance care planning; however, it differs in that it is led by clinicians (JRCALC 2022, p.132)	There are two ways a DNACPR can be issued: 1. Agreed in advance by the patient This has no legal standing however the patient can make a legally compliant by completing an advance decision to refuse life-sustaining treatment 2. Agreed in advance by a doctor - This can be decided even if the patient doesn't agree - The patient must be told that a DNACPR has or is going to be completed - The patient should be given sufficient information to understand the process and the reasons for the DNACPR - The patient should be asked about their wishes and preferences - If a patient disagrees with the DNACPR, they can request a second opinion and a review - The patient is not required to provide their consent in law, they are required to be informed and involved in the decision - If the patient lacks capacity, a doctor should check to see if there are any advance decisions made or if there is a Lasting Power of Attorney (health and care decisions) (NHS 2021)	**Not applicable**
Recommended summary plan for emergency care and treatment (ReSPECT)	ReSPECT is a process that offers a summary of personalised recommendation for a patient's future care in an emergency and when they do not have the mental capacity to make their own decisions. It also contains information about CPR/DNACPR	ReSPECT involves conversations with one or more healthcare professionals involved in the patients care and consists of the following (RCUK 2023): • A discussion and reaching a shared understanding of the patient's current state of health and how it may change in the foreseeable future • Identifying what is important to the person in relation to goals of care in the event of a future emergency • Using the information to record an agreed focus of care (either more towards life-sustaining treatments or more towards prioritising comfort over efforts to sustain life)	**Not applicable**

(*Continued*)

TABLE 33.7 ***(Continued)***

	• The making and recording of shared recommendations about specific types of care and the realistic treatment that should/shouldn't be given, and explaining sensitively recommendations about treatments that would clearly not work int their situation • Making and recording a shared recommendation about whether or not CPR is recommended

provides a summary of the types of advance care planning (that may be seen in clinical practice.

Sources of support and advice

The paramedic has a number of sources of advice for their patient's available including those in Table 33.8.

TABLE 33.8 Sources of advice for patients.

Internal	External
Clinical advice line	NHS 111
Advanced paramedics in urgent/critical care	GP
Specialist paramedics in urgent/critical care	Hospice clinical advice line
Palliative care paramedics	District nurse
Clinical managers	

Conclusion

This chapter has provided an overview of end-of-life care for paramedics. The role of a frontline paramedic will involve supporting patients who may require palliative care and might be receiving end-of-life care. Supporting patients requires the paramedic to use their knowledge and skills in a different way to caring for emergency patients.

The paramedic needs to be proactive and seek advice and support from other healthcare professionals wherever possible to help them make an informed decision. Palliative and end-of-life care is a developing speciality within paramedicine with new roles such as the clinical paramedic specialist and hospice paramedics. The paramedic's actions will have a long-lasting effect not just for the patient, but their families and carers, but the paramedic must always remember Dame Cicely Saunders's words: 'How someone dies lives on in the memory of those left behind.' Whatever you do and say will be remembered.

Activities

Now review your learning by completing the learning activities in this chapter. The answers to these appear at the end of the book. Further self-test activities can be found at **www.wileyfundamentalseries.com/paramedic/3e.**

Test your knowledge

1. What is an adjuvant?
   (a) A category of drugs used to maintain fluid balance.
   (b) A category of drugs used to prevent the vomiting.
   (c) A medicine designed for other conditions but is also effective for treating pain.
   (d) A medicine designed for somatic pain but is also effective for treating nausea.
2. Which of these medications would be appropriate analgesia for an end-of-life patient in severe pain?
   (a) Paracetamol
   (b) Ibuprofen
   (c) Aspirin
   (d) Oxycodone

3. Under the Human Rights Act, which article covers the right to life?
   (a) Article 2
   (b) Article 3
   (c) Article 5
   (d) Article 8
4. Which of these medications is an example of NSAID's?
   (a) Morphine
   (b) Ibuprofen
   (c) Paracetamol
   (d) Codeine
5. An antiemetic medication is used to:
   (a) Relieve the symptoms of pain.
   (b) Relieve the symptoms of nausea.
   (c) Treat a patient who is having indigestion.
   (d) Treat a patient who is having constipation.
6. How many different stages of cancer are there?
   (a) 1
   (b) 2
   (c) 3
   (d) 4
7. Which of these is the preferred route of administration for medication to an end-of-life patient?
   (a) Oral
   (b) Subcutaneous
   (c) Intravenous
   (d) Transdermal patch
8. Which of these is **NOT** part of the biopsychosocial model of health and illness?
   (a) Biological
   (b) Psychological
   (c) Social
   (d) Environmental
9. Which of these is legally binding for a patient over 18 years old who has decided not to consent to receiving CPR?
   (a) A recommended summary plan for emergency care and treatment.
   (b) A do not attempt cardiopulmonary resuscitation (DNACPR) form.
   (c) Advance decision to refuse treatment (ADRT).
   (d) Advance decision to refuse life-sustaining treatment.
10. Which of these is covered by the Mental Capacity Act 2005?
   (a) An advance directive.
   (b) Advance decision to refuse treatment (ADRT).
   (c) A do not attempt cardiopulmonary resuscitation (DNACPR) form.
   (d) A recommended summary plan for emergency care and treatment.

Glossary

Antidiuretic: A category of drugs used to maintain fluid balance.

Analgesic/ Analgesia: A category of drugs used to relieve pain.

Antiemetic: A category of drugs preventing nausea.

Adjuvants: An adjuvant is a medicine which has been designed for other medical conditions but is also effective for certain types of pain.

Tumour: An abnormal growth of tissue.

End-of-life care: The provision of care in the last year of life.

Life-limiting illness: An incurable condition that will shorten a person's life.

NSAID: Non-steroidal anti-inflammatory drugs are a category of drugs used to manage pain, reduce inflammation, and reduce fever.

ReSPECT: Recommended summary plan for emergency care and treatment is a personalised recommendation for the provision of care in an emergency when the person no longer has mental capacity to make their own decisions.

DNACPR: Do not attempt cardiopulmonary resuscitation is a decision recorded on a special form made by the person and/or a doctor for CPR to not be given in the event of a cardiac arrest.

A power of attorney: for health and welfare: A person who is trusted by the patient to makes decisions about health and welfare on their behalf if they no longer have mental capacity.

Further reading

Organisation	Website
Isabel Hospice	www.isabelhospice.org.uk
Mare Curie	www.mariecurie.org.uk
ReSPECT	www.respectprocess.org.uk
Cancer Research UK	www.cancerresearchuk.org
St Christopher's Hospice	www.stchristophers.org.uk
Advance Care Plan	www.advancecareplan.org.uk
Resuscitation Council UK	www.resus.org.uk
Palliative Care Australia	https://palliativecare.org.au/
End-of-Life Directions for Aged Care	https://www.eldac.com.au/
Care Search	https://www.caresearch.com.au/caresearch/tabid/579/Default.aspx

References

Advance Care Plan. (2016). Jargon buster. [Online]. Available at: http://advancecareplan.org.uk/ (accessed 18 June 2023).

Anekar, A., Maxwell Hendrix, J., and Cascella, M. (2023). *WHO Analgesic Ladder*. [Online]. National Library of Medicine. Available at: https://www.ncbi.nlm.nih.gov/books/NBK554435/ (accessed 10th June 2023).

Blackmore, T.A. (2022). What is the role of paramedics in palliative and end of life care? *Palliative Medicine* **36** (3): 402–404. [Online]. Available at: https://www.ncbi.nlm.nih.gov/pmc/articles/PMC8972948/pdf/10.1177_02692163211073263.pdf (accessed 28th April 2023).

British Institute of Human Rights. (Unknown). *End of Life Care and Human Rights: A Practitioner's Guide*. London: British Institute of Human Rights.

Campbell, H. (2012). *Nursing and Health Palliative Care Survival Guide*. London: Routledge.

Cancer Research UK. (2020). About cancer pain. [Online]. Cancer Research UK. Available at: https://www.cancerresearchuk.org/about-cancer/coping/physically/cancer-and-pain-control/about-cancer (accessed 18 June 2023).

Cancer Research UK. (2020). Causes and types of cancer pain. [Online]. Cancer Research UK. Available at: https://www.cancerresearchuk.org/about-cancer/coping/physically/cancer-and-pain-control/causes-and-t (accessed 18 June 2023).

Cancer Research UK. (2023). Stages of cancer. [Online]. Available at: https://www.cancerresearchuk.org/about-cancer/what-is-cancer/stages-of-cancer?gad=1&gclid=CjwKCAjwo7 (accessed 30 April 2023).

Charles, A. and Nicholls, T. (2012). End-of-life patients and their pain management. In: Pain: An Ambulance Perspective (ed. T. Nicholls and L. Hawkes-Frost, L.), p. 88–92. Bridgewater: Class Health.

Gangaram, P., Alinier, G., and Dippenaar, E. (2021). Paramedic adult pain assessment: pilot study. [Online]. *Journal of Paramedic Practice 2*. Available at: https://www.paramedicpractice.com/features/article/paramedic-adult-pain-assessment-pilot-study (accessed 18 June 2023).

Graves, J. (2020). The importance of human rights in end of life care. [Online]. Hospice UK. Available at: https://www.hospiceuk.org/latest-from-hospice-uk/importance-human-rights-end-life-care (accessed 2nd April 2023).

Health Education England. (2023). Person-centred care. [Online]. Health Education England. Available at: https://www.hee.nhs.uk/our-work/person-centred-care (accessed 2nd April 2023).

Joint Royal Colleges Ambulance Liaison Committee, Association of Ambulance Chief Executives. (2022). *JRCALC Clinical Guidelines 2022*. Bridgwater: Class Professional Publishing.

Macmillan Cancer Support. (2019). Advance directive. [Online]. Macmillan Cancer Support. Available at: https://www.macmillan.org.uk/cancer-information-and-support/treatment/if-you-have-an-advanced-cancer (accessed 18 June 2023).

Mallinson, T. (2022). Analgesics. In: *Fundamental of Pharmacology for Paramedics* (ed. I. Peate, S. Evans, and L. Clegg), pp. 125–148. Oxford: Wiley-Blackwell.

Marie Curie. (2022). Communication needs in palliative care. [Online]. Available at: https://www.mariecurie.org.uk/professionals/palliative-care-knowledge-zone/individual-needs/communic (accessed 21 April 2023).

Marie Curie. (2022). Pain management in palliative care. [Online]. Available at: https://www.mariecurie.org.uk/professionals/palliative-care-knowledge-zone/symptom-control/pain-cont (accessed 2nd June 2023).

Marie Curie. (2022). Syringe pumps in palliative care. [Online]. Available at: https://www.mariecurie.org.uk/professionals/palliative-care-knowledge-zone/symptom-control/syringe-d (accessed 18 June 2023).

Marie Curie. (2022). What is a terminal illness? [Online]. Available at: https://www.mariecurie.org.uk/who/terminal-illness-definition (accessed 21 May 2023).

Mc Inerney, S. (2002). Introducing the Biopsychosocial Model for good medicine and good doctors. [Online]. *The British Medical Journal*. Available at: https://www.bmj.com/rapid-response/2011/10/29/introducing-biopsychosocial-model-good-medicine-and-go (accessed 17 June 2023).

McCann, L. (2022). *The Paramedic at Work a Sociology of a New Profession*. Oxford: Oxford University Press.

Mencap. (2023). What is a learning disability? [Online]. Available at: https://www.mencap.org.uk/learning-disability-explained/what-learning-disability?gclid=CjwKCAjwgqejB (accessed 20 April 2023).

Murphy-Jones, G. and Timmons, S. (2016). Paramedic's experiences of end-of-life care decision-making with regard to nursing home residents: an exploration of in. *Emergency Medical Journal* **33** (10): 722–726.

National Health Service (NHS). (2020). Managing pain and other symptoms. [Online]. Available at: https://www.nhs.uk/conditions/end-of-life-care/controlling-pain-and-other-symptoms/ (accessed 20 April 2023).

National Health Service (NHS). (2021). Do not attempt cardiopulmonary resuscitation (DNACPR) decisions. [Online]. Available at: https://www.nhs.uk/conditions/do-not-attempt-cardiopulmonary-resuscitation-dnacpr-decisions/ (accessed 22 June 2023).

National Institute for Health and Clinical Excellence. (2015). Care of dying adults in the last days of life. [Online]. Available at: https://www.nice.org.uk/guidance/ng31/ifp/chapter/medicines-prescribed-in-advance-just-in-case-medic (accessed 18 June 2023).

NHS England. (2023). Palliative and end of life care. [Online]. Available at: https://www.england.nhs.uk/eolc/ (accessed 21 May 2023).

Patterson, R., Standing, H., Lee, M. et al. (2019). Paramedic information needs in end-of-life care: a qualitative interview study exploring access to a shared electronic r. *BMC Palliative Care* **108** (18): 1–8. doi: 10.1186/s12904-019-0498-2.

Resuscitation Council UK. (2023). *FAQs: Recommendations about CPR. [Online]. Resuscitation Council UK*. Available at: https://www.resus.org.uk/home/faqs/faqs-decision-making-cpr (accessed 10 June 2023).

Rezaie, P. (ND). *The Biopsychosocial Model of Mental Health*. [Online]. *The Open University.* Available at: https://www.open.edu/openlearn/science-maths-technology/exploring-the-relationship-between-anxiety-a (accessed 17 June 2023).

Ventafridda, V., Saita, L., Ripamonti, C. et al. (1985). WHO guidelines for the use of analgesics in cancer pain. *Int J Tissue React* **7** (1): 93–96. PMID: 2409039.

World Health Organisation (WHO). (2020). *Palliative Care. [Online]. Last Updated*: August 2020. Available at: https://www.who.int/news-room/fact-sheets/detail/palliative-care (accessed 21 May 2023).

Answers

Chapter 1

Test your knowledge

1. (a) Professional parameters (e.g. legal and ethical aspects).
   (b) Professional behaviours (e.g. discipline-related knowledge and skills).
   (c) Professional responsibilities (e.g. responsibility to clients, oneself, employers, and the public).
2. Understanding of professional identity, response to socialisation, integration into professional culture, professional development and learning, professional body codes and ethics, organisational policies, and procedures.
3. Both.
4. (a) No case to answer.
   (b) Minor breaches of conduct.
   (c) Significant breaches of conduct.
   (d) Serious breaches of conduct.
   (e) Major breaches of conduct.

Activity 1.1

Whilst it may seem that this is a conversation intended to be humorous, and therefore harmless, it is implying that John thinks it is acceptable to commit fraud. Honesty, integrity, and trustworthiness are integral to professionalism.

Activity 1.2

(a) Inform the paramedic driver in clear, specific, and assertive style of their need for urgent assistance. Apply performance-enhancing psychological model (e.g. B: Breathe, T: Talk, S: See and F: Focus) strategy to the situation.

(b) Reflective on their practice using a model (e.g. Gibbs 1998) and consider implementing positive help-seeking behaviour in their professional practice.

Chapter 2

Test your knowledge

1. An independent body of individuals that self-regulate in accordance with prevailing legislation, regulations, evidence, and societal expectations.
2. Quality and safety in healthcare; research and evidence-based practice; regulation and law.
3. Practice is any role, whether remunerated or not, in which the individual uses their skills and knowledge as a practitioner in their regulated health profession. Practice is not restricted to the provision of direct clinical care. It also includes using professional knowledge in a direct nonclinical relationship with patients or clients, working in management, administration, education, research, advisory, regulatory, or policy development roles, and any other roles that have an impact on the safe, effective delivery of health services in the health profession.
4. Self-regulation, assessment by peers, standardised curricula, discretionary decision-making supported by the profession.
5. Conduct where the registered health practitioner has:
   - practised their profession whilst intoxicated by alcohol or drugs, or
   - engaged in sexual misconduct in connection with the practice of their profession, or
   - placed the public at risk of substantial harm in their practice of the profession because the practitioner has an impairment, or
   - placed the public at risk of harm because they have practised the profession in a way that constitutes a significant departure from accepted professional standards.

Activity 2.2

1. True.
2. True.

Fundamentals of Paramedic Practice: A Systems Approach, Third Edition. Edited by Sam Willis and Ian Peate.

Companion website: www.wiley.com/go/willis/paramedic3e

3. True.
4. False – clinical incompetence.
5. False.

Chapter 3

Test your knowledge

1. (i) Patient capacity
   (ii) Consent being provided voluntarily
   (iii) The nature of the treatment being understood (broadly) by the patient

Chapter 4

1. c) Cultural competency
2. c) To enhance patient satisfaction and trust.
3. d) Cultural background may influence a patient's willingness to express pain.
4. c) Develop cultural sensitivity and competence.
5. b) To provide equitable and patient-centred care.

Chapter 5

Test your knowledge

1. Those factors within the paramedic's working environment which affect patient care by influencing the ambulance crew, either directly or indirectly.
2. Fatigue, crew/team working, stress, situational awareness, hazardous attitudes.
3. (a) Palpitations.
   (b) Rapid breathing.
   (c) Chest tightness.
   (d) Sweating.
   (e) Unnecessary shouting.
   (f) Use of bad language that would not normally be used.
4. Work overload, crew conflict, poor communication, lack of promotional opportunities, attending distressing scenes.
5. Lack of preparation for the shift, e.g. not getting enough rest before for the shift; an inability to adapt to shift work, e.g. not taking sufficient nourishment before the shift; not having enough rest between shifts as well as job demands placed on the paramedic during the shift. In addition, the paramedic may also have to drive long distances to and from work; might undertake several shifts in a row; might have a student working alongside them for the shift, thus placing additional demands on energy; as well as the possibility of having to undertake alternative roles between calls.
6. Attitudes held by the paramedic that can cause risk to the patient, such as being anti-authority, complacency, machismo, impulsiveness, and resignation.

Activity 5.1

1. The task: recording a 12-lead ECG.
2. Organisational factors: no training provided for a new piece of equipment.
3. Environmental factors: at this time, Jim does not have the luxury of an ambulance saloon in which to conduct his assessment. He and his patient are out in the street.
4. Tools and technology: new cardiac monitor.

Activity 5.2

1. The task will not change; Jim still needs to undertake a 12-lead ECG if this is indicated by the history.
2. The organisation should ensure that staff are adequately trained to perform their duties. This is not an issue that Jim can solve today, by himself. However, he does have a duty to make his employer aware if he is not adequately trained.
3. Jim cannot control the weather! All he can do is request back-up and provide an adequate rationale for his request.
4. On this occasion Jim would have been safer to swap the new device for an older cardiac monitor with which he was familiar until such time as he had completed his training.

Chapter 6

Test your knowledge

1. The scientific and systematic study of society.
2. Learning to see yourself and others within the context of history and the social environment and considering the influence of individual agents in shaping society.

3. Depending upon your background and context, relevant answers include family, culture, religion, workplace, community resources, educational experiences, professional and medical associations, the media, the economic micro- and macro-environments, and global institutions such as the World Health Organization or the United Nations.
4. Social interaction can lead to stigmatisation and social rationing where individuals are perceived to have agency or responsibility for a health condition – e.g. if societal norms promote the view that a smoker has encouraged their own asthma or other smoking-related condition by their own actions, this may influence the quality of relationship we establish with the patient and thus affect the quality of care provided.
5. Medicalisation can affect how people view personal responsibility for a condition, and how they view the individual affected by the condition. For example, a person labelled with the term schizophrenia may isolate themselves and tacitly accept the erroneous social stigma that people with this condition are dangerous and unpredictable. This will further restrict the individual's social network.

Chapter 7

Activity 7.1

Q: How might you, as a provider of healthcare, adapt the below communicative behaviours to reduce the social distance between provider and patient, flatten provider- patient authority gradients, and create a safe space for patients to use their own communicative cues?

- Rate of speech
- Tone of voice
- Gestures
- Position of self vs position of patient
- Eye contact (noting cultural cue dependence)

A: Exemplar only.

- **Rate of speech – see page 71.**
  There are clear healthcare benefits when providers use moderately paced speech. Pausing and using silence are important vocalic tools that invite patients to comprehensively tell their story.
- **Tone of voice – see page 71.**
  There are clear healthcare benefits when providers use empathetic and friendly tones.
- **Gestures – see page 70.**
  Kinesics refers to the role of hand, arm, body, and face movements in non-verbal communication. Positive use of body language is known to enhance provider–patient rapport and thus patient safety.
  - *Subtle head nods*
  - *Leaning slightly forward and keeping hands visible with an open chest*
  - *Shoulders back*
- **Position of self vs position of patient – see page 71 and 72.**
  Work in the 'social space' zone.

Eye contact (noting cultural cue dependence) – see page 71.

Eye contact as a non-verbal communication tool differs depending on a person's cultural identity and norms. Where culturally appropriate, maintaining good eye contact can be interpreted as a willingness to listen, can help make a patient feel heard, and demonstrates respect. Typically, Western culture's view eye contact as a positive non-verbal communication cue, whilst some East Asian cultures consider too much eye contact as disrespectful. Similarly, eye contact amongst some Indigenous and First Nations persons makes said persons feel uncomfortable and can be viewed as rude or even aggressive. Some First Nation's persons interpret respect by the lowering of one's eyes during conversation. As a healthcare provider, managing the non-verbal communication behaviour of eye contact requisites educating oneself on cultural safety concepts, seeking cultural competency advice from experts, and accommodating for an individual's eye-contact needs by observing and responding to their cultural identity and body language.

Activity 7.2

Q: As a healthcare provider, how will you explicitly acknowledge the presence of private patient information? How will you, together with the patient, establish privacy rules and boundaries?

A: Exemplar only.

A: "Successful communication is more likely when those involved explicitly acknowledge the existence of private information and together determine privacy rules and boundaries" (Bylund et al. 2012, p. 265).

Activity 7.3

Q: As a healthcare provider, how will you communicate to a patient your role in obligatory disclosure to regulatory bodies or law enforcement? (For instance, communicable diseases in keeping with reporting requirements; child abuse in keeping with legislation.)

A: Exemplar answers only.

A: As a provider of healthcare, creating a therapeutically beneficial relationship with a patient involves pairing **honesty with compassion.** Information should be delivered in a straightforward manner whilst adopting previously discussed non-verbal communication techniques.

Activity 7.4

Q: Can you think of a time when you felt disregarded or unheard by a healthcare provider?

- **Describe this experience? (Description)**
- **How did this experience make you feel? (Feelings)**
- **How did this affect your healthcare experience? (Evaluation)**
- **How did this impact your relationship with your healthcare engagement? (Analysis)**
- **What did this experience teach you? (Conclusion)**
- **As a healthcare provider, how will you ensure that clients feel heard and validated? (Action Plan)**

A: As per participants own critical reflection (following subheadings as provided).

Activity 7.5

Q: What will your script be when required to deliver 'bad news' to a patient, bystanders, family members? What language will you use? What language will you avoid?

A: Exemplar only.

A:

A health professional does not only provide care to the patient, but also to those directly or indirectly impacted by the patient's health event. Bystanders, family, friends etc. Regardless of audience, delivering 'bad' news should ensure utilisation of Chapter highlighted verbal and non-verbal communication cues. An empathetic and respectful tone whilst delivering moderately paced truths obliging of body language should seek to minimise authority gradients (perceived or otherwise). Consider delivering bad news whilst positioned at level with or lower to the recipient. Maintain an open chest, eye contact in keeping with recipient culture, pause routinely etc. When delivering 'bad news', there should be no indirect or convoluted wording. Messaging should be clear, i.e., 'person has died', not, 'person is no longer with us' (as an example). Wherever possible, delivering 'bad' news should coincide with arranging psychosocial healthcare for recipients. For example, arranging GP follow up, arranging social services follow up, arranging transport for recipients immediately after an event, contacting recipient next-of-kin etc (consensual). There are a number of pneumonic-led scripts for health professionals to aid with delivering 'bad news' directly to a patient. See: Kumar, Vinay; Sarkhel, Sujit1. Clinical Practice Guidelines on Breaking Bad News. Indian Journal of Psychiatry 65(2):p 238–244, February 2023. | DOI: 10.4103/indianjpsychiatry.indianjpsychiatry_498_22.

Chapter 8

Test your knowledge

1. By integrating classroom learning with real-world experiences.
2. Hands-on training in real care settings.
3. Apply classroom knowledge to clinical scenarios.
4. It allows students to analyse their experiences and learn from them.
5. Participating in real world patient scenarios.

Chapter 9

Test your knowledge

1. Mindfulness is a mental state characterised by being fully present and engaged in the current moment, without judgment or distraction. It involves paying attention to one's thoughts, feelings and surroundings in a non-reactive and accepting manner. Often it is associated with meditation and various contemplative practices.
2. It is important to acknowledge that the effectiveness of coping mechanisms can vary from person to person. Experimenting with different strategies and combining several approaches often brings about the best results. Additionally, creating a supportive workplace culture and addressing systemic sources

of stress can contribute to a healthier work environment for everyone.

Physiological Responses:

Increased Heart Rate
Dilated Pupils
Bronchodilation
Increased Blood Pressure
Muscle Tension
Sweating
Inhibition of Digestive Processes
Release of Glucose

Psychological Responses:

Heightened Awareness: Attention becomes focused and alert enhancing perception and vigilance for potential threats.
Increased Alertness: Mental alertness and cognitive functions are heightened, processing information quickly and efficiently.
Emotional Changes: There may be a surge of emotions such as fear, anxiety or excitement, depending on the nature of the perceived threat.
Impaired Concentration on Non-Essential Tasks: Attention is diverted away from non-essential tasks, as the individual's focus shifts to the immediate threat or challenge.
Memory Formation: The encoding of memories may be enhanced, particularly for the details surrounding the stressful event.
Suppression of Non-Essential Functions: Non-essential functions, such as the reproductive and immune systems, may be temporarily suppressed to allocate resources to immediate survival needs.
Preparation for Action: The individual may experience a strong urge to either confront the threat (fight) or escape from it (flight), depending on the circumstances.

3. Cortisol is a steroid hormone that plays a crucial role in the body's response to stress. It is often referred to as the "stress hormone" as its release is triggered by stress and it is involved in various physiological processes that help the body cope with challenges.
4. Depression is a mental health disorder that can be characterised by persistent feelings of sadness, hopelessness and a lack of interest or pleasure in activities. It can vary widely in severity, ranging from mild, temporary episodes to more severe and chronic forms. The causes of depression are multifaceted, involving a complex interplay of biological, psychological and environmental factors.

Chapter 10

Activity 10.1

This activity is subjective. That means the notes you make and how they relate to your own personal work experience. We all have protective factors, family, supportive networks, work interventions, these help build and strengthen resilience.

Activity 10.2

This activity is subjective.
Reflection opens up opportunity to see what you would say or do differently. How can you improve a situation. Ask for support when you need it.

Activity 10.3

This activity is subjective. By spending time to complete this activity at the start and the end of a shift will offer some guidance of where you are and provide evidence of the actions that help you.

Chapter 11

Test your knowledge

1. What is the primary intention and function of the mental health legislation in Australia?
   - To protect the rights and dignity of people experiencing mental health difficulties affecting their capacity to make sound decisions.
2. What is the difference between mental illness, psychopathology, and positive mental health?
   - Mental illness is the experience of mental health symptoms, while psychopathology refers to the presence of a psychiatric diagnosis. Positive mental health refers to the overall subjective psychological well-being.
3. Discuss the difference between positive and negative symptoms and provide examples.
   - Positive symptoms
     - Hallucinations:
       - Visual and tactile – seeing a dozen spiders racing towards oneself and crawling up their arm.

- Auditory – hearing derogatory voices that are not a person's inner voice
    - Olfactory and gustatory – smelling and tasting rotten fish
  - Delusions:
    - The food that your family is cooking for you is poisoned.
  - Thought disorder:
    - Sitting in a waiting room and believing that all other people can hear what one is thinking about.
  - Disorganised speech:
    - Speaking very fast and erratically about several things (flight of ideas)
- Negative
  - Blunted affect (lack variability in facial expression)
  - Anhedonia (reduced/lack of enjoyment)
  - Responding in one-word answers when prompted (reduced/lack of speech)
  - Has not showered and brushed their teeth for four days (neglecting personal hygiene)
  - Not doing the dishes for days (difficulty in completing activities of daily living)
  - Hiding in fear behind the curtain and not answering the door when someone knocks (social withdrawal).

4. Identify and discuss physiological symptoms that could present as psychosis.
   - Psychosis is a condition whereby a person loses touch with reality. It includes a combination of positive and negative symptoms affecting thinking patterns, behaviour, and perceptions.
5. Discuss the main practical steps in attending to a person who presents in mental distress.
   - Addressing priorities (dispatching of attendees, assessment of the scene and first impressions)
   - Engagement, rapport building and de-escalation skills to complete assessment
   - Managing potential intoxication.
   - Being alert to and managing unpredictable situations.
   - Assessing and reducing risk.
   - Initiating required interventions.
6. Describe the common symptoms of depression, bipolar disorder, schizophrenia, and dementia.
   - **Depression:** may include low mood, tearfulness, changes (increase or decrease) in appetite and sleep patterns, social isolation or withdrawal, loss of libido and interest in previously enjoyable activities, low self-esteem, reduced confidence, and hopelessness. Some people, but not all, may experience suicidal thoughts and engage in self-harm behaviour. However, people with depression are not 'down, sad, and depressed' all of the time. Some may still be able to engage in humour, smile, or exhibit traits that could appear inconsistent with popular expectation of depression.
   - **Bipolar disorder**: A mental health disorder characterised by extreme mood shifts from mania which be experienced as feeling intensely upbeat, jumpy, or wired, with a marked increase in energy, activity, or agitation. Some people experience an exaggerated sense of self or self-confidence (grandiosity), excitement or happiness (euphoria). Periods of mania tend to precede periods of depression. However, despite common extreme mood shifts, symptoms will vary between individuals.
   - **Schizophrenia:** loss of touch with reality that includes a combination of symptoms affecting thinking patterns, behaviour, and perceptions that are either new or added to a person's usual presentation (positive symptoms) or represent a reduction in normal affect or functioning (negative symptoms)
   - **Dementia:** Umbrella term comprising several symptoms relating to progressive neurological conditions affecting the brain. Some examples are (but not limited to): memory loss, disorientation, thinking/planning/executing difficulties, problems with language and comprehension, reduced motivation, walking and movement challenges, behavioural changes, voiding/elimination issues and incontinence, change in mood or behaviour, impulsivity, decline in self-care, reduced appetite, reduced/lack of insight, repetitive behaviours.
7. Identify and discuss factors considered in conducting a risk assessment.
   - Obtaining background/historical information (e.g. past suicide attempts, family history of mental health conditions)
   - Obtaining and assessing current events and difficulties (e.g. medical psychiatric conditions, current self-harm attempts)
   - Identification of circumstantial factors (e.g. loss of dwelling)
   - Identification of protective factors (e.g., children, pets)

8. What constitutes intimate partner violence?
    - Aggression and abuse committed in the context of a current or former romantic relationship. Other family members may also inflict abuse or commit violent acts towards others in the household. The violence or abuse perpetrated may be physical, verbal, sexual, emotional, financial, or social and aims to instil fear in the partner or family member to maintain, or gain, control over them.
9. What type of exposure could lead to PTSD?
    - **Direct:** person directly affected by the trauma.
    - **Vicarious:** as a witness to the traumatic event.
    - **Indirect:** learning that a relative/friend/close person was exposed to a trauma, or being exposed to the details of trauma, often through work duties (first responders, crime scene investigators, medics).
10. What could be the advantages and disadvantages of using humour in paramedicine?
    - It may be helpful in engaging and defusing tension but can be out of place or misinterpreted.

Chapter 12

Activity 12.2

De-escalation techniques implemented by Carl:

- Introductions. Carl introduced himself his partner and his qualifications.
- Remained calm. Despite Irene being in a heightened emotional state and yelling at people, Carl kept his emotions calm.
- Position within the room. Carl did not block the exit to the room.
- Language. Carl chose easy to understand language to enhance communication with Irene.

Activity 12.3

De-escalation techniques NOT implemented by Carl:

- Stood over Irene creating a power imbalance.
- Poor body language with hands on hips.
- Carl did not attempt to build rapport through finding common interests.
- Carl did not have spatial awareness and did not consider removing the staff member who Irene was yelling at.

Chapter 13

1. Both.
2. To improve the effectiveness of the public health policy implementation.
3. Eleven.
4. Due to the profession's evolutionary history from 'ambulance drivers' with basic first aid qualifications to OOH care professionals.
5. Health outcomes assessed through this model are more likely to result in system-wide and system-level responses.
6. Five
7. Any waking behaviour with very reduced energy expenditure, for example prolonged sitting.
8. Constitutional factors including age, biological sex and genetics.
9. Any social and environmental factor that influences health experience and / or outcomes.
10. Six.

Chapter 14

Test your knowledge

1. The Old English etymology of the verb *to lead* can be traced back to the word *lædan,* which means 'to show the way'.
2. Staying flexible and adaptable according to context.
3. Any 3 of the following: transformational leadership, transactional leadership, servant leadership, authentic leadership, autocratic leadership, democratic leadership, laissez-faire leadership, distributed leadership.
4. Any 5 of the following: Resource Investigator, Teamworker, Co-ordinator, Plant, Monitor/Evaluator, Specialist, Shaper, Implementer and Completer/Finisher.

Activities 14.1 and 14.2

These questions were set in the previous version of the book and they did not provide any answers for the previous version. The answers to these questions are very dependant on the readers own situation.

Chapter 15

Test your knowledge

1. Research produces evidence through systematic investigation and scientific evaluation. This can be evidence for best practice, but also evidence towards the answers for other questions about the world.
2. Think about words that identify the issue you are interested in or select key words from your research question. Identify synonyms (words meaning the same thing). Use Boolean operators (particularly AND, OR) to turn your search terms into a search strategy.
3. The allocation to treatment/control group is by chance in a randomised controlled trial. Each participant has the same chance of being allocated to a treatment or control group as any other participant. This is called randomisation and it is done to avoid systematic differences between treatment and control groups.

Activity 15.1

The main differences are in the type of data (information) collected and in the methods (techniques) used to collect this data. Quantitative research will produce numerical data for the purpose of measurement. Qualitative research seeks understanding through words or observation data.

Chapter 16

Test your knowledge

1. A component placed at the start of a word – e.g. peri-.
2. A component placed at the end of a word – e.g. -itis.
3. Inflammation.
4. The heart.

Activity 16.1

1. Swift/accelerated beating of the heart.
2. Inflammation of the stomach.
3. Bad breathing.
4. The heart's circulation.

Chapter 17

Test your knowledge

1. **a)** Sympathomimetic toxidrome
   b) Amphetamines, cocaine, MAOI's or other stimulants
   c) Possible ongoing release due to concealment of drugs in body cavities
2. **a)** Cholinergic toxidrome
   b) Chemical nerve agents or orthophosphates
   c) Acetylcholinesterase inhibitor
3. **a)** Neuroleptic malignant syndrome
   b) Stop the antipsychotics, supportive care and active cooling. Consider benzodiazapines for agitation.
4. **a)** Sedative toxidrome
   b) Conscious state assessment, vital sign survey, ECG, history taking, assessment of quantity of medication consumed.
5. **a)** Malignant hyperthermia
   b) First action is to remove the methoxyflurane from the patient.
   c) Move the patient to a cool location and begin actively cooling the patient.

Activity 17.1

1. Increased cardiac workload and oxygen consumption.
2. Metoprolol is a beta blocker. It is listed as a '1 or 2 pill can kill' due to the bradycardia it will cause.
3. Intra-cerebral haemorrhage.
4. Increased bleeding from her skin tears. Increased risk of bleeding from further falls.

Chapter 18

Test your knowledge

1. Hypertension (high blood pressure), bradycardia (slow heart), altered respirations.
2. Swelling, loss of movement, irregularity, pain, deformity, unnatural movement, crepitus, tenderness, bruising.
3. Flail segment.
4. Pneumothorax is air in the pleural space that has not yet built up. Tension pneumothorax is when that

air has built up and starts to compress the other side, including the heart, causing a life-threatening situation.
5. Neck of femur.
6. Crush injuries.

Chapter 19

Test your knowledge

1. Atrial depolarisation
2. Ventricular depolarisation
3. Ventricular repolarisation
4. An abnormal (non-sinus) rhythm
5. AV blocks.
6. A slowed conduction where the left bundle branch is blocked, resulting in depolarisation of the left ventricle via cell-to-cell conduction rather than down the fast Purkinje fibres.

Activity 19.1

1. 1, standard paper speed rate is 25 mm/second.
2. 1 large square = 0.2 seconds.
3. 300-method, where you take 300 and divide it by the number of large squares between the QRS complexes to get the heart rate.

Activity 19.2

Unstable angina, non-ST elevation AMI, and ST elevation AMI (STEMI).

Activity 19.3

Because the largest ventricle is not depolarised fast and reliably, but rather cellularly through the signal travelling from myocyte to myocyte. In the right clinical context, a LBBB may be considered a STEMI equivalent meaning it should be treated with the same degree of seriousness and attention as a STEMI. This will vary from service to service.

Chapter 20

Test your knowledge

1. False. Only STEMI, NON-STEMI, and Unstable Angina are types of ACS
2. False. Aspirin is an antiplatelet drug which reduces clots by preventing platelet aggregation in a clot.
3. Myocardium.

Activity 20.1

Blood enters the right atria from the superior and inferior vena cava. It travels to the right ventricle through the tricuspid valve and enters the pulmonary circulation through the pulmonary valve for oxygenation following contraction of the right ventricle. It then leaves the pulmonary vein (the only vein to carry oxygenated blood) and enters the left atria through the mitral valve and into the left ventricle. When the left ventricle contracts it sends blood through the aortic valve and into the aorta for distribution around the body.

Chapter 21

Test your knowledge

1. False
2. False
3. True
4. False
5. False
6. True

Activity 21.1

1. Signs of ischaemic stroke can include numbness or weakness to the face, arms and/or legs, and is often on one side of the body. Patients may also present with confusion, dysphagia, aphasia, loss of balance and coordination.

   Haemorrhagic strokes can also present with all of the above. Patients may also complain of a sudden onset thunderclap 'worse headache ever', vomiting, neck stiffness, vision changes and photophobia, seizures, and coma.

Ischaemic strokes are a loss of blood supply to a part of the brain due to thrombus formation or embolism. This is the most common type of stroke.

Haemorrhagic strokes are caused by bleeding into the brain due to blood vessel rupture. Haemorrhagic stroke can be further subdivided into intracerebral haemorrhage (bleeding into the brain parenchymal tissue) and subarachnoid haemorrhage (bleeding into the subarachnoid space).

Ischaemic and haemorrhagic strokes present differently. Ischaemic strokes reduce blood supply to the brain, however, do not cause bleeding into brain tissue, brain and meningeal irritation, and raised intracranial pressure. Haemorrhagic strokes are often more severe than ischaemic strokes because they don't just disrupt blood flow to the brain tissue, but also cause bleeding and subsequent haematoma which compresses the brain tissue and raises the intracranial pressure

2. Asking open-ended questions at the beginning of history taking allows the patient to explore their concerns in their own words. This will provide a broad overview of the patient's current issues and allows them to speak freely about what they believe is important regarding their health. Once we have gathered information from open-ended questions, we can then ask more specific questions which aim to support or refute our differential diagnosis, and aid in our clinical decision making.

Chapter 22

Test your knowledge

1. Method 1: Divide into quadrants:
   - **(a)** Right upper quadrant: liver, gall bladder, common bile duct and cystic ducts, head of pancreas and pancreatic duct, small bowel (parts of duodenum, ileum, jejunum), colon (hepatic flexure), right kidney.
   - **(b)** Left upper quadrant: stomach, spleen, tail of pancreas, small bowel (mostly jejunum), colon (splenic flexure), left kidney.
   - **(c)** Right lower quadrant: terminal ileum, caecum, appendix, ascending colon, right ovary (females).
   - **(d)** Left lower quadrant: small bowel (mostly ileum), descending colon, sigmoid colon, left ovary (females).

   Method 2: Divide into nine regions:
   - **(a)** Right hypochondrium: right lobe of the liver, gall bladder, hepatic flexure of the colon, and part of the right kidney.
   - **(b)** Epigastrium: stomach, left lobe of the liver, pancreas, duodenum, superior part of the kidneys (including adrenals), oesophagus, transverse colon.
   - **(c)** Left hypochondrium: splenic end of the stomach, spleen and extremity of pancreas, splenic flexure of the colon, and part of the left kidney.
   - **(d)** Right lumbar: ascending colon, part of the right kidney, and some convolutions of the small intestines.
   - **(e)** Umbilical: transverse colon, part of the great omentum and mesentery, transverse part of the duodenum, some sections of jejunum and ileum, and part of both kidneys and ureters.
   - **(f)** Left lumbar: descending colon, part of the omentum, part of the left kidney, and some convolutions of the small intestines.
   - **(g)** Right iliac (inguinal): caecum, appendix, ovary and fallopian tube in females.
   - **(h)** Hypogastrium: convolutions of the small intestines, the bladder in children (adults if distended), the uterus during pregnancy, right and left ovary and fallopian tubes in females, vas deferens in males.
   - **(i)** Left iliac (inguinal): sigmoid flexure of the colon, ovary and fallopian tube in females.

2. **(a)** Visceral pain originates from within an organ. It is most often poorly localised, centralised to the midline, and referred to other regions that are also supplied by that same division of the splanchnic system (that is, anywhere from upper chest down to lower abdomen). Discomfort tends to begin gradually as a dull, vague, mostly central, aching pain. It may be accompanied by autonomic response to pain, such as tachycardia, tachypnoea, nausea and vomiting, diaphoresis, and pallor. Relieving factors will depend on the underlying cause.
   - **(b)** Parietal pain originates from stimulation of somatic nociceptors within the parietal peritoneum. In contrast to visceral pain, parietal pain is sharp, localised, often more severe, and tends not to be referred unless there is accompanying underlying visceral pain. Patients will often

sit still, have shallow breathing, and guard the painful region. This type of pain may also have the same associated autonomic responses as visceral pain, although they may tend to be more pronounced in severe parietal pain.

3. The 'acute abdomen' refers to any nontraumatic, sudden, severe abdominal pain of unclear aetiology and for which an urgent operation may be necessary.

   Conditions include (but are not limited to) acute cholecystitis, appendicitis, bowel obstruction, cancer, and acute vascular conditions (leading to gut ischaemia or bleeding).

   History will likely include descriptions of gradually worsening pain, or perhaps a very sudden onset of immediately severe pain. Careful note of the evolution of pain to include different regions may guide diagnosis.

   A higher level of suspicion should be reserved for the elderly, the immunocompromised, children, and women of childbearing age.

   There are often systemic signs of shock, such as tachycardia, tachypnoea, diaphoresis, hypotension, pallor, and decreased conscious state, and thus treatment of the acute abdomen focuses on immediate resuscitation, analgesia, and prompt transport to a hospital capable of providing emergency laparotomy.

4. Differential diagnoses (more likely in, or specific to, females) could include pelvic inflammatory disease, or urinary tract infection. Obstetric and gynaecological issues to consider would include menstrual cycle pain (especially 'mittelschmerz', a German term meaning 'middle pain', which is pain experienced by many females midway through their menstrual cycle), ectopic pregnancy, acute salpingitis (inflammation of the fallopian tubes), ruptured/haemorrhagic cyst, or ovarian torsion.

Chapter 23

1. Gas exchange.
2. Initial assessment of a patient.
3. Acute asthma.
   Inhalation burn.
   Foreign body obstruction.
   Pulmonary oedema.
   Pulmonary embolus.
   Pneumothorax.
4. History taking.
   Clinical examination – inspection, palpation, percussion and auscultation.

Chapter 24

Case 3

68-year-old male who's got crushing central chest pain. which radiates into their left arm. They are sweating and look pale. They have a bradycardic pulse at 40 beats per minute and perfusing their peripheral organs as they have a radial pulse.

They are alert because they are communicating with us therefore have a patent airway. Their breathing rate is elevated at 24 breaths per minute.

Working impression is an ACS to which we would complete a 12 lead ECG to further examine the heart.

Case 4

28-year-old female who's sustained a traumatic injury. They are unresponsive therefore have a reduced GCS. Breathing rate is slow at 8 breaths per minute and a tachycardic pulse at 120 beats per minute. They feel waxy and clammy and have an injury to their femur and bleeding externally. These injuries suggest the patient is in hypovolaemic shock and they have sustained a head injury from the fall. The airway will need to be maintained, initially with a jaw thrust and then adjuncts and their injuries and bleeding need treating.

Chapter 25

1. 37–42 weeks.
2. Two – latent phase: the period of irregular contractions which build in intensity and that prepare the cervix to dilate and permit the passage of the foetus out of the uterus; active phase: the beginning of active child delivery.
3. Three.
4. Shoulder dystocia.

Chapter 26

Test your knowledge

1. Possible answers:

   Fewer alveoli.
   Prominent use of diaphragm.
   Poorly developed accessory muscles.
   Compliant chest wall.
   Immature respiratory control centre.

2. • Fewer alveoli - Less capacity for gaseous exchange.
   • Prominent use of diaphragm – any abdominal distention can impact upon ability to breathe.
   • Poorly developed accessory muscles – rapid respiratory muscle fatigue, increased attempts to use accessory muscles will result in signs of respiratory distress like head bobbing.
   • Compliant chest wall – chest expansion limited. Intercostal, subcostal, and sternal recession all signs of increased work of breathing. Likelihood of chest wall collapse greater.
   • Immature respiratory control centre – irregular breathing patterns and apnoea may occur in the presence of respiratory conditions, particularly in preterm and small infants.

3. Possible answers:

Haemorrhage	Rapid loss of > 25% circulating blood volume Signs of poor perfusion and circulatory compromise Bradycardia Reduced level of consciousness
Intestinal obstruction (intussusception, volvulus, paralytic ileus)	Bile-stained vomiting Abdominal distension Severe colicky abdominal pain (drawing up of knees in infants) Inconsolability 'Redcurrant jelly' stools
Gastroenteritis	Less than half normal input and output in preceding 24 hours (<4 wet nappies in infants) Estimated severe dehydration Oliguria Signs of poor perfusion and circulatory compromise Bradycardia Reduced level of consciousness
Burns	Children <12 months old at higher risk Burn or scold estimated at >10% Full thickness burns Any burn involving face, mouth, or airway (suspected smoke inhalation) Circumferential burns Chemical or electrical burns
Distributive shock	
Sepsis	Children <12 months at higher risk Non-blanching rash (petechiae or purpura) Temperature with 'toxic' signs Signs of poor perfusion and circulatory compromise Bradycardia Reduced level of consciousness
Anaphylaxis	History of previous anaphylaxis Respiratory difficulties Presence of stridor and/or wheeze Signs of poor perfusion and circulatory compromise Reduced level of consciousness

4. Dry mucous membranes
   Lethargy
   Reduced skin turgor
   PLUS
   Poor perfusion (pale, mottled, slow capillary refill)
   Deeply sunken eyes/fontanelle
   Reduced level of consciousness
   Thready or absent peripheral pulses
   Marked tachycardia
   Hypotension
   Markedly prolonged capillary refill time

Chapter 27

What are the management priorities for a patient experiencing a hypoglycaemic episode?
Consider airway management as necessary, either changing the patient's position or using airway adjuncts. The secondary priority is then achieving normoglycaemia, by choosing an appropriate way to deliver glucose to the patient or using a hyperglycaemic agent such as glycogen. Paramedics should also be prepared for the risk of a seizure. Providing reassurance to the patient, family.

What factors should the paramedic consider as potential causes leading to an episode of autonomic dysreflexia?
Paramedics should do a full exposure and examination to look for causes along with good history taking, especially asking about previous triggers the patient has experienced. Common causes include blocked catheters; urinary retention; bowel impaction; constipation; boils; pressure sores; ingrown toenails; and unidentified injuries or fractures below the patient's spinal cord injury.

In your own words describe sepsis.
Sepsis is a life-threatening organ dysfunction as a result of a heightened host response to an infection. During sepsis, the body reacts to a pathogen such as bacteria through the activation of innate immune cells. The reaction between these immune cells and the pathogen leads to the release of proinflammatory cytokines and it is these cytokines that cause the vasodilation and increased vascular permeability leading to hypovolaemic shock, as well as activation of the clotting cascade leading to disseminated intravascular coagulopathy.

Describe the difference between an ischaemic and haemorrhagic stroke.
Strokes occur when the blood supply to the brain is interrupted. In an ischaemic stroke, this blood supply interruption is caused by a blocked artery; and in a haemorrhagic stroke, it is due to a rupture of a weakened artery. The impairment of blood supply to the brain leads to a lack of essential oxygen and nutrients resulting in damaged brain cells.

What are some specific considerations when looking after a paediatric patient with suspected sepsis?
Parental concern or multiple interactions with healthcare providers within 48 hours should act as a red flag to paramedics that a child is at risk of having sepsis. The non-specific and unwell presentation of a child such as reduced muscle tone or level of consciousness, mottled or discoloured skin, non-blanching rash and potentially long pauses in their breathing should increase clinician concern for sepsis. Hypotension is a late and fatal sign; normal blood pressure can provide false reassurance.

What are some causes of a seizure?
Beyond epilepsy other causes of seizures include pregnancy, diabetes, dementia, migraines, lesions, recreational drug use, new or poor adherence to medications, persistent fevers, alcohol withdrawal, or head trauma.

Outline the symptoms required to meet the criteria for anaphylaxis and how would you manage a patient with anaphylaxis?

1. Rapid onset of illness (minutes to several hours) involving the skin and/or mucosal tissue with at least one of the following:
   a. Respiratory compromise (dyspnoea, wheeze, stridor, hypoxaemia)
   b. Reduced blood pressure or signs associated with end organ dysfunction (collapse, syncope, incontinence)
   c. Severe gastrointestinal symptoms (severe cramping abdominal pain, repetitive vomiting), especially when exposure was to a non-food allergen.
2. Rapid onset illness (minutes to several hours) without skin or mucosal involvement, after exposure to a known or highly probable allergen with any of the following:
   a. Acute hypotension (SBP reduction greater than 30% of pts baseline or SBP <90mmHg in adults)
   b. Bronchospasm (wheeze, persistent cough)
   c. Laryngeal involvement (stridor, vocal changes, painful swallow)

Prompt administration of Intramuscular (IM) adrenaline is required, multiple doses may be needed. Patients then should not be walked post adrenaline administration. Following this, the paramedic can then target normoxia, with an appropriate oxygen delivery system; hypotension should be addressed with the administration of isotonic crystalloid solutions. Paramedics may also consider managing any ongoing wheezing with beta-2 agonists and bronchodilators such as salbutamol and ipratropium bromide, either via MDI or nebuliser. Persistent stridor can be managed with nebulised adrenaline to assist with ongoing laryngeal and pharyngeal oedema.

How would a person experiencing an adrenal crisis present?
The patient may present with vague non-specific symptoms such as acute abdominal pain; hyponatremia; hypoglycaemia and pyrexia; nausea; vomiting; headaches; generalised body aches; fatigue and postural hypotension. Due to this adrenal crisis is defined in adults as an acute deterioration with a systolic blood pressure <100 mmHg or a decrease in systolic blood pressure equal to or greater than 20 mmHg.

Chapter 28

1. **(a)** False
   (b) False
   (c) False
   (d) False
   (e) True

Chapter 29

Test your knowledge

1. Mechanism of injury is the 'how, what, when, why' of the injury in question, considering the direction, magnitude, and duration of force. Establishing these details is an essential part of the paramedic's history-taking process.
2. The characteristics of a *Look, Feel, Move* assessment are:

   Look:
   - Compare with the unaffected side.
   - Bleeding, swelling, bruising.
   - Wounds, scars.
   - Look from all angles/aspects.
   - Foreign bodies.
   - Deformity, wasting.
   - Colour – cyanosis, pallor, erythema.
   - Tracking, lymphangitis.

   Feel:
   - Start palpating in the proximal joint away from the site of pain.
   - Feel one area at a time, using a single finger.
   - Identify the anatomical landmarks in a systematic manner.
   - Relate surface anatomy to underlying structures and try to identify specific areas of tenderness.
   - Observe for facial expressions and gestures, as well as verbal expressions of pain.
   - Skin temperature.
   - Crepitus.
   - Check sensation (two-point discrimination).
   - Feel for distal pulses/capillary refill time (CRT).

   Move:
   - Know how the joint is supposed to move.
   - Compare range of movement to the unaffected side.
   - Active movement – the patient performs the movement, without assistance and using their own power.
   - Passive movement – movement of the limb is performed on the patient by the clinician.
   - Resisted movement – in testing resisted movement, the joints do not move and the integrity of the musculotendon is tested, e.g. the straight leg raise testing the extensor mechanism in the knee.
3. The Ottawa Ankle Rules were developed and clinically tested by Stiell et al. (1994) to show that application of the rules led to a decrease in the use of ankle radiography, waiting times, and costs, without patient dissatisfaction or missed fractures. Using the Ottawa Ankle Rules as an aid to examination will allow for safe diagnosis and appropriate treatment of ankle injury.
4. Stage treatment:
   - Cooling – Cool the affected body area for a minimum of 20 minutes, ideally with cool running water.
   - Analgesia – Burns are very painful and it is important to administer appropriate analgesics as soon as possible.

- Assessment - Assess the burn thoroughly. Does the burn require further assessment or treatment? If so, be guided by your local referral guidelines.
- Cover – Cover the burn with cling film and cover the cling film with a wet dressing to keep the affected area cool. You may have to continue cooling en route to hospital using 0.9% sodium chloride.
- Consideration – Consider complications such as ABCs, hypothermia, IV fluid challenge, nonaccidental injury.
- Review – Continually review and assess.

5. You should contact your local MIU to confirm what they are able to offer in the way of services, but below are some common grounds:
   - Musculoskeletal and ligamentous injury.
   - Mild head injury (GCS 15).
   - Eye injury.
   - Burns.
   - Foreign body removal.
   - Bites and stings.
   - Wound care.
   - Limb fractures.
   - X-ray facility.
6. The five wound-closure methods available in the prehospital setting are:
   - Tissue/skin adhesive.
   - Staples.
   - Steristrips.
   - Sutures.
   - Skin link.
7. The five considerations during a nose injury assessment are:
   - Is the airway compromised?
   - Is there a septal haematoma?
   - Is there a severe epistaxis?
   - Is there severe displacement?
   - Are there associated fractures to the face?

Activity 29.2

1. This is a subcutaneous collection of blood giving rise to a fluctuant swelling.
2. This is a wound with a fine path made by a pointed object, for example railing spike, knife, or nail.
3. This is a breach in the skin, with surrounding bruising.

Activity 29.4

1. Falls.
2. Yes.
3. Ottawa Ankle Rules.

Chapter 30

Test your knowledge

1. Any incident where the location, number, severity, or type of live casualties requires extraordinary resources.
2. - Major incident.
   - Exact location.
   - Type of incident.
   - Hazards.
   - Access.
   - Number of casualties.
   - Emergency services.
3. The patient is a Priority 1. As the patient cannot walk, they are immediately ruled out of the Priority 3 category. The patient is breathing and therefore they cannot be assigned as deceased. The patient is breathing at a rate of 8, a respiratory rate that immediately assigns the patient to a Priority 1 regardless of pulse rate.
4. Priority 2.
5. Performing life-saving clinical interventions; providing stabilisation of the patient to allow for safe transportation.
6. False. Transport timing should align with the patient triage and treatment priority. However, in clinical practice, treatment and stabilisation together with the complexities of the transport decision-making process may permit those of a lesser priority to be transported first.
7. False. Command relates to the internal direction of personnel within an organisation.
8. - Major incident declared – Yes.
   - Exact location – Serves You Right Café, Ravenshoe.
   - Type of incident – Vehicle collision with premises resulting in explosion.
   - Hazards present – Potential issues include fire, structural damage to building, unstable vehicle, gas leak, electrical hazards.

- Access and egress – Vehicular access via main street, helicopter access via nearby school oval.
- Number and type of casualties – 21 people injured.
- Emergency services:
  - On scene – Police, fire, ambulance, medical.
  - Required – Additional ambulances, aeromedical transfer.

9. True. There may be multiple bronze commanders allocated to different geographical areas within an incident scene, or allocated to specialist functions. These bronze commanders will report to a single silver commander.

10. Prevention, preparedness, response, and recovery (PPRR).

Chapter 31

1. Falls, medication compliance, social welfare/living conditions.
2. More.
3. Marfan's syndrome and is also associated with congenital heart disease.
4. Lung cancer, congenital heart disease, cirrhosis, endocarditis.
5. Hyperinflation of the lungs.
6. Major back pain and restrictive respiratory insufficiency.
7. Ultrasound, point-of-care testing, telemedicine.
8. Excess thyroid hormone production and has a classic thyroid stare appearance.

Activity 31.1

A red flag. It denotes the possibility that this symptom could mean a diagnosis of an urgent or dangerous problem with the patient that requires your immediate attention and care.

Chapter 32

1. c) Neglect
2. b) Allowing a child to be exposed to FDV is considered a form of CAN.
3. d) The majority of the most damaging FDV is perpetrated by males against women.
4. True
5. a) Intimate partner violence.
6. Recognise, Respond, Refer, Record
7. d) The patient has more than four children.
8. c) Do you feel safe at home?
9. d) All of the above.

Chapter 33

1. c) A medicine designed for other conditions but is also effective for treating pain
2. d) Oxycodone
3. a) Article 2
4. b) Ibuprofen
5. b) relieve the symptoms of nausea.
6. d) 4
7. a) Oral
8. d) Environmental
9. d) Advance Decision to Refuse Life-sustaining Treatment
10. Which of these is covered by the Mental Capacity Act 2005?
    b) Advance Decision to Refuse Treatment (ADRT).

Index

Note: Page numbers in *italics* refer to figures and those in **bold** to tables.

Fundamentals of Paramedic Practice: A Systems Approach, Third Edition. Edited by Sam Willis and Ian Peate.

Companion website: www.wiley.com/go/willis/paramedic3e

Printed in the USA/Agawam, MA
October 9, 2024

874236.002